Pathology of Melanocytic Nevi and Malignant Melanoma

RAYMOND L. BARNHILL, M.D.

Associate Professor of Pathology
Harvard Medical School;
Director, Dermatopathology Division,
Department of Pathology
Brigham and Women's Hospital
Children's Hospital and
Harvard Community Health Plan
Boston, Massachusetts

with contributions by

KLAUS J. BUSAM, M.D.

Dermatopathology Fellow
Harvard Medical School;
Department of Pathology
Brigham and Women's Hospital
Boston, Massachusetts

in Chapters 1, 2, 6, 11

BUTTERWORTH–HEINEMANN

Boston Oxford Melbourne Singapore Sydney Toronto Munich New Delhi Tokyo

Every effort has been made to ensure that the drug dosage schedules within this text are accurate and conform to standards accepted at time of publication. However, as treatment recommendations vary in the light of continuing research and clinical experience, the reader is advised to verify drug dosage schedules herein with information found on product information sheets. This is especially true in cases of new or infrequently used drugs.

Recognizing the importance of preserving what has been written, Butterworth–Heinemann prints its books on acid-free paper whenever possible.

Library of Congress Cataloging-in-Publication Data

Barnhill, Raymond L.
Pathology of melanocytic nevi and malignant melanoma/Raymond L. Barnhill.
p. cm.
Includes bibliographical references and index.
ISBN 0-7506-9504-8 (alk. paper)
1. Melanoma—Pathophysiology. I. Title.
[DNLM: 1. Nevus—pathology. 2. Skin Neoplasms—pathology. 3. Melanocytes—pathology. 4. Melanoma—pathology. QZ 310 B262p 1994]
RC280.M37B37 1994
616.99'477—dc20
DNLM/DLC for Library of Congress 94-33338
CIP

British Library Cataloguing-in-Publication Data
A catalogue record for this book is available from the British Library.

Butterworth–Heinemann
313 Washington Street
Newton, MA 02158-1626

10 9 8 7 6 5 4 3 2 1

Printed in the United States of America

To MAB and ARB
who have provided continued encouragement,
strength, love, and inspiration.

Foreword

This important monograph clearly describes the many variations of benign pigmented lesions of the skin as well as cutaneous melanoma. Principally written from a pathological perspective, this scholarly text describes the spectrum of benign and malignant melanocytic lesions of the skin while correlating the histopathologic findings with clinical outcome and the biology of metastatic disease. There are extensive discussions of clinical features. Dr. Barnhill carefully details the distinguishing pathological features of these conditions based on the extensive experience of the Pigmented Lesion Clinic at the Massachusetts General Hospital. He effectively blends his perspective as a clinical dermatologist and as a dermatopathologist in a manner that provides useful information for dermatologists, pathologists, and surgeons treating skin cancer. The most salient features of each entity are summarized in the form of a précis (in tables) for quick reference. Much other information is also summarized in tables for easy access. There is particular emphasis on differential diagnosis. Dr. Barnhill's book has clarity in writing style, is superbly organized, and the figures, tables, and photographs (including over 250 color photomicrographs) nicely enhance the text. It is a valuable resource to all physicians interested in the biology of benign and malignant melanocytic skin conditions.

Charles M. Balch, MD

Foreword

The global incidence of malignant melanoma is increasing dramatically. Cutaneous melanoma currently represents approximately 3 percent of cancers by incidence (excluding non-melanoma skin cancer) and although this incidence is increasing more rapidly than the mortality rate, melanoma is the leading fatal illness arising in the skin, accounting for approximately 1 percent of all cancer deaths. Contrasting with this rather disillusioning scenario, large multicenter studies show an average five-year survival rate of approximately 80 percent in patients with localized (stage I and II) disease. When compared to internal cancers this reflects an excellent prognosis which can be almost completely ascribed to early recognition of the tumor. Thus early diagnosis of melanoma both clinically and histopathologically, is the most important single prognostic determinant. It is therefore most timely that Dr. Raymond L. Barnhill, a leading expert in the field, has embarked on writing this most informative, highly concise, and beautifully illustrated volume.

Since melanoma results from the malignant transformation of melanocytes in the epidermis, dermis or mucosal epithelium and nevus cells in certain precursor lesions, it always has to be considered in the context of and vis à vis other benign or premalignant melanocytic lesions. Bearing this in mind, the author has therefore not only focused on melanoma but has also produced a much needed state-of-the-art description of all melanocytic lesions. The strength of this volume is that it is based primarily on the outstanding expertise and vast experience of the author. The logical sequence of its chapters will lead the reader to understand the sequence of benign to malignant lesions and its emphasis on diagnosis and differential diagnosis and procedures currently employed to distinguish between benign and malignant melanocytic lesions will make it invaluable to all interested in dermatologic oncology and pathology. Dr. Barnhill's didactic skills in presenting the material make me predict that this book will be a classic in the field.

Klaus Wolff, MD, FRCP

Preface

The histopathologic interpretation of melanocytic lesions of the skin remains one of the most frustrating and difficult areas in dermatopathology and surgical pathology. The continued increase in incidence of cutaneous melanoma coupled with earlier diagnosis will undoubtedly present even greater challenges in histologic diagnosis. Thus, there is an unquestioned need for more information on this subject.

The goal of this book is to provide a comprehensive description of melanocytic lesions occurring in the skin. Considerable effort has also been made to provide detailed clinical descriptions of the lesions in order to assist histopathologists in differential diagnosis. A thorough knowledge of the clinical features of the various melanocytic lesions is essential in histologic diagnosis but is often neglected in textbooks of histopathology. The most important aspects of differential diagnosis are presented, and for most of the entities in the book, a concise description (précis) of the neoplasm has been provided in tables. Much other information useful to the practicing clinician, dermatopathologist, and surgical pathologist has also been summarized in numerous other tables in each of the chapters. Because of the importance of illustrating histopathologic criteria for diagnosis, over 250 color photomicrographs are included in the book.

The author is grateful for the kind and generous help provided by many friends and colleagues. The major sources of material used in this book are from the Dermatopathology Division, Harvard Medical School (the Brigham and Women's Hospital, Children's Hospital, Massachusetts General Hospital, and Harvard Community Health Plan). However, the author also gratefully acknowledges the use of other material from consultations, friends and colleagues, and from the Pigmented Lesion Clinic, Massachusetts General Hospital.

With particular reference to the completion of this book, the author is especially indebted to his secretary, Miss Michelle Wood. Without her highly skilled assistance and dedication to the project, undoubtedly the book would not have been completed. The author also acknowledges the contributions of Klaus J. Busam, M.D. Dr. Busam provided assistance in writing some chapters and advice on the manuscript at a critical time in the evolution of the book. The author is also highly appreciative of the support provided by his chairman, Ramzi Cotran, M.D., in pursuing projects such as this. The author is also grateful to other colleagues for critical analysis of portions of the manuscript.

Raymond L. Barnhill, MD

Contents

Pathology of Melanocytic Nevi and Malignant Melanoma

1

Melanocytes

MELANIN PIGMENT

Melanocytes are dendritic cells, whose unique property is the production of melanin pigments,[1] which allow a wide range of colors, as seen, for example, in mammalian hair, which may be black, brown, yellow, reddish brown, or carroty red. The type of pigmentation is under genetic control, involving a number of interacting gene products, some of which have been identified recently.[2] While in many animals melanin pigments play an important role in camouflage and mimicry, their major function in humans is protection against the potentially toxic or carcinogenic effects of sunlight. Their broad spectral absorbance makes them suitable for light-shielding purposes. Melanins also have been suggested to be involved in radiant heat loss and detoxification of oxygen radicals or metals.[3–6] In addition to their protective role against damage from ultraviolet (UV) light, recent evidence shows that melanocytes also participate in the inflammatory response. Melanocytes have been found to be the source of and responsive to a variety of inflammatory mediators.[7]

Two prototypes of melanin have been described traditionally: *eumelanin*, which is brown-black and insoluble, and *pheomelanin*, which is reddish yellow and alkali-soluble.[8] However, this classification represents an oversimplification of the actual variety of natural melanins, because each of the two groups includes pigments with different physical and chemical properties. Typical eumelanins such as those of dark human hair are a mixture of high-molecular-weight polymers consisting mainly of 5,6-dihydroxyindole units, which are derived from multiple enzymatic and nonenzymatic reactions.[8,9] Pheomelanin is a polymer formed via cysteinyldopas through reactions of dopaquinone with cysteine or glutathione.[10] Pheomelanin is more photolabile than eumelanin. Irradiation of pheomelanin may lead to the formation of potentially toxic hydroxyl radicals, which are thought to play a role in carcinogenesis.[11,12] They may contribute to the higher incidence of melanoma in red-haired individuals.

The metabolic pathways of both eumelanin and pheomelanin biosynthesis were established by Raper,[13] Mason,[14] and Prota and Nicolaus.[10] L-tyrosine is the initial substrate for the melanin pathway. It is oxidized by the enzyme tyrosinase to L-dopa (3,4-dihydroxyphenylalanine) and then dehydrogenized to dopachinone. While in the Raper-Mason scheme of melanin synthesis melanogenesis is primarily regulated at the level of the enzyme tyrosinase, recent evidence suggests that additional regulatory sites exist, for which a novel pigmentation gene family has been identified (pmel 17 gene family).[2,9]

Melanin synthesis is stimulated by melanocyte-stimulating hormone (MSH) and a variety of other hormones, including adrenocorticotropic hormone (ACTH) and sex steroids,[15] as well as by a number of inflammatory mediators.[7] While melanin is produced by many melanocytes during embryonic life, only melanocytes of the epidermis and hair follicles form measurable amounts of melanin in adult life.[1] Epidermal melanocytes connect to neighboring keratinocytes, to which they transfer melanin pigment particles—a relationship that has been named the *epidermal melanin unit.*[16] The melanocytes in hair follicles have a similar relationship with cells of the hair matrix.[1] They actively synthesize and transfer melanin into matrix cells during the anagen phase of the hair cycle.[17] No melanin synthesis, however, is observed in the telogen stage of the hair cycle.

Because epidermal and hair follicle melanocytes transfer melanin to neighboring cells, they have been called *secretory melanocytes.*[16] In contrast, other melanocytes, such as dermal melanocytes, which retain the melanin they have produced, have been called *continent melanocytes.*[16]

Melanin pigment is not always apparent in sections stained with hematoxylin and eosin (H&E). It may be present intracellularly within melanocytes, keratinocytes, or macrophages, or it may be found extracellularly. When melanin pigment is seen within melanocytes, it is usually finely granular or dustlike. Within keratinocytes, macrophages, or extracellularly, melanin pigment granules appear coarser and more uneven in size and shape.[18] When melanin pigment granules assume unusually large dimensions (up to 6 μm), they are called *macromelanosomes.*[19] These giant granules very rarely occur in normal melanocytes. They have been described, however, as an occasional finding in association with a variety of melanocytic lesions, such as simple lentigo, café-au-lait spots, especially in cases of neurofibromatosis,[19] and in a number of different types of melanocytic nevi.[20]

Melanin needs to be distinguished from other brown pigments. Melanin is the only endogenous brown-black pigment besides *homogentisic acid pigment,* which is deposited in various tissues, including the skin in ochronosis.[21] *Hemosiderin,* a hemoglobin-derived pigment, usually presents as golden-yellow to brown granular pigment[21] and occasionally may be confused with melanin. Hemosiderin can easily be identified by its iron content (see also Chap. 2). *Lipofuscin,* which appears as a yellow-brown, finely granular intracytoplasmic pigment on H&E-stained sections, also referred to as *wear-and-tear pigment,* contains insoluble material of lipids complexed with protein, which is thought to derive from indigestible residues of autophagic vacuoles. Lipofuscin is seen in cells undergoing slow, regressive changes. It may be confused with melanin, since it also stains when silver stains are used to identify melanin.[22] However, lipofuscin is positive on fat stains and is resistant to bleaching—unlike melanin (see also Chap. 2). Moreover, lipofuscin has a characteristic appearance on electron microscopy. Lipofuscin granules are highly electron dense, often surround membranous structures, and are located typically around the nucleus.[21] *Bilirubin,* which appears as green-brown to black deposits, usually can readily be distinguished from melanin by microscopy because of its green color and the amorphous globular composition of the pigment.[21] The pigment of *pseudomelanosis coli* is not melanin but rather related to lipofuscin.[23] It is found as fine brown granules of variable size within macrophages of the lamina propria of the large bowel, most often affecting the right colon. It is thought to be due to anthracene-containing laxatives. Similar pigment also can be seen in various storage diseases and in chronic granulomatous disease.

Neuromelanin is a melanin pigment that accumulates in catecholaminergic neurons during aging.[24] It is particularly prominent at the substantia nigra and the locus ceruleus. Electron paramagnetic resonance spectroscopy has shown that neuromelanin is indeed a melanin pigment, although with some unusual features in its mode of formation (auto-oxidation rather than enzymatically) and its composition (it has been suggested to be a copolymer derived from dopamine and glutathione). Its function in the brain is still unknown. It is thought to have a cytoprotective role under normal conditions, but it may be involved in neurocytotoxicity at advanced ages and in patients with Parkinson's disease.[25]

ANATOMIC DISTRIBUTION OF MELANOCYTES

The majority of melanocytes reside in the skin, in particular within the epidermis and hair follicles.[1] Some of them reside in the dermis and may be found around sebaceous glands or near the lactiferous ducts of the nipple.[26] Melanocytes also have been identified in visceral organs, the orbital cavity, the leptomeninges, and the inner ear.[27]

Epidermal melanocytes are present in all regions of the body. Estimations of the volume of melanocyte mass in an adult human range between 1 and 1.5 ml.[28] Their population density varies, depending on the region.[1] The ratio of melanocytes to keratinocytes of the basal layer ranges from approximately 1:4 to 1:10. The population density of melanocytes is highest on the face and genitalia (more than 2000/mm^2) and lowest on the skin of the trunk and upper arm (about 800 to 1000/mm^2).[29] Aging results in a decreased number of melanocytes as well as a decline in the activity of melanin synthesis.[27] The relative concentration of melanocytes appears to be independent of race and sex.[30] Racial differences in skin coloration result primarily from differences in the production and packaging of melanin pigment, but not from differences in the number of melanocytes.[31,32]

MORPHOLOGY OF MELANOCYTES

Light Microscopy

Melanocytes of the human epidermis exhibit a territorial behavior.[33] They are distributed at a distance from each other in a network located along the dermoepidermal

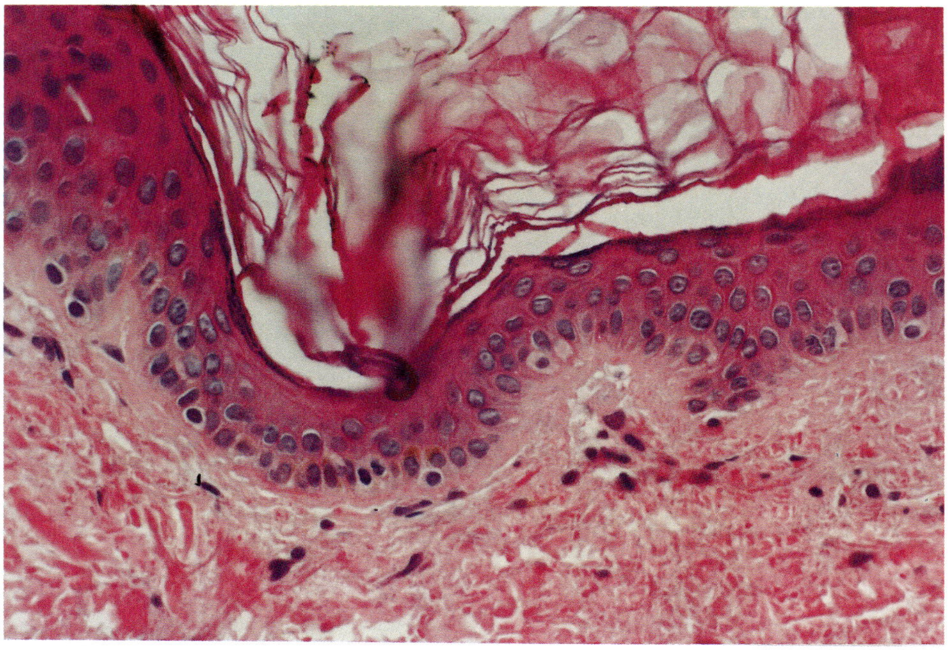

FIGURE 1-1
Epidermal melanocytes. Solitary cells with pale cytoplasm and round or ovoid nuclei are situated at the dermoepidermal junction, just below basal layer keratinocytes (H&E, × 400).

junction.[28] Melanocytes appear as small round or oval cells with pale cytoplasm in and immediately beneath the basal cell layer of the epidermis (Fig. 1-1). Their dendrites are usually invisible in H&E-stained paraffin sections, unless they are packed with melanin. In hair follicles, melanocytes are located at the epithelial side of the basement membrane bordering the central hair papilla.

The nucleus of melanocytes, whose contour often appears polygonal or indented, is somewhat smaller and more hyperchromatic than the nucleus of nearby keratinocytes.[34] The chromatin pattern is uniform with no apparent nucleoli. Thin cytoplasmic dendrites project from the cell body and extend in all directions (Fig. 1-2). Their visualization usually requires special histochemical stains (see Fig.1-2; see also Chap. 2).

Adult resident epidermal melanocytes may proliferate in response to UV light or growth factors released during tissue regeneration.[35] Three proliferative patterns have been described.[36] *Lentiginous melanocytic hyperplasia* refers to a pattern of single-cell melanocytic proliferation along the dermoepidermal junction. *Nesting* describes presumed clonal proliferation of clusters of melanocytes. If single-cell growth is discohesive and seen throughout the entire epidermis, a pattern of *pagetoid proliferation* is present. Lentiginous hyperplasia is often a feature of lentigines or "lentiginous" forms of melanocytic nevi. Nesting is typical of melanocytic nevi. Pagetoid spread, although often associated with melanoma, also may be observed in both acquired and congenital nevi of children, Spitz nevi, pigmented spindle cell nevi, and common acquired nevi of acral skin. The pattern of benign melanocytic proliferation is typically symmetrical and shows in vertical growth a gradient of cytologic development that is referred to as *maturation*.

Electron Microscopy

Electron micrographs of melanocytes typically show a prominent Golgi complex and rough endoplasmatic reticulum as well as numerous mitochondria—features characteristic of metabolically active cells. Melanocytes lack tonofilaments and desmosomes. They contain, however, intermediate filaments (vimentin). Where melanocytes appose the epidermal basal lamina, half-desmosome-like structures are seen.[18] The nucleus of melanocytes may be smooth or lobulated. Nuclear lobation has been suggested to be a feature of metabolically active melanocytes.[37]

The ultrastructural hallmark of melanocytes is a unique organelle, the melanosome.[38] Melanosomes originate

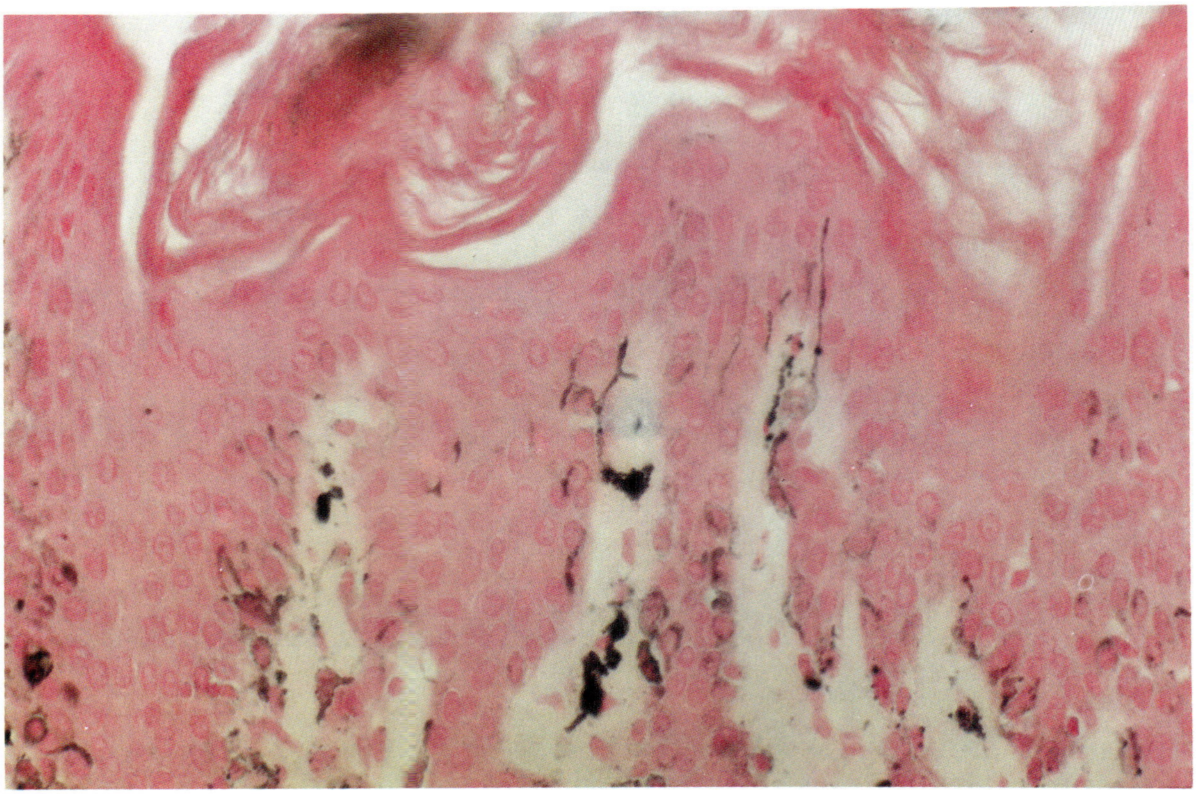

FIGURE 1-2
Silver-stained melanocytes. The dendritic processes of melanocytes become apparent (Masson-Fontana, × 400).

from the Golgi apparatus and contain enzymes involved in melanogenesis.[39]

In the formation of eumelanosomes, four stages have been described.[40] Premelanosomes comprise stage I and II melanosomes, while stages III and IV represent mature melanosomes. Stage I melanosomes are spherical structures that contain vesicular inclusions with histochemically detectable tyrosinase activity or occasionally few filaments that have a distinct periodicity (Fig. 1-3*A*). Stage II melanosomes are oval organelles with a characteristic internal lamellar structure (see Fig. 1-3*B*). These membranous filaments have a distinctive periodicity with or without regular cross-striations. They are more extensively developed in stage II than in stage I melanosomes. Granular deposits of melanin pigment appear on early stage III melanosomes (see Fig. 1-3*C*). These pigment granules are more developed in late stage III (see Fig. 1-3*D*) when they partly obliterate the organelle. Stage IV melanosomes are completely melanized (see Fig. 1-3*E*). While stage I melanosomes measure approximately 0.3 μm in length, stage II to IV melanosomes measure 0.4 to 1.0 μm in greatest dimension. As melanosomes mature, they gradually move from the cytoplasm of the melanocyte into the dendritic processes. The tips of the dendrites, filled with mature melanosomes, are snipped off (apocopated) and are phagocytosed by neighboring keratinocytes, wherein melanosomes fuse with lysosomes.[1]

The development of pheomelanosomes also has been discerned in four stages.[18] Pheomelanosomes are round rather than oval throughout all stages. In stage I, a vacuole is present, which contains small microvesicles. These microvesicles become more numerous in stage II. Deposition of melanin pigment on microvesicles and in the matrix characterizes stage III. When the matrix is completely filled with melanin, stage IV is reached.

Skin pigmentation depends on the number and maturation of melanosomes as well as their packaging.[1] In whites, melanosomes are less numerous than in blacks. While in the former, melanosomes are present mainly in stages I and II, most melanosomes are stage IV in blacks.

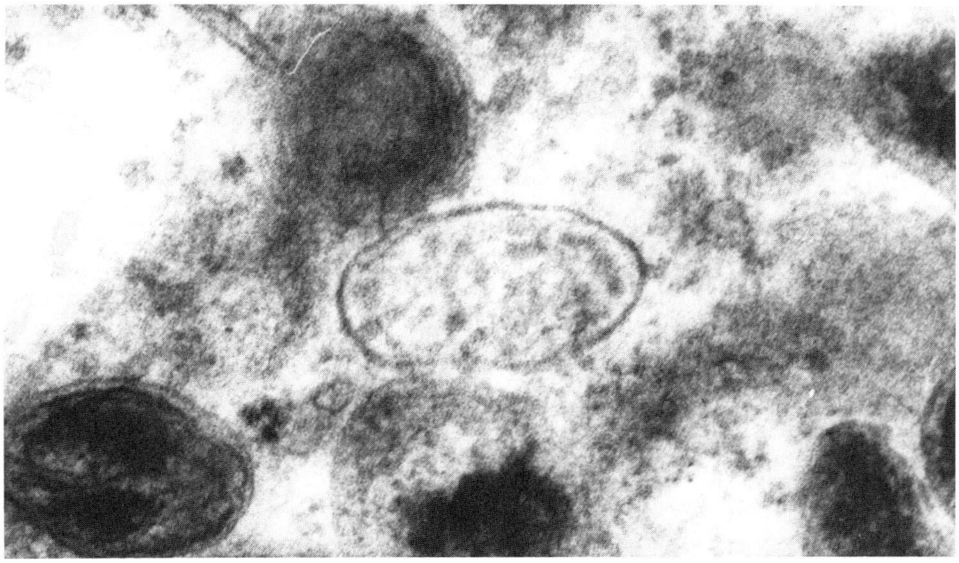

A

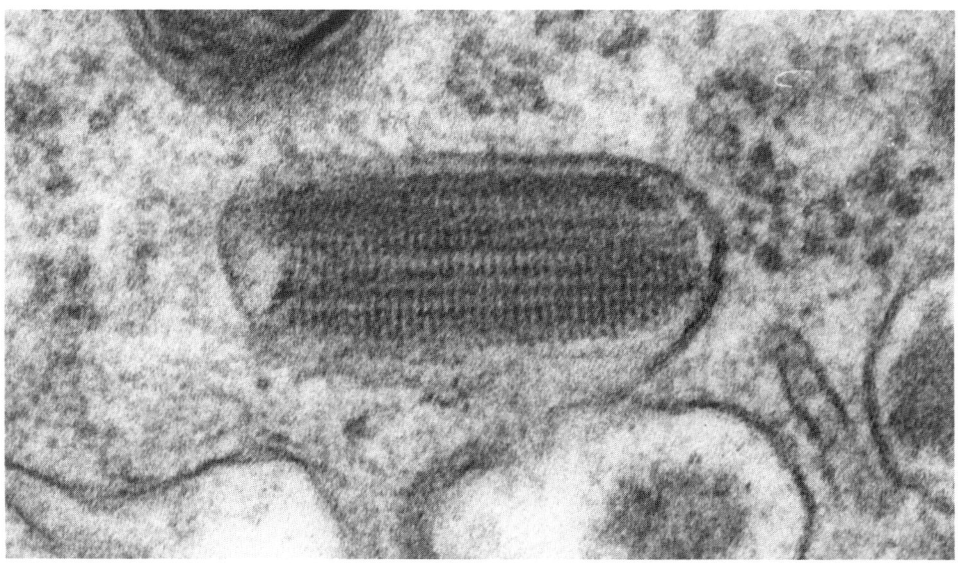

B

FIGURE 1-3

Ultrastructure of eumelanosomes. The four stages of eumelanosome formation are illustrated in electron micrographs: (A) stage I: vesicular inclusions (× 100,000); (B) stage II: striated inclusions (× 100,800); (C) early stage III: granular deposits on striated inclusions (× 130,100); late stage III: more granular deposits (× 94,000); (E) stage IV: fully melanized organelles (× 96,000). (Courtesy of Dr. M. Seiler, West Roxbury VA Medical Center, West Roxbury, Mass.)

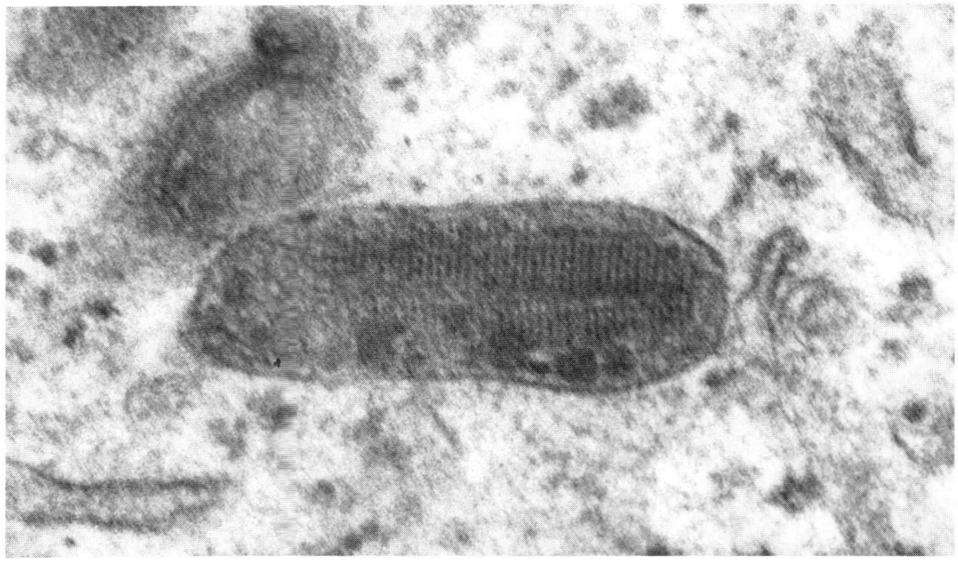

C

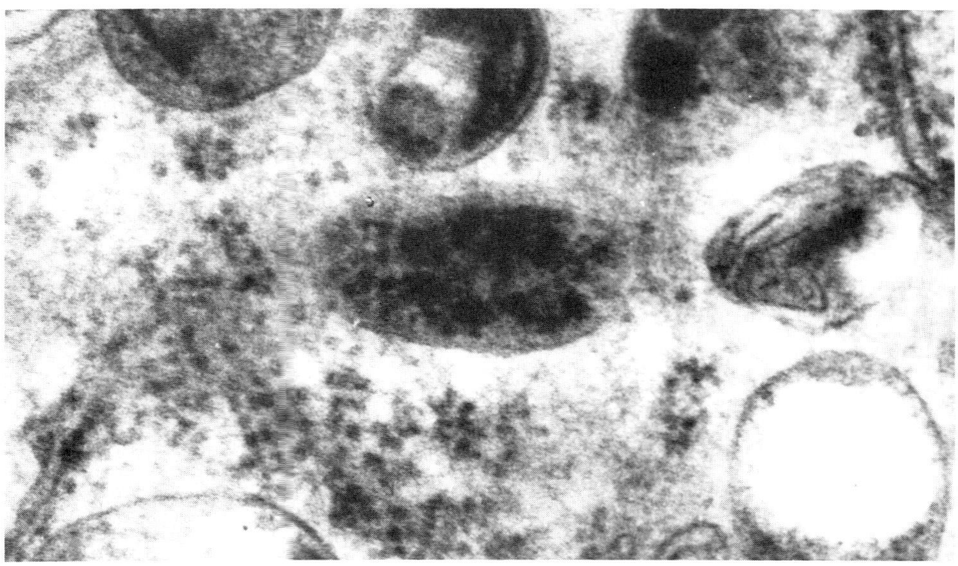

D

FIGURE 1-3 *(Continued)*

Sun-induced darkening of the skin corresponds to an increase in stage III and IV melanosomes in keratinocytes. In blacks, melanosomes lie individually rather than grouped together in melanosome complexes and are degraded more slowly.[31,32]

HISTOGENESIS OF MELANOCYTES

Melanocytes are thought to be of neural crest origin based on in vivo studies of ablation and transplants of the neural crest, which produced changes in patterns of cutaneous pigmentation.[41,42] This theory is supported also by in vitro studies demonstrating that neural crest cells from various species can give rise directly to melanocytes.[43,44]

Much controversy still exists about when and where along the migration of neural crest–derived cells commitment toward melanocytic differentiation occurs.[45] In the center of this debate is the concept of a *melanoblast*, which has been defined as a melanocytic stem cell.[1] Although it seems possible that such stem cells undergo commitment

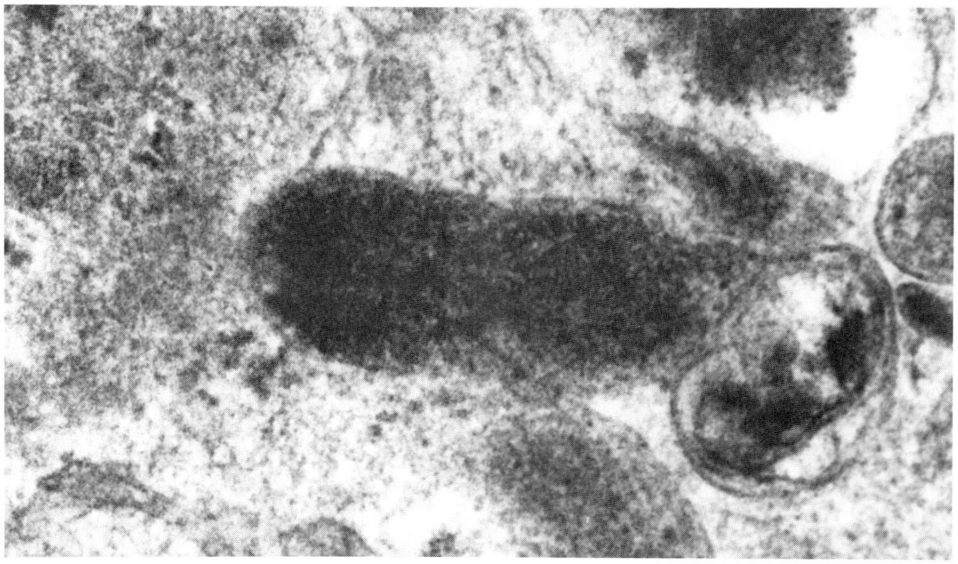

E

FIGURE 1-3 *(Continued)*

toward melanocytic differentiation prior to or early during migration with other primitive cells from the neural crest, to date, no direct evidence for the existence of nonpluripotential melanocytic stem cells has been provided.[45] Alternatively, it has been postulated that melanocytes might derive from pluripotential cells that travel from the neural crest to the skin via the paraspinal ganglia and their peripheral nerves and become committed only late, i.e., after migration to the local microenvironment of dermis and epidermis.[44,46,47] This view has been supported by several studies showing that explants of peripheral developing nerves or embryonic paraspinal ganglia can be manipulated to give rise to melanocytes.[48,49] It is also interesting to note in this context that embryonic nerves have extended close to the human epidermis by 8 weeks of gestation, which coincides with the earliest time that melanocytes have been identified in human skin.[46,50] Commitment late during migration is furthermore suggested by the observation that it is only in the periderm that the first characteristic melanocytic features such as dendrites and melanosomes usually become detectable.[36]

Once commitment to melanocytic differentiation has occurred after arrival of the pluripotential cells in the periderm and dermis, immature melanocytes mature as they migrate through the dermis and dermoepidermal junction to become terminally differentiated resident melanocytes in the epidermis.[45]

Despite their migratory potential, the location of mature melanocytes in the basal cell layer of the epidermis is quite stable. Proliferation and migration of melanocytes may be observed in epidermal regeneration and repigmentation after tissue injury. The principal reservoir for melanocytes repopulating reepithelialized epidermis is thought to be melanocytes normally dispersed along the basal layer of hair follicles and/or melanocytes derived from pluripotential perineural stem cells.[51]

MORPHOLOGY OF NEVUS CELLS

The cells of nevocellular nevi, which are thought to be melanocytic, are typically grouped in nests with apposition of individual cells to each other.[36] Nesting can occur along the dermoepidermal junction (junctional nevus) or within the dermis (dermal nevus). Both patterns are often present simultaneously (compound nevus). The dermal component may extend deep and involve adnexal or neural structures (congenital features).

Three different cytologic variations of melanocytes have been described in nevi.[36] The intraepidermal or intradermal melanocytes, which typically have an epithelioid appearance with prominent cytoplasm containing moderately coarse melanin pigment, are also historically referred to as *type A cells* (Fig. 1-4*A*). They contain a round to oval nucleus, slightly smaller in size than the nucleus of a keratinocyte, with uniformly dispersed chromatin and occasionally an inconspicuous nucleolus. Type B melanocytes resemble lymphocytes (see Fig. 1-4*B*). Their nuclei are small, round to oval, and are surrounded by scant cytoplasm. The nuclear chromatin is uniformly dispersed

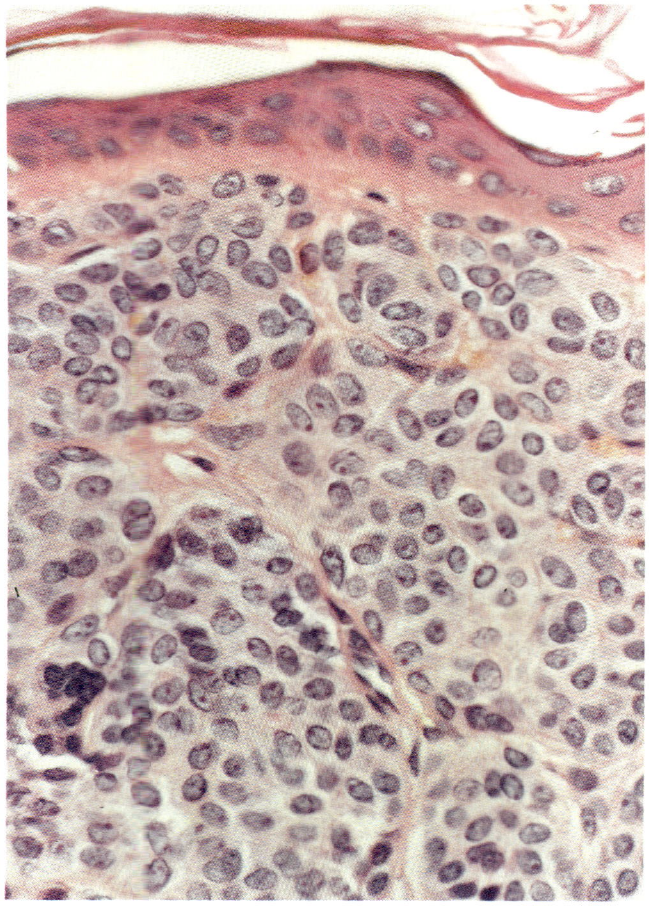

A

FIGURE 1-4

Cytology of melanocytes in nevi: (A) epithelioid or type A cells (H&E, × 400); (B) lymphoid or type B cells (H&E, × 400); and (C) Schwannian or type C cells (H&E, × 400).

with no apparent nucleoli. Type B cells are usually part of the dermal component or compound nevi. The neural or type C cell is spindle-shaped and typically present in the deeper layers of a melanocytic lesion. It resembles fibroblasts or peripheral nerve sheath cells (see Fig. 1-4C).

HISTOGENESIS OF NEVUS CELLS

The histogenesis of melanocytes in nevi (nevus cells) is still not entirely resolved.[45] It has been suggested that nevocytes represent a distinct cellular entity which arises from a nevoblast, a pluripotential precursor that migrates from the neural crest.[52] However, no such nevoblast with distinctive phenotypic characteristics has ever been identified.[45] Alternatively, it is currently widely accepted that nevocytes are melanocytes.[53] In this view, their nesting pattern may be interpreted as a melanocytic response to a distinct local microenvironment, a functionally altered state, or injury.

It is contingent to the concept of neural crest origin that precursors of epidermal melanocytes must actually migrate from the dermis to the epidermis during development. With this in mind, there are two ways to explain the dermal presence of melanocytes. Melanocytes may come to reside in the dermis after a process of "dropping off" (*Abtropfung*) from proliferating epidermal melanocytes.[54] Alternatively, they may stay in the dermis because they are unable to complete upward migration (*Hochsteigerung*) into the epidermis.[45] In this latter view, if incomplete upward migration occurs during development, congenital nevi arise. Acquired nevi result in this interpretation from increasing loss of migratory capability of

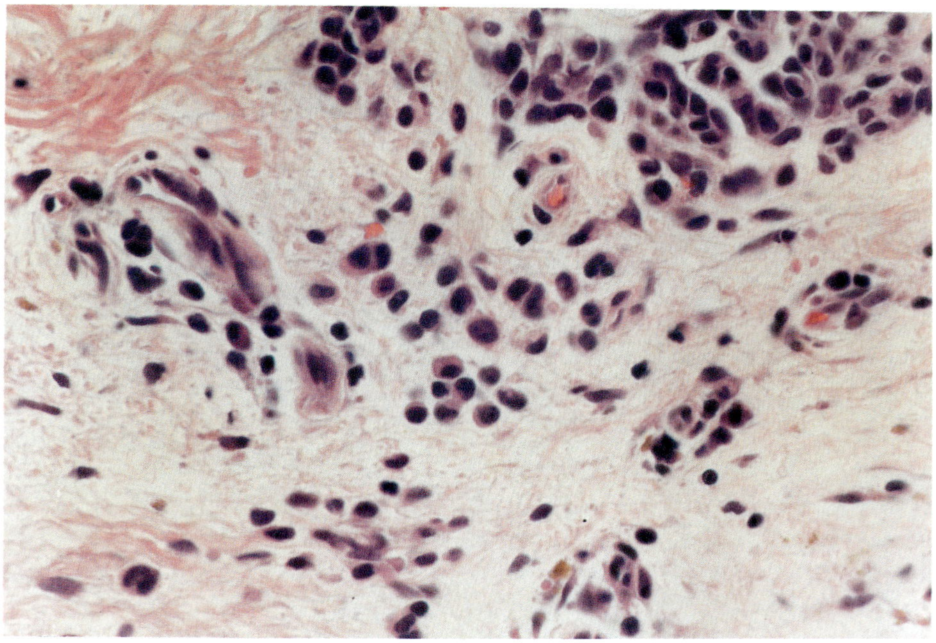

B

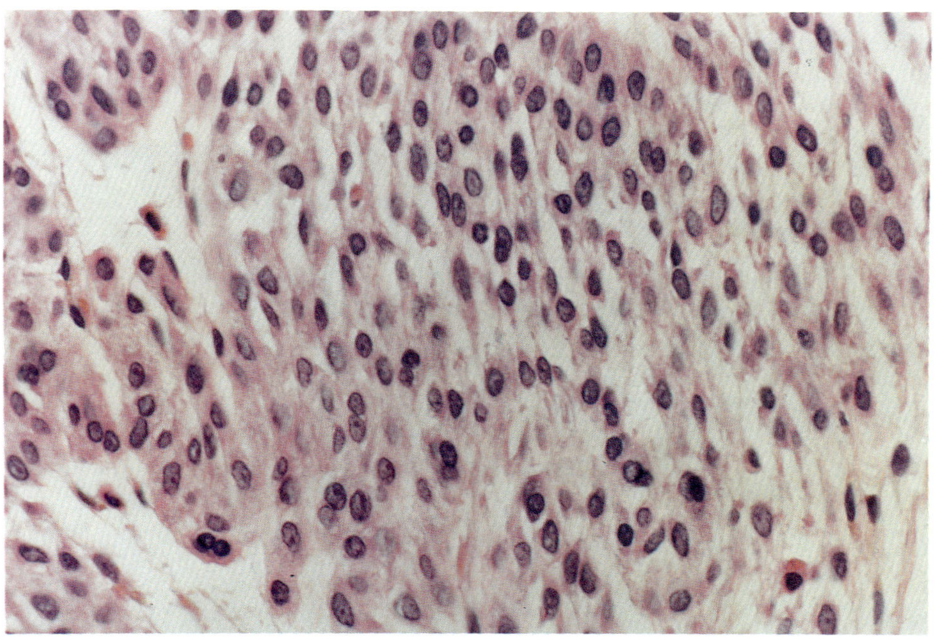

C

FIGURE 1-4 *(Continued)*

melanocytes derived from proliferating pluripotential peripheral nerve-sheath precursor cells. Both theories, however, remain speculative, since to date no direct evidence for either direction of cell movement exists.

Acquired melanocytic nevi are thought to reflect a melanocytic response to chronic growth stimulation by UV light or inflammatory mediators and may represent an early stage in the process of melanocytic carcinogenesis.[35]

EMBRYOLOGY OF MELANOCYTES

During development of human skin, melanocytes appear first in the vicinity of nerves and blood vessels of the dermis at approximately 4 to 10 weeks of fetal life.[55] They reach the epidermis by the end of the second month of gestational age.[56] Production of melanin is first observed in the skin of the eyelids, the external auditory canal, and the labial mucosa. Pigment synthesis in fetal body skin begins between the third and fifth month depending on the racial background.[56-58] During this period of time, the number of melanocytes increases approximately threefold.[59]

While initially melanocytes are randomly distributed throughout all epidermal layers,[60,61] a stable population residing near the basal cell layer with bipolar dendritic processes is established by 6 months.[58] Melanosome transfer to keratinocytes begins at this time. Morphologically, fetal melanocytes are more uniform in size, structure, and number of dendritic processes than adult melanocytes.[59]

REFERENCES

1. Quevedo WC Jr, Fitzpatrick TB, Szabo G, Jimbow K: Biology of melanocytes, in Fitzpatrick TB, Eisen AZ, Wolff K, Freedberg IM, Austen KF (eds): *Dermatology in General Medicine*, ed 3. New York, McGraw-Hill, 1987, pp 224–251.
2. Kwon BS: Pigmentation genes: The tyrosinase gene family and the pmel 17 gene family. *J Invest Dermatol* 100:134S–140S, 1993.
3. Morison WL: What is the function of melanin? *Arch Dermatol* 121:1160–1163, 1985.
4. Nordlund JJ, Abdel-Malek ZA, Boissy RE, Rheins CA: Pigment cell biology: A historical review. *J Invest Dermatol* 92:53S–60S, 1989.
5. Proctor PH, McGinnis JE: The function of melanin. *Arch Dermatol* 122:507–508, 1986.
6. Riley PA: Materia melaninca: Further dark thoughts. *Pigment Cell Res* 5(3):101–106, 1990.
7. Morelli JG, Norris DA: Influence of inflammatory mediators and cytokines on human melanocyte function. *J Invest Dermatol* 100:191S–196S, 1993.
8. Prota G: Recent advances in the chemistry of melano genesis in mammals. *J Invest Dermatol* 75:122–127, 1980.
9. Prota G: Regulatory mechanisms of melanogenesis: Beyond the tyrosinase concept. *J Invest Dermatol* 100:156S–161S, 1993.
10. Prota G, Nicolaus RA: On the biogenesis of phaeomelanins, in Montagna W, Hu F (eds): *Advances in Biology of Skin*. New York, Pergamon Press, 1966, pp 323–328.
11. Chedekel MR, Smith SK, Post PW, et al: Photodestruction of pheomelanin: Role of oxygen. *Proc Natl Acad Sci USA* 75:5395–5399, 1978.
12. Tomita Y, Hariu A, Kato C, Seiji M: Radical production during tyrosine reaction, dopa-melanin formation, and photoirradiation of dopa-melanin. *J Invest Dermatol* 16:573–576, 1984.
13. Raper HS: The aerobic oxidases. *Physiol Rev* 8:245–282, 1928.
14. Mason HS: The chemistry of melanin: III. Mechanism of oxidation of dihydroxyphenylalanine by tyrosinase. *J Biol Chem* 172:83–99, 1948.
15. Thody AJ, Smith AG: Hormones and skin pigmentation. *Int J Dermatol* 16:657–664, 1977.
16. Masson P: Pigment cells in man, in Miner RW, Gordon M (eds): *The biology of melanomas*. New York, New York Academy of Sciences, 1948, pp 15–51.
17. Kukita A: Changes in tyrosinase activity during melanocyte proliferation. *J Invest Dermatol* 28:273–274, 1957.
18. Mooi WJ, Krausz T: Melanin and melanocytes, in Mooi WJ, Krausz T (eds): *Biopsy Pathology of Melanocytic Disorders*. London, Chapman and Hall, 1991, pp 1–16.
19. Jimbow K, Szabo G, Fitzpatrick TB: Ultrastructure of giant pigment granules (macromelanosomes) in the cutaneous pigmented macules of neurofibromatosis. *J Invest Dermatol* 61:300–309, 1973.
20. Konrad KK, Wolff K, Hoenigsmann H: The giant melanosome: A model of deranged melanosome-morphogenesis. *J Ultrastruct Res* 48:102–123, 1974.
21. Cotran RS, Kumar V, Robbins SL: Pigments, in Cotran RS, Kumar V, Robbins SL (eds): *Pathologic Basis of Disease*, ed 4. Philadelphia, WB Saunders, 1989, pp 24–26.
22. Burck HC: Pigmentnachweis, in Burck HC (ed): *Histologische technik*, ed 3. Stuttgart, Thieme, 1973, pp 141–151.
23. Goldman H: Effects of laxative and enemas, in Ming SC, Goldman H (eds): *Pathology of the Gastrointestinal Tract*. Philadelphia, WB Saunders, 1992, p 706.
24. Enochs WS, Nilges MJ, Swartz HM: Purified human neuromelanin, synthetic dopamine melanin as a potential model pigment, and the normal human substantia nigra: Characterization by electron paramagnetic resonance spectroscopy. *J Neurochem* 61:68–79, 1993.
25. Kastner A, Hirsch EC, Lejeune O, et al: Is the vulnerability of neurons in the substantia nigra of patients with Parkinson's disease related to their neuromelanin content? *J Neurochem* 59:1080–1089, 1992.
26. Montagna W: Histology and cytochemistry of human skin: XXXV. The nipple and areola. *Br J Dermatol* 83:2–13, 1970.
27. Nordlund JJ: The lives of pigment cells. *Clin Geriatr Med* 5(1):91–108, 1989.

28. Rosdahl I, Rorsman H: An estimate of the melanocyte mass in humans. *J Invest Dermatol* 81:278–281, 1983.
29. Fitzpatrick TB, Szabo G: The melanocyte: Cytology and cytochemistry. *J Invest Dermatol* 32:197–209, 1959.
30. Szabo G: The number of melanocytes in human epidermis. *Br Med J* 1:1016–1017, 1954.
31. Szabo G, Gerald AB, Pathak MA, Fitzpatrick TB: Racial differences in human pigmentation at the ultrastructural level. *J Cell Biol* 39:132–133, 1968.
32. Szabo G, Shelburne J, Linder J, Klintworth GK: Racial differences in the fate of melanosomes in human epidermis. *Nature* 222:1081–1082, 1969.
33. Cochran AJ: The incidence of melanocytes in normal skin. *J Invest Dermatol* 57:38–43, 1970.
34. Hu F: Melanocyte cytology in normal skin, melanocytic nevi, and malignant melanomas: A review, in Ackerman AB (ed): *Pathology of Malignant Melanoma.* New York, Masson, 1981, pp 1–21.
35. Medrano EE, Farooqui JZ, Boissy RE, et al: Chronic growth stimulation of human adult melanocytes by inflammatory mediators in vitro: Implications for nevus formation and initial steps in melanocyte oncogenesis. *Proc Natl Acad Sci USA* 90:1790–1794, 1993.
36. Imber MJ, Mihm MC: Benign melanocytic tumors, in Farmer ER, Hood AF (eds): *Pathology of the Skin.* Norwalk, Conn: Appleton and Lange, 1990, pp 663–683.
37. Szabo G, Flynn E: Morphological aspects of normal human melanocytes, in Veronesi U, Cascinelli N, Santinami M (eds): *Cutaneous Melanoma: Status of Knowledge and Future Perspective.* London, Academic Press, 1987, pp 127–138.
38. Seiji M, Fitzpatrick TB, Birbeck MSC: The melanosome: A distinctive subcellular particle of mammalian melanocytes and the site of melanogenesis. *J Invest Dermatol* 36:243–252, 1961.
39. Seiji M, Iwashita S: Intracellular localization of tyrosinase and site of melanin formation in melanocytes. *J Invest Dermatol* 45:305–314, 1965.
40. Jimbow K, Kukita A: Fine structure of pigment granules, in Kawamura (ed): *Biology of Normal and Abnormal Melanocytes.* Tokyo, University of Tokyo Press, 1971, pp 171–193.
41. Rawles ME: Origin of melanophores and their role in development of color patterns in vertebrates. *Physiol Rev* 28:383–408, 1948.
42. LeDouarin NM: *The Neural Crest.* New York, Cambridge University Press, 1982, pp 108–133.
43. Barrofino A, Dupin E, LeDouarin NM: Clone forming ability and differentiation potential of migratory (quail) neural crest cells. *Proc Natl Acad Sci USA* 85:5325–5329, 1988.
44. Perris von Boxberg Y, Lofberg J: Local embryonic matrices determine region-specific phenotypes in (axolotl) neural crest cells. *Science* 241:86–89, 1988.
45. Cramer SF: The origin of epidermal melanocytes. *Arch Pathol Lab Med* 115:115–119, 1991.
46. Cramer SF: The histogenesis of acquired melanocytic nevi: Based on a new concept of melanocytic differentiation. *Am J Dermatopathol* 6(Suppl 1):289–298, 1984.
47. Cramer SF: The melanocytic differentiation pathway in congenital melanocytic nevi: Theoretical considerations. *Pediatr Pathol* 8:253–265, 1988.
48. Weston JA: Neural crest cell development. *Prog Clin Biol Res* 85:359–379, 1982.
49. Ciment G, Glimelius B, Nelson DM, Weston JA: Reversal of a developmental restriction in neural crest cells of avian embryos by a phorbol ester drug. *Dev Biol* 118:392–398, 1986.
50. Sagebiel RW, Odland GF: Ultrastructural identification of melanocytes in early human embryos, in Riley V (ed): *Pigmentation: Its Genesis and Biologic Control.* East Norwalk, Conn: Appleton and Lange, 1969, pp 43–50.
51. Staricco RG: Mechanism of migration of the melanocyte from the hair follicle into the epidermis following dermabrasion. *J Invest Dermatol* 36:99–104, 1961.
52. Mishima Y: Macromolecular changes in pigmentary disorders. *Arch Dermatol* 91:519–557, 1965.
53. Magna-Garcia M, Ackermann B: What are nevus cells? *Am J Dermatopathol* 12:93–102, 1990.
54. Unna PG: Naevi and naevocarcinome. *Berl Klin Wochenschr* 30:14–16, 1893.
55. Zimmermann AA, Becker SW Jr: Precursors of epidermal melanocytes in the Negro fetus, in Gordon M (ed): *Pigment Cell Biology.* Orlando, Fla: Academic Press, 1959, pp 159–170.
56. Holbrook KA, Vogel AM, Underwood RA, Foster CA: Melanocytes in human embryonic and fetal skin: A review and new findings. *Pigment Cell Res* 1(Suppl):6–17, 1988.
57. Breathnach AS, Wyllie LM: Electron microscopy of melanocytes and Langerhans cells in human fetal epidermis at 14 weeks. *J Invest Dermatol* 44:51–60, 1965.
58. Zimmermann AA, Cornbleet T: The development of epidermal pigmentation in the Negro fetus. *J Invest Dermatol* 11:383–395, 1948.
59. Becker SW, Zimmermann AA: Further studies on melanocytes and melanogenesis in human fetus and newborn. *J Invest Dermatol* 25:103–112, 1955.
60. Mishima Y, Widlan S: Embryonic development of melanocytes in human hair and epidermis. *J Invest Dermatol* 46:263–277, 1966.
61. Barla-Szabo L: Ejection of melanocytes and melanin from fetuses and newborn mammalian animals. *Acta Morphol Acad Sci Hung* 18:213–225, 1970.

2

Biopsies, Tissue Processing, and Special Studies

TYPES OF BIOPSIES

Excisional Biopsies

The specimen submitted for histopathologic examination needs to provide critical diagnostic and prognostic information, such as symmetry and lateral and deep extension. Therefore, the proper procedure for most pigmented cutaneous lesions is an *excisional biopsy.* The biopsy should not be too large so as to avoid unnecessary removal of normal skin if the lesion is benign, in which case the biopsy constitutes definitive treatment. When the lesion is malignant, excision of the whole lesion becomes necessary, with margins appropriate for tumor thickness.

A skin excision usually provides an ellipse of skin with some subcutaneous fat. The biopsy should be oriented in such a way that a reexcision, when indicated, can be done with minimal skin loss. Generally, the excision is best performed with the long axis in the direction of cutaneous lymphatics. Orientation by the clinician or the pathologist handling the specimen can be accomplished by attaching suture material to a designated margin.

The skin excision is fixed whole. A macroscopic description of the lesion itself should be provided by the pathologist, with particular attention paid to the proximity of the lesion to the respective margins (Table 2-1). If there is suspicion for malignancy, the surgical margins are inked prior to dissection of the specimen. Orientation of the surgical margins is facilitated by applying two different colors of ink to each half of the lateral and deep margins of the excisional biopsy. Scoring of the specimen for orientation by superficial incisions with razor blades is not recommended because it often leads to separation of fragments from the remainder of the specimen. Sections are taken such that the minimal distance of the lesion to a resection margin, maximal thickness of the lesion, and any unusual features such as ulceration are demonstrated (Fig. 2-1). Small excisional biopsies (<1 cm in greatest dimension) may be bisected along their longitudinal axes and the two halves processed separately if orientation is important.

Punch Biopsies

Punch biopsies of cutaneous pigmented lesions are indicated only in a few situations: (1) to establish a diagnosis with minimal loss of tissue and to guide further therapy, if any is needed, for large lesions such as lentigo maligna or large congenital nevi, (2) for cosmetic reasons, (3) for certain anatomic sites, e.g., the face or subungual locations, and (4) to treat lesions sufficiently small that a punch biopsy includes the entire lesion and a rim of surrounding normal skin. Otherwise, punch biopsies are not recommended for pigmented lesions because they generally do not provide adequate information on symmetry and extension of the lesion.

The macroscopic description should include the diameter of the specimen, its depth, and the presence of subcutaneous fat. A brief description of the surface should be recorded. The punch biopsy is bisected through its center with a sharp razor blade. Small punch biopsies (diameters of 4 mm or less) should be embedded intact.

Shave or Saucerization Specimens

The use of shave biopsy for removal of atypical melanocytic lesions is to be discouraged. The most disastrous result from such a procedure is the partial removal or

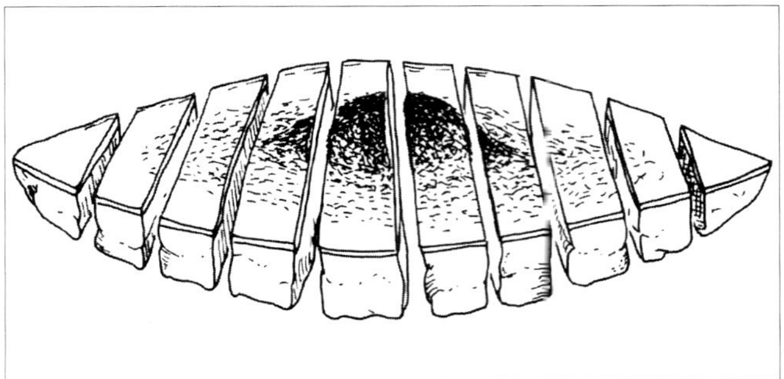

FIGURE 2-1
Handling of excisional specimens. The initial transverse section should be taken through the thickest or darkest portion of the pigmented lesion. Serial sections should then be taken at 2- to 3-mm intervals through the remainder of the specimen.

disruption of a primary melanoma. Thus both histopathologic diagnosis and important prognostic features may be rendered suboptimal or compromised altogether. However, it must be pointed out that dermatologists or other physicians sufficiently knowledgeable about melanocytic lesions are able to optimize the use of this technique for the appropriate indications.

TISSUE PROCESSING

Frozen sections are generally not recommended for melanocytic lesions for a number of reasons: the histologic appearance is inferior, the study of multiple levels is more difficult, and a portion of the tissue is lost in the cutting of sections. Moreover, measurements of tumor thickness on frozen sections are not comparable with those on paraffin-embedded tissue, which has been used for standardization of tumor thickness as a prognostic marker. These considerations do not apply to frozen section diagnoses of metastatic lesions.

Tissue for Research

In general, obtaining tissue for research is only acceptable if the lesion exceeds 1 cm in greatest dimension and if only a thin slice of the lesion, excluding its thickest part and relevant margins, is taken. Tissue may be frozen in either liquid nitrogen or another suitable fluid for immediate tissue freezing, such as dry-ice-cooled 2-methylbutane. Tissue for cytogenetic studies or for experimental therapy using tumor infiltrating lymphocytes requires handling of the specimen under sterile conditions.

Fixation

Most melanocytic lesions are small skin biopsies which are fixed in toto by immersion in neutral buffered formalin. Larger specimens (> 1 cm) and lymph nodes should be incised to secure adequate penetration by the fixative. Paraffin sections are adequate for most routine diagnostic purposes. Most antibodies available to distinguish melanocytic from nonmelanocytic lesions are applicable on paraffin-embedded tissue. Frozen tissue and occasionally fresh sterile tissue for cytogenetics should be saved if the diagnosis is uncertain and sarcomas or lymphomas are considered.

SPECIAL STUDIES IN THE EVALUATION OF MELANOCYTIC LESIONS

Melanin Stains

In the histologic and cytologic diagnosis of melanocytic lesions, the correct identification of melanin is important. If a pigment cannot be identified readily as melanin on routine histologic sections by morphologic criteria alone, a number staining procedures can enable one to confirm the presence of melanin. The most widely used methods are reducing silver stains, such as the Masson-Fontana and Schmorl stain or the more sensitive Warthin-Starry stain.[1] These stains, however, are not entirely specific, since they also highlight some lipofuscins and argentaffin endocrine cells. It is prudent to use an iron stain in parallel with a melanin stain if melanin is to be distinguished from hemosiderin. Bleaching also might be useful for the latter distinction; melanin pigment can be removed by bleaching, e.g., in 0.5% potassium permanganate, while hemosiderin and lipofuscin are resistant to bleaching. The

TABLE 2-1
Routine Handling of Skin Excisions for Pigmented Lesions

1. Record dimensions of specimen: length, width, depth.
2. Record gross morphologic features of pigmented lesion:
   a. Length and width in mm or cm and proximity to surgical margins.
   b. Symmetry or asymmetry.
   c. Regularity or irregularity of borders.
   d. Coloration, uniform or variegated.
   e. Colors present: pink, tan, brown, black, blue, gray, white.
   f. Topography: flat, raised, nodular, ulcerated, presence of crust or hemorrhage.
3. In general, specimen is inked for surgical margins.
4. Transverse sections should be taken through thickest or darkest area or through the center of lesion.
5. Serial sections every 2 to 3 mm may be taken through the remainder of the specimen or the "rule of halves" applied, i.e., the subsequent transverse sections are taken to bisect each half of the residual specimen until one has tissue sections 2 to 3 mm in thickness after the initial transverse section.

TABLE 2-2
Immunohistochemical Evaluation of Melanoma

	Type of Specimen	Sensitivity	Specificity
S-100 protein	Frozen, paraffin	High	Low
HMB-45	Frozen, paraffin	High	High
NKI/beteb	Frozen	High	High
NKI/C3	Paraffin	Moderately high	Low
HMW-MAA	Frozen only	High	Low
Vimentin	Frozen, paraffin	High	None
Neuron-specific enolase	Frozen, paraffin	Moderately high	Low

brown pigment of pseudomelanosis coli is generally PAS-positive, whereas melanin is negative.

Occasionally, formalin pigment, a hemoglobin-derived pigment, may cause confusion. The pigment forms if formalin is not buffered to a neutral pH. It does not stain with silver stains[2] and can be distinguished rapidly by incubating the slide in a picric acid solution.

Enzyme Histochemistry
Tyrosinase activity can be demonstrated by the dopa oxidase technique, which may be useful in identifying traces of melanin synthesis in hypomelanotic lesions. This reaction can be performed on frozen sections, as well as on paraffin sections of adequately fixed tissue.[3] False-positive results may be seen in the presence of mast cells, since their granules also stain with this technique. However, because of their metachromatic properties, this should not generate diagnostic problems.

Immunomarkers
A number of immunomarkers are available to aid in identifying a lesion as melanocytic (Table 2-2). Their most important applications include the evaluation of poorly differentiated (generally amelanotic) primary or metastatic malignant tumors, in particular in the absence of a known primary neoplasm, that suggest melanoma. Examples of diagnostic uncertainties in which melanocytic lesions need to be considered are spindle cell tumors (e.g., squamous cell carcinoma, atypical fibroxanthoma, leiomyosarcoma), small round cell tumors (e.g., lymphoma, neuroendocrine carcinoma), intraepidermal neoplasms (such as extramammary Paget's disease, squamous cell carcinoma in situ), and signet-ring cell neoplasms (e.g., adenocarcinoma, lymphoma). Whenever the melanocytic origin of a lesion needs to be confirmed, it is critical to apply a panel of markers and to weigh the pattern of immunoreactivities against the clinical and histologic impression (Table 2-3). It is also prudent to include markers positive for those nonmelanocytic cell types which enter into the differential diagnosis.[4] For the diagnosis of melanocytic versus nonmelanocytic tumors, we recommend the use of a combination of antibodies to S-100 protein, HMB-45, vimentin, low- and high-molecular-weight keratins, epithelial membrane antigen (EMA), leukocyte common antigen (LCA), and possibly neuron-specific enolase (NSE), all of which can be used on formalin-fixed and paraffin-embedded tissue.

TABLE 2-3
*Use of Immunomarkers in the Differential Diagnosis of Melanoma**

	Melanoma	Paget's Disease	Carcinoma	Lymphoma	Sarcoma
S-100 protein	+	−	±	−	Peripheral nerve-sheath tumors Chondrosarcoma Osteosarcoma Histiocytosis-X
HMB-45	+	−	−	−	−
Neuron-specific enolase	+	−	±	−	±
Cytokeratin	±	+	+	−	±
Epithelial membrane antigen	±	+	+	±	±
Carcinoembryonic antigen	−	+	±	−	−
Leukocyte common antigen	−	−	−	+	−
Vimentin	+	−	±	±	+

*The immunostaining patterns outlined represent the *usual* outcome, but there are many exceptions. It is safe to say that no tumor is uniformly negative or positive for an individual marker.

Anti–S-100 protein antibodies are important in the diagnosis of melanocytic tumors because of their high sensitivity; the vast majority of melanocytic lesions (>95 percent), including amelanotic melanoma and its metastases, is immunoreactive with these antibodies.[5] Both nuclear and cytoplasmic staining are seen. Usually, the majority of melanocytes stain, although a heterogeneous distribution can be observed.[6] S-100 protein comprises a family of calcium-binding proteins (S-100a, S-100ab, and S-100b) that consist of α-α, α-β and β-β subunits, respectively.[7] S-100 protein was first isolated from brain extract and acquired its name from its solubility in saturated ammonium sulfate at neutral pH.[6] The protein is abundantly expressed in astrocytes and oligodendrocytes within the central nervous system and in Schwann cells in the peripheral nervous system but is also present in a diverse set of nonneural cells, e.g., melanocytes, Langerhans cells, cells of chondroid derivation, sustentacular cells of the adrenal medulla, and myoepithelial cells.[6,8–10] Rabbit polyclonal antibody against S-100 protein is commercially available. Recently, monoclonal antibodies against the α and β subunits have been developed and are also commercially available.[11] Melanocytes have been reported to contain only α subunits, while Schwann cells express only β subunits.[12] The high sensitivity of S-100 protein expression in melanocytic lesions is paralleled by a low specificity. S-100 protein is detectable in a number of nonmelanocytic tumors, such as schwannoma, chordoma, granular cell tumor, chondroma, chondrosarcoma, chondroblastoma, osteosarcoma, glioma, benign and malignant myoepithelial tumors, and some carcinomas.[6,10,13,14] Since the majority of S-100 protein–positive nonmelanocytic tumors can be distinguished easily from melanocytic tumors on morphologic grounds alone, the lack of specificity of S-100 protein antibodies is usually not a problem.

HMB-45 is a monoclonal antibody that was developed against human melanoma cells.[15] It recognizes a premelanosomal glycoprotein,[16] which explains its relative specificity for melanin-producing cells. The staining pattern is intracytoplasmic and often heterogeneous. The antibody is commercially available. HMB-45 is particularly helpful in the evaluation of a nonmelanocytic S-100 protein–positive tumor. The degree of sensitivity of HMB-45 antigen was reported to be less than that of S-100 protein in one study[17] and found to be slightly higher in two others.[18,19] Normal epidermal melanocytes of adults or melanocytes in common dermal nevi do not generally react with HMB-45, whereas the majority of epidermal and dermal melanomas are immunoreactive. HMB-45, however, stains not only melanomas but also melanocytes in fetal skin, the junctional component of common and dysplastic nevi, intraepidermal melanocytes overlying scars and hemangiomas, as well as dermal melanocytes within Spitz, deep penetrating, and blue nevi.[15,20–22] HMB-45 is not entirely specific for melanocytes. HMB-45 positivity has been reported for a number of nonmelanocytic tumors, including, for example, some breast carcinomas,[23] peripheral nerve sheath tumors,[24] gliosarcomas,[24] primitive neuroectodermal tumors,[24] malignant schwannomas,[24] some ependymomas,[24] adrenal pheochromocytomas,[25] angiomyolipomas,[26] lymphangiomyomatosis of the lung,[27] and some plasmacytomas.[24,28] It should be noted that the vast majority of desmoplastic melanomas are negative for HMB-45, except for perhaps the intraepidermal or superficial dermal components of some tumors.[29] Fortunately, almost all desmoplastic melanomas are immunoreactive with S-100 protein.

Other monoclonal antibodies have been developed using a similar approach as for HMB-45. NKI/beteb was prepared against membranes from a human melanoma metastasis and reacts with an epitope of a 100- to 107-kD glycoprotein located on the inner side of membranes of premelanosomes, which is different from the one recognized by HMB-45.[30] The monoclonal antibody is commercially available. The specificity is comparable with that of HMB-45 when frozen sections are used. Its sensitivity is greatly reduced in paraffin-embedded material.[30] In frozen sections, the antigens of HMB-45 and NKI/beteb have a similar distribution with a cytoplasmic staining pattern. The degree of sensitivity is less than that of S-100 protein.

NKI/C3 is another commercially available monoclonal antibody that was developed against melanomas and found to react with melanocytic lesions in paraffin-embedded tissue.[31] It recognizes a cytoplasmic glycoprotein with a molecular weight ranging from 25 to 110 kDa. While normal adult melanocytes are not immunoreactive with this antibody, the cytoplasm of melanocytic tumor cells is markedly stained. The staining of melanocytes is often heterogeneous. Junctional and subepidermal melanocytes are preferentially stained in melanocytic nevi or primary melanoma.[32,33] In particular, areas of necrosis are highlighted. The specificity of this antibody for melanocytic lesions is lower than that of HMB-45. In paraffin sections of the normal skin, immunoreactivity can be seen in the acinar cells of sweat glands and in mast cells. In frozen sections, its specificity is even lower. NKI/C3 is less sensitive for melanocytic lesions in comparison with antibodies against S-100 protein.[34]

High-molecular-weight melanoma-associated antigen (HMW-MAA) is also known as *melanoma proteoglycan*—a chondroitin sulfate proteoglycan that consists of two chains with a molecular weight of 420 and 250 kD.[35] HMW-MAA is thought to play a role in cell-cell or cell-matrix interactions. A number of monoclonal antibodies against this molecule have been developed by various investigators.

The antibody can be used reliably only in frozen-section material. While its sensitivity for melanocytic tumors, primary or metastatic, is high, it lacks sufficient specificity to be a useful marker in a routine diagnostic setting.[6] A large number of other monoclonal antibodies have been reported as melanocytic differentiation markers. However, they are not discussed here because they lack sufficient sensitivity or specificity for diagnostic purposes or have not yet been evaluated completely for their diagnostic utility.

Neuron-specific enolase (NSE) is the most acidic isoform of the glycolytic enzyme enolase and marks neuronal and peripheral endocrine cells as well as benign and malignant melanocytic tumors.[36] Although NSE lacks specificity, it is a useful marker if used in a panel of other antibodies.[37]

Antibodies recognizing intermediate filaments are used in the distinction of melanomas from carcinomas. Melanomas are usually immunoreactive for vimentin, whereas most carcinomas are not. Instead, they are typically positive for keratin filaments, whereas most melanomas are negative. Keratin positivity, however, also may be noted in some melanomas, when the antibodies applied recognize low-molecular-weight keratins.[16]

In the distinction of melanomas from sarcomas, antibodies against epithelial membrane antigen (EMA) may be useful, since EMA is almost always negative in melanomas, whereas it is positive in a large majority of epithelial and spindle cell tumors, plasmacytomas, T-cell lymphomas, and Ki-1 lymphomas.[38]

The not infrequent differential diagnosis between lymphoma and melanoma can be approached readily using antibodies against leukocyte common antigen (LCA) and other lymphoid or monocytoid markers for which melanomas are typically negative.

Immunohistochemistry has been applied not only to aid in the differential diagnosis of melanocytic lesions from other tumors but also on an investigational basis for prognostic purposes.[6] As tumors progress from precursor lesions to early invasion or metastases, a number of nuclear, cytoplasmic, or cell-surface molecules become increasingly expressed, and these might be used as indicators of the malignant (i.e., invasive) or metastatic potential of this tumor. These molecules have been termed *progression-associated melanoma antigens* (PAMAs).[6] Such PAMAs are oncogenes and growth factors,[39] growth factor receptors (e.g., the nerve growth factor receptor[40] or the epidermal growth factor receptor[41]), or adhesion molecules (e.g., the integrin VLA-2[42] or the intracellular adhesion molecule-1[43]). The function of many PAMAs on melanoma cells, like HLA-DR, whose expression in melanomas has been said to indicate a poor prognosis,[44] is not yet clear. The usefulness of these factors for prognostic purposes is still under investigation. However, it is already apparent that probably more than a single factor will be required to allow a reliable prognosis on the progression of a melanoma. It is also clear, based on experience with the currently available panel of PAMAs, that an immunohistologic distinction between Spitz nevus and primary melanoma will be difficult and is not feasible so far.

Electron Microscopy

With the advent of melanocytic differentiation markers, immunohistochemistry has become the central aide in solving differential diagnostic problems.[45] At present, electron microscopy is only rarely needed in the diagnosis of melanocytic lesions (Table 2-4). It has been used to identify premelanosomes, melanosomes, and atypical melanosomes such as spherical forms with irregular granular material, which are more likely found in melanoma or dysplastic nevi and rarely seen in normal melanocytes or common acquired nevi.[46,47]

A diagnostic dilemma in which electron microscopy may still be required is the differential diagnosis of a pigmented HMB-45–positive schwannoma from a melanoma. While melanosomes may be found in both schwannoma and melanoma, schwannomas would be distinguished ultrastructurally by the following features: (1) spindle cells with intertwining processes, (2) basal lamina covering processes and cell bodies, and (3) long-spacing collagen (Luse bodies).[45]

Cytogenetics

Chromosome analyses of human melanocytic tumors have demonstrated a variety of nonrandom abnormalities involving chromosomes 1, 3, 6, 7, 9, 10, and 11.[49-51] The most frequent cytogenetic rearrangements of malignant cutaneous melanomas affect chromosomal regions

TABLE 2-4
Ancillary Techniques Used in the Evaluation of Melanoma

Electron microscopy	Demonstration of premelanosomes, melanosomes, schwannian features
Cytogenetics	Experimental at present; chromosomal abnormalities of 1p36,6q27,7,9p21, and 11
DNA ploidy	Abnormal DNA content correlates with tumor thickness, but many melanomas are diploid
Nucleolar organizer regions	No reliable distinction of melanoma from nevi
Proliferation markers PCNA, Ki-67	Potential use for tumor grading

1p36,[52] 6q27,[53,54] and 9p21.[55] Forty percent of melanomas show loss of heterozygosity on chromosome 6q.[53] Approximately 46 percent of melanomas have cytogenetically detectable loss or rearrangement of chromosome 9p.[55] However, while these studies are important in understanding the biology of melanomas, they also indicate that human cutaneous melanomas are genetically very heterogeneous. Analysis of chromosomal abnormalities might help to predict the biologic behavior of melanomas. Preliminary results have suggested that chromosomal abnormalities located on chromosomes 7 and 11 are associated with a poor prognosis.[56]

Cytogenetic analysis also might aid in the differential diagnosis of a soft-tissue tumor that shows many phenotypic features in common with cutaneous melanoma, i.e., malignant melanoma of soft parts (MMSP) or clear cell sarcoma, from metastatic cutaneous malignant melanoma. MMSP exhibits a recurrent chromosome translocation involving chromosome 22, specifically t(12;22)(q13;q12).[57–59] The resulting chimeric protein consists of the *N*-terminal domain of EWS linked to the bZIP domain of ATF-1, a transcription factor that normally may be regulated by cyclic AMP.[60] This chromosomal aberration clearly distinguishes this soft-tissue tumor from cutaneous melanoma and supports the concept that MMSP represents a true soft-tissue tumor entity that is distinct from cutaneous melanoma.

OTHER TECHNIQUES IN THE DIAGNOSIS OF MELANOMA

A number of other techniques have been used in tumor pathology to measure parameters that might assist in the evaluation of the malignant potential of a lesion (see Table 2-4). Such parameters are DNA ploidy[61] and angiogenesis (microvessel density).[62,63] The utility of either parameter for diagnostic or prognostic purposes is still under investigation. Another parameter, the number of nucleolar organizer regions, which are segments of DNA encoding ribosomal RNA, has been said to be too variable among melanomas to allow a reliable distinction from dysplastic or Spitz nevi.[64]

Proliferative activity has been shown to correlate with the degree of malignancy of a number of neoplasms. Proliferative cell nuclear antigen (PCNA) and Ki-67 are antibodies that are currently being evaluated for their usefulness in quantitative immunohistochemical studies. PCNA is a nuclear protein that was identified as cofactor of DNA polymerase δ.[65] Its maximal expression is in the S phase of the cell cycle.[66] Ki-67 recognizes a nuclear antigen of 395- and 345-kDa size that is expressed in late G_1, S, G_2, and M phases but not in early G_1 and G_0 phases of the cell cycle.[67,68] Preliminary data suggest that these markers might be useful for tumor grading in melanocytic lesions.[69] Their relevance as prognostic parameters, however, remains to be evaluated in long-term follow-up studies.

REFERENCES

1. Warkel R, Luna L, Helwig E: A modified Warthin-Starry procedure at low pH for melanin. *Am J Clin Pathol* 73:812–815, 1980.
2. Ackerman A, Penneys N: Formalin pigment in skin. *Arch Dermatol* 102:318–321, 1970.
3. Rodriguez H, McGavran M: A modified dopa reaction for the diagnosis and investigation of pigmented cells. *Am J Clin Pathol* 52:219–227, 1969.
4. Gatter K, Ralfkaier E, Skinner J, et al: An immunohistochemical study of malignant melanoma and its differential diagnosis from other malignant tumors. *J Clin Pathol* 38:7–15, 1985.
5. Gaynor RB, Herschman HR, Irie R, et al: S-100 protein: A marker for malignant melanoma. *J Clin Pathol* 38:1353–1357, 1981.
6. Ruiter D, Broecker E-B: Immunohistochemistry in the evaluation of melanocytic tumors. *Semin Diagn Pathol* 10(1):76–91, 1993.
7. Cochran A, Wen DR, Herschman HR, Gaynor RB: Detection of S-100 protein as an aid to the identification of melanocytic tumors. *Int J Cancer* 30:295–297, 1982.
8. Cooper M, Hutchins G, Israel M: Histogenesis of the human adrenal medulla: An evaluation of the ontogeny of chromaffin and nonchromaffin lineages. *Am J Pathol* 137(3):605–615, 1990.
9. Schmitt F, Bacchi C: S-100 protein: Is it a useful marker in diagnostic immunocytochemistry? Histopathology 15:281–288, 1989.
10. Smoller B: Immunohistochemistry in the diagnosis of malignant melanoma. *Clin Dermatol* 9: 235–241, 1991.
11. Hyun Cho K, Hashimoto K, Taniguchi J: Immunohistochemical study of melanocytic nevus and malignant melanoma with monoclonal antibodies against S-100 subunits. *Cancer* 66:765–771, 1990.
12. Nakajima T, Sato Y, Watanabe S: Immunoelectron microscopical demonstration of S-100 protein in epidermal Langerhans cells. *Biomed Res* 3:226–231, 1982.
13. Jabi M, Dardick I, Cardigos N: Adenomyoepithelioma of the breast. *Arch Pathol Lab Med* 112(1):73–76, 1988.
14. Okajima K, Honda I, Kitagawa T: Immunohistochemical distribution of S-100 protein in tumors and tumor-like lesions of bone and cartilage. *Cancer* 61(4):792–799, 1988.
15. Gown A, Vogel A, Hoak D, et al.: Monoclonal antibodies specific for melanocytic tumors distinguish subpopulations of melanocytes. *Am J Pathol* 123:195–203, 1986.
16. Zarbo R, Gown A, Visscher D, Crissman J.: Anomalous cytokeratin expression in malignant melanoma: One- and two-dimensional Western blot analysis and immunohistochemical survey of 100 melanomas. *Mod Pathol* 3:494–501, 1990.

17. Colombari R, Bonetti F, Zambone G, et al: Distribution of melanoma specific antibody (HMB-45) in benign and malignant melanocytic tumors: An immunohistochemical study on paraffin sections. *Virchows Arch [A]* 413:17–24, 1988.
18. Ordonez N, Ji X, Hickey R: Comparison of HMB-45 monoclonal antibody and S-100 protein in the immunohistochemical diagnosis of melanoma. *Am J Clin Pathol* 90(4):385–390, 1988.
19. Thomson W, MacKie R: Comparison of five antimelanoma antibodies for identification of melanocytic cells on tissue sections in routine dermatopathology. *J Am Acad Dermatol* 21:1280–1284, 1989.
20. Palazzo J, Duray P: Congenital agminated Spitz nevi: Immunoreactivity with a melanoma associated antibody. *J Cutan Pathol* 15:166–170, 1988.
21. Smoller B, Hsu A, Krueger J: HMB-45 monoclonal antibody recognizes an inducible and reversible melanocytic cytoplasmic protein. *J Cutan Pathol* 18:315–322, 1991.
22. Wood W, Tron V: Analysis of HMB-45 immunoreactivity in common and cellular blue nevi. *J Cutan Pathol* 18:261–263, 1991.
23. Bonetti F, Colombari E, Zamboni G, et al: Breast carcinoma positive for melanoma marker (HMB-45). *Am J Clin Pathol* 22:491–495, 1989.
24. Zimmer C, Gottschalk J, Goebel S, Cercos-Navarro J: Melanoma-associated antigens in tumors of the nervous system: An immunohistochemical study with the monoclonal antibody HMB-45. *Virchows Arch [A]* 420(2):121–126, 1992.
25. Unger P, Hoffman K, Thung S, et al: HMB-45 reactivity in adrenal pheochromocytomas. *Arch Pathol Lab Med* 116:151–153, 1992.
26. Tsui W, Yuen A, Ma K, and Tse C: Hepatic angiomyolipomas with a deceptive trabecular pattern and HMB-45 reactivity. *Histopathology* 21:569–573, 1992.
27. Bonetti F, Chiodera P, Pea M, et al: Transbronchial biopsy in lymphangiomatosis of the lung. *Am J Surg Pathol* 17:1092–1102, 1993.
28. Pelosi G, Bonetti F, Colombardi R, et al: Use of monoclonal antibody HMB-45 in the cytological diagnosis of melanoma. *Acta Cytol* 34:382–384, 1990.
29. Bruijn J, Mihm MC Jr, Barnhill RL: Desmoplastic melanoma. *Histopathology* 20:197–205, 1992.
30. Vennegoor C, Hageman P, Van Nouhuijs H, et al: A monoclonal antibody specific for cells of the melanocytic lineage. *Am J Pathol* 130:179–192, 1988.
31. Vennegoor C, Calafat J, Hageman P, et al: Biochemical characterization and cellular localization of formalin-resistant melanoma-associated antigen reacting with monoclonal antibody NHI/C3. *Int J Cancer* 35:287–295, 1985.
32. MacKie R, Campbell L, Turbitt M: Use of NKI/C3 monoclonal antibody in the assessment of benign and malignant melanocytic lesions. *J Clin Pathol* 37:367–372, 1984.
33. Van Duinen S, Ruiter D, Hageman P: Immunohistochemical and histochemical tools in the diagnosis of amelanotic melanoma. *Cancer* 35:1566–1573, 1984.
34. Hagen E, Vennegoor C, Schlingemann R, et al: Correlation of histopathologic characteristic with staining patterns in human melanoma assessed by (monoclonal) antibodies reactive on paraffin sections. *Histopathology* 10:689–700, 1986.
35. Garin-Chesa P, Beresford HR, Carrato-Mena A, et al: Cell surface markers of human melanoma: Immunohistochemical analysis of the gp57, GD3, and mel-CSPG antigenic system. *Am J Pathol* 135:295–305, 1989.
36. Schmechel D, Marangos P, Brightman M: Neuron specific enolase is a marker for the peripheral and central neuroendocrine cells. *Nature* 276:834–836, 1978.
37. Hachisuka H, Sakamoto F, Nomura H, et al: Immunohistochemical study of S-100 protein and neuron-specific enolase in melanocytes and related tumors. *Acta Histochem* 89:215–223, 1986.
38. Pinkus G, Kurtin P: Epithelial membrane antigen—A diagnostic discriminant in surgical pathology: Immunohistochemical profile in epithelial, mesenchymal and hematopoietic neoplasms using paraffin sections and monoclonal antibodies. *Hum Pathol* 16:929–940, 1985.
39. Albino A: The role of oncogenes and growth factors in progressive melanoma-genesis. *Pigment Cell Res* 2:199–218, 1992.
40. Broecker E, Magiera H, Herlyn M: Nerve growth and nerve growth factor expression in tumors of melanocytic origin. *J Invest Dermatol* 96:662–665, 1991.
41. DeWit P, Moretti S, Weterman M: Epidermal growth factor receptor is a progression marker in human melanocytic lesions. *J Invest Dermatol* 99:168–173, 1992.
42. Klein C, Steinmeyer T, Kaufmann D, et al: Identification of a melanoma progression antigen as integrin VLA-2. *J Invest Dermatol* 96:281–284, 1991.
43. Johnson JP, Stade BG, Holzmann B, et al: De novo expression of intercellular adhesion molecule 1 in melanoma associated with increased risk of metastasis. *Proc Natl Acad Sci USA* 86:641–644, 1989.
44. Broecker E, Suter L, Sorg C: HLA-DR antigen expression in primary melanomas of the skin. *J Invest Dermatol* 82:244–247, 1984.
45. Jundt G, Schultz A, Paul E, et al: S-100 protein in amelanotic melanoma: A convenient immunocytochemical approach compared to electron microscopy. *Pathol Res Pract* 181:37–44, 1986.
46. Rhodes A, Seki Y, Fitzpatrick T, Stern R: Melanosomal alterations in dysplastic melanocytic nevi: A quantitative, ultrastructural investigation. *Cancer* 61:358–369, 1988.
47. Dickersin GR: Schwannoma and other nerve sheath neoplasms, in Dickersin GR (ed): *Diagnostic Electron Microscopy. New York,* Igaku-Shoin, 1988, p 238.
48. Fletcher J, Kozakewich H, Hoffer E, et al: Diagnostic relevance of clonal cytogenetic aberrations in malignant soft-tissue tumors. *N Engl J Med* 324:436–442, 1991.
49. Parmiter A, Nowell P: The cytogenetics of human malignant melanoma and premalignant lesions. *Cancer Treat Res* 43:47–61, 1988.
50. Parmiter A, Nowell P: Cytogenetics of melanocytic tumors. *J Invest Dermatol* 100(3):254S–258S, 1993.
51. Trent J: Cytogenetics of malignant melanoma. *Cancer Metastasis Rev* 10(2):103–113, 1991.

52. Bale S, Dracopoli N, Tucker M, et al: Mapping of the gene for hereditary cutaneous malignant melanoma—dysplastic nevus to chromosome 1 p. *N Engl J Med* 320:1367–1372, 1989.
53. Millikin D, Meese E, Vogelstein B, et al: Loss of heterozygosity for loci on the long arm of chromosome 6 in human malignant melanoma. *Cancer Res* 51:5449–5453, 1991.
54. Trent J, Rosenfeld S, Meyskens F: Chromosome 6q involvement in malignant melanoma. *Cancer Genet Cytogenet* 9:177–180, 1989.
55. Cannon-Albright L, Goldgar D, Meyer L, et al: Assignment of a locus for familial melanoma, MLM, to chromosome 9p13-p22. *Science* 258:1148–1152, 1992.
56. Trent JM, Meyskens FL, Salmon SE, et al: Relation of cytogenetic abnormalities and clinical outcome in metastatic melanoma. *N Engl J Med* 322:1508–1511, 1990.
57. Bridge JA, Borek DA, Neff JR, Huntrakoon M: Chromosomal abnormalities in clear cell sarcoma: Implications for histogenesis. *Am J Clin Pathol* 93:26–31, 1990.
58. Bridge J, Srrekantaiah C, Neff J, Sandberg A: Cytogenetic findings in clear cell sarcoma of tendons and aponeuroses. *Cancer Genet Cytogenet* 52:101–106, 1991.
59. Fletcher J: Translocation (12;22) (q13-14;q12) is a nonrandom aberration in soft tissue clear cell sarcoma. *Genes Chrom Cancer* 5:184, 1992.
60. Zucman J, Delattre O, Desmaze C, et al: EWS and ATF-1 gene fusion induced by t(12;22) translocation in malignant melanoma of soft parts. *Nature Genet* 4:341–345, 1993.
61. Herzberg A: Significance of DNA ploidy in cutaneous lesions. *Arch Dermatol* 128:663–678, 1992.
62. Barnhill RL, Fandrey K, Levy M, et al: Angiogenesis and tumor progression of melanoma. *Lab Invest* 3:331–337, 1992.
63. Srivastava A, Laidler P, Davies RP, et al: The prognostic significance of tumor vascularity in intermediate-thickness (0.76–4.0 mm thick) skin melanoma: A quantitative histologic study. *Am J Pathol* 133:419–423, 1988.
64. Fallowfield M, Cook M: The value of nuclear organizer region staining in the differential diagnosis of borderline melanocytic lesions. *Histopathology* 14:229–304, 1989.
65. Bravo R, Frank R, Blundell P, MacDonald-Bravo H: Cyclin/PCNA is the auxiliary protein of DNA polymerase-δ. *Nature* 326:515, 1987.
66. Kurki P, Vanderlaan M, Dolbeare F, et al: Expression of proliferating cell nuclear antigen (PCNA)/cyclin during the cell cycle. *Exp Cell Res* 166:209, 1986.
67. Gerdes J, Li L, Schlueter C, et al: Immunohistochemical and molecular biological characterization of the cell proliferation-associated nuclear antigen that is defined by monoclonal antibody Ki-67. *Am J Pathol* 138:867, 1991.
68. Gerdes J, Lemke H, Baisch H, et al: Cell cycle analysis of a cell proliferation-associated human nuclear antigen defined by the monoclonal antibody Ki-67. *J Immunol* 133:1710–1715, 1984.
69. Rieger E, Hofmann-Wellenhof R, Soyer H, et al: Comparison of proliferative activity as assessed by proliferating cell nuclear antigen (PCNA) and Ki-67 monoclonal antibodies in melanocytic lesions. *J Cutan Pathol* 20:229–236, 1993.

3

Circumscribed Pigmented Lesions Composed of Basilar Melanocytes

FRECKLE

Synonym: ephelis.

Ephelides are small, well-circumscribed pigmented macules found only on sun-exposed skin. Ephelides are common in individuals with fair skin color (phototypes I and II),[1] especially in combination with blond or red hair. They are not present at birth but usually appear in the first few years of life. Ephelides darken with exposure to sunlight and fade when shielded from insolation. However, the tendency to develop ephelides decreases with advancing age. An autosomal dominant inheritance is possible, since freckling can be seen in some families over generations.[2]

Recently, Rhodes et al.[3] have suggested that some ephelides may overlap or represent a subtype of solar lentigo (Table 3-1). Lesions studied by these authors exhibited melanocytic hyperplasia and occasional cytologic atypia, features shared with solar lentigo. Further studies are needed to clarify the significance of the latter findings. Clinically, ephelides become less prominent with age, but even when they are clinically inapparent in older individuals with ordinary light, they remain visible on Wood's lamp examination.[4]

Clinical Features

Ephelides occur only on sun-exposed areas of the body, mainly on the face, the dorsal aspects of the arms, and the upper part of the chest and the back (see Table 3-1). Ephelides are well demarcated, round, oval, or irregular in shape; they are usually 1 to 3 mm in diameter, but some may be several millimeters in diameter. Depending on the intensity of sun exposure, they vary in color from light to dark brown, but they almost never become as dark as lentigines or junctional nevi; they may increase in number and distribution and show a tendency to confluency.

Histopathology

The epidermis exhibits a normal configuration. The keratinocytes show an increase in melanin content, predominantly in the basal cell layer (Fig. 3-1). Occasionally, melanophages are seen in the papillary dermis. The number of melanocytes in ephelides does not differ significantly from normal. However, examination of dopa-stained sections has been reported to show both significantly fewer melanocytes[5] and an increased number of melanocytes per unit area in ephelides.[3] The differences in the latter results are probably related to examination of epidermal sheets en face[5] versus standard vertical histologic sections.[3] The melanocytes in ephelides are larger and have more branching of dendrites and a higher dopa positivity than those in adjacent normal epidermis, apparently indicating greater functional activity.

Differential Diagnosis

Histologically, the freckle cannot be distinguished from a café-au-lait macule, melanotic macule of Albright, and melasma. Discrimination of freckle from the latter entities must be based solely on clinical findings. The solar and simple lentigines also may enter into the differential diagnosis of freckle (see Table 3-1). The simple lentigo differs from the freckle by showing elongated epidermal rete ridges and melanocytic hyperplasia. The solar lentigo usually has prominently club-shaped rete; melanocytic hyperplasia may or may not be present.

TABLE 3-1
Précis: Freckle, Solar Lentigo, Lentigo Simplex

Freckle (Ephelis)	*Solar Lentigo*	*Lentigo Simplex*
	Clinical Features	
Onset early childhood	Onset often over age 30 years	Onset childhood, adolescence, later
Skin phototypes I, II ("Celtic") common	More common in skin phototypes I, II, III	All phototypes
Responsive to sun exposure and tendency to fade	Follows repeated sun exposure; persistent	Some probably related to sun exposure; persistent
1- to 3-mm macules	5- to 15-mm or larger macules	Usually 1- to 5-mm macules
Light to medium brown	Medium to dark brown	Light, medium, dark brown, black
Round, polycyclic	Round, oval, polycyclic	Homogeneous pigment pattern
Jagged border	Regular or slightly irregular border	Round, oval, symmetrical, regular borders, well circumscribed
On all sun- exposed areas, face, forearms, back	Sun- exposed skin, face, neck, forearms, dorsal hands	Anywhere, including sun-protected skin
	Histopathologic Features	
Normal configuration of epidermis	Elongated, club-shaped epidermal rete ridges, often anastomosing	Elongated, club-shaped epidermal rete ridges
Basal layer hyperpigmentation of epidermis	Basal layer hyperpigmentation of epidermis, accentuated on lower poles of rete ridges	Basal layer hyperpigmentation, accentuated lower poles of rete
Reduced, normal, or slightly increased numbers of melanocytes in basal layer	Basilar melanocytes normal or increased in frequency	Increased numbers of basilar melanocytes concentrated on tips of rete ridges
Melanophages in papillary dermis		Melanophages in papillary dermis
	Solar elastosis common	
	Some degree of cytologic atypia of melanocytes occasionally present	
	Transition to large cell acanthoma occasionally	
	Transition to reticulated seborrheic keratosis in some instances	
	Transition to lichenoid keratosis occasionally	
	Differential Diagnosis	
Café-au-lait macule	Freckle	Freckle
Melasma	Pigmented actinic keratosis	Café-au-lait macule
Solar lentigo	Lentigo simplex	Becker's nevus (melanosis)
Simple lentigo	Lentigo maligna	Solar lentigo
		Melanocytic dysplasia

CAFÉ-AU-LAIT MACULE

Café-au-lait macules (CALMs) are well-circumscribed, uniformly light to dark brown spots. CALM can occur as an isolated lesion or as multiple lesions; the latter may be a marker for multisystem disease and occur in various syndromes.[6–17] Single CALMs are found in 10 to 20 percent of the normal population, and about 1 percent of all healthy young adults have up to three CALMs. They may be present at birth but usually develop in early childhood and increase in size with age. CALMs grow proportionately to body growth and remain stable in size after body growth has ceased. They demonstrate no tendency toward malignancy.

Clinical Features

The term *café-au-lait* refers to the characteristic uniform color of coffee with milk of such lesions, which may vary from light to dark brown. CALMs are completely flat,

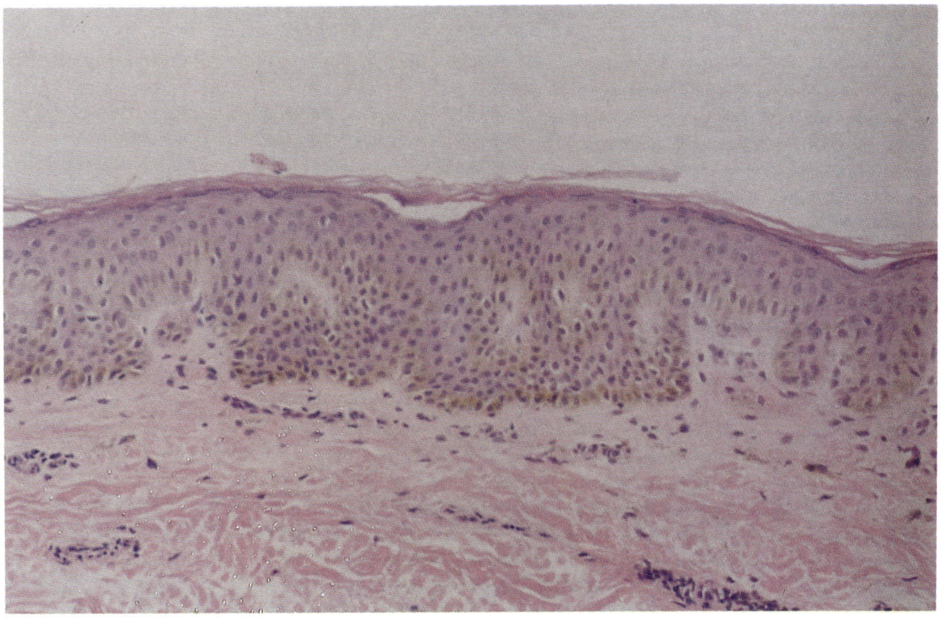

FIGURE 3-1
Freckle. There is basal layer hyperpigmentation of an otherwise unremarkable epidermis. The number of basilar melanocytics does not appear to be significantly increased (H&E, × 200). (Courtesy of Arthur R. Rhodes, M.D.).

often have an oval morphology, and the margins are well defined and usually regular. They may be located anywhere on the body, except the mucous membranes. CALMs are usually 2.0 to 5.0 cm in diameter in adults but may vary from freckle-like lesions of less than 2.0 mm to macules of greater than 20 cm in size (Table 3-2).

Histopathology

The epidermis has a normal configuration with slightly increased melanin content in the basilar keratinocytes (Fig. 3-2). The number of melanocytes is normal or slightly increased. The adnexal epithelium is spared of hyperpigmentation, and only rarely does one see melanophages in the upper dermis. In dopa-stained epidermis from most patients with neurofibromatosis, the density of melanocytes is higher in both CALMs and normal adjacent skin in comparison with healthy individuals.[9] The melanocytic density in isolated CALMs of otherwise normal persons, however, is usually less than in surrounding skin.[10] Melanin macroglobules (large pigment particles) which may be found in CALMs are not specific for neurofibromatosis, since they are occasionally found in isolated CALMs without underlying disease and occur in several other conditions such as simple lentigines, Becker's nevus, congenital nevi, and dysplastic nevi and sometimes even in normal skin.[10,18–20]

On electron microscopy, the melanosomes are usually dispersed singly in melanocytes and are usually homogeneous, electron-dense, and ellipsoidal when fully melanized.[18]

Associated Diseases and Syndromes

Neurofibromatosis (von Recklinghausen's disease) is an autosomal dominant disease of neural crest-derived cells.[6,7,11,12] Its cutaneous manifestations may occur in conjunction with systemic manifestations that mainly affect the central nervous system. Besides neurofibromata and multiple freckle-like macules in the axillae and other intertriginous areas, multiple CALMs are the leading cutaneous features in neurofibromatosis; they are present in more than 99 percent of all patients with neurofibromatosis (Table 3-3). Usually they are present at birth, but they can occur months later. The presence of six or more CALMs greater than 1.5 cm in diameter in adults or five or more such macules that are 0.5 cm or more in diameter in children younger than 5 years has been considered diagnostic, but more reliable are the pigmented hamartomas of the iris called *Tisch nodules.*[11,12]

Albright's syndrome includes polyostotic fibrous dysplasia of the bones, endocrine dysfunction causing precocious puberty (more often in females than in males), and melanotic macules that are present in nearly two-thirds

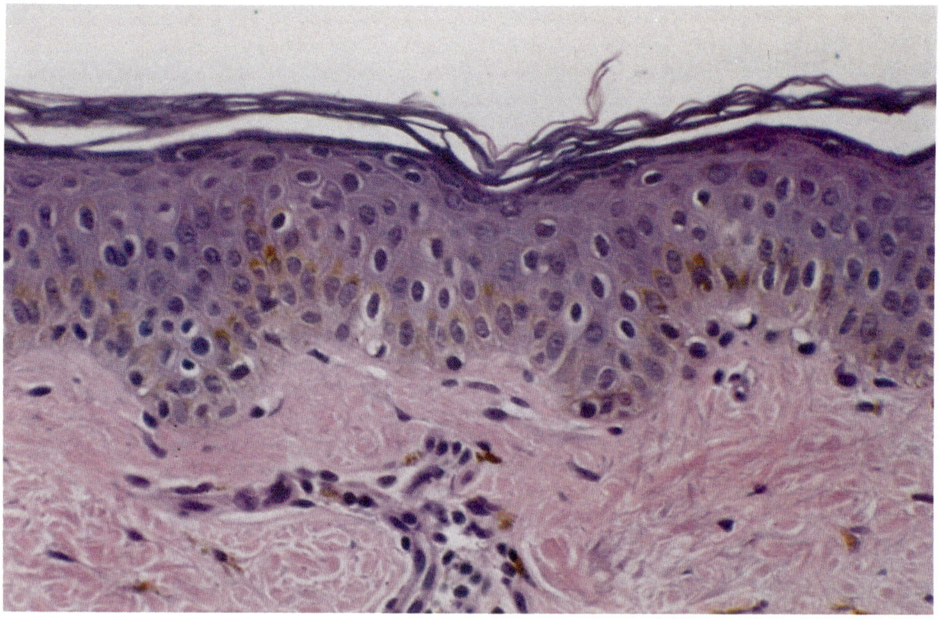

FIGURE 3-2
Café-au-lait macule. The lesion is characterized by a normal configuration of the epidermis and basal layer hyperpigmentation (H&E, × 400).

of patients with this disease.[9,12] The macules may be present at birth but more commonly develop in the first few years of life. They are usually several centimeters in diameter, few in number, and may be indistinguishable both clinically and histologically from CALMs in neurofibromatosis. However, the distribution of the lesions may be somewhat helpful for diagnosis: they favor the forehead, nuchal area, sacrum, and buttocks. They also tend to be unilateral in a linear or segmented arrangement with irregular margins, often involving the same side as the bone lesions and situated directly above them. Axillary freckling does not occur in Albright's disease.

TABLE 3-2
Précis: Café-au-Lait Macule

Clinical Features
Onset in childhood
Single CALM in 10 to 20 percent of population
Associated with neurofibromatosis and other multisystem diseases
2- to 5-cm oval macules
Well defined
Usually regular borders
Homogeneous light to dark brown
Histopathology
Normal configuration of epidermis
Increased melanin in basilar keratinocytes
Normal or slightly increased number of basilar melanocytes
Differential Diagnosis
Freckle
Melasma

Differential Diagnosis

Hyperpigmented macules potentially confused with CALMs histologically include freckle, melasma, postinflammatory hyperpigmentation, and occasionally Becker's melanosis. Clinical findings should allow separation of CALMs from the latter entities in most instances. In general, melasma has a distinctive clinical appearance, commonly involving the face in a symmetrical pattern, particularly the malar areas, but also the forehead and upper lip. Women are affected most commonly, and there is a relationship to pregnancy and oral contraceptives, suggesting an endocrine factor. Histologically, one generally observes varying degrees of basal layer hyperpigmentation and numbers of melanophages in the papillary dermis. Basilar melanocytes are normal or slightly increased in number, but the epidermal morphology is otherwise unchanged. Epidermal forms of melasma may be indistinguishable from CALMs. Otherwise, melasma differs

TABLE 3-3
Diseases and Syndromes Associated with Café-au-Lait Macules (CALMs)

Disease/Syndrome	*Pertinent Features*
Neurofibromatosis	See text
Albright's syndrome	See text
Tuberous sclerosis (epiloa)[13]	Autosomal dominant Epilepsy Mental retardation Adenoma sebaceum Shagreen patch Periungual fibromas "Ash-leaf" (hypopigmented) macules
Silver-Russell syndrome[14]	CALM in 45 percent of patients Short stature Skeletal asymmetry Shortened, incurved fifth fingers Abnormal sexual development
Watson's syndrome[15]	Pulmonary stenosis Mental retardation Perineal freckling
Westerhof's syndrome[16]	Mental retardation Growth retardation Hypopigmented macules
Bloom's syndrome[17]	CALM in over 50 percent of patients Growth retardation Congenital facial telangiectactic erythema Photosensitivity

from CALMs because of greater numbers of melanophages. Postinflammatory hyperpigmentation is also distinguished from CALMs by prominent pigment incontinence (melanophages) but also delicate fibroplasia, often in the papillary dermis.

Becker's melanosis (see below), in addition to clinical differences such as hypertrichosis, usually is characterized by variable papillomatosis, elongation of rete ridges, and often slight melanocytic hyperplasia.

LENTIGO SIMPLEX

SOLAR LENTIGO

Synonyms: lentigo senilis, liver spot, "ink spot" lentigo

The solar lentigo occurs on sun-exposed skin generally in somewhat older individuals[22–25] (see Table 3-1). Solar lentigines are observed in more than 90 percent of the Caucasian population over the age of 60 years.[22] Such lesions and the relatively flat seborrheic keratoses are referred to as *liver spots.* Some solar lentigines have resemblance to freckles but are distinguished from common freckles by their persistence despite absence of sun exposure. Solar lentigines are a prominent finding in xeroderma pigmentosum.

The photochemotherapy-induced (PUVA) lentigo has been observed in patients receiving long-term methoxsalen photochemotherapy (PUVA) for psoriasis.[26–29]

Clinical Features

Solar lentigines are well-circumscribed, round, oval, or irregularly bordered macules of yellow, tan, or brown color. More lightly pigmented lesions are usually homogeneous, whereas darker ones tend to have a mottled appearance. Solar lentigines usually appear as multiple lesions; they vary in size from about 5 to 15 cm in diameter, with a tendency to confluency. Solar lentigines occur on sun-exposed areas, predominantly the dorsal aspects of hands and forearms, the face, and the upper chest and back. A particular variant that may be termed *"sunburn," hypermelanotic,* or *"ink spot" solar lentigo* is characterized by a striking jet-black color and a stellate outline.[30] The PUVA lentigo has a close clinical resemblance to the solar lentigo, particularly the hypermelanotic type. The latter macules occur on light-exposed skin and range from 3 to 8 mm in greatest diameter.[26–29]

Histopathology

In general, the solar lentigo is notable for elongated, club-shaped epidermal rete ridges, basal layer hyperpigmentation most prominent at the tips of the rete, and an increased frequency of basilar melanocytes; however, in some instances, the melanocytes are not increased in number[22,25] (Fig. 3-3). The epidermis between rete ridges is usually atrophic. On occasion, there is slight cytologic atypia of basilar melanocytes.[3] There also may be hyperkeratosis and rather prominent elongation and anastomosis of epidermal rete ridges. Some varieties of solar lentigo are characterized by an effaced epidermis; i.e., epidermal rete ridges are diminished in length or absent. Varying degrees of solar elastosis are almost always present in the dermis. Accumulation of melanin-laden macrophages and slight lymphocytic infiltration are also frequent findings.

The solar lentigo may show transitions to reticulated seborrheic keratosis, large cell acanthoma, and lichenoid keratosis.[31,32] Sometimes there are two or more patterns of these various entities in the same lesion. Reticulated seborrheic keratosis is in reality an exaggerated form of solar lentigo; the epidermal rete ridges are more elongated and exhibit a greater degree of anastomosis compared with solar lentigo. The large cell acanthoma is a

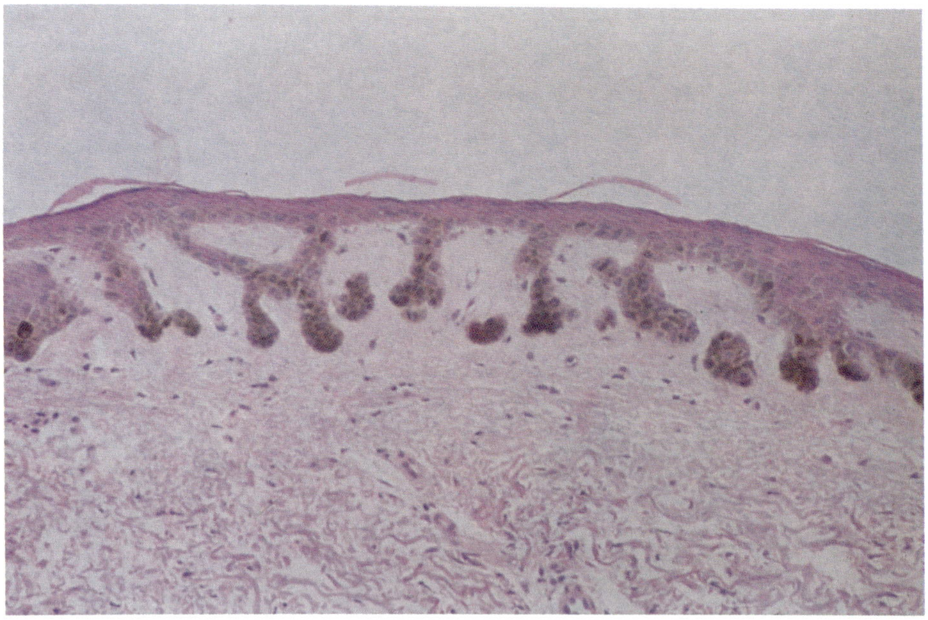

A

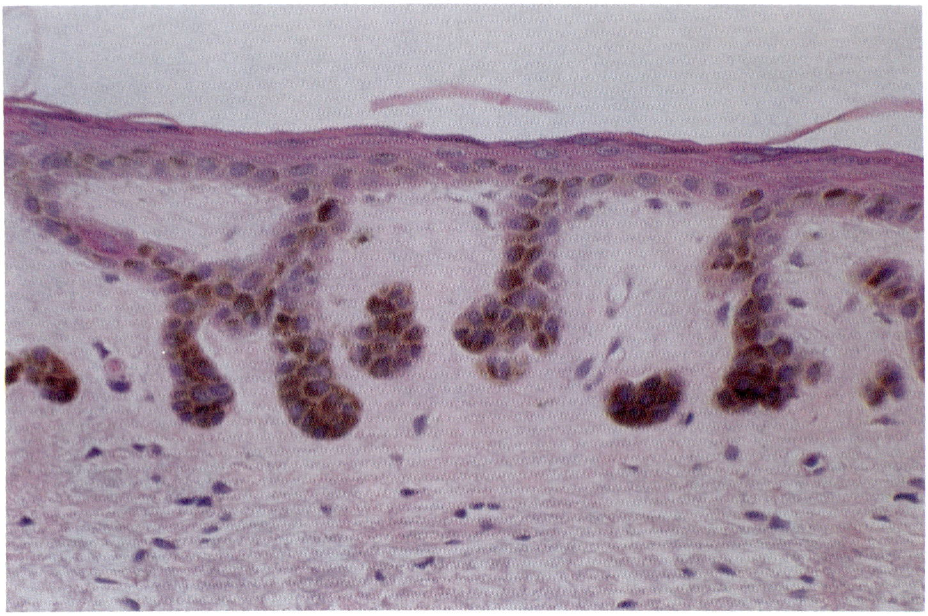

B

FIGURE 3-3

Solar lentigo. (A) The lesion exhibits elongated club-shaped epidermal rete ridges with prominent basal layer hyperpigmentation (H&E, × 200). (B) There is anastomosis of the elongated rete ridges. The basilar melanocytes are not increased in frequency in this lesion (H&E, × 400).

TABLE 3-4
Comparison of Solar Lentigo and Lentigo Maligna

Solar Lentigo	*Lentigo Maligna*
	Clinical Features
Onset over age 30–40 years	Onset generally over age 50 years
Sun-exposed skin, face, dorsal hands	Sun-exposed skin, cheek most common site
5- to 15-mm or larger macule	10- to 200-mm or larger macule
Medium to dark brown	Tan, brown, dark brown, black
Slightly rough surface	"Varnish-like" stain
Some variation in color	Often marked variegation
Some asymmetry	Prominent asymmetry
Regular or slightly irregular border	Irregular or notched border
	Histopathology
Usually well circumscribed	Usually poorly circumscribed
Symmetry	Usually some asymmetry
Elongated, club-shaped rete ridges	Often effacement of epidermis
Increased number of basilar melanocytes often	Increased frequency of basilar melanocytes
Melanocytes more frequent on tips of retes	No particular affinity for rete ridges
Intraepidermal nests of melanocytes usually not present	Formation of intraepidermal nests with diminished cohesion
Basilar melanocytes usually not involving adnexae	Basilar melanocytes often involve adnexal epithelium
Occasional variable cytologic atypia of melanocytes	Greater cytologic atypic
	Melanocytes often slightly pleomorphic, with high nuclear to cytoplasmic ratio, spindle-shaped

relatively flat pigmented lesion on sun-exposed skin that histologically contains enlarged monotonous keratinocytes either in the lower half or throughout most of the epidermis. The basilar epidermis is often hyperpigmented and thus often overlaps to some degree with solar lentigo. Some solar lentigines develop an associated lichenoid dermatitis and hence are termed *lichenoid* or *lichen planus–like keratosis.* Such lesions usually undergo regression and may show considerable resemblance to or be indistinguishable from a regressing melanocytic nevus.

Similar to solar lentigines, the PUVA lentigo exhibits lentiginous melanocytic hyperplasia, and a low-grade cytologic atypia of melanocytes is occasionally noted.[27,28]

Differential Diagnosis

The most common differential diagnosis for the solar lentigo includes distinction from lentigo maligna (Table 3-4) and pigmented actinic keratosis. In general, lentigo maligna, particularly when present on the central face, is characterized by absence or diminution of the epidermal rete pattern in contrast to solar lentigo. In addition, there is usually a greater frequency of basilar melanocytes and also prominent involvement of adnexal epithelium by the lentiginous proliferation of melanocytes in lentigo maligna compared with solar lentigo. Finally, lentigo maligna is characterized by a striking cytologic atypia of basilar melanocytes that should not be seen in solar lentigo. Nonetheless, on occasion, one may encounter lesions transitional between solar lentigo and lentigo maligna.

Pigmented actinic keratosis is distinguished from solar lentigo by the presence of disorder and cytologic atypia of basilar keratinocytes, "budding" of the dysplastic epidermis, and overlying parakeratosis in most instances. It should be borne in mind that occasional pigmented actinic keratoses may be difficult to separate from large cell acanthoma or solar lentigines with features or a component of large cell acanthoma. Actinic keratosis usually can be distinguished by the presence of "crowding," pleomorphism, and nuclear atypia of basilar keratinocytes versus the monomorphous enlarged keratinocytes typical of large cell acanthoma.

BECKER'S MELANOSIS

Synonyms: Becker's nevus, Becker's pigmentary hamartoma, nevoid melanosis, pigmented hairy epidermal nevus

Becker's melanosis (BM) is a unilateral, hyperpigmented, and often hypertrichotic macule or slightly elevated patch.[33-38] Although it is usually acquired, some cases are congenital. The lesions mostly occur in the second and third decades of life and are six times more common in males than in females. Familial occurrence has been reported. The prevalence among 19,302 army recruits aged 17 to 26 was 0.52 percent.[33]

Becker's melanosis is believed to be an organoid hamartoma of ectodermally and mesodermally derived tissues, and a segmental increase in androgen receptors and probable heightened sensitivity to androgens have been postulated.[38] The latter characteristics would explain its onset during or after puberty, leading to its clinical and histologic manifestations, which include hirsutism, acanthosis, dermal thickening, acne, and hypertrophic sebaceous glands. Androgen stimulation also would explain the accentuated smooth-muscle elements often found in the dermis of BM patients. Hyperpigmentation, similar to that found in "sexual skin," is due to increased melanin content in the epidermal keratinocytes and is often preceded by extensive sun exposure that has resulted in sunburns.

After development, BM enlarges slowly for 1 or 2 years, but then it remains stable in size. The color may fade with time, but hypertrichosis usually persists. Becker's melanosis is a benign lesion, and malignant transformation has not been reported.

In contrast to the hyperplasia of the ectodermal and mesodermal tissues in BM, occasional developmental abnormalities have been found associated with BM and are generally hypoplastic in nature. These abnormalities include hypoplasia of the ipsilateral breast, areola, nipple, and arm, ipsilateral arm shortening, lumbar spina bifida, thoracic scoliosis, and pectum carinatum, as well as enlargement of the ipsilateral foot.[37] In cases of BM with associated abnormalities, the male–female ratio is reversed 2:5 in comparison with patients with BM without abnormalities.

Clinical Features

The onset of BM is usually noted in the second or third decade of life, often following intense sunbathing. The lesions commonly have a unilateral distribution on the shoulders, the submammary area, and the back, but they also have been described on the forehead, cheeks, eyelids, neck, abdomen, hips, lower leg, and buttocks.[33] Normally, BM appears as a single lesion, but multiple lesions have been reported. The arrangement may be linear or zosteriform. Becker's melanosis ranges in size from a few centimeters in diameter to palm size or larger. There may be slow centrifugal extension of pigmentation. Hyperpigmentation varies from uniformly tan to dark brown. The lesions are well demarcated, but the margins are usually irregular. The center of the lesion may show slight thickening and corrugation of the skin. Hairiness usually develops after pigmentation, and the hairs become coarser and darker with time. Sometimes hypertrichosis is subtle and can only be appreciated by comparison with the contralateral side. The hypertrichosis and pigmentation may not overlap completely. In some cases, perifollicular papules may be a marker for coexistent proliferation of the muscular arrectores pilorum. Acneiform lesions strictly limited to the area of hyperpigmentation also have been reported.[34]

Histopathology

The configuration of the epidermis may vary from virtually normal to having variable degrees of papillomatosis, elongation of the epidermal rete ridges, or both[33] (Table 3-5). Thus the epidermal pattern may resemble an epidermal nevus or lentigo simplex (Fig. 3-4). The melanin content of the basilar keratinocytes is increased, whereas the number of melanocytes is normal or only slightly increased. Melanophages may be found in the papillary dermis. There may be prominence or hypertrophy of pilosebaceous units. A concomitant smooth-muscle hamartoma is often but not invariably present in the dermis.[35]

TABLE 3-5
Précis: Becker's Melanosis

Clinical Features
Onset in childhood, adolescence
Congenital on occasion
Unilateral location: shoulder, back, inframammary area, other sites
Usually solitary macular or slightly raised lesion
A few centimeters to palm size or larger
Tan to dark brown
Usually has prominent coarse hair
Usually irregular borders
Histopathology
Epidermal configuration varies from almost normal to papillomatous or lentiginous (elongated rete ridges)
Increased melanin in basal layer
Melanocytes normal or slightly increased in frequency
Smooth-muscle elements often increased in dermis (smooth-muscle hamartoma)
Prominent pilosebaceous units
Differential Diagnosis
Café-au-lait macule
Lentigo simplex
Epidermal nevus
Congenital melanocytic nevus

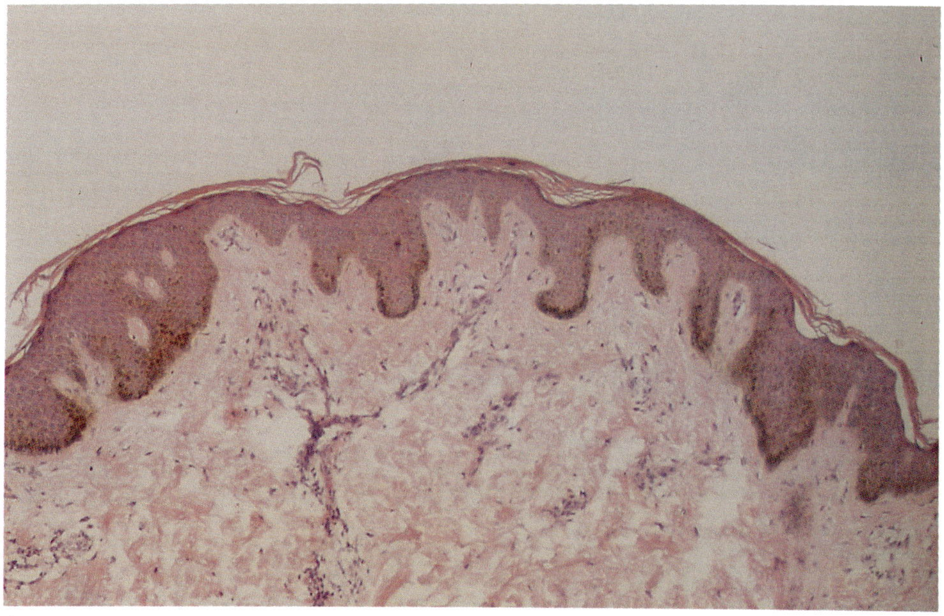

A

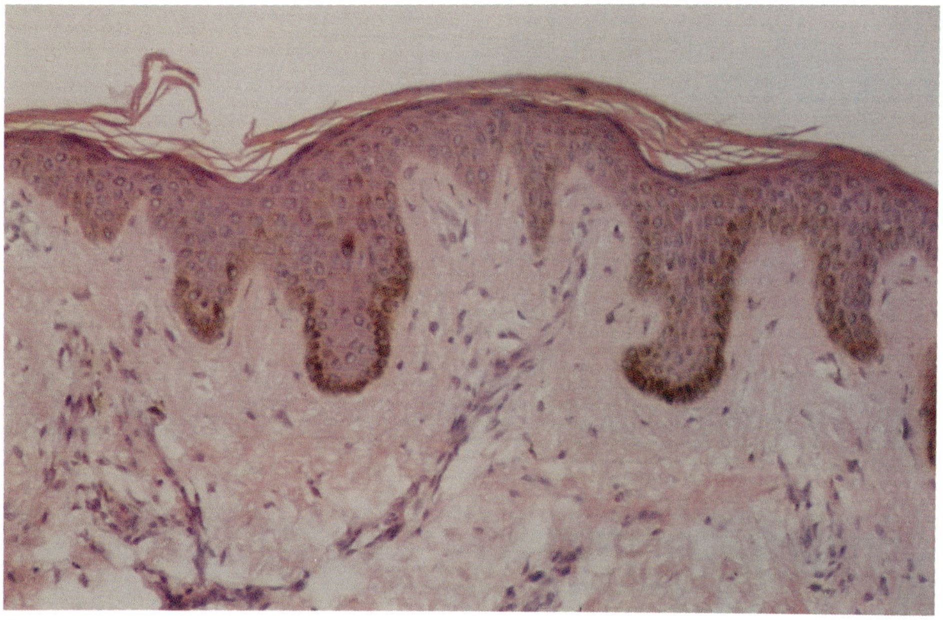

B

FIGURE 3-4

Becker's melanosis. (A) The epidermis is characterized by elongated hyperplastic epidermal rete ridges (H&E, × 200). (B) There is also significant basal layer hyperpigmentation, most prominently involving the lower-most aspects of the rete ridges. Although the basilar melanocytes are not increased in number, the overall histologic pattern resembles a lentigo (H&E, × 200).

Differential Diagnosis

The principal entities to be considered in the histologic differential diagnosis include café-au-lait macule, lentigo simplex, epidermal nevus, and congenital melanocytic nevus (see Table 3-5). In general, BM is distinguished histologically from CALM based on epidermal changes, i.e., papillomatosis and elongated rete ridges, and dermal findings such as prominent pilosebaceous and smooth-muscle components that are not observed in CALM. Both entities may or may not have slight basilar melanocytic hyperplasia. Clinical findings also should allow rapid discrimination in most instances, since BM is often raised and displays hypertrichosis. Histologic overlap may occur between Becker's nevus and lentigo, but gross morphologic features are usually distinctly different. Large (often congenital) varieties of lentigo may be difficult to distinguish from some forms of BM, i.e., those which are macular and lack hypertrichosis. Becker's melanosis may potentially be discriminated clinically from such lentigines by irregular borders and histologically by the presence of papillomatosis and other hamartomatous features, such as smooth-muscle hamartoma. Lesions showing only features of lentigo are probably best designated as such.

Both BM and epidermal nevus are cutaneous hamartomas that show some degree of clinical and histologic similarity. Epidermal nevus differs from BM by usually having more exaggerated epidermal changes, i.e., acanthosis and papillomatosis, the absence of melanocytic hyperplasia, and usually the absence of dermal hamartomatous features (e.g., smooth-muscle hamartoma).

The congenital melanocytic nevus may resemble BM clinically but is immediately discriminated from BM by the presence of nevus cells histologically.

MELANOTIC MACULES AND LENTIGINES OF MUCOCUTANEOUS SITES

Certain pigmented macules may involve mucosal sites such as the conjunctivae, oral mucosa and vermilion border of the lip, and genitalia.[39–54] Multiple lentigines may involve the oral mucosa and vermilion border as part of the Peutz-Jeghers syndrome.[55–57]

Clinical Features

These lesions are usually solitary or multiple macules measuring 1 to 5 mm and are often characterized by uniform light to dark brown or black homogeneous color[39–54] (Table 3-6). The borders are generally regular and well defined. However, occasional lesions on the genitalia in particular are notable for a mottled appearance and large size, measuring up to 50 mm in greatest diameter.[45–48,50–53] The latter clinical appearance suggests melanoma, but such lesions generally do not show atypical changes histologically (see below) or eventuate in melanoma on subsequent follow-up examination.[47,48]

TABLE 3-6
Précis: Melanotic Macules, Lentigines, and Lentiginosis of Mucocutaneous Sites

Clinical Features
Onset almost any age
Any mucosal site involved, especially lower lip, vulva, penis
Solitary, occasionally multiple
Usually 1- to 5-mm macule but occasionally up to 40 to 50 mm
Light to dark brown, or black
Sometimes mottled
Usually regular, well-defined borders
Round, oval
Occasionally polycyclic with irregular borders
Usually symmetric
Histopathology
Well-circumscribed
Symmetrical
Variable acanthosis
Tendency to elongated rete (lip, penis, vulva)
Basal layer hypermelanosis
Normal to increased numbers of solitary basilar melanocytes
Usually no melanocytic atypia
Melanophages usually present
Sparse lymphocytic infiltrates
Differential Diagnosis
Melanocytic nevus
Atypical melanocytic proliferations
Melanoma

Histopathology

The histologic spectrum of these lesions may vary from slight acanthosis of the epithelium, to presence or absence of club-shaped rete ridges, to presence or absence of basilar melanocytic hyperplasia (Fig. 3-5). The lesions without melanocytic hyperplasia may be designated as a *melanotic macule* or *melanosis.* The presence of melanocytic hyperplasia is best termed a *lentigo.* As with other simple lentigines, there is hyperpigmentation of the basilar epithelium. Melanophages and little or no lymphocytic infiltrate are present in the stroma.

Differential Diagnosis

The differential diagnosis includes melanocytic nevi of mucosal sites, atypical melanocytic proliferations, and

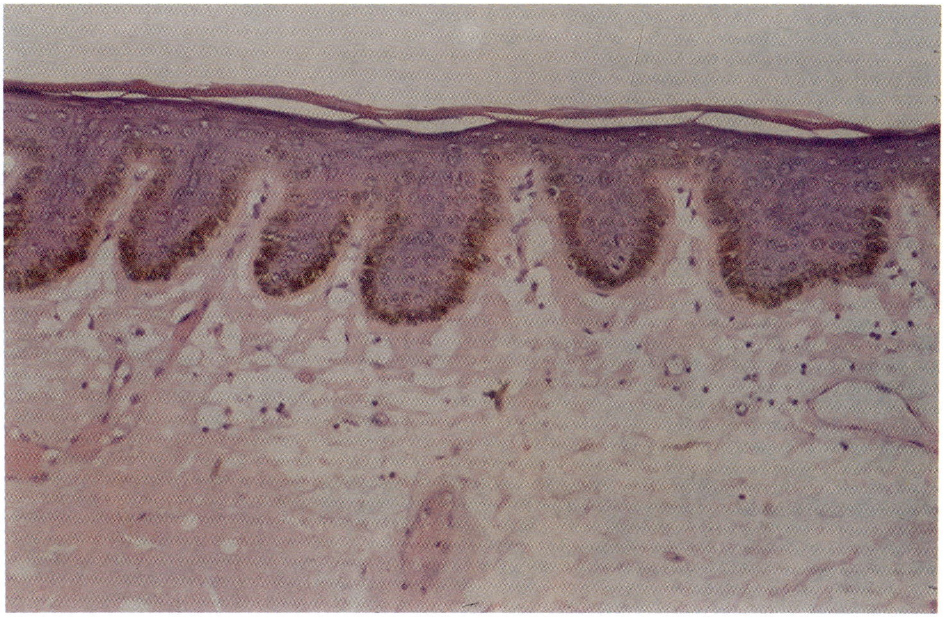

FIGURE 3-5
Vulvar lentigo. The lesion is notable for elongated rete ridges, basal layer hyperpigmentation, and slightly increased numbers of basilar melanocytes (H&E, × 200).

melanoma. In general, as with melanocytic lesions located in other sites, progressively greater clinical atypicality raises concern about atypical histologic changes and melanoma. For example, asymmetry, size greater than 5 to 6 mm, irregular borders, irregularity and complexity of color, blue-black color, and bleeding should raise concern about melanoma.

Histologically atypical melanocytic lesions and melanoma on mucosae are characterized by progressively greater frequency of basilar melanocytes and prominent cytologic atypia. In the case of melanoma, the basilar melanocytes often reach confluence along the basal layer in a lentiginous pattern. The melanocytes exhibit continuous marked cytologic atypia. Pagetoid spread is variable and may be absent, minimal, or prominent.

REFERENCES

1. Fitzpatrick TB: Soleil et peau. *J Med Esthet* 2(7):33–34, 1975.
2. Brues AM: Linkage of body build with sex, eye color and freckling. *Am J Hum Genet* 2:215–239, 1950.
3. Rhodes AR, Albert L, Barnhill RL, Weinstock MA: Sun-induced freckles in children and young adults: A correlation of clinical and histopathologic features. Cancer 67:1990–2001, 1991.
4. Gilchrest BA, Fitzpatrick TB, Anderson RR, Parrish JA: Localization of melanin pigmentation in the skin with Wood's lamp. *Br J Dermatol* 96:245–248, 1977.
5. Breathnach AS: Melanocyte distribution in forearm epidermis of freckled human subjects. *J Invest Dermatol* 29:253–261, 1957.
6. Crowe FW, Schull WJ: Diagnostic importance of café-au-lait spot in neurofibromatosis. *Arch Intern Med* 91:758–766, 1953.
7. Crowe FW, Schull WJ, Noel JV: *A Clinical, Pathological and Genetic Study of Multiple Neurofibromatosis.* Springfield, Ill, Charles C. Thomas, 1956.
8. Whitehouse D: Diagnostic value of the café-au-lait spot in children. *Arch Dis Child* 41:316–319, 1966.
9. Benedict PH, Szabó G, Fitzpatrick TB: Sinesi SJ. Melanotic macules in Albright's syndrome and in neurofibromatosis. *JAMA* 205:72–80, 1968.
10. Johnson BL, Charneco DR: Café-au-lait spot in neurofibromatosis and in normal individuals. *Arch Dermatol* 102:442–446, 1970.
11. Riccardi VM: Von Recklinghausen neurofibromatosis. *N Engl J Med* 305:1617–1627, 1981.
12. Mosher DB, Fitzpatrick TB, Hori Y, Ortonne J-P: Disorders of pigmentation, in Fitzpatrick TB, Eisen AZ, Wolff K, Freedberg IM, Austen KF (eds): *Dermatology in General Medicine,* ed 4. New York, McGraw-Hill, 1993, pp 903–995.
13. Bell SD, MacDonald DM: The prevalence of café-au-lait patches in tuberous sclerosis. *Clin Exp Dermatol* 10:562–565, 1985.
14. Silver HK: Asymmetry, short stature, and variations in sexual development: A syndrome of congenital malformations. *Am J Dis Child* 107:495–515, 1964.
15. Watson GH: Pulmonary stenosis, café-au-lait spots, and dull intelligence. *Arch Dis Child* 42:303–307, 1967.

16. Westerhof W, Beemer FA, Cormane BH, et al: Hereditary congenital hypopigmented and hyperpigmented macules. *Arch Dermatol* 114:931–936, 1978.
17. Bloom D: Congenital telangiectatic erythema resembling lupus erythematosus in dwarfs: Probably a syndrome entity. *Am J Dis Child* 88:754–758, 1954.
18. Jimbow K, Szabó G, Fitzpatrick TB: Ultrastructure of giant pigment granules (macromelanosomes) in the cutaneous pigmented macules of neurofibromatosis. *J Invest Dermatol* 61:300–309, 1973.
19. Silvers DN, Greenwood RS, Helwig EB: Café-au-lait spots without giant pigment granules: Occurrence in suspected neurofibromatosis. *Arch Dermatol* 110:87–88, 1974.
20. Nakagawa H, Hori Y, Sato S, et al: The nature and origin of the melanin macroglobule. *J Invest Dermatol* 83(2):134–139, 1984.
21. Sanchez WP, Pathak MA, Sato S: Melasma: A clinical, light microscopic, ultrastructural, and immunofluorescence study. *J Am Acad Dermatol* 4:698–710, 1981.
22. Hodgson C: Senile lentigo. *Arch Dermatol* 87:197–207, 1963.
23. Braun-Falco O, Schoefinius H-H: Lentigo senilis. Übersicht und eigene Untersuchungen. *Hautarzt* 7:277–283, 1971.
24. Bean WB: Senile freckles. *JAMA* 234(10):1059, 1975.
25. Montagna W, Hu F, Carlisle K: A reinvestigation of solar lentigines. *Arch Dermatol* 116:1151–1154, 1980.
26. Miller RA: Psoralens and UVA-induced stellate hyperpigmented freckling. *Arch Dermatol* 118:619–620, 1982.
27. Rhodes AR, Harrist TJ, Momtaz KT: The PUVA-induced pigmented macule: A lentiginous proliferation of large, sometimes cytologically atypical, melanocytes. *J Am Acad Dermatol* 9:47–58, 1983.
28. Rhodes AR, Stern RS, Melski JW: The PUVA lentigo: An analysis of predisposing factors. *J Invest Dermatol* 81:459–463, 1983.
29. Kanerva L, Niemi K-M, Lauharanta J: A semiquantitative light and electron microscopic analysis of histopathologic changes in photochemotherapy-induced freckles. *Arch Dermatol Res* 276:2–11, 1984.
30. Bolognia JL: Reticulated black solar lentigo ("ink spot" lentigo). *Arch Dermatol* 128:934–940, 1992.
31. Roewert HJ, Ackerman AB: Large-cell acanthoma is a solar lentigo. *Am J Dermatopathol* 14:122–132, 1992.
32. Mehregan AH: Lentigo senilis and its evolutions. *J Invest Dermatol* 65:429–433, 1975.
33. Copeman PM, Wilson Jones E: Pigmented hairy epidermal nevus (Becker). *Arch Dermatol* 92:249–251, 1965.
34. Burgreen BL, Ackerman AB: Acneiform lesions in Becker's nevus. *Cutis* 21:617–619, 1978.
35. Urbanek RW, Johnson WC: Smooth muscle hamartoma associated with Becker's nevus. *Arch Dermatol* 114:104–106, 1978.
36. Tymen R, Forrestier JF, Bontet B, Colomb B: Nevus tardif de Becker. *Ann Dermatol Venereol* 108:41–46, 1981.
37. Glinick, SE, Alper JC, Bogaars H, Brown JA: Becker's melanosis: Associated abnormalities. *J Am Acad Dermatol* 9:509–515, 1983.
38. Person JR, Longcope C: Becker's nevus: An androgen-mediated hyperplasia with increased androgen receptors. *J Am Acad Dermatol* 10:235–238, 1984.
39. Shapiro L, Zegarelli DJ: The solitary labial lentigo: A clinicopathologic study of 20 cases. *Oral Surg Oral Med Oral Pathol* 31:87–92, 1971.
40. Weathers DR, Corio RL, Crawford BE, et al: The labial melanotic macule. *Oral Surg Oral Med Oral Pathol* 42:196–205, 1976.
41. Page LR, Corio RL, Crawford BE, et al: The oral melanotic macule. *Oral Surg Oral Med Oral Pathol* 44:219–226, 1977.
42. Powell JP, Cummings CW: Melanoma and the differential diagnosis of oral pigmented lesions. *Laryngoscope* 88:1252–1267, 1978.
43. Buchner A, Hansen LS: Melanotic macule of the oral mucosa: A clinicopathologic study of 105 cases. *Oral Surg* 48:244–249, 1979.
44. Spann CR, Owen CG, Hodge SJ: The labial melanotic macule. *Arch Dermatol* 123:1029–1031, 1987.
45. Tsukada Y: Benign melanosis of the vagina and cervix. *Am J Obstet Gynecol* 124:211–212, 1976.
46. Jackson R: Melanosis of the vulva. *J Dermatol Surg Oncol* 10:119–121, 1984.
47. Sison-Torre EQ, Ackerman AB: Melanosis of the vulva: A clinical simulator of malignant melanoma. *Am J Dermatopathol* 7(Suppl):51–60, 1985.
48. Barnhill RL, Albert LS, Shama SK, et al: Genital lentiginosis: A clinical and histopathologic study. *J Am Acad Dermatol* 22:453–460, 1990.
49. Cullen SI: Incidence of nevi: Report of survey of the palms, soles, and genitalia of 10,000 young men. *Arch Dermatol* 86:41–43, 1962.
50. Landthaler M, Stolz W, Braun-Falco O: Lentigo der Glans penis. *Hautarzt* 40:221–225, 1989.
51. Kopf AW, Bart RS: Tumor conference 43: Penile lentigo. *J Dermatol Surg Oncol* 8:637–639, 1982.
52. Bhawan J, Cahn TM: Atypical penile lentigo. *J Dermatol Surg Oncol* 10:99–100, 1984.
53. Revuz J, Clerici T: Penile melanosis. *J Am Acad Dermatol* 20:567–570, 1989.
54. Folberg R, McLean IW: Primary acquired melanosis and melanoma of the conjunctiva: Terminology, classification and biologic behavior. *Hum Pathol* 16:129–135, 1985.
55. Jeghers H, McKusick BA, Katz KH: Generalized intestinal polyposis and melanin spots of the oral mucosa, lips and digits. *N Engl J Med* 241:993–1005, 1949.
56. Utsunomiya J, Gocho H, Miyanaga T, et al: Peutz-Jeghers syndrome: Its natural course and management. *Johns Hopkins Med J* 136:71–82, 1975.
57. Blank AA, Schneider BV, Panizzon R: Pigmentfleckenpolypose (Peutz-Jeghers-Syndrom). *Hautarzt* 32:296–300, 1981.

4

Common Acquired Melanocytic Nevi

As discussed in Chapter 1, the cutaneous melanocyte originates from the neural crest, taking residence in the epidermis and potentially giving rise to melanocytic proliferations such as lentigines and melanocytic nevi. The subject of this chapter is a description of the common acquired melanocytic nevi of skin.

HISTOGENESIS OF MELANOCYTIC NEVI

The origin of melanocytic nevi is poorly understood. Although these proliferations originate from neural crest–derived cells, little else is known about their histogenesis.[1-3] Most authors currently believe that melanocytic nevi arise from the proliferation of intraepidermal melanocytes with formation of growth centers (junctional nests or theques) and subsequent "dropping off" (*Abtropfung* of Unna[4]) of cells into the dermis. The latter hypothesis is based on the resemblance of the cells in melanocytic nevi to melanocytes[8] and cross-sectional observations correlating histologic findings in nevi with age.[5-16]

Alternative theories about the origin of nevi include derivation of all cells from cutaneous nerves or a pluripotential cell of nerve-sheath origin[17] or only a portion of the dermal component having a neural origin.[18-19] The difficulty in providing final proof for any of these theories is related to the fact that cells derived from the neural crest may exhibit both melanocytic and neural differentiation to varying degrees.[7,20,21]

There also has been a long-standing debate as to whether melanocytic nevi are hamartomas versus neoplasms.[7,18,22] The presence of other elements of the skin in excess in nevi, such as epidermal hyperplasia, hypertrophy of adnexal structures, and connective-tissue alterations, has suggested to some authors that the lesions are indeed developmental malformations—hence use of the term *nevus* as synonymous with *malformation*.

On the other hand, there are growing data that the melanocytic nevus is a neoplasm and perhaps the first stage in tumor progression of the melanocytic system.[3,23-27] In addition to gross morphologic and cytologic differences, experimental evidence suggests that the cells in melanocytic nevi exhibit distinct differences from intraepidermal melanocytes. Antigenic phenotyping with monoclonal antibodies has demonstrated that nevus cells express markers of tumor progression not present on intraepidermal basilar melanocytes.[27] Nevus cells in cell culture also have been shown to have growth advantages over typical melanocytes in culture.[25-27]

Both genetic[28,29] and environmental factors may influence the development of melanocytic nevi.[30-34] Increased numbers of nevi are known to aggregate in families, and this occurrence has been especially well documented in melanoma-prone families.[28,29,32] However, development of nevi may be influenced by sun exposure, particularly at an early age.[30] The distribution of melanocytic nevi generally conforms to sites receiving sun exposure. Some authors have postulated that melanocytic nevi are the result of sunlight acting as an initiator. Thus nevi could be viewed as clonal proliferations of initiated cells with a growth advantage over intraepidermal basal melanocytes.[7]

Lentigines and melanocytic nevi are thought to represent progressive stages of melanocyte migration and proliferation in the skin.[7,10,13] Melanoblasts (or a related

TABLE 4-1
Events in the Involution of Melanocytic Nevi

Diminished intraepidermal proliferative activity of nevus cells
Decreased proliferative activity of nevus cells with descent into the dermis
Loss of cellularity
Terminal differentiation with descent into dermis to neural-appearing cells (neurotization)
Gradual replacement of nevus cells by fibrous tissue, mucin, and fat

precursor cell) are believed to migrate from the neural crest, taking residence in the epidermis early in development.[1-3] Proliferation of these cells in the basilar epidermis may give rise sequentially to lentigo and the three subsequent stages of the melanocytic nevus. The proliferation of melanocytes as clusters or nests within the epidermis defines the junctional nevus.[5-7] The term *nevus cell* has been used to designate the cells within these nests or clusters. These cells are believed to be closely related to melanocytes but perhaps functionally somewhat altered by the aggregative pattern of growth.[8] These cells tend to lose the dendritic processes that are characteristic of solitary basilar melanocytes and to assume a more rounded morphology. In general, these cells have more abundant cytoplasm, somewhat larger nuclei, and somewhat more prominent nucleoli compared with the basilar melanocyte. Ultrastructurally, nevus cells contain single melanosomes in all stages of development similar to melanocytes.[8] Thus many authors consider nevus cells to be melanocytes and dismiss the need for alternative nomenclature.

The presumptive natural history of melanocytic nevi is characterized by proliferation within the epidermis as junctional nests and subsequent migration or "dropping off" of nevus cells into the papillary dermis, where proliferation results in nests of cells.[4,5] According to this hypothesis, eventually all intraepidermal proliferation of melanocytes ceases, and the nevi become entirely intradermal.[5,6] Nevus cells entering the dermis are usually characterized by a reduction in both proliferation and metabolic activity, except for the formation of melanosomes[5,6,35] (Table 4-1). Thus the cellularity of a nevus tends to decrease with age; because of this cessation of replication, the nevus cells are gradually replaced by mesenchymal elements—fibrous matrix, mucin, and fat.[6] Most dermal nevi are believed to undergo progressive involution, perhaps via acrochordons and eventual shedding.[11] It is also believed, however, that this developmental sequence may be arrested at any point such that a lentigo, junctional nevus, or compound nevus may persist indefinitely.[7]

An alternative hypothesis suggesting the reverse order of development has been presented recently.[17] According to this model, the progenitor cells first take residence in the dermis, resulting in proliferation and formation of a dermal nevus. There is subsequent migration of cells to the epidermis, resulting in proliferation and development of a compound nevus. All nevus cells may migrate from the dermis, taking residence in the epidermis and giving rise to a junctional nevus. According to this hypothesis, the final stage of differentiation is that of a lentigo.[17]

CLASSIFICATION OF MELANOCYTIC NEVI

As elaborated in Tables 4-2 and 4-3, melanocytic nevi may be classified according to a number of clinical and histologic attributes. A detailed discussion of clinical features of melanocytic nevi is beyond the scope of this chapter. However, it should be emphasized that clinical characteristics are important in arriving at a pathologic diagnosis. For example, conclusive documentation of a small nevus (e.g., 5 mm in greatest diameter) being present at birth enables the pathologist to designate the lesion as a congenital nevus. Similarly, the presence of a predominantly bluish color in a nevus strongly argues for a diagnosis of blue nevus, unless the histologic features are unusual, as in a tattoo or regressed melanocytic lesion.

TABLE 4-2
Clinical Criteria for the Classification of Melanocytic Nevi

A. Age of onset, e.g., congenital or acquired
B. Size
   1. Small congenital nevus < 1.5 cm
   2. Medium-sized congenital nevus > 1.5–19.9 cm
   3. Large congenital nevus > 20 cm
   4. Garment or bathing-trunk nevus
   5. Segmental nevus
C. Anatomic location, e.g., acral, genital
D. Appearance
   1. Borders regular or irregular, well-defined or ill-defined (hazy)
   2. Surface topography, e.g., macular, papular, papillomatous
   3. Symmetry
   4. Coloration homogeneous or haphazard
   5. Colors present: flesh, tan, brown, black, blue, gray, white, pink, red
   6. Speckled, targetoid, agminated, zosteriform

HISTOLOGIC CRITERIA FOR MELANOCYTIC LESIONS

Location of Melanocytes in the Skin

A primary criterion for histologic classification is the location of melanocytes in the skin (see Table 4-3). An arbitrary but useful subclassification is to designate nevi as superficial, superficial and deep, or deep according to the criteria in Table 4-3. Such a categorization is useful in indicating the extent of the lesion and also general categories; most common acquired nevi are superficial, whereas many congenital nevi are superficial and deep.[20]

Disposition of Melanocytes

The disposition or spatial relationship of melanocytes in various compartments of the skin is a major criterion for their classification. For example, the arrangement of melanocytes in a basilar single-cell pattern within the epidermis (alone) is found in only a limited number of conditions, e.g., the lentigines and atypical lentiginous melanocytic proliferations on acral or sun-damaged skin. A so-called pagetoid pattern refers to a dispersion of single and small aggregates of melanocytes throughout the epidermis, resulting in an appearance reminiscent of Paget's disease of the breast. Although an important histopathologic feature of melanoma, pagetoid spread is often observed in other settings, such as nevi of children, nevi on acral surfaces, Spitz and pigmented spindle cell nevi, and atypical nevi.

Nested arrangements of melanocytes are characteristic of melanocytic nevi. Further categorization is based on depth, architecture, stroma, and cytologic characteristics.

Particular arrangements of melanocytes are found in certain types of nevi. For example, interstitial disposition of melanocytes between collagen bundles of the reticular dermis, perivascular cuffing by melanocytes, and nests of melanocytes within sebaceous glands are features typical of congenital nevi (see Chap. 5).

Stroma

Stromal alterations in melanocytic nevi are poorly understood but may reflect the diverse phenotypic expressions of cells derived from the neural crest. Certain melanocytic nevi exhibit sclerosis of their dermal elements with some regularity.[6] Such nevi include the Spitz nevi (the sclerosing or desmoplastic variant; see Chap. 6), blue nevi, and their closely related variants.

Cell Type

In addition to the attributes referred to above, the cytologic characteristics of the melanocytes themselves are fundamental to the classification of melanocytic lesions. Although there is often both maturation/differentiation(or atrophy) and some degree of heterogeneity in the vast majority of nevi, most nevi are composed of essentially one nevus cell type. In the case of most acquired and congenital nevi, this cell type is a relatively small, round, oval, or polygonal "nevus" cell.

TABLE 4-3
Histologic Criteria for the Classification of Melanocytic Nevi

I. Location of melanocytes in the skin (depth)
   A. Superficial
      1. Intraepidermal
      2. Papillary dermis
      3. Upper half of reticular dermis
   B. Deep
      1. Lower half of reticular dermis
      2. Subcutaneous
      3. Fascial
II. Disposition of melanocytes
   A. Intraepidermal
      1. Basilar melanocytes (single cell pattern)
         a. Normal numbers
         b. Increased frequency
            (1) With elongated rete (lentiginous)
            (2) Without elongated rete
      2. Pagetoid pattern
      3. Nested pattern
         a. With lentiginous pattern
         b. Without lentiginous pattern
   B. Dermal
      1. Diffuse, interstitial
      2. Inverted wedge (deep apex of nests, fascicles of melanocytes extend into reticular dermis or subcutaneous fat)
      3. Patchy or plexiform pattern (discreet nests, fascicles associated with neurovascular or adnexal structures of reticular dermis with intervening normal dermis)
      4. Bulbous aggregates, nodules (cellular nests or fascicles with rounded contours, usually extending into reticular dermis, subcutis)
      5. Alveolar pattern
      6. Maturation/differentiation
III. Stroma, e.g., desmoplasia, sclerosis
IV. Cell type
   A. Small, round or oval cells
   B. Fusiform/spindle cell
   C. Epithelioid cell (abundant cytoplasm, overall enlarged)
   D. Dendritic cell (lengthy, delicate cellular processes)
   E. Intermediate, difficult to classify cell types
   F. All with varying degrees of melanization

LENTIGO SIMPLEX

Synonyms: simple lentigo, nevoid lentigo

Lentigo simplex is a sharply demarcated macule of uniform or variegate hyperpigmentation located anywhere on the body (without predilection for sun-exposed skin).[7,36] The frequency of lentigo simplex in children and adults is unknown; these lesions are found in all races and seem to occur equally in both sexes. Isolated lesions are often present at birth, more commonly in black than in white newborns.[37] In darkly pigmented races, lentigo simplex is the most common histologic pattern of pigmented lesions on acral cutaneous sites.[38] Lentigines simplex may increase in number during childhood or puberty and sometimes occur in an eruptive form as so-called lentiginosis with or without obvious precipitating factors.[39,40]

Pigmented bands on the nails showing the histology of a lentigo simplex are common in dark-skinned races, especially black individuals.[41] They are found in up to 11 percent of Japanese,[42] whereas they are extremely rare in white individuals.[43]

Clinical Features

The simple lentigo is defined clinically as a regular, well-circumscribed macule measuring 1 to 5 mm in diameter and having a uniform light brown, brown, or dark brown color[36] (see Table 3-1). The simple lentigo may occur in a localized or a widespread pattern as in lentiginosis profusa or in association with certain syndromes, such as, for example, LEOPARD (multiple lentigines), LAMB, or Peutz-Jeghers syndrome[44–48] (Table 4-4).

Histopathology

The simple lentigo is defined histologically by three features (see Table 3-1): (1) increased frequency of basilar melanocytes compared with adjacent normal skin, (2) elongated, club-shaped epidermal rete, and (3) basilar hyperpigmentation of the epidermis (see Fig. 12-1) that may extend into the upper portion of the epidermis and stratum corneum.[7,10,13] A characteristic feature of the lentigo pattern is the increased frequency of melanocytes at the tips of the elongated epidermal rete ridges with diminished frequency proceeding upward along the sides and between the epidermal rete ridges. Thus the greatest concentration of melanocytes is usually on the tips and lower-most sides of the rete ridges and the lowest frequency of cells in the epidermis overlying the dermal papillae. Similar to the concentration of melanocytes, melanin content tends to be located in the same distribution. Melanin-containing macrophages and sparse perivascular lymphocytic infiltrates are also commonly observed in the papillary dermis. The overall architecture of the lesion is that of a well-circumscribed process.

Differential Diagnosis

A simple lentigo must first of all be discriminated from a freckle and a solar lentigo, and this is discussed in Chapter 3 (see Table 3-1). Briefly, a simple lentigo differs histologically from a freckle because of elongated epidermal rete ridges and an increased frequency of basilar melanocytes. The simple lentigo does not usually have rete ridges as elongated and showing anastomosis or solar elastosis to the degree observed in solar lentigo. In addition, melanocytic hyperplasia may not be present in solar lentigo.

A common dilemma is differentiating a simple lentigo from a typical melanocytic nevus or dysplastic nevus. The melanocytic nevus is distinguished by the presence of junctional nests.[13] One occasionally observes lesions that have features of lentigo and only a rare small junctional cluster of cells. Such lesions in the past have been termed *nevoid lentigo* or even *"jentigo."* Our current practice is to

TABLE 4-4
Syndromes Associated with Multiple Lentigines

Syndrome	*Onset*	*Distribution*	*Associations*	*Inheritance*
Lentiginosis profusa	Birth to adulthood	Widespread, mucosa spared	None	None
Multiple lentigines (LEOPARD)	Infancy	Widespread, mucosa spared	Cardiac conduction defects, ocular hypertelorism, pulmonary stenosis, genital abnormalities (hypoplasia of gonads or ovaries), growth retardation, neural deafness	Autosomal dominant
LAMB		Genital mucosa	Atrial myxoma, cutaneous myxomas, blue nevi	
Peutz-Jeghers		Perioral, vermilion border, oral mucosa, dorsal fingers	Multiple gastrointestinal polyps, adenocarcinoma	Autosomal dominant

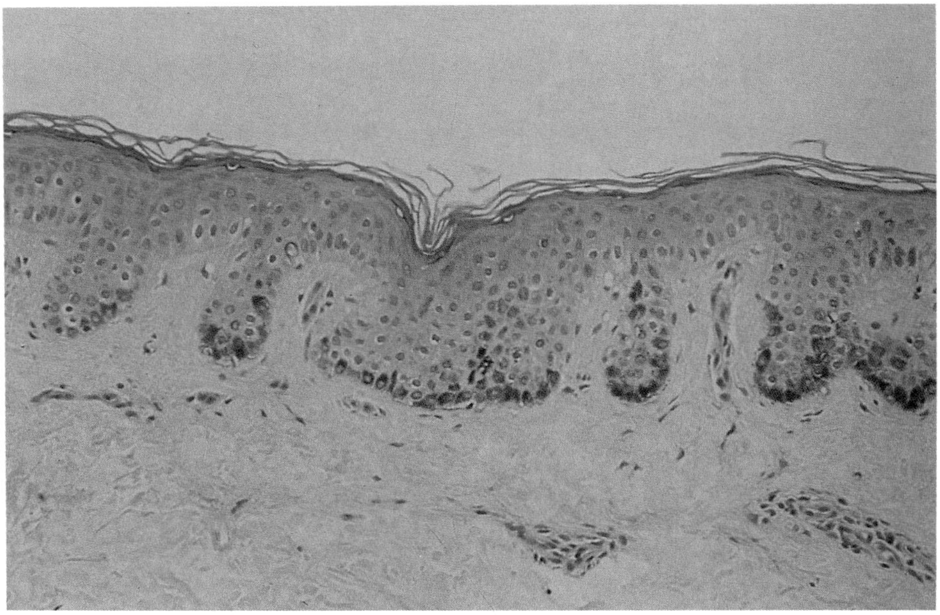

FIGURE 4-1
Lentigo simplex. Note elongated epidermal rete and basal layer hyperpigmentation, most prominently involving the lower-most aspects of the rete (H&E, × 200).

designate a lesion as a lentiginous junctional nevus if junctional nests are observed and otherwise to use the term *lentigo.* Lentigo is distinguished from dysplastic nevus by the lack of increased frequency of basilar melanocytes resulting in a multilayered confluence of cells and cytologic atypia of the intraepidermal cells (see Chap. 9).

COMMON ACQUIRED MELANOCYTIC NEVI

Synonyms: nevocellular nevus, mole

Common acquired nevi range from small, well-circumscribed pigmented macules to raised, flesh-colored lesions defined by the location of aggregations of "nevus cells" in the skin; junctional nevi have intraepidermal collections of nevus cells, dermal (intradermal) nevi have nevus cells in the dermis, and compound nevi have nevus cells in both areas.[5,6]

The natural history of acquired melanocytic nevi is poorly documented.[4–7] The prevalence of nevi is related to age, race, and perhaps genetic and environmental factors.[28–34] Very few nevi are present in early childhood, but they increase in number, reaching a peak in the third decade of life, and tend thereafter to disappear with increasing age.[5,7,10,11,14–16] There is a period of particularly rapid development of nevi at puberty. In general, the greatest numbers of nevi are noted among individuals aged 20 to 29 years.[16] A study in Scotland noted that in the first decade of life females had an average of 3 moles and males 2 moles. For the age interval 20 to 29 years, women and men had mean nevus counts of 33 and 22, respectively. There was a progressive decline thereafter, with females having a mean of 6 nevi and males 4 nevi in the seventh decade. No substantial differences between men and women have been noted for prevalence of nevi.[15,16] Caucasians in general have greater numbers of nevi than darker-skinned groups, i.e., blacks and Asians.[49] Furthermore, a greater prevalence of nevi is associated with lighter skin color in Caucasians.[50] The frequency of melanocytic nevi on the palms and soles, nail beds, and conjunctivae is also related to race; nevi on these surfaces are more prevalent in blacks than in whites.[38] Mean acral nevus counts for blacks in Uganda were 11[51] versus 2 to 8 for American blacks.[38,52]

Genetic factors may be operative in the prevalence of nevi; increased numbers of nevi have been noted to cluster in families, especially in families associated with familial melanoma.[29] Although an autosomal dominant mode of inheritance has been postulated for clinically atypical nevi in hereditary melanoma families,[53] the pattern of inheritance may be more complex.[29] Environmental factors such as sun exposure also may influence the development of melanocytic nevi.[30] There is some evidence that individuals residing in sunny climates have a greater prevalence of melanocytic nevi compared with persons living in more temperate zones, but more objective evidence is needed to establish this relationship.[30]

Clinical Features

Melanocytic nevi are well-circumscribed, round or ovoid lesions, generally measuring from 2 to 6 mm in diameter[54,55] (Table 4-5). They appear orderly and symmetrical overall. Although many nevi display slight asymmetry, the borders are usually regular and well defined. The natural history of melanocytic nevi is believed to be a progression from a junctional nevus to a compound nevus, then to a dermal nevus, and subsequent involution.[4-7,11] However, this model is based on cross-sectional histologic observations and has not actually been observed. It is also believed that the evolution of a nevus may halt at any point, with a particular lesion remaining a junctional nevus, compound nevus, or dermal nevus. The junctional nevus is a macular lesion with slight accentuation of skin markings visible with sidelighting. Junctional nevi are also characterized by a uniform medium to dark brown color. Compound nevi show variable degrees of elevation and in general somewhat lighter shades of brown than do junctional nevi. Dermal nevi are usually more elevated and show lighter shades of brown or even flesh tones compared with compound nevi. However, it should be emphasized that there is considerable clinical

TABLE 4-5
Précis: Common Acquired Melanocytic Nevi

Junctional Nevus	*Compound Nevus*	*Dermal Nevus*
	Clinical Features	
Onset childhood, adolescence	Onset childhood, adolescence, third decade	Onset first, second, third decades, or later
2- to 5-mm macule	3- to 6-mm papule (slight to clear elevation)	3- to 6-mm papule, often dome-shaped, globoid, polypoid, or papillomatous
Round, oval	Round, oval	Round, oval
Symmetrical	Symmetrical	Symmetrical
Well-defined regular borders	Well-defined regular borders	Well-defined regular borders
Homogeneous brown, dark brown	Homogeneous tan, brown, dark brown	Uniform flesh color, light brown
Slight accentuation of skin cleavage lines with oblique lighting	Slight accentuation of skin cleavage lines with oblique lighting	Slight accentuation of skin cleavage lines with oblique lighting
	Histopathology	
Symmetry	Symmetry	Symmetry
Well circumscribed	Well circumscribed	Well circumscribed
Regular arrangement of junctional nests of nevus cells	Regular arrangement of junctional nests of nevus cells	Dome-shaped or papillomatous configuration
Fairly uniform size, shape, position of nests	Fairly uniform size, shape, position of nests	Orderly arrangement of nevus cells in dermis
Nests usually at tips of epidermal rete ridges	Nests usually at tips of epidermal rete ridges	Usual transition (maturation) from epithelioid to lymphocytoid to spindle cells with increasing depth of nevus.
Cohesive nests usually	Cohesive nests usually	
Lentiginous melanocytic proliferation common	Generally no pagetoid spread	
Generally no pagetoid spread	Nevus cells usually confined to papillary dermis or superficial reticular dermis	Nevus cells usually confined to papillary dermis or superficial reticular dermis
	Usual transition or maturation from epithelioid to lymphocytoid to spindled nevus cells	Usual transition or maturation from epithelioid to lymphocytoid to spindled nevus cells
	Mitotic figures uncommon or rare in dermis	Mitotic figures uncommon or rare
	Usually only minimal nuclear pleomorphism	Usually minimal nuclear pleomorphism

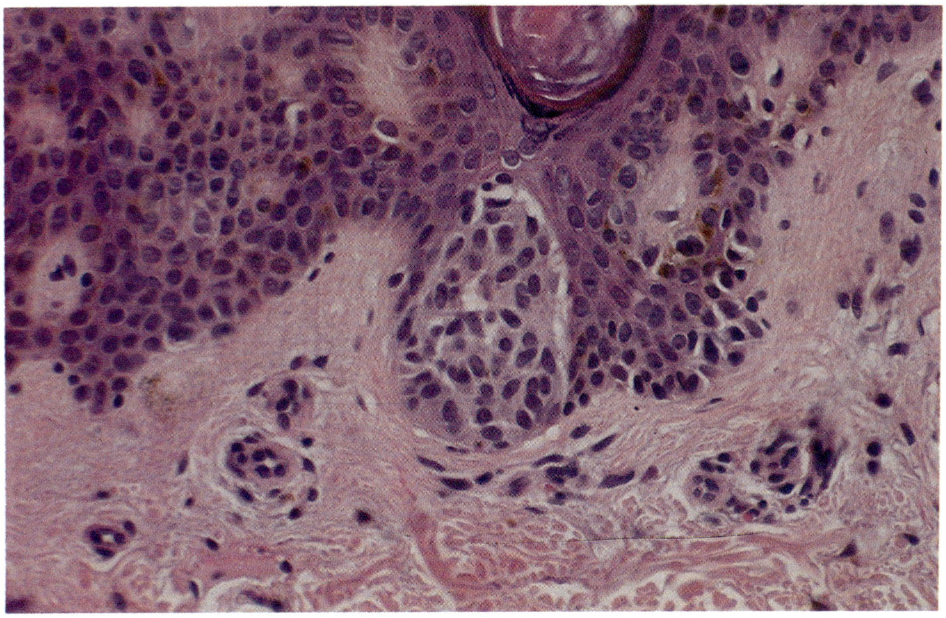

FIGURE 4-2
Junctional nevus. Cohesive nest of type A nevus cells (H&E, × 400).

overlap among all three types of nevi.[12] Dermal nevi and, to a lesser degree, compound nevi may be dome-shaped or papillomatous. Nevi may have a verrucous surface simulating that of seborrheic keratosis. Many nevi contain hairs that are coarse and dark compared with those in surrounding skin.

Nevi on the palms and soles usually are macular or only slightly raised, have regular and well-defined borders, and show uniform brown or dark brown coloration. Melanocytic nevi of the nail bed usually present as uniformly pigmented brown or dark brown longitudinal bands (melanonychia striata) with regular and distinct margins.[41–43]

Histopathology

The junctional nevus is defined by the nesting of nevus cells within the epidermis.[4–6] A junctional nest or *theque* contains five or more nevus cells in close apposition, usually above the basement membrane[12,13] (Fig. 4-2). The characteristics of these nests, such as size, shape, location, and spacing within the epidermis, tend to be regular and similar within a given nevus. The nevus cells within these nests are typified by a cohesion of cells such that the nest has a syncytial appearance[18] (Fig. 4-3). Another common feature is the location of junctional nests on the tips of elongated epidermal rete ridges rather than on the sides or between rete ridges.

The compound nevus has nevus cells within the dermis as well as junctional nesting, whereas the dermal (or intradermal) nevus has no intraepidermal component[5] (Figs. 4-4 to 4-8); (see also Table 4-5). It should be emphasized that most nevi are compound. Kopf and Andrade[12] examined a series of otherwise typical dermal nevi and found that on serial sectioning, 80 percent of these nevi had junctional nests.

The pattern of dermal involvement in common acquired nevi is essentially confined to the adventitial dermis (the finely textured collagenous stroma comprising the papillary dermis and surrounding adnexal structures and blood vessels)[5] (see Fig. 4-5). Dermal nevi mainly proliferate in and expand the papillary dermis, resulting in progressive elevation of nevus contours commensurate with the volume of nevus cells (see Figs. 4-7 and 4-8).

MATURATIONAL SEQUENCE AND CYTOLOGY OF NEVUS CELLS

Nevus cells within the intraepidermal component or superficial dermis exhibit a pattern of cohesive rounded nesting of cells, tendency to synthesis of melanin, and cytologic characteristics of epithelial cells[5–7,18,20,35] (see Fig. 4-3). The latter features refer to the abundant cytoplasm in the cells, frequently with slightly eosinophilic staining properties and the rounded or polygonal configuration

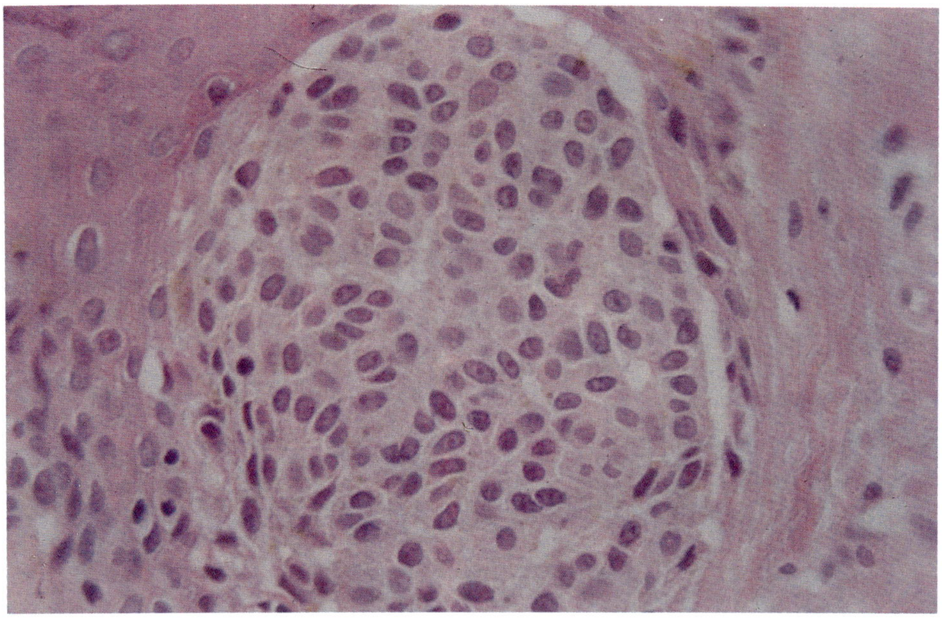

FIGURE 4-3

Junctional nevus containing syncytial aggregate of type A nevus cells. Note round, oval, and slightly elongate nuclei with even dispersed "ground glass" chromatin. Occasional small nucleoli are also present in some nuclei (H&E, × 600).

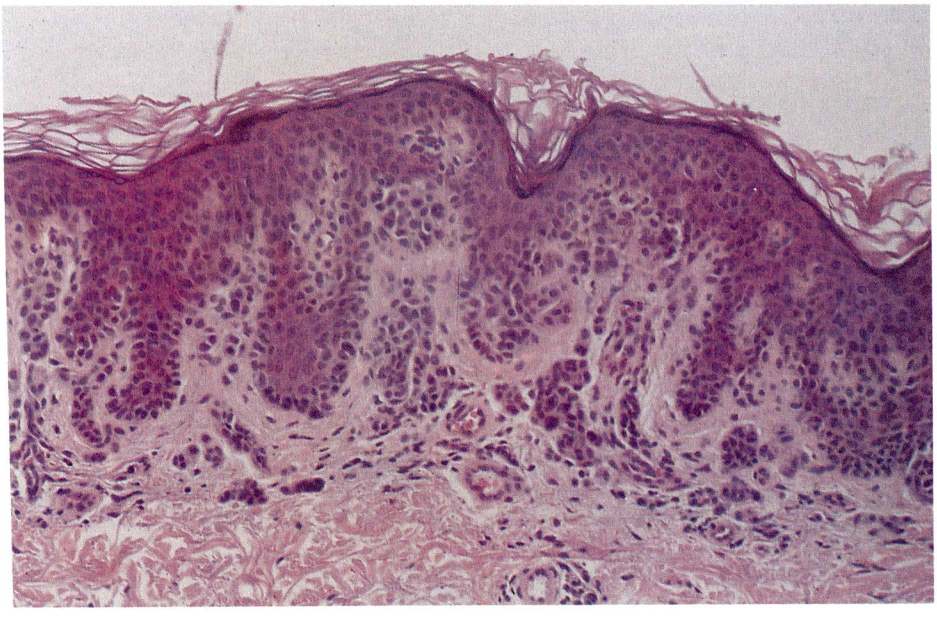

FIGURE 4-4

Lentiginous compound nevus. Epidermis shows lentiginous and junctional nested pattern of melanocytes (H&E, × 200).

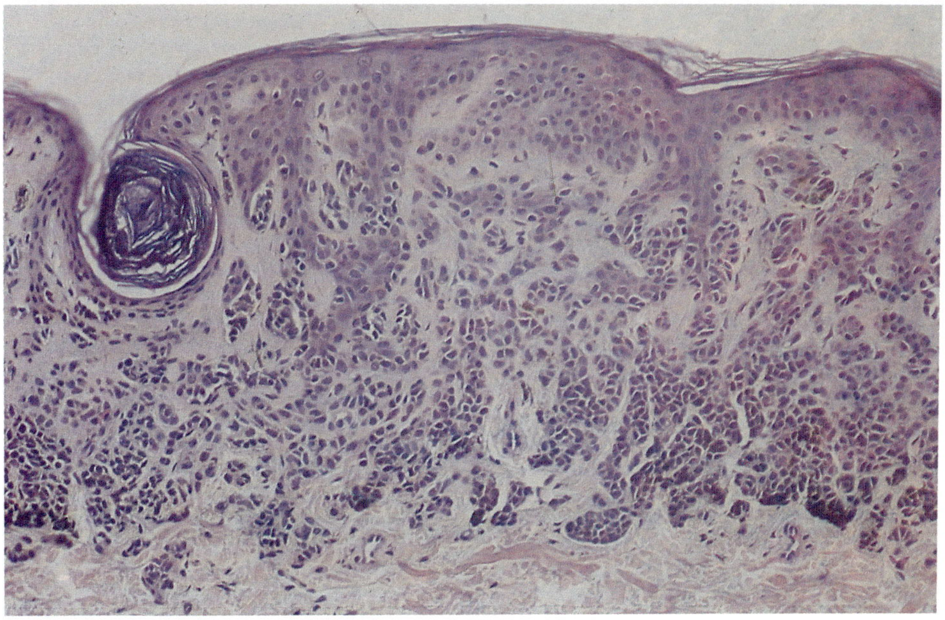

FIGURE 4-5
Compound nevus. Most nevus cells are disposed in cords in the papillary dermis (H & E, × 200).

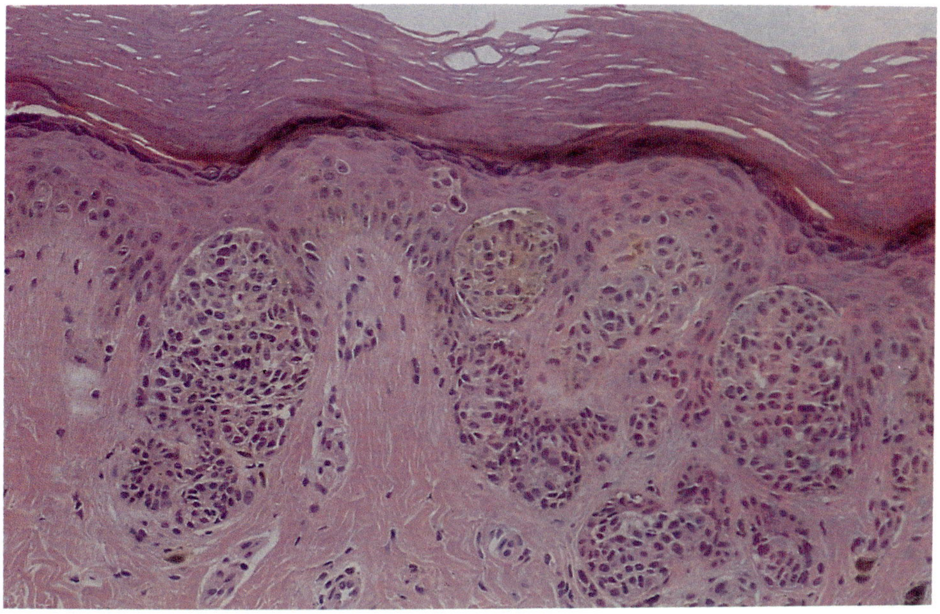

FIGURE 4-6
Compound nevus of acral skin. Nests of type A cells in both epidermis and dermis. Note focal upward migration of melanocytes in the epidermis, a finding commonly observed in acral nevi (H&E, × 200).

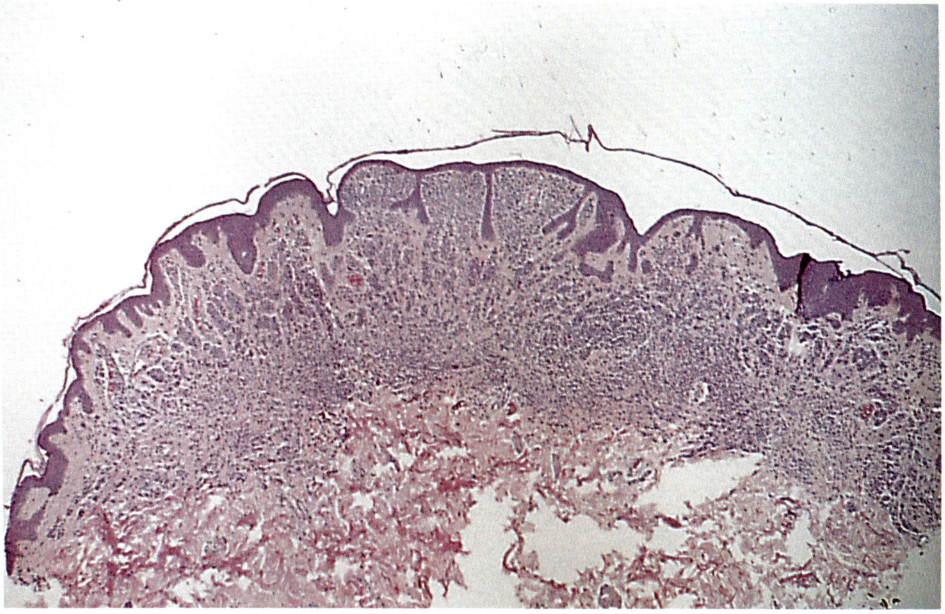

A

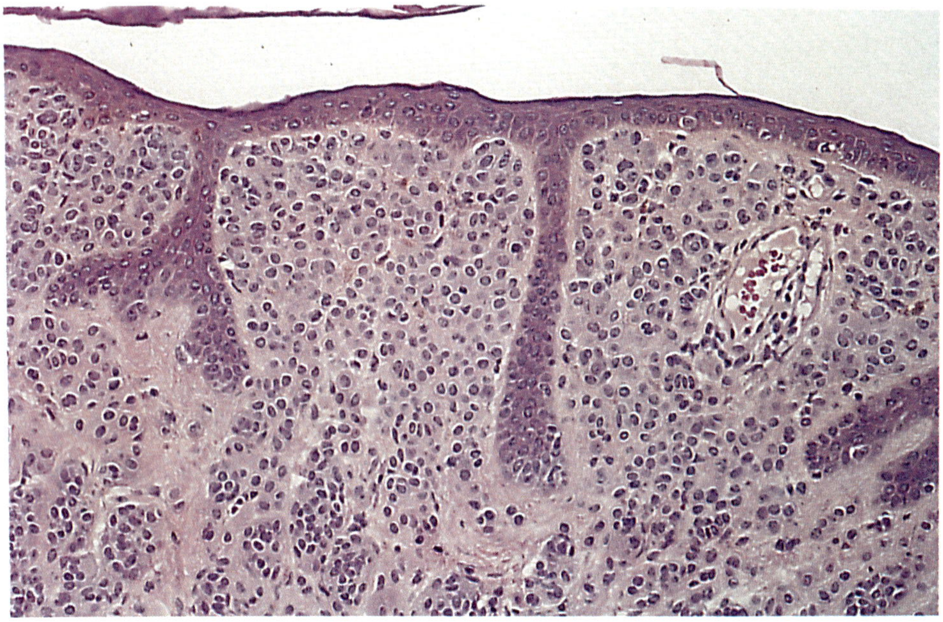

B

FIGURE 4-7

Dermal nevus. (A) Note dome-shaped surface and overall symmetry (H&E, × 40). (B) Orderly disposition of nevus cells in papillary dermis (H&E, × 200).

of the cells. In general, the nuclei of these cells are slightly greater in size than those of basilar melanocytes.[8] The cells are also characterized by a uniform disposition of chromatin generally having a ground glass basophilic appearance and delicate nuclear membranes[5,8,18,35] (see Fig. 4-3). Small nucleoli also may be observed within the nuclei. Some authors have designated nevus cells with the latter attributes as *epithelioid* or *type A* nevus cells.[18,35] Nevus cells in the papillary dermis usually subjacent to the type A cells have an appearance resembling lymphocytes[18,35] (Fig. 4-9). This is due to a smaller amount of cytoplasm and the tendency to form more compacted cords and nests of cells (see Fig. 4-9B). Generally, the latter type of nevus cell does not have the capacity to synthesize melanin or to form

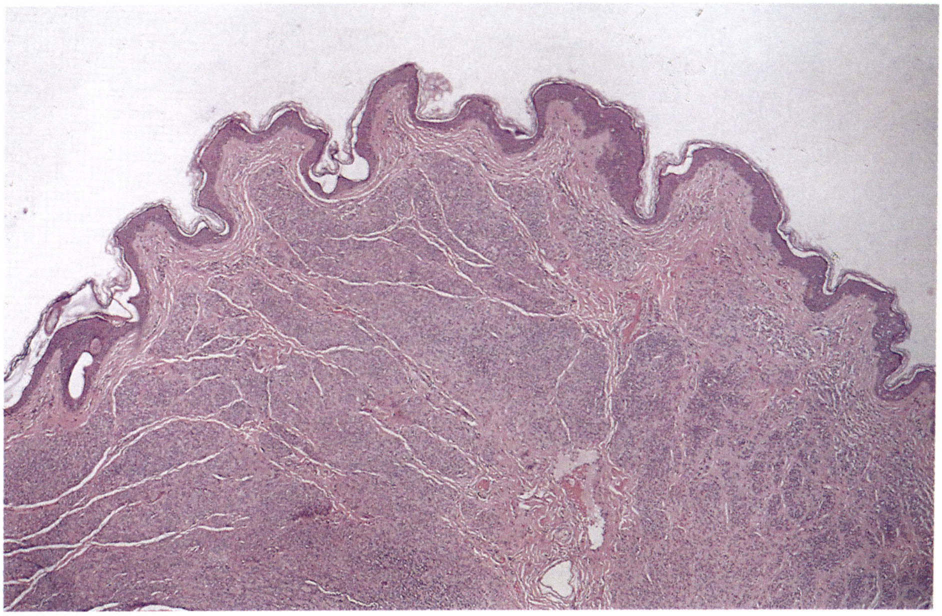

FIGURE 4-8
Papillomatous dermal nevus. The epidermal surface has a papillary topography (H & E, × 40).

rounded nests.[5-7,18,35] These cells also have been referred to as *lymphocytoid* or *type B* nevus cells.[35] The final stage of maturation is that of nevus cells with an elongate or spindle-shaped morphology and separation by delicate fibrous tissue[5-7,18,19,35] (see Fig. 4-9C and D). The latter cells have considerable resemblance to fibroblasts or Schwann cells, as in peripheral nerve sheath tumors.[5-7,18,19,35]

Nevus cells in general exhibit some degree of pleomorphism (i.e., anisokaryosis or variation in nuclear size and shape) and variation in staining of chromatin.[20] These findings must be interpreted in the overall context of the lesion. A certain degree of cytologic variation is permissible, particularly if other histologic characteristics such as proliferative architectural abnormalities and host response are absent. The same caveat applies to the cytologic features of nevi in infants and young children (see Chap. 5).

Nevus giant cells are a frequent finding in melanocytic nevi but also may be found in atypical nevi and melanoma.[5] These giant cells are principally of two types. One type is characterized by tightly packed nuclei with scant cytoplasm and has been called a *mulberry-type giant cell* (see Fig. 4-9E). The molding of nuclei in such a cell may lead to misinterpretation as a bizarre, atypical nevus cell. This cell type is often present in the dermal component of a nevus. The second type of giant cell is typified by a peripheral, wreathlike arrangement of nuclei with central pink or slightly bluish cytoplasm. The latter cell type may closely simulate or on occasion be identical to a Touton giant cell observed in histiocytic proliferations such as juvenile xanthogranuloma. This particular giant cell is commonly observed in junctional nests (see Fig. 4-19B).

Another common cytologic feature of nevus cells is the presence of pseudonuclear inclusions[56] (see Fig. 4-9B). This finding results from an invagination of cytoplasm that on cross section seems to lie within the nucleus and has the same staining properties as the nevus cell cytoplasm, often a pale or "dusty" ground glass appearance.

HISTOLOGIC VARIATIONS IN COMMON ACQUIRED NEVI

General Architecture

Melanocytic nevi in general have an overall histologic symmetry and usually a well-circumscribed configuration (see Fig. 4-7A). The junctional component as a general rule does not extend peripherally beyond a dermal component,[7] if present (see Chap. 9). The surface profile of a nevus may vary from being almost flat to dome-shaped, polypoid, or papillomatous.[55] This surface profile has a general correlation with type of nevus; e.g.,

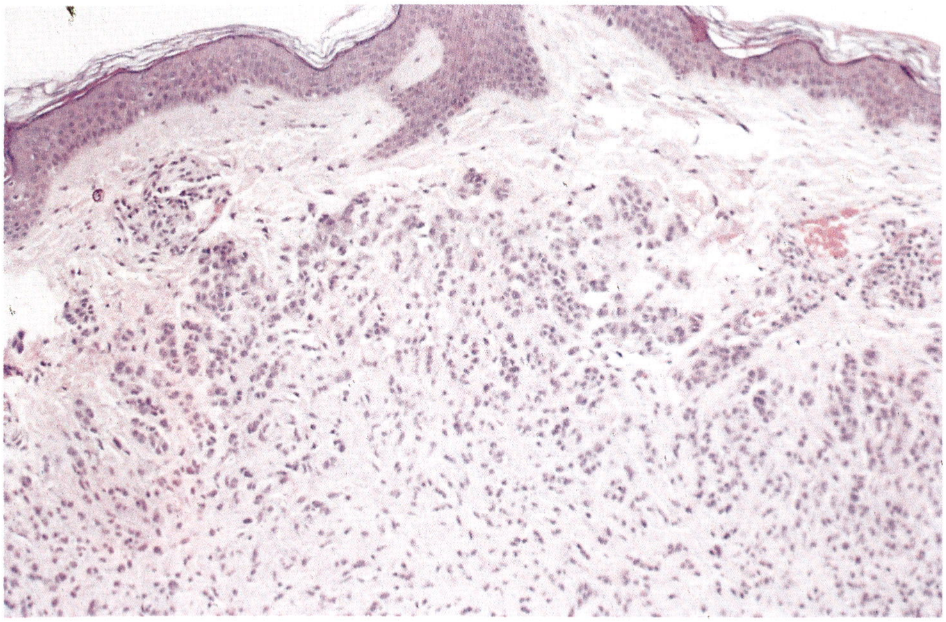

A

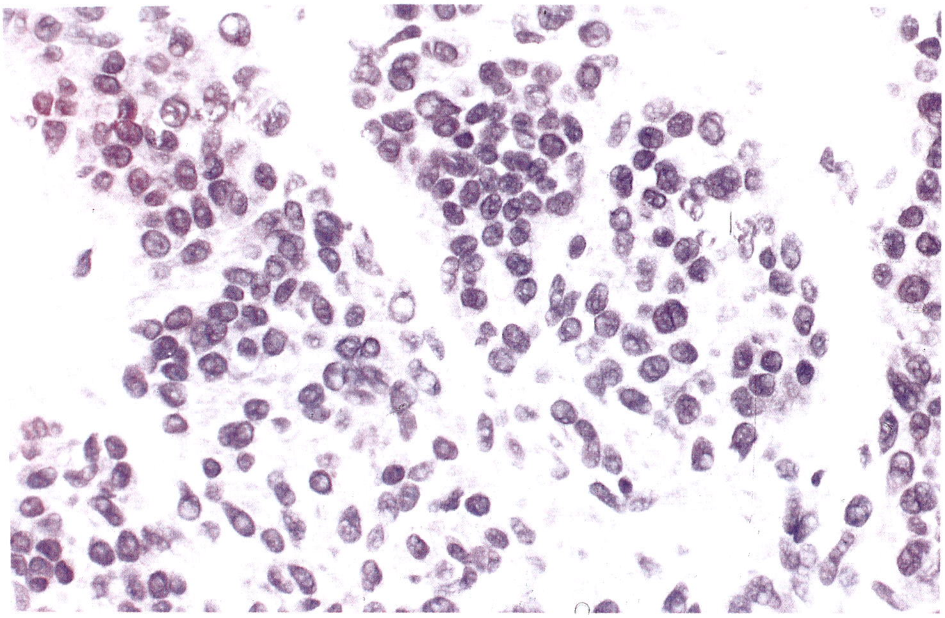

B

FIGURE 4-9

Dermal nevus. (A) Maturation of type B (superficial) nevus cells to type C (deeper) nevus cells. (B) Type B (lymphocytoid) nevus cells in dermis. The cells contain minimal cytoplasm and uniform round or oval nuclei (H&E, × 400). (C) Type C (spindled) nevus cells. The cells resemble Schwann cells and are separated by delicate connective tissue (H&E, × 400). (D) Marked neurotization in dermal nevus. These cellular structures resemble Wagner-Meissner corpuscles. (E) Multinucleate ("mulberry-type") nevus giant cells in dermal nest of type A cells (H & E, × 600).

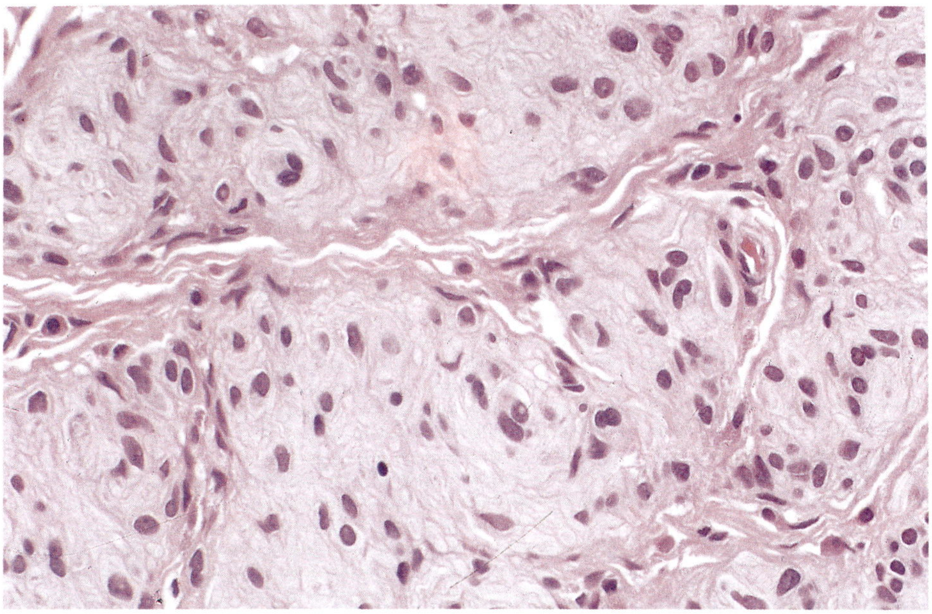

C

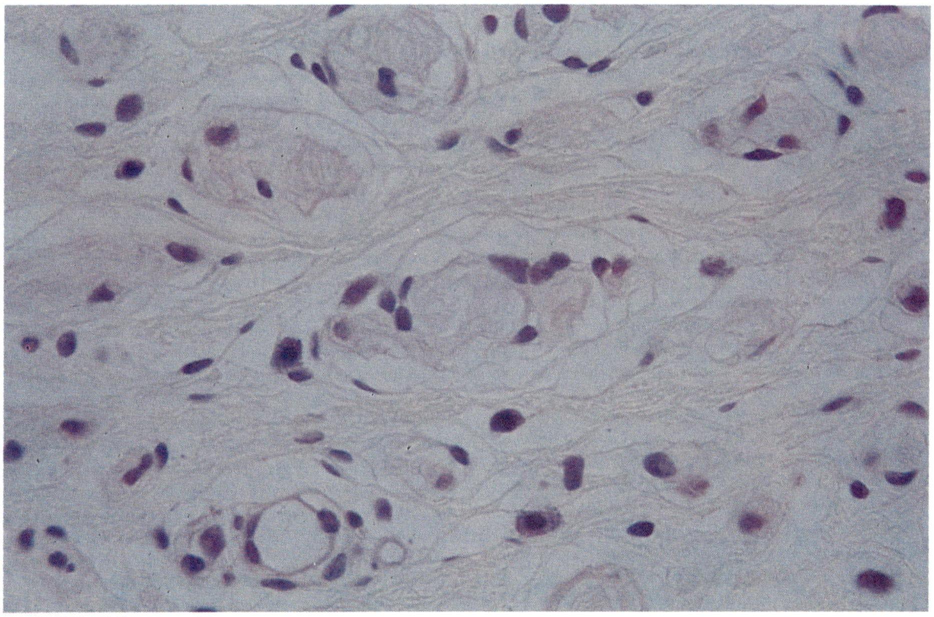

D

FIGURE 4-9 *(Continued)*

junctional nevi are usually relatively flat, compound nevi are slightly raised, and dermal nevi are often dome-shaped, polypoid, or papillomatous. This surface configuration also correlates with anatomic location of the nevus. Most nevi on acral sites are relatively flat or slightly raised, junctional or compound nevi[5,6,12–14] (see Fig. 4-6). In contrast, many nevi on the head and neck and to a lesser extent on the trunk are dome-shaped or polypoid compound or usually dermal nevi (see Fig. 4-8). The latter observations must of course be interpreted with the age of the individual and the natural history of nevi in mind.

Epidermal Changes

The epidermis in common acquired nevi may demonstrate considerable variation in histologic pattern, e.g., little or no acanthosis, elongation of the epidermal rete ridges in the pattern of a lentigo, papillomatous epidermal hyperplasia (in some instances resembling seborrheic

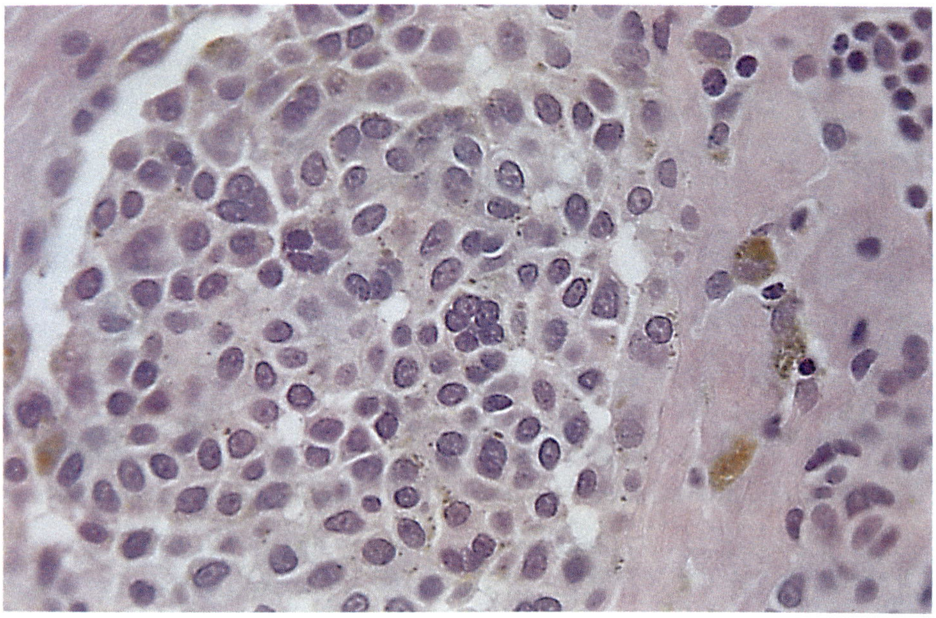

E

FIGURE 4-9 *(Continued)*

keratosis), and effacement of the epidermal rete ridges as in some dermal nevi.[57]

VARIATIONS IN THE DERMAL COMPONENT

Maturational Variations

The proportion of nevus cells that are type A, B, and C varies within nevi and may be related to the age of the nevus and other poorly understood factors[5-7,18,35] (see Fig. 4-9). The failure of the dermal component to progress beyond type A cells is believed to be a maturational disturbance and will be discussed in the context of dysplastic nevus. Thus the dermal component of some nevi may be largely type A, type B, or type C cells.[5-7,18,35]

Balloon Cell Alteration

This type of cytologic alteration is believed to be a degenerative or senescent change of nevus cells seen focally in approximately 2 percent of nevi.[58-60] The balloon cells are considerably enlarged with abundant vacuolated cytoplasm and small, centrally placed nuclei (see below). Based on ultrastructural findings, the balloon cell change is thought to originate from vacuolar degeneration of melanosomes.[61,62]

Congenital Nevus Pattern

Some common acquired nevi may exhibit changes that have been attributed to congenital nevi in the past but are currently recognized as nonspecific.[63] The changes include involvement of the superficial reticular dermis with nevus cells dispersed interstitially between collagen bundles and/or in discrete aggregates associated with blood vessels or adnexal structures. Other features also suggesting congenital origin but probably nonspecific are large junctional nests and a diffuse, cohesive plaque of nevus cells filling the papillary dermis.

Desmoplasia (Sclerosis)

This feature refers to increased density of fibrous tissue in the stroma of nevi[6] (Fig. 4-10). The nevus cells are often disposed interstitially in this fibrotic matrix.

Fibrous Involution

Melanocytic nevi are believed to undergo gradual involution with progressive replacement of dermal nevus cells by delicate fibrous tissue or in some instances fat.[5,6,11] Thus the final stages of some nevi may be fibroepithelial polyps or possibly angiofibromas.[6,11,64]

Lipomatous Alteration

Progressive accumulation of fat may occur in dermal nevi and generally correlates with age[6] (Fig. 4-11). This change is thought to represent involution or regression of a nevus. At one time, this histologic pattern was believed to be a combination of nevus lipomatosus and melanocytic nevus.[65]

Mucinous Alteration

The deposition of mucin is a common finding in many nevi.[6] The latter feature is noted most often in dermal

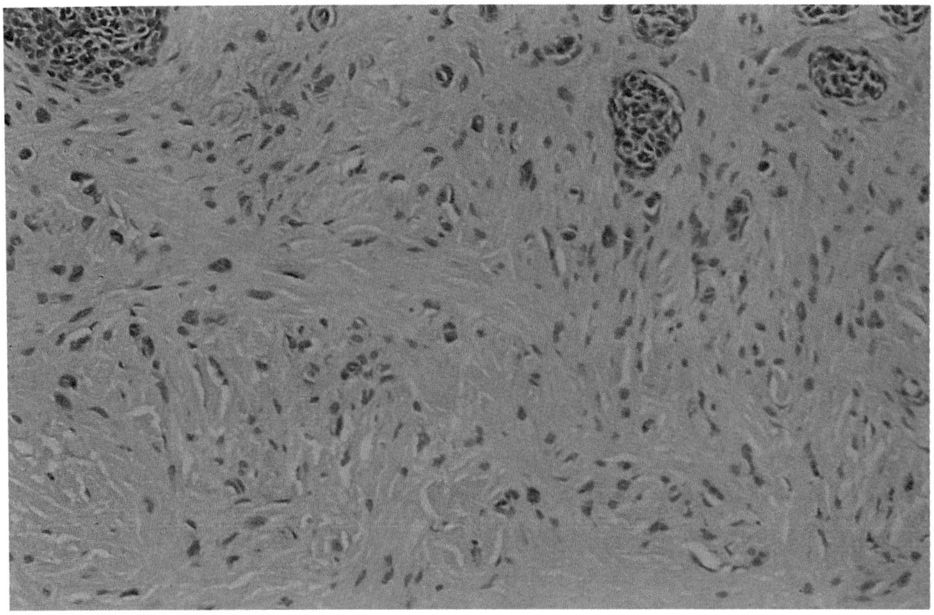

FIGURE 4-10
Desmoplasia (sclerosis) in dermal nevus (H&E, × 200).

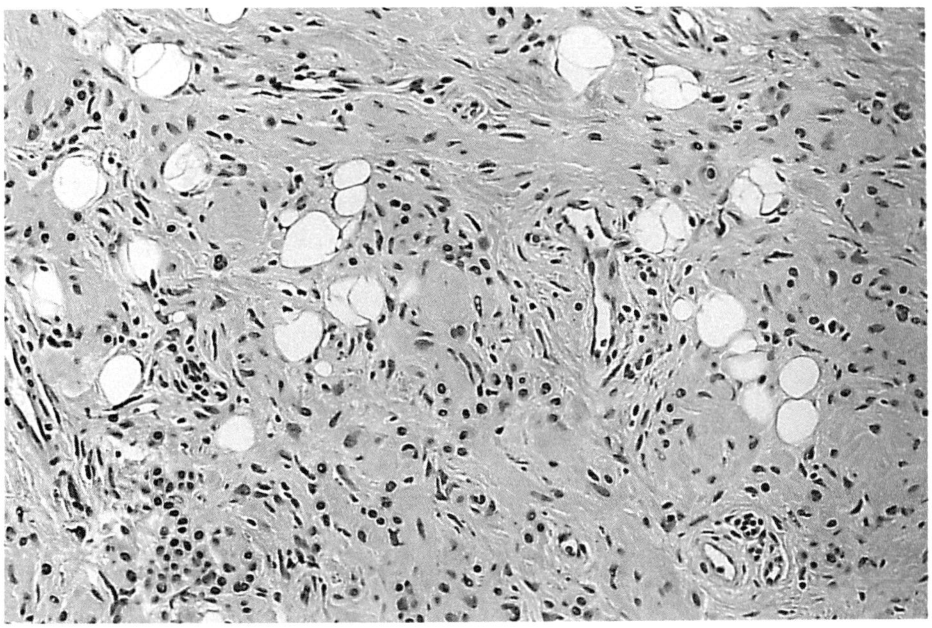

FIGURE 4-11
Lipomatous alteration in dermal nevus (H&E, × 200).

TABLE 4-6
Uncommon Findings in or Presentations of Melanocytic Nevi

Agminated (speckled) lentiginosis or melanocytic nevi[97]	Circumscribed grouping of hyperpigmented macules and/or papules equivalent tonevus spilus but with absence of background macule; hyperpigmented foci are lentigines, junctional or compound nevi.
Amyloid deposition[98]	Degenerative nevus cells.
Angiomatous, pseudovascular pattern[99,100]	Nevus cell pattern resembles vascular or lymphatic spaces, possibly secondary to tissue shrinkage, processing (see Fig. 4-12).
Cockarde (Cockade) nevus[101–104]	Peripheral pigmented halo (junctional nevus usually) with intervening nonpigmented annulus about central nevus (junctional or compound nevus).
Keratinous cyst rupture, folliculitis, abscess formation[105–108]	Enlargement, change in color, suggesting melanoma.
Meyerson's nevus[109–111]	Subacute eczematous epidermal changes associated with nevus, often forming eczematous halo.
Nevus (osteonevus) of Nanta[112,113]	Bone formation in nevus (metaplastic ossification).
Perinevoid alopecia[114]	Hair loss associated with scalp nevi; inflammatory reaction resembling halo nevus but associated with hair follicles.
Psammoma bodies[115]	Probably associated with degenerative nevus cells.

nevi and uncommonly may result in confluent pools of the basophilic material.

Neurotization (Peripheral Nerve Sheath Differentiation)
Neurotization refers to the histologic pattern of neural differentiation or prominence of type C cells in the dermal component of a nevus[5–7,14,18,19,35] (see Fig. 4-9C). The constituent cells are usually spindle shaped and may form neuroidal structures resembling Wagner-Meissner corpuscles[5,6,18,19,35] (see Fig. 4-9D). Both schwannian and perineurial differentiation may be observed. The cells are usually separated by a delicate fibrous stroma that on occasion also may be slightly myxoid, as in a neurofibroma.[18] Other uncommon histologic changes observed in melanocytic nevi are listed in Table 4-6.[66]

VARIANTS OF MELANOCYTIC NEVI

There are a number of distinctive variants of melanocytic nevi that merit specific discussion.

MELANOCYTIC NEVUS OF ACRAL SKIN

As previously discussed, nevi of acral skin frequently have junctional components in patients of all ages. Such nevi have always been of particular concern to both clinicians and pathologists. However, the same guidelines as for other melanocytic lesions should be applied to acral nevi.

Clinical Features
Acral nevi are usually macular or only slightly elevated (Table 4-7). In general, they display uniform brown or dark brown color. Clinically, they are often indistinguishable from simple lentigines. The same clinical parameters as outlined in Table 4-5 apply to acral nevi.

Histopathology
Many of the same features as described for common acquired nevi of other sites (see Table 4-5) are also applicable for acral nevi. They are usually relatively small (<5 to 6 mm), well-circumscribed, and symmetrical compound nevi (see Table 4-7). On occasion, the junctional nests of

TABLE 4-7
Précis: Melanocytic Nevus of Acral Skin

Clinical features
- All ages
- Size 3 to 6 mm
- Macular or only slightly elevated
- Uniform brown or dark brown
- Symmetry
- Regular and well-defined borders

Histopathology
- Overall symmetry
- Well demarcated
- Often prominent but regular junctional nests, uniform size, shape, spacing
- Often lentiginous melanocytic proliferation but confined to rete ridges
- Pagetoid spread commonly present but orderly
- Usually no host response
- Often rounded papillary dermal nests of nevus cells

Differential diagnosis
- Dysplastic nevi
- Acral lentiginous melanoma

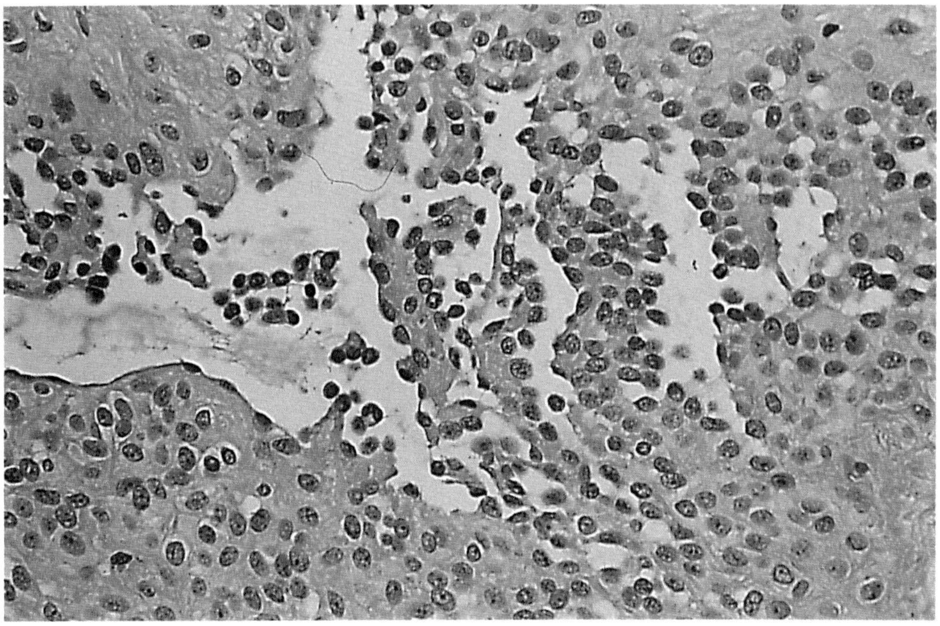

FIGURE 4-12
Pseudovascular pattern. Dermal nevus cells line clear spaces suggesting vascular lumina (H&E, × 400).

acral nevi are somewhat enlarged, but they usually have a fairly uniform round or oval shape and are similar in size and spacing (see Fig. 4-6). Lentiginous melanocytic proliferation and some degree of upward migration of melanocytes are features commonly observed in acral nevi (see Fig. 4-6). One should be cautious in overinterpreting the latter changes unless prominent architectural disorder and cytologic atypia are also present. The dermal component of acral nevi is often characterized by round nests of type A cells.

Differential Diagnosis

Acral nevi must be distinguished from atypical or dysplastic nevi and melanoma. Both atypical nevi and melanoma demonstrate progressively greater architectural and cytologic atypicality. In particular, an increased frequency of basilar melanocytes is an important feature of both atypical nevi and acral lentiginous melanoma. Irregular nesting patterns, discohesion of nests, prominent pagetoid spread, poor lateral demarcation, and mononuclear cell infiltrates are also features of atypical acral (dysplastic) nevi (see Chap. 9).

The atypical basilar melanocytes in acral nevi and melanoma often have enlarged, hyperchromatic nuclei with prominent pleomorphism. Such cells show a contiguous basilar disposition in acral lentiginous melanoma. The dendritic processes of such cells often extend throughout the epidermis and reach the granular layer.

ACQUIRED MELANOCYTIC NEVUS WITH SUPERFICIAL CONGENITAL PATTERN

As discussed above, some common acquired nevi have involvement of the superficial reticular dermis in a pattern historically ascribed to congenital nevi.[63] However, in most instances, a congenital onset is not verified, and the size of the nevus, usually less than 1 cm in diameter, argues against a congenital basis.

BALLOON CELL NEVUS

Balloon cell nevus is a rare variant of melanocytic nevus in which over half the nevus cell population is composed of balloon cells.[58–62] Nevi composed entirely of balloon cells are exceedingly rare.

Clinical Features

Balloon cell nevi do not appear to have any distinctive gross morphologic features, although one was reported to have a faint yellow halo surrounding an otherwise ordinary brown nevus[59] (Table 4-8). Most balloon cell nevi measure under 5 mm, and they are located most commonly in the head and neck area.[60] The majority of cases have been reported in persons less than 30 years of age; they affect men and women equally.[58,60]

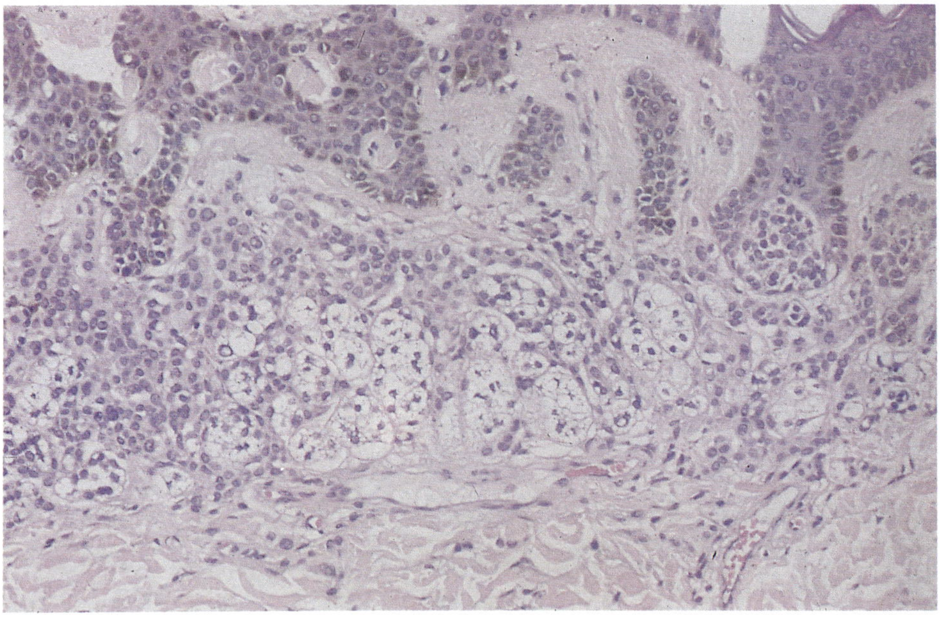

A

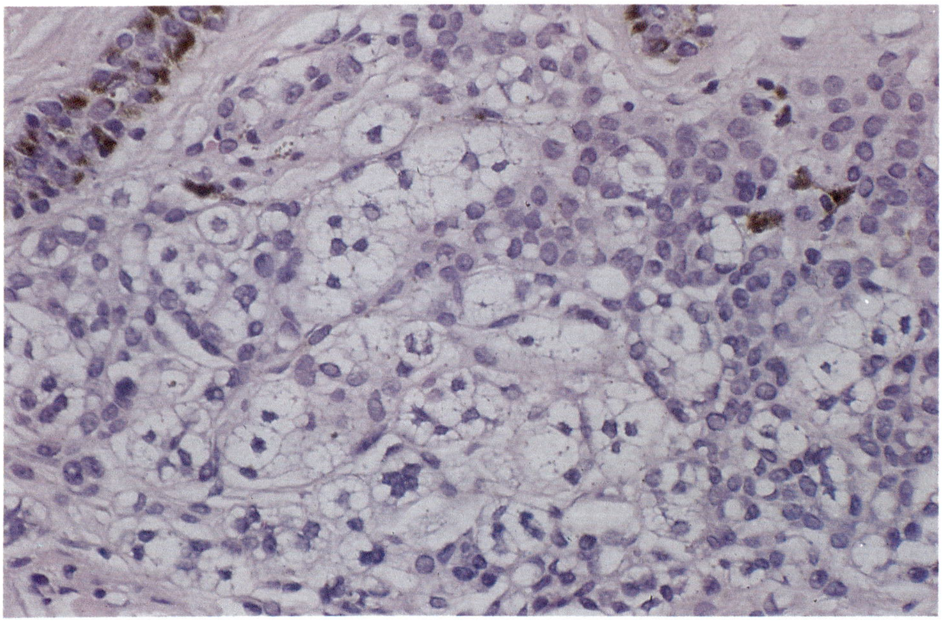

B

FIGURE 4-13

Balloon cell nevus. (A) Note enlarged vacuolated nevus cells in dermal component (H&E, × 200). (B) Balloon nevus cells contain a small, centrally placed nucleus surrounded by clear vacuolated space (H&E, × 400).

Histopathology

The balloon cell nevus contains balloon cells admixed with typical nevus cells, and cells transitional between ordinary nevus cells and balloon cells are noted[58–60] (Fig. 4-13A; see also Table 4-7). The balloon cells are enlarged with clear, foamy, or vacuolated cytoplasm[58] (see Fig. 4-13B). The cells contain relatively small, centrally located, round nuclei with uniform basophilic chromatin. Multinucleate balloon giant cells are commonly observed. Typically maturation is noted with increasing depth of the nevus.

Melanin may be present to varying extent and may be finely or coarsely granular or clumped.[60] Electron microscopy of balloon cells has demonstrated progressive

TABLE 4-8
Précis: Balloon Cell Nevus

Clinical features
- None distinctive
- Usually < 5 mm

Histopathology
- Balloon cells admixed with regular nevus cells
- More than half of nevus composed of balloon cells
- Balloon cells enlarged with clear, foamy, or vacuolated cytoplasm

Electron microscopy
- Enlargement and lysis of melanosomes

Differential diagnosis
- Balloon cell melanoma (see Chap. 10)
- Xanthoma
- Sebaceous neoplasms

vacuolization of melanocytes resulting from the enlargement and lysis of melanosomes.[61,62] The latter phenomenon is considered to be a degenerative process, but the pathogenesis for these changes has not been established.[61]

Differential Diagnosis

The primary entity to be distinguished from balloon cell nevus is balloon cell melanoma (BCM)[60] (see Chap. 10). As with balloon cell nevus, BCM may be composed of any proportion of balloon cells. In contrast to balloon cell nevus, BCM occurs in older patients and is histologically characterized by prominent cytologic atypia (i.e., the nuclei are larger, more pleomorphic, and contain less cytoplasm than balloon nevus cells) and mitotic activity. Other entities entering into the differential diagnosis include xanthomas, granular cell tumors, and sebaceous neoplasms.[58,60]

HALO NEVUS

Synonyms: leukoderma acquisitum centrifugum, Sutton's nevus, perinevoid vitiligo, perinevoid leukoderma

The halo nevus is defined clinically as a melanocytic nevus surrounded by a white (hypo- or depigmented) band or halo and histologically by a dense mononuclear cell infiltrate filling the papillary dermis.[67–70] The central nevus is almost always a common acquired nevus, but other nevi such as congenital nevi and blue nevi may develop halos.[67–71]

Halo nevi generally affect individuals under age 20, with a mean age of approximately 15 years.[69,70] In one series, the ages ranged from 3 to 42 years.[69] The overall incidence of halo nevi in individuals under age 20 is probably less than 1% percent.[72] There is no difference in incidence between males and females.[69] Approximately 20 percent of individuals with halo nevi have vitiligo, and halo nevi have an association with malignant melanoma and atypical (dysplastic) nevi.[73]

The natural history of halo nevi has not been well documented. However, in general, the onset of a ring of depigmentation is thought to occur over a period of weeks to months.[68–70] The central nevus may persist or, more likely, undergoes involution over a matter of months to years.

Etiology

The development of a halo of depigmentation is thought to result from either (1) an immune response against antigenically altered nevus cells associated with tumor progression (dysplasia)[20,74,75] or (2) cell-mediated and/or humoral (antibody-mediated) reaction against nonspecifically altered nevomelanocytes and possible cross-reactivity with nevomelanocytes at a distant site or sites.[76] The first hypothesis holds that all halo nevi are atypical and thus the immunologic response is one associated with tumorigenesis. The second notion holds that halo nevi are the result of host response directed against nonspecifically altered nevomelanocytes in response to physical, chemical, or other insult or perhaps from an autoimmune etiology, as in vitiligo.[76]

The basis for nevus cell destruction in halo nevi is poorly understood. Both humoral and cellular immunologic factors have been implicated.[73–75,77,78] Copeman and colleagues[74,75] were the first to show that individuals with regressing halo nevi have antibodies directed against the cytoplasm of melanoma cells. These antibodies also have been noted in patients with primary melanoma who have not developed metastases, but not in individuals with other types of conventional nevi. It also has been found that lymphocytes isolated from patients with halo nevi and from melanoma patients are cytotoxic to melanoma cells in culture.[78] It is not known whether the preceding observations are important in the pathogenesis of halo nevi or are merely epiphenomena.

As discussed below, the central nevus component in active halo nevi is usually associated with dense lymphocytic infiltrates, while the peripheral white halo has little or no such infiltrate.[69,70] The mechanisms responsible for the white halo are even less well understood than other aspects of the pathogenesis of halo nevi. Presumably, the destruction of melanocytes in this zone is secondary to the diffusion of a cytotoxic factor such as a cytokine.

Clinical Features

Halo nevi are characterized by a central melanocytic nevus component that may be relatively flat or raised and dark brown to pink in color[68–70] (see Table 4-9). The nevus

TABLE 4-9
Comparison of Halo Nevus and Malignant Melanoma

	Halo Nevus	*Malignant Melanoma*
Clinical features	Central nevus 3- to 6-mm in size	Usually > 6 mm
	Symmetry of central nevus and halo	Asymmetry
	Regular borders	Irregular borders
	Uniform color of central nevus—tan, brown, or pink, and halo—hypo- or depigmentation	Haphazard or irregular color
Histopathologic features	Symmetry	Asymmetry
	Usually well circumscribed	Poorly circumscribed
	Mononuclear cell infiltrate orderly with well-defined inferior margin	Often variation in pattern of infiltrate
	Maturation/differentiation of nevus elements	Usually no maturation
	Apoptosis of nevus cells common	Apoptosis may be observed
	Rete ridges maintained	Effaced rete ridges common
	Little or no cytologic atypia commonly	Prominent cytologic atypia
	Few mitoses in dermal component	Mitoses in dermal component frequent
	Atypical mitoses usually absent	Atypical mitoses may be observed

may exhibit surface scale or crusting. The central nevus is surrounded by a well- circumscribed annulus of hypo- or depigmented skin. In typical halo nevi, the central nevus commonly measures 3 to 6 mm in longest diameter, has regular and well-defined borders, and has homogeneous coloration. The white halo is usually symmetrical with a uniform width that may vary from a few millimeters up to several centimeters (uncommon).[68-70]

Halo nevi are most typically located on the upper back but may be found in any location.[68-70] Approximately 25 to 50 percent of affected individuals have two or more halo nevi. Rarely, large numbers of halo nevi occur, sometimes with rapid onset.[68-70]

After the development of a halo nevus, its subsequent course is variable. The central nevus may persist indefinitely or regress completely, with the area of hypo- or depigmentation persisting, often indefinitely.[68-70] The coloration of the central nevus may not change, or it may become irregular or pink or red. Probably over half of all halo nevi undergo complete regression.[68] The period of time associated with nevus regression varies from months to as long as several years.

Histopathology

The halo nevus may be junctional, compound, or dermal.[68-70] In the fully evolved stages, the central nevus is associated with a well-circumscribed, dense, almost bandlike infiltrate of mononuclear cells, almost exclusively lymphocytes and histiocytes, that occupies the papillary dermis and permeates nests of nevus cells (Fig. 4-14 and Table 4-9). The latter change is so prominent that nevus cells are difficult to distinguish from surrounding mononuclear cells. Degenerating nevus cells can sometimes be identified in this zone (Fig. 4-15A). Homogeneous eosinophilic (apoptotic) bodies, representing degenerated cells, are often observed near the dermoepidermal junction. Occasional nevus cells within the infiltrate show prominent eosinophilic cytoplasm and slightly enlarged nuclei. Although most halo nevi demonstrate no obviously atypical nevus cells, some display varying degrees of cytologic atypia.[20] The peripheral zones of the nevus, corresponding to the clinical halo, are characterized by diminished or absent basilar melanocytes and melanin in the basal layer.[70] The papillary dermis in this annulus also may demonstrate slight reparative alteration of the stroma, but usually no inflammatory cell infiltrates are found.[70]

With complete regression, all nevus cells are destroyed in halo nevi. At this stage, the central part of the nevus is typified by thickening of the papillary dermis, occasional delicate fibroplasia and frequent mucinous alteration, vascular ectasia, variable residual mononuclear cell infiltrates, and melanophages (see Fig. 4-15B). There may be complete depigmentation of the epidermis in this central zone, in addition to the peripheral annulus.

It should be noted that occasional nevi with typical hypopigmented halos present clinically do not exhibit cellular infiltrates histologically.[71,79] The absence of a mononuclear cell infiltrate might be related to the timing of biopsy in the natural history of a halo nevus (i.e., possibly after resolution of the infiltrate).

Characterization of the mononuclear cell infiltrates in halo nevi has shown that most of the cells are T lymphocytes and monocyte/macrophages[73] (see Table 4-9). There are approximately equal numbers of helper/

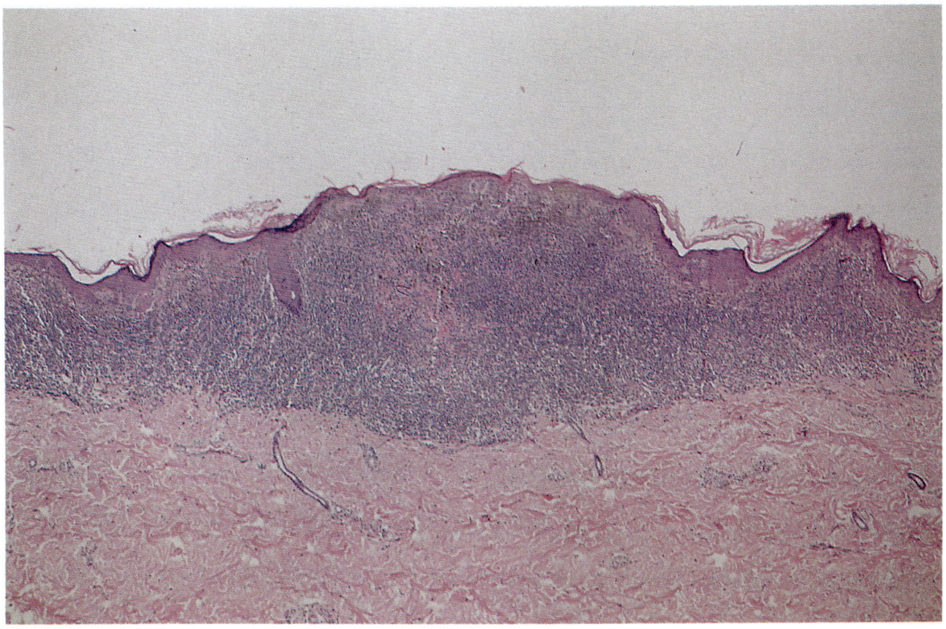

A

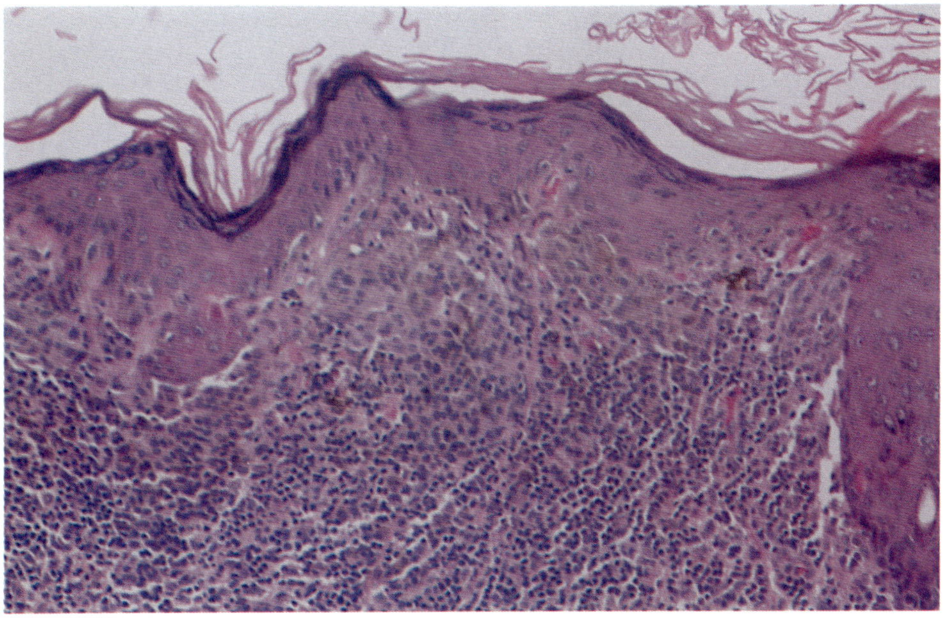

B

FIGURE 4-14

Halo nevus. (A) Scanning magnification shows symmetry and well-defined inferior margin of infiltrate. (B) Dense mononuclear cell infiltrate almost obscures junctional and papillary dermal nests of nevus cells (H&E, × 200).

inducer (CD4+) and cytotoxic/suppressor (CD8+) T cells. The nevus cells within dense mononuclear cells also express class I HLA antigens to a much greater extent than class II antigens (see Table 5-6). These findings are similar to the immunophenotype of dysplastic nevi and melanoma[73] and suggest a specific cell-mediated immune response in halo nevi.

Differential Diagnosis

The halo nevus must be distinguished primarily from malignant melanoma. This distinction is not a significant problem for halo nevi showing little or no cytologic atypia (see Table 4-8). Such halo nevi generally are characterized by a relatively small size (i.e., <5 to 6 mm), an overall symmetry, and an orderly appearance compared with

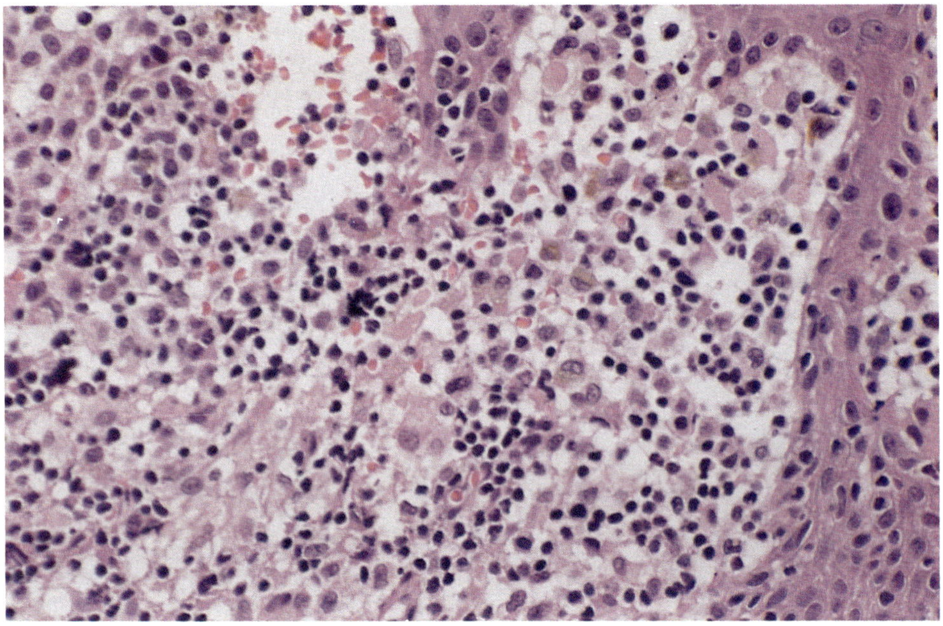

A

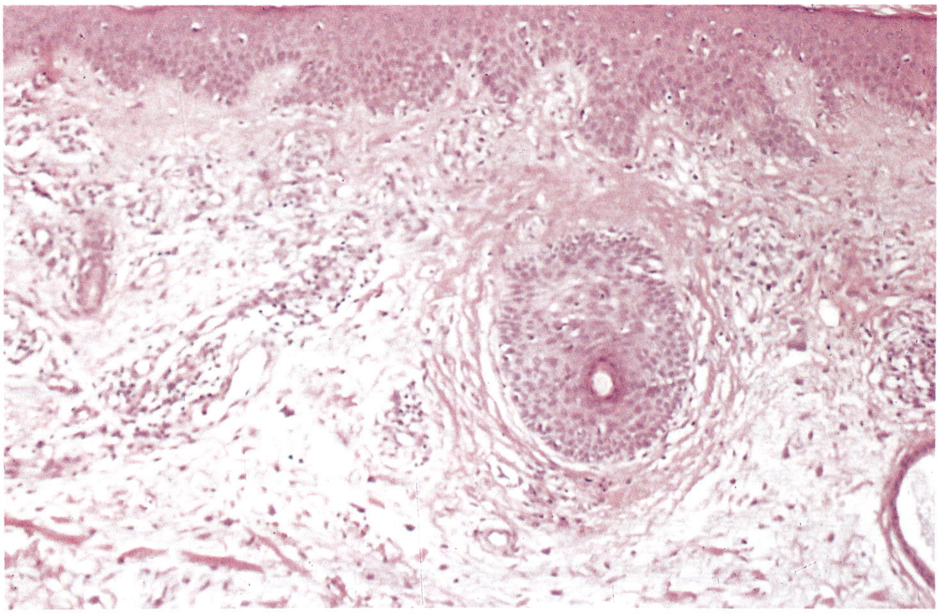

B

FIGURE 4-15

Halo nevus. (A) Lymphocytes form rosettes around nevus cells. Apoptotic and degenerative cells are present. These features are consistent with active regression (H&E, × 400). (B) Complete regression of halo nevus. There are no residual nevus cells (H&E, × 100).

TABLE 4-10
Immunophenotype of Halo Nevi

Nevus cell expression of HLA antigens
Class I (HLA-A,B,C) > > class II (HLA-DR)
Mononuclear cell infiltrate
T lymphocytes (~80%) > > B lymphocytes
T lymphocytes express HLA-DR
CD8+ = CD4+ T cells
Monocyte/macrophages present

melanoma. Halo nevi are notable for the symmetry and well-defined inferior margin of the mononuclear cell infiltrate contained in the papillary dermis. A feature important to look for is the maturation of nevus cells from the superficial elements to those more deeply situated. Although mitotic figures may be noted in the dermal component of any melanocytic lesion, more than a few mitoses, mitoses in the deepest dermal cells, and atypical mitoses are of particular concern.

LENTIGINOUS JUNCTIONAL NEVUS (NEVOID LENTIGO, "JENTIGO") AND LENTIGINOUS COMPOUND NEVUS

These nevi are characterized by a prominent lentiginous pattern of the epidermis, i.e., an elongated epidermal rete, lentiginous melanocytic hyperplasia, and basal layer hypermelanosis (Figs. 4-4 and 4-16). The degree of junctional nesting may vary from almost none (nevoid lentigo) to prominent nesting.

Differential Diagnosis

The importance of recognizing lentiginous nevi is their distinction from dysplastic nevi and lentigo maligna. As will be discussed later (see Chap. 9), lentiginous nevi lack the increased frequency of melanocytic proliferation and the cytologic atypia found in dysplastic nevi and lentigo maligna. In addition, lentigo maligna generally exhibits an effacement of the epidermal rete and pronounced involvement of adnexal structures in contrast to lentiginous nevi.

NEURAL NEVUS (NEUROTIZED NEVUS)

This term indicates complete or nearly complete neurotization (maturation to type C cells) of a dermal nevus[5,6,18,35] (see Fig. 4-9C). In some instances, it may not be possible to distinguish this lesion from a solitary cutaneous neurofibroma. However, the presence of nesting of cells suggests a nevus.

NEVUS SPILUS (SPECKLED LENTIGINOUS NEVUS)

The nevus spilus is a slightly hyperpigmented (tan) macular lesion that contains hyperpigmented foci or speckles that may be either flat or raised.[80-87] The nevus spilus may be present at birth but more often develops in childhood.[80] Approximately 2.3 percent of white adults have a nevus spilus according to one study.[86] Males and females are equally affected. These lesions most commonly affect the trunk and extremities.

In general, the nevus spilus persists indefinitely; however, increased degrees of speckling over time have been documented by serial photography,[87] and the specks become more prominent after solar exposure.[80] There are several reports of malignant melanoma arising in association with a nevus spilus.[88-90] In two instances, melanocytic dysplasia has been noted in the nevus spilus adjacent to the site of melanoma development.[88,90]

Clinical Features

The tan macular area commonly varies from under 1 to 10 or 20 cm in greatest diameter[80-87] (Table 4-11). This area is completely flat without any distortion of skin markings. The hyperpigmented speckles are approximately 1 to 6 mm in greatest diameter and may be macular or papular. Large varieties of nevus spilus may be unilateral, segmental, or zosteriform (speckled zosteriform lentiginous nevus) and involve a substantial portion of skin, e.g., an entire extremity or half the trunk.[83-85]

TABLE 4-11
Précis: Nevus Spilus

Clinical features
Tan café-au-lait macule, 1 to 20 cm or larger
Hyperpigmented speckles, macules, and papules present on tan macule
Speckles 1 to 6 mm in diameter
Uncommon segmental or zosteriform variants
Histopathology
Tan macule: lentiginous melanocytic proliferation (lentigo simplex)
Speckles:
Macule: lentiginous melanocytic proliferation or junctional nevus
Papule: junctional or compound nevus
Occasional features of Spitz nevus
Occasional atypical features in dysplastic variants
Occasional congenital features
Differential diagnosis
Large or congenital lentigo
Congenital nevus
Dysplastic nevus

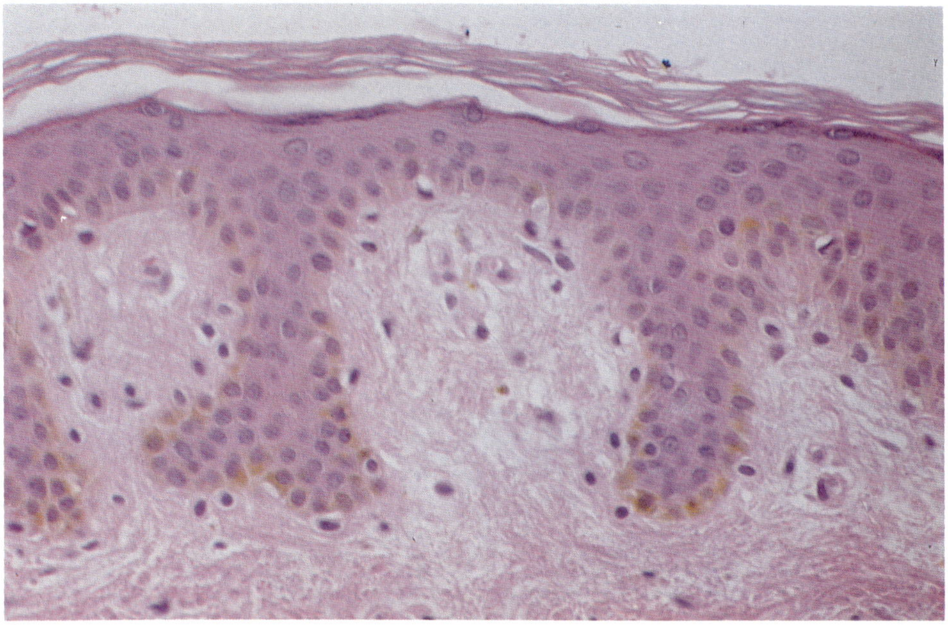

A

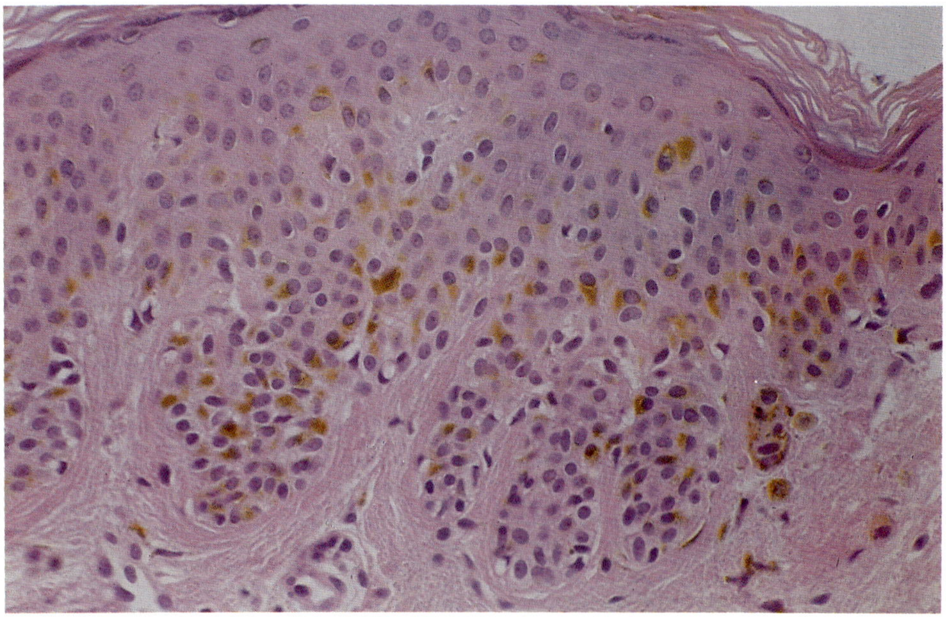

B

FIGURE 4-16

Nevus spilus. (A) Tan macule shows histologic features of lentigo simplex, i.e., elongated rete, basilar melanocytic hyperplasia, and increased melanin content of basilar epidermis (H&E, × 400). (B) Histologic examination of hyperpigmented papule demonstrates lentiginous junctional nevus (H&E, × 400).

Histopathology
The tan macule or patch of nevus spilus is characterized by lentiginous melanocytic hyperplasia associated with elongated epidermal rete ridges (see Fig. 4-16*A* and Table 4-11). The hyperpigmented macular foci are also characterized by lentiginous melanocytic hyperplasia or junctional nevus, whereas the papular foci contain junctional or compound nevus elements (see Fig. 4-16*B*). In rare instances, the histologic changes of spindle and epithelioid cell (Spitz) nevi have been noted in the raised speckled area. Varying degrees of architectural disorder and/or cytologic atypia may be observed in nevus spilus, comparable with that noted in dysplastic nevi (see Chap. 9).

Differential Diagnosis
The histologic differential diagnosis includes large or congenital lentigo, congenital nevus, and dysplastic nevus. In reality, the background macule of nevus spilus is a lentigo. Therefore, unless the dark speckles that usually show junctional or compound nevus are present in the biopsy, the histology of nevus spilus may be indistinguishable from lentigo. The clinical features should, however, enable one to discriminate nevus spilus from lentigo. A certain proportion of nevi spili are in fact congenital and thus simply a curious subtype of congenital nevus. As has been mentioned, uncommonly, some nevi spili exhibit architectural disorder and cytologic atypia (melanocytic dysplasia), as do all nevi. Such nevi have been designated *dysplastic nevus spilus*. The same guidelines for evaluating dysplastic nevi (see Chap. 9) should be applied to these atypical variants of nevus spilus.

RECURRENT MELANOCYTIC NEVUS

Synonyms: pseudomelanoma, recurrent/persistent melanocytic nevus

Recurrent melanocytic nevus is defined as the recurrence of a nevus at the site of previous nevus removal.[91-94] The primary concern with this phenomenon is the possibility of recurrent melanoma. The prevalence of recurrent melanocytic nevi has not been clearly established. The phenomenon appears to be relatively common among individuals with incompletely removed nevi. Most recurrent nevi have been reported in relatively young females,[91-94] resulting from the fact that greater numbers of nevi are generally removed from women. The trunk is the most common site for recurrent nevi, followed by the head and neck area.[94] Most of the recurrences have followed a shave excision. Approximately half the cases recur within 6 months.[91,94] As might be expected, dysplastic nevi also recur and generally do so within a 6-month interval. However, on occasion, this interval to recurrence may be as long as 1 to 2 years for dysplastic nevi (R. L. Barnhill, personal observations, 1994).

TABLE 4-12
Précis: Recurrent Melanocytic Nevus

Clinical features
Onset about 6 weeks to 6 months after previous surgery
Macular pigmentation
Limited to scar
4 to 6 mm (usually < 1.5 cm)
Some irregularity of borders often
Histopathology
Effacement of epidermis
Dermal scar
Intraepidermal melanocytic proliferation limited to area above scar
Lentiginous or nested pattern of intraepidermal melanocytes
Variable cytologic atypia, usually low grade
Differential diagnosis
Dysplastic nevus
Melanoma

The recurrence of melanocytic nevi is thought to result from an intraepidermal proliferation of residual melanocytes, possibly from nearby sweat ducts, hair follicles, or intraepidermal melanocytes.[94] Trophic factors stimulating either melanocyte migration, proliferation, or both may be related to mechanisms of wound healing or scar formation. Most recurrent nevi are stable after development and persist indefinitely. No increased melanoma risk has been associated with recurrent nevi.

Clinical Features
These lesions are characterized by circumscribed hyperpigmentation within a scar from the previous surgical procedure for nevus removal[91-94] (Table 4-12). The lesion is usually macular and exhibits variable irregularity of borders and pigment pattern.[91-94] Stippling, mottling, and loss of pigment may be observed.[93,94] Most recurrent nevi measure 4 to 6 mm in diameter and almost all are less than 1.5 cm.

Histopathology
Histologic examination usually reveals intraepidermal melanocytic proliferation confined to the area above a dermal scar[91-94] (Fig. 4-17*A* and Table 4-12). There is effacement of the epidermal rete ridge pattern and variable lentiginous or nested intraepidermal proliferation of melanocytes (see Fig. 4-17*B*). The melanocytes often contain abundant melanin and relatively uniform nuclei. Occasionally, low-grade cytologic atypia is noted. Dysplastic nevi tend to recur with fairly similar grades of cytologic

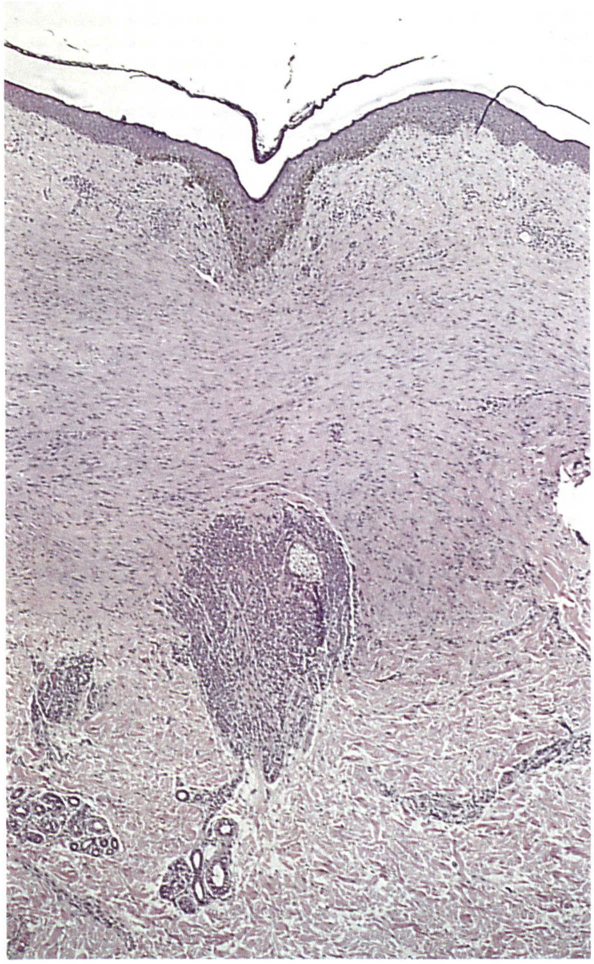

A

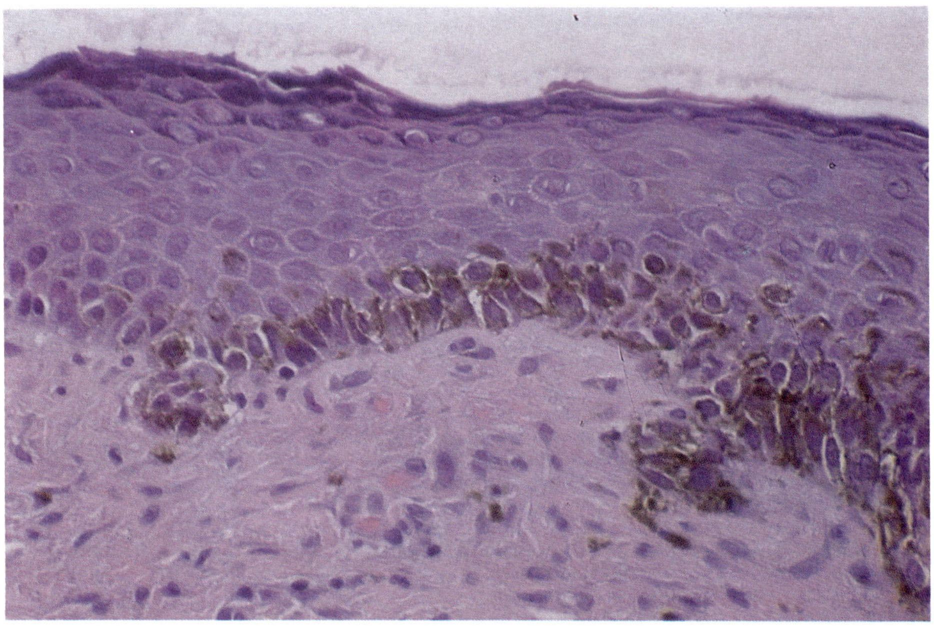

B

FIGURE 4-17

Recurrent melanocytic nevus. (A) Dermal scar between epidermis and aggregate of residual dermal nevus cells (lower center of field) (H&E, × 40). (B) The epidermis shows two small nests of melanocytes along dermoepidermal junction, as well as basilar melanocytic hyperplasia and prominent basilar hyperpigmentation (H&E, × 400). (C) Recurrent dysplastic nevus with irregular junctional and dermal nests and cytologic atypia suggesting melanoma. However, the latter changes were limited to the scar and the lesion was benign (H&E, × 200).

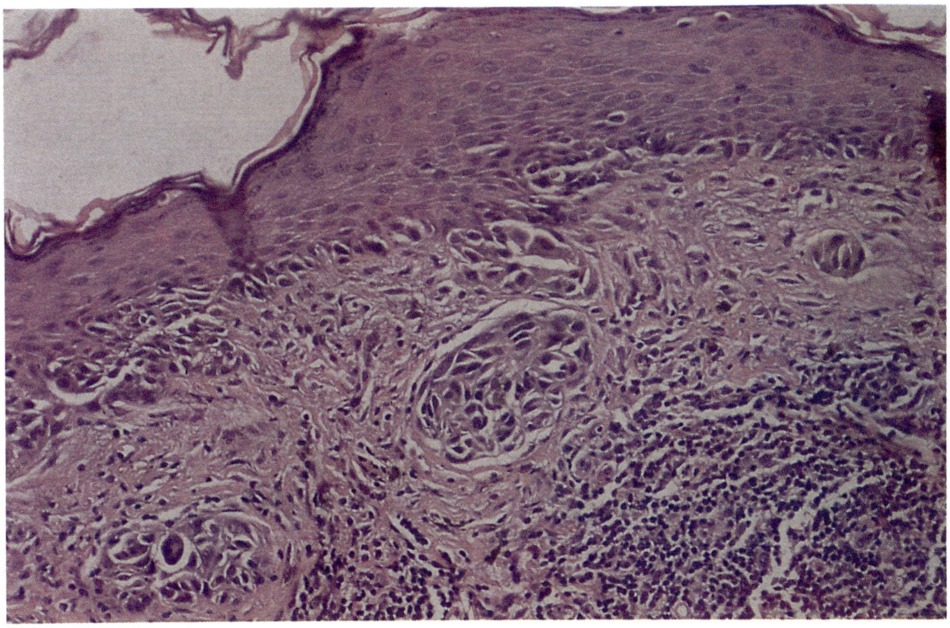

C

FIGURE 4-17 *(Continued)*

atypia compared with the original lesion removed (see Fig. 4-17C). However, it is important that the recurrent and original lesions be examined carefully to rule out progression to melanoma and also to avoid overdiagnosis of melanoma. Frequently, there are residual dermal nevus cells beneath the superficial dermal scar.

Differential Diagnosis

The differential diagnosis of recurrent nevus includes recurrent atypical (dysplastic) nevus, lentiginous melanocytic proliferations developing in melanoma scars, and recurrent melanoma. In general, recurrent melanocytic nevus is confined to the area of the surgical scar, appears within 6 months after surgery, and exhibits well-defined margins and a banal histologic picture. Recurrent dysplastic nevi may have greater cytologic atypia than conventional recurrent nevi. Clinical features suggesting melanoma include irregular pigmentation, recurrence beyond the confines of the surgical scar, and a longer interval until recurrence (> 6 months).

Establishing that a previous surgical procedure has occurred is integral to the diagnosis. Review of the previous biopsy is mandatory in order to establish a diagnosis for the original lesion and to rule out an atypical proliferation, particularly melanoma. Reexcision of a recurrent nevus is not necessary unless abnormal features are present, such as extension of the lesion beyond the surgical scar or substantial cytologic atypia.

UNUSUAL (OR ATYPICAL) MELANOCYTIC NEVI OF GENITAL (VULVAR) SKIN

Particular melanocytic nevi occurring on the vulva are thought to have distinctive histopathologic features compared with most nevi from this site and those from nongenital sites.[95,96] However, similar nevi may occur in other locations, such as the scrotum or umbilicus (R. L. Barnhill, personal observations, 1994). As with all melanocytic lesions, how such nevi are selected for removal may influence these observations. The significance of the histologic features of such nevi in terms of melanoma risk and association with an atypical nevus phenotype has not been elucidated and requires further study. As reviewed below, it is apparent that some of the unusual vulvar nevi previously reported exhibit features intermediate between ordinary nevi and melanoma and thus share features with dysplastic nevi.

Clinical Features

The small number of cases thus far reported have occurred in premenopausal women (ages 14 to 40)[95,96] (see Table 4-13). These unusual nevi appear to be uncommon among all vulvar nevi, perhaps accounting for less than 10 percent of nevi removed, but these data could be biased by selectional factors.[96]

Careful documentation of clinical features of such nevi has not been reported. However, it is the impression of this author from personal examination of such nevi and

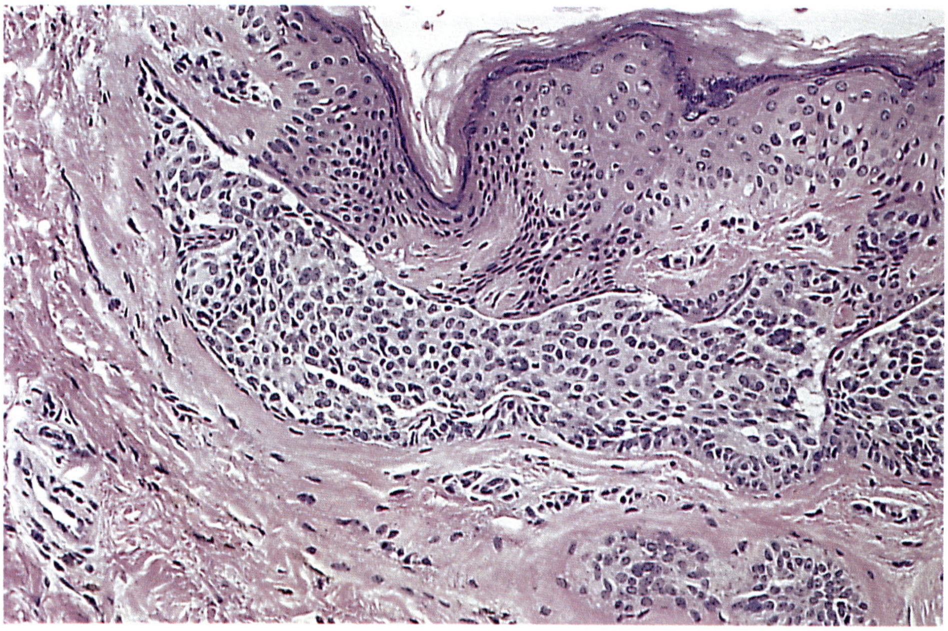

FIGURE 4-18

Vulvar nevus. Note large confluent nests of nevus cells along dermoepidermal junction (H&E, × 200).

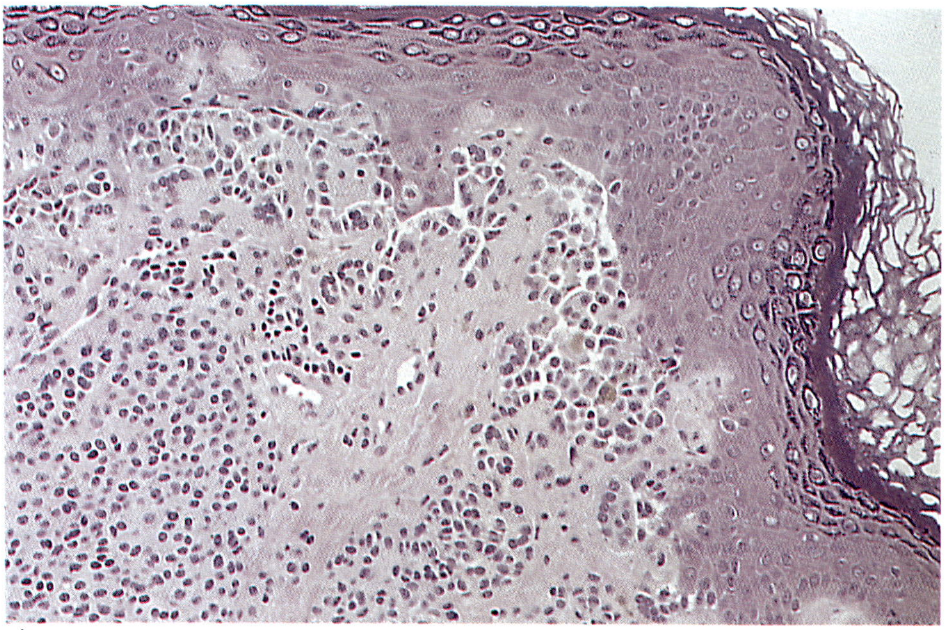

A

FIGURE 4-19

Scrotal nevus. (A) Irregular, confluent, and bridging nests along dermoepidermal junction. (B) The individual nevus cells tend to have abundant cytoplasm. Multinucleate nevus giant cells are also evident (H&E, × 400).

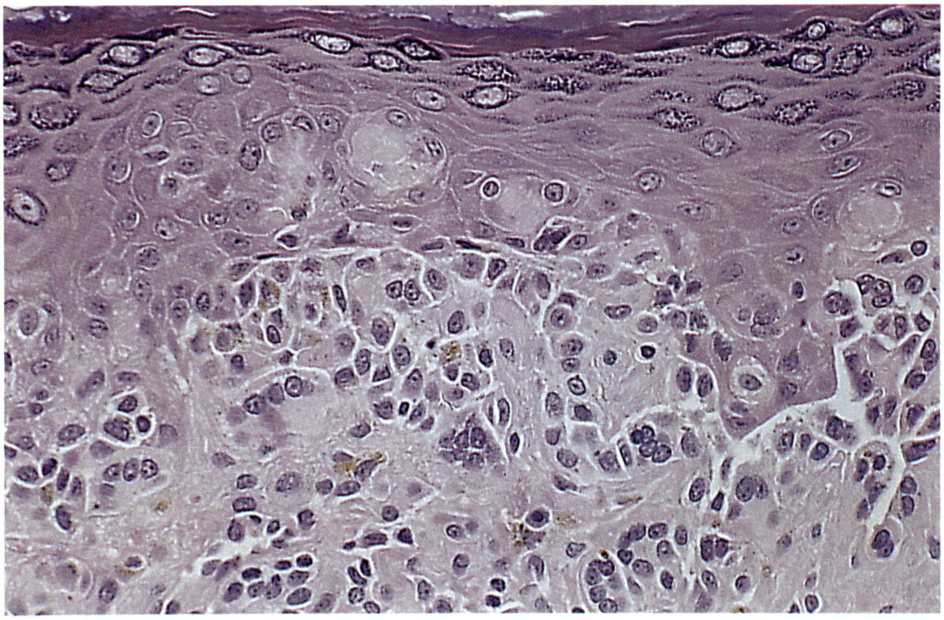

B

FIGURE 4-19 *(Continued)*

previous accounts[95,96] that such nevi are often larger in size (up to 10 to 12 mm) than nongenital ordinary nevi, are often relatively flat but not necessarily so, generally have fairly regular borders, and often present with a complex mahogany color (i.e., an admixture of tan, brown, and red).

Histopathology

The histologic features of these nevi are listed in Table 4-13. In general, these nevi are characterized by an overall symmetry, frequent absence of lateral extension of intraepidermal melanocytic components beyond the dermal nevus elements (if present), and well-circumscribed borders.[95,96] The most notable features are those shared with dysplastic nevi, namely, prominent lentiginous melanocytic proliferation, enlarged junctional nests, variation in the size, shape, position, and cohesion of junctional nests, confluence and bridging of nests, and often cytologic atypia of melanocytes (generally low grade).[95,96] The horizontal confluence and discohesion of junctional nests may be pronounced in these nevi (Fig. 4-18). The basilar proliferation or confluence of nests also frequently extends along the dermoepithelial junction of adnexal structures (Fig. 4-19A). In general, pagetoid spread is not observed. The confluent intraepidermal melanocytes are often slightly enlarged with abundant cytoplasm, to some extent resembling the epithelioid cells in Spitz ne-

TABLE 4-13
Précis: Unusual Genital (Vulvar) Melanocytic Nevus

Clinical features
Occurrence in premenopausal women (range 14 to 40 years of age)
Often enlarged, up to 10 mm in diameter
Other features not well studied

Histopathology
- Symmetrical
- Well circumscribed usually
- Enlarged junctional nests with diminished cohesion
- Lentiginous melanocytic proliferation
- Confluence of cells, nests along dermoepidermal junction
- Variation in size, shape, position of junctional nests
- Extension of intraepidermal component along adnexal epithelium
- Generally no pagetoid spread
- Generally no lateral extension (variable)
- Fibroplasia common, often lamellar
- Lymphocytic infiltrates
- Cytologic atypia, often slight to moderate
- Somewhat enlarged intraepidermal melanocytes, often with abundant cytoplasm
- Multinucleate nevus giant cells
- Maturation of nevus cells common

Differential diagnosis
- Vulvar melanoma
- Spindle and epithelioid cell (Spitz) nevus
- Dysplastic nevus

vus (see Fig. 4-19B). The cells may contain dusty-appearing cytoplasm.

The papillary dermis may show striking lamellar fibroplasia with entrapment of nests of nevus cells therein.[95,96] The latter feature may suggest invasion by melanoma, but careful study will disclose maturation of nevus cells. Perivascular lymphocytic infiltrates are also present in most of these nevi.

Differential Diagnosis

The differential diagnosis of these unusual vulvar and related nevi is primarily that of melanoma, spindle and epithelioid cell (Spitz) nevus, and dysplastic nevus. Although abnormal architecture and cytologic atypia may be present in these peculiar nevi, these features are not as developed as in melanoma. Melanoma usually demonstrates asymmetry, contiguous proliferation of basilar intraepidermal melanocytes, prominent pagetoid spread, poorly defined margins, greater cytologic atypia, and more developed host response. It is all-important to point out that vulvar melanoma tends to occur in older women (average age approximately 65 years) compared with these unusual genital nevi (see Table 4-13). Spindle and epithelioid cell (Spitz) nevi are recognized by the presence of typical enlarged monomorphous epithelioid/fusiform cells. Although these unusual nevi are not considered dysplastic by many, this issue is debatable. In a general sense, they may qualify as nevi exhibiting architectural disorder and cytologic atypia (see Table 4-12). It seems reasonable to conclude that the biologic significance of these nevi has not been fully delineated and requires further study.

REFERENCES

1. Weston JA: The migration and differentiation of neural crest cells. *Adv Morphol.* 8:41–114, 1971.
2. LeDouarin N: Migration and differentiation of neural crest cells. *Curr Top Dev Biol* 16:31–85, 1980.
3. Quevedo WC, Fleischman RD: Developmental biology of mammalian melanocytes. *J Invest Dermatol* 75:116–120, 1980.
4. Unna PG: Naevi and naevo-carcinoma. *Berl Klin Wochenschr* 30:14, 1893.
5. Lund HZ, Stobbe GD: The natural history of the pigmented nevus: Factors of age and anatomic location. *Am J Pathol* 25:1117–1155, 1949.
6. Maize JC, Foster G: Age-related changes in melanocytic naevi. *Clin Exp Dermatol* 4:49–58, 1979.
7. Clark WH Jr, Elder DE, Guerry D IV, et al: A study of tumor progression: The precursor lesions of superficial spreading and nodular melanoma. *Hum Pathol* 15:1147–1165, 1984.
8. Hu F. Melanocyte cytology in normal skin, melanocytic nevi, and malignant melanomas, in Ackerman AB (ed): *Pathology of Malignant Melanoma.* New York, Masson, 1981, pp 1–21.
9. Pack GT, Lenson N, Gerber DM: Regional distribution of moles and melanomas. *AMA Arch Surg* 65:862–870, 1952.
10. Stegmaier OC, Montgomery H: Histopathologic studies of pigmented nevi in children. *J Invest Dermatol* 20:51–62, 1953.
11. Stegmaier OC: Natural regression of the melanocytic nevus. *J Invest Dermatol* 32:413–419, 1959.
12. Kopf AW, Andrade R: A histologic study of the dermoepidermal junction in clinically "intraepidermal" nevi, employing serial sections: I junctional theques. *Ann NY Acad Sci* 100:200–222, 1960.
13. Stegmaier OC, Becker SW Jr: Incidence of melanocytic nevi in young adults. *J Invest Dermatol* 34:125–129, 1960.
14. Winkelmann RK, Rocha G: The dermal nevus and statistics: An evaluation of 1200 pigmented lesions. *Arch Dermatol* 86:310–315, 1962.
15. Nicholls EM: Development and elimination of pigmented moles and the anatomical distribution of primary malignant melanoma. *Cancer* 32:192–195, 1973.
16. MacKie RM, English J, Aitchison TC, et al: The number and distribution of benign pigmented moles (melanocytic naevi) in a healthy British population. *Br J Dermatol* 113:167–174, 1985.
17. Cramer SF: The histogenesis of acquired melanocytic nevi: Based on a new concept of melanocytic differentiation. *Am J Dermatopathol* 6(Suppl 1):289–298, 1984.
18. Masson P: My conception of cellular nevi. *Cancer* 4:9–38, 1951.
19. Masson P: Melanogenic system: Nevi and melanomas. *Pathol Annu* 2:351–397, 1967.
20. Reed RJ, Ichinose H, Clark WH Jr, Mihm MC Jr: Common and uncommon melanocytic nevi and borderline melanomas. *Semin Oncol* 2:119–147, 1975.
21. Aso M, Hashimoto K, Eto H, et al: Expression of Schwann cell characteristics in pigmented nevus. *Cancer* 62:938–943, 1988.
22. Whimster IW: What are moles? *Am J Dermatopathol* 7 (Suppl):A8–A15, 1985.
23. Herlyn M, Herlyn D, Elder DE, et al: Phenotypic characteristics of cells derived from precursors of human melanoma. *Cancer Res* 43:5502–5508, 1985.
24. Balaban G, Herlyn M, Elder DE, et al: Cytogenetics of human malignant melanoma and premalignant lesions. *Cancer Genet Cytogenet* 11:429–439, 1984.
25. Herlyn M, Thurin J, Balaban G, et al: Characteristics of cultured human melanocytes isolated from different stages of tumor progression. *Cancer Res* 45:5670–5676, 1985.
26. Herlyn M, Clark WH, Rodeck U, et al: Biology of tumor progression in human melanocytes. *Lab Invest* 56:461–474, 1987.
27. Mancianti ML, Herlyn M, Weil D, et al: Growth and phenotypic characteristics of human nevus cells in culture. *J Invest Dermatol* 90:134–141, 1988.
28. Easton DF, Cox GM, MacDonald AM, Ponder BA: Genetic susceptibility to naevi–A twin study. *Br J Cancer* 64:1164–1167, 1996.
29. Goldgar DE, Cannon-Albright LA, Meyer LJ, et al: Inheritance of nevus number and size in melanoma and dysplastic

nevus syndrome kindreds. *J Natl Cancer Inst* 83:1726–1733, 1991.

30. Armstrong BK, de Klerk NH, Holman CDJ: The etiology of common acquired melanocytic moles: Constitutional variables, sun exposure, and diet. *J Natl Cancer Inst* 77:329–335, 1986.
31. Green A, Bain C, MacLennan R, et al: Risk factors for cutaneous melanoma in Queensland, in Gallagher RP (ed): *Recent Results in Cancer Research: Epidemiology of Malignant Melanoma,* vol 102. Berlin, Springer-Verlag, 1986, pp 76–97.
32. Armstrong BK, English DR: The epidemiology of acquired melanocytic naevi and their relationship to malignant melanoma, in Elwood JM (ed): *Melanoma and Naevi.* Basel, Karger, 1988, pp 27–47.
33. Hughes BR, Cunliffe WJ, Bailey CC: Excess benign melanocytic naevi after chemotherapy for malignancy in childhood. *Br Med J* 299:88–91, 1989.
34. de Wit PEJ, de Vaan GAM, de Boo ThM, et al: Prevalence of nevocytic nevi after chemotherapy for childhood cancer. *Med Pediatr Oncol* 18:336–338, 1990.
35. Mishima Y: Macromolecular changes in pigmentary disorders. *Arch Dermatol* 91:519–557, 1965.
36. Lucky PA, Nordlund JA: The biology of the pigmentary system and its disorders. *Dermatol Clin* 3:197–224, 1985.
37. Alper J, Holmes LB: The incidence and significance of birthmarks in a cohort of 4641 newborns. *Pediatr Dermatol* 1:58–64, 1983.
38. Coleman WP III, Gately LE III, Krementz AB, et al: Nevi, lentigines, and melanomas in blacks. *Arch Dermatol* 116:548–551, 1980.
39. Coskey RJ. Eruptive nevi (letter). *Arch Dermatol* 111:1658, 1975.
40. Eady RAJ, Gilkes JJH, Wilson Jones E: Eruptive nevi: Report of two cases, with enzyme histochemical, light and electron microscopic findings. *Br J Dermatol* 97:267–278, 1977.
41. Leyden JJ, Spott DA, Goldschmidt H: Diffuse and banded melanin pigmentation in nails. *Arch Dermatol* 105:548–551, 1972.
42. Kawamura T, Nishihara K, Kawasakiya S, et al: Pigmentatio longitudinalis striata unguium and the pigmentation of nail plate in Addison's disease (abstract). *Jpn J Dermatol* 68:10, 1958.
43. Kopf AW, Waldo E: Melanonychia striata. *Australas J Dermatol* 21:59–70, 1980.
44. Voron DA, Hatfield HH, Kalkhoff RK: Multiple lentigines syndrome: Case report and review of the literature. *Am J Med* 60:447–456, 1976.
45. Rhodes AR, Silverman RA, Harrist TJ, Perez-Atayde AR: Mucocutaneous lentigines, cardiomucocutaneous myxomas, and multiple blue nevi: The "LAMB" syndrome. *J Am Acad Dermatol* 10:72–82, 1984.
46. Carney JA, Gordon H, Carpenter PC, et al: The complex of myxomas, spotty pigmentation, and endocrine overactivity. *Medicine* 64:270–283, 1985.
47. Jeghers H, McKusick VA, Katz KH: Generalized intestinal polyposis and melanin spots of the oral mucosa, lips, and digits: A syndrome of diagnostic significance. *N Engl J Med* 241:993–1005, 1949.
48. Utsunomiya J, Gocho H, Miyanaga T, et al: Peutz-Jeghers syndrome: Its natural course and management. *Johns Hopkins Med J* 136:71–82, 1975.
49. Rampen FHJ, de Wit PEJ: Racial differences in mole proneness. *Acta Derm Venereol (Stockh)* 69:234–236, 1989.
50. Sigg C, Pelloni F: Frequency of acquired melanocytic nevi and their relationship to skin complexion in 939 schoolchildren. *Dermatologica* 179:123–128, 1989.
51. Lewis MG, Johnson K: The incidence and distribution of pigmented naevi in Ugandan Agricans. *Br J Dermatol* 80: 362–366, 1968.
52. Pack GT, Davis J: The relation of race and complexion to the incidence of moles and melanomas. *Ann NY Acad Sci* 100:719–742, 1963.
53. Greene MH, Goldin LR, Clark WH Jr, et al: Familial cutaneous malignant melanoma: Autosomal dominant trait possibly linked to the Rh locus. *Proc Natl Acad Sci USA* 80:6071–6075, 1983.
54. Shaffer B: Pigmented nevi: A clinical appraisal in the light of present-day histopathologic concepts. *Arch Dermatol* 72: 120–132, 1955.
55. Pack GT, Davis J: The pigmented mole. *Postgrad Med* 27:370–382, 1960.
56. Barr RJ, King DF: The significance of pseudoinclusions within the nuclei of melanocytes of certain neoplasms, in Ackerman AB (ed): *Pathology of Malignant Melanoma.* New York, Masson, 1981, pp 269–272.
57. Bentley-Phillips CB, Marks R: The epidermal component of melanocytic naevi. *J Cutan Pathol* 3:190–194, 1976.
58. Schrader WA, Helwig EB: Balloon cell nevi. *Cancer* 20:1502–1514, 1967.
59. Lewis BL: Clinical appearance of a balloon cell nevus. *Arch Dermatol* 100:312–313, 1969.
60. Goette DK, Doty RD: Balloon cell nevus: Summary of the clinical and histologic characteristics. *Arch Dermatol* 114:109–111, 1978.
61. Hashimoto K, Bale GF: An electron microscopic study of balloon cell nevus. *Cancer* 30:530–540, 1972.
62. Okun MR, Donnellan B, Edelstein L: An ultrastructural study of balloon cell nevus: Relationship of mast cells to nevus cells. *Cancer* 34:615–625, 1974.
63. Rhodes AR, Silverman RA, Harrist TJ, Melski JW: A histological comparison of congenital and acquired nevomelanocytic nevi. *Arch Dermatol* 121:1266–1273, 1985.
64. McGibbon DH, Jones EW: Fibrous papule of the face (nose): Fibrosing nevocytic nevus. *Am J Dermatopathol* 1:345–348, 1979.
65. Lever WF, Schaumberg-Lever G: *Histopathology of the Skin,* ed 5. Philadelphia, Lippincott, 1975, p 650.
66. Weedon D: Unusual features of nevocellular nevi. *J Cutan Pathol* 9:284–292, 1982.
67. Sutton RL: An unusual variety of vitiligo (leucodermal acquisitum centrifugum). *J Cutan Dis* 34:797–800, 1916.
68. Frank SB, Cohen HJ: The halo nevus. *Arch Dermatol* 89:367–373, 1964.
69. Kopf AW, Morrill SD, Silberberg I: Broad spectrum of leukoderma acquisitum centrifugum. *Arch Dermatol* 92:14–35, 1965.

70. Wayte DM, Helwig EB: Halo nevi. *Cancer* 22:69–90, 1968.
71. Brownstein MH, Kazam BB, Hashimoto K: Halo congenital nevus. *Arch Dermatol* 113:1572–1575, 1977.
72. Larsson PA, Liden S: Prevalence of skin diseases among adolescents 12–16 years of age. *Acta Derm Venereol (Stockh)* 60:415–423, 1980.
73. Bergman W, Willemze R, de Graaff-Reitsma C, Ruiter DJ: Analysis of major histocompatibility antigens and the mononuclear cell infiltrate in halo nevi. *J Invest Dermatol* 85:25–29, 1985.
74. Copeman PWM, Lewis MG, Phillips TM, Elliott PG: Immunological associations of the halo naevus with cutaneous malignant melanoma. *Br J Dermatol* 88:127–137, 1973.
75. Bennett C, Copeman PWM: Melanocyte mutation in halo naevus and malignant melanoma? *Br J Dermatol* 100:423–426, 1979.
76. Whimster I: The halo naevus and cutaneous malignant melanoma. *Br J Dermatol* 90:111–113, 1974.
77. Roenigk HH, Deodhar SD, Krebs JA, Barna B: Microcytotoxicity and serum blocking factors in malignant melanoma and halo nevus. *Arch Dermatol* 111:720–725, 1975.
78. Mitchell MS, Nordlund JJ, Lerner AB: Comparison of cell-mediated immunity to melanoma cells in patients with vitiligo, halo nevi or melanoma. *J Invest Dermatol* 75:144–147, 1980.
79. Gauthier Y, Surlève J–E, Texier L: Halo nevi without dermal infiltrate (letter). *Arch Dermatol* 114:1718, 1978.
80. Cohen HJ, Minkin W, Frank SB: Nevus spilus. *Arch Dermatol* 102:433–437, 1970.
81. Matsudo H, Reed WB, Homme D, et al: Zosteriform lentiginous nevus. *Arch Dermatol* 107:902–905, 1973.
82. Stewart DM, Altman J, Mehregan AH: Speckled lentiginous nevus. *Arch Dermatol* 114:895–896, 1978.
83. Port M, Courniotes J, Podwal M: Zosteriform lentiginous naevus with ipsilateral rigid cavus foot. *Br J Dermatol* 98:693–698, 1978.
84. Pritchett RM, Pritchett PS: Zosteriform speckled lentiginous nevus with giant melanosomes. *Cutis* 30:329–334, 1982.
85. Nguyen KQ, Pierson DL, Rodman OG: Mosaic speckled lentiginous nevi. *Cutis* 30:65–68, 1982.
86. Kopf AW, Levine LJ, Rigel DS, et al: Prevalence of congenital-nevus-like nevi, nevi spilus, and café-au-lait spots. *Arch Dermatol* 121:766–769, 1985.
87. Falo LD Jr, Sober AJ, Barnhill RL: Evolution of nevus spilus. *Dermatology* (in press).
88. Rhodes AR, Mihm MC Jr: Origin of cutaneous melanoma in a congenital dysplastic nevus spilus. *Arch Dermatol* 126:500–505, 1990.
89. Stern JB, Haupt HM, Aaronson CM: Malignant melanoma in a speckled zosteriform lentiginous nevus. *Int J Dermatol* 29:583–584, 1990.
90. Kurban RS, Preffer FI, Sober AJ, et al: Occurrence of melanoma in "dysplastic" nevus spilus: Report of case and analysis by flow cytometry. *J Cutan Pathol* 19:423–428, 1992.
91. Schoenfeld RJ, Pinkus H: The recurrence of nevi after incomplete removal. *Arch Dermatol* 78:30–35, 1958.
92. Cox AJ, Walton RA: The induction of junctional changes in pigmented nevi. *Arch Pathol* 79:428–434, 1965.
93. Kornberg R, Ackerman AB: Pseudomelanoma. *Arch Dermatol* 111:1588–1590, 1975.
94. Park HK, Leonard DD, Arrington JH, Lund HZ: Recurrent melanocytic nevi: Clinical and histologic review of 175 cases. *J Am Acad Dermatol* 17:285–292, 1987.
95. Friedman RJ, Ackerman AB: Difficulties in the histologic diagnosis of melanocytic nevi on the vulvae of premenopausal women, in Ackerman AB (ed): *Pathology of Malignant Melanoma*. New York, Masson, 1981, pp 119–127.
96. Christensen WN, Friedman KJ, Woodruff JD, Hood AF: Histologic characteristics of vulvar nevocellular nevi. *J Cutan Pathol* 14:87–91, 1986.
97. Thompson GW, Diehl AK: Partial unilateral lentiginosis. *Arch Dermatol* 116:356, 1980.
98. MacDonald DM, Black MM: Secondary localized cutaneous amyloidosis in melanocytic naevi. *Br J Dermatol* 103:553–556, 1980.
99. Söderström K-O: Angiomatous type of intradermal nevi (letter). *Am J Dermatopathol* 9:549–551, 1987.
100. Collina G, Eusebi V: Naevocytic naevi with vascular-like spaces. *Br J Dermatol* 124:591–595, 1991.
101. Mehregan AH, King JR: Multiple target-like pigmented nevi. *Arch Dermatol* 105:129–130, 1972.
102. Happle R: Kokardennaevus. *Hautarzt* 25:594–596, 1974.
103. Warin AP: Cockarde naevus. *Clin Exp Dermatol* 1:221–224, 1976.
104. James MP, Wells RS: Cockade naevus: An unusual variant of the benign cellular naevus. *Acta Derm Venereol (Stockh)* 60:360–363, 1980.
105. Saunders TS: Abscess formation in pigmented nevi: Report of three cases. *Arch Dermatol* 76:189–192, 1957.
106. Freeman RG, Knox JM: Epidermal cysta associated with pigmented nevi. *Arch Dermatol* 85:590–594, 1962.
107. Haber H: Some observations on common moles. *Br J Dermatol* 74:224–228, 1962.
108. Canizares O: Subnevic folliculitis resembling melanoma. *Arch Dermatol* 97:363, 1968.
109. Meyerson LB: A peculiar papulosquamous eruption involving pigmented nevi. *Arch Dermatol* 103:510–512, 1971.
110. Krivanek JFC, Cains GD, Paver K: Halo eczema and junctional naevi: A case report. *Australas J Dermatol* 18:81–83, 1977.
111. Weedon D, Farnsworth J: Spongiotic changes in melanocytic nevi. *Am J Dermatopathol* 6(Suppl):257–259, 1984.
112. Burgdorf W, Nasemann T: Cutaneous osteomas: A clinical and histopathologic review. *Arch Dermatol Res* 260:121–135, 1977.
113. Delacrétaz J, Frenk E: Zur pathogenese des osteo-naevus nanta. *Hautarzt* 15:487–489, 1964.
114. Yesudian P, Thambiah AS: Perinevoid alopecia: An unusual variant of alopecia areata. *Arch Dermatol* 112:1432–1434, 1976.
115. Weitzner S: Intradermal nevus with psammoma body formation. *Arch Dermatol* 98:287–289, 1968.

5

Congenital Melanocytic Nevi and Associated Neoplasms, Congenital and Childhood Melanoma

By definition, the term *congenital nevus* denotes presence at birth[1,2] (Table 5-1). However, *congenital melanocytic nevi* (CMN) are also defined by striking differences from common acquired nevi. In general, these differences include (1) overall size, (2) depth of cutaneous involvement by nevus cells, (3) adnexal and vascular involvement, and (4) diversity of neurocristic differentiation.[3] Most melanocytic nevi greater than 1.5 cm in diameter are probably congenital,[1] if not acquired dysplastic nevi or melanoma. However, smaller CMN may be indistinguishable from acquired nevi.[2,4–6] Thus documentation at birth by reliable observers such as physicians or parents, photography, or medical records is necessary to confirm a congenital onset for such nevi less than 1.5 cm. The larger varieties of CMN are distinctive because of their size.[1,6–8] A small subset of nevi are remarkable for clinical and histologic features indistinguishable from typical CMN but are associated with onset several months to 2 years after birth. Such nevi have been termed *congenital nevi tardive*.[9]

A number of methods have been used to classify CMN according to size: surface area, the relationship to other anatomic structures such as the palm, longest diameter of the nevus, and difficulty of surgical removal.[9–16] All are arbitrary, and none are entirely satisfactory. Kopf et al.[15] have classified nevi less than 1.5 cm as small, nevi 1.5 to 19.9 cm as medium sized, and nevi greater than 20 cm as large or giant (Tables 5-2, 5-3, and 5-4). The terms *giant, gigantic, bathing trunk,* and *garment-type nevus* refer to CMN that occupy a major anatomic region or significant portion of the cutaneous surface.[7] Some authors have classified CMN based on their ease of surgical removal.[13] Small CMN are those which may be removed by simple surgical excision and primary closure. Intermediate- or medium-sized CMN often require a skin graft or flap. Giant CMN may prove difficult to remove altogether or require staged excision. It should be pointed out that CMN tend to enlarge proportionately with growth of the individual, and thus the category of CMN may change.[3,9]

INCIDENCE AND MELANOMA RISK

The significance of CMN, particularly the larger varieties, relates to their risk for progression to melanoma and cosmetic disfigurement.[7,12–21] There has been and continues to be considerable controversy surrounding the melanoma risk and management of CMN of all sizes, but especially relatively small CMN. Accurate estimates of melanoma risk associated with CMN are difficult to obtain. The prevalence of relatively small CMN is approximately 1 percent, and thus these nevi are fairly common.[2,22,23] However, one particular problem associated with estimating melanoma risk in these nevi is the lack of specificity of histologic features for CMN of this size.[5] At present, a general estimate of melanoma risk associated with small CMN is approximately 5 percent.[9] However, it should be emphasized that this may be an overestimate, and the melanoma risk may be lower and may more closely approximate that of common acquired nevi. Giant CMN are rare, with an incidence of approximately 1 in 20,000 births.[22] Very high estimates of melanoma risk associated with large/giant CMN are largely explained by referral bias. Perhaps the most accurate figures of melanoma risk have been associated with studies

TABLE 5-1
Summary of Congenital Melanocytic Nevi, Congenital and Childhood Melanoma

1. Prevalence
   a. All congenital nevi 1.1%
   b. Giant congenital nevi 0.005%
2. Classification
   a. Small < 1.5 cm
   b. Medium > 1.5 to 19.9 cm
   c. Large/giant ≥ 20 cm
   d. Congenital nevus "tardive"—onset between 1 month and 2 years of age
3. Familial aggregation
   a. Familial aggregation of small congenital nevi (prevalence rate 11 times the population-based prevalence)
   b. Familial aggregation of large and medium CMN
   c. Autosomal dominant inheritance with incomplete penetrance or polygenic inheritance possible
4. Association of large CMN of head and neck or posterior midline and underlying leptomeningeal melanocytosis of cranium, spine, or both
5. Lifetime melanoma risk
   a. Relatively small CMN—5% (estimate)
   b. Very large CMN—6.3%

   Congenital melanoma
   a. Incidence exceedingly rare
   b. Subtypes:
      (1) Transplacental spread of maternal metastatic melanoma
      (2) De novo primary melanoma
      (3) Primary melanoma arising in association with congenital melanocytic nevi
7. Childhood melanoma incidence:
   a. Prepubertal—0.4% (of total melanomas)
   b. Under age 20 years—2%

from the Danish Birth Registry.[11] A lifetime risk of approximately 6.3 percent has been estimated from the latter database.[11,18] It is possible that melanoma risk is directly related to size of the cellular population of the nevus and thus would be greatest for giant CMN and lowest for small CMN (again, perhaps comparable with common acquired nevi). It is obvious that frequency and size have a direct bearing on the management of CMN; small CMN are relatively common and fairly easy to remove, while large/giant CMN are rare and exceedingly difficult to excise.

TABLE 5-2
Précis: Small Congenital Nevus

Clinical features
- Symmetry
- < 1.5 cm
- Round, oval
- Tan, brown, dark brown
- Slightly raised, dome-shaped, papillomatous
- Pebbled surface topography common
- Coarse hairs often

Histopathology
- Lentiginous melanocytic proliferation common
- Junctional, compound, or dermal nevus
- Plaque of nevus cells in papillary dermis common
- Involvement of upper half of reticular dermis common
  - Interstitial pattern
  - Perivascular, periadnexal pattern

Differential diagnosis
- Common acquired nevus
- Dysplastic nevus

TABLE 5-3
Précis: Medium-Sized Congenital Nevus

Clinical features
- May occur anywhere, but head and neck common
- Symmetry
- 1.5 to 19.9 cm
- Round, oval, elongate
- Tan, brown, dark brown, often mahogany; or black
- Slightly raised plaque
- Pebbled or rugose surface
- Coarse hairs often

Histopathology
- Lentiginous melanocytic proliferation common
- Junctional, compound, or dermal
- Involvement of reticular dermis, particularly lower half
- Diffuse dermal involvement by nevus cells often
- Interstitial pattern
- "Inflammatory" pattern
- Nevus cells within appendages, blood vessels, nerves

Differential diagnosis
- Becker's nevus
- Dysplastic nevus
- Epidermal nevus
- Congenital lentigo
- Melanoma

HISTOGENESIS

Acquired nevi and CMN demonstrate many of the same histopathologic features: lentiginous melanocytic proliferation, unctional nesting, and maturation in the dermis.[1-8] However, there are substantial differences in size, depth, adnexal/vascular infiltration, and neurocristic differentiation.[3,8] As has been mentioned already, little is known about the histogenesis of nevi in general, but this is especially true for CMN. Thus there is no information available on the developmental biology of nevi that might account for the differences between acquired nevi and CMN. Cramer[3] has suggested that all nevi may

TABLE 5-4
Précis: Large or Giant Congenital Nevus

Clinical features
- Symmetry
- > 20 cm
- Involvement of major anatomic area, segmental
- Often dorsal involvement
- Occasional congenital deformities
- Well-defined borders
- Brown, dark brown, black
- "Animal pelt" feature, rugose, doughy
- Soft tissue hypertrophy
- Hypertrichosis
- Scattered satellite nevi distant from giant nevus
- Involvement of meninges common for head and neck nevi

Histopathology
- Lentiginous melanocytic proliferation common
- Usually compound or dermal
- Reticular dermal involvement, superficial and deep
  - Diffuse
  - Interstitial
  - Perivascular, periadnexal
- Subcutaneous involvement, septal > > lobular
- Maturation
- Neural differentiation, neuroid or neurofibroma-like pattern, on occasion
- Wagner-Meissner-like corpuscles
- Fascial or muscle involvement
- Cellular nodules in reticular dermis, on occasion
- Blue nevus component, on occasion
- Spindle and epithelioid cell nevus component, on occasion
- Hamartomatous elements
  - Cartilaginous differentiation
  - Adipose differentiation

Differential diagnosis
- Becker's nevus
- Neurofibromatosis
- Melanoma
- Peripheral nerve-sheath tumors

originate from nerve sheath precursor cells that migrate to the skin associated with peripheral nerves. These pluripotential cells may then differentiate and migrate to the dermis and epidermis, giving rise to nevi. If this differentiation to nevus cells occurs in larger, more proximal nerves, the migration of nevus cells to the area of innervation of such a nerve might account for the large surface area of many CMN. Presumably, acquired nevi would develop from differentiation and migration of precursor cells associated with small distal cutaneous nerves. Such a hypothesis has merit but has not been verified.[3]

By definition, all CMN develop in utero, but the time of their appearance or full development may vary. For example, as mentioned, nevi with the gross morphologic features of CMN ("tardive" nevi) may be CMN with migratory cells reaching the superficial skin and achieving full development after birth.[9] The congenital divided nevus of the eyelid provides some information on the development of CMN. Because such nevi appear (intact) at a time when the eyelids are fused and before the eyelids reopen, one can estimate that these nevi probably develop between approximately 8 and 24 weeks of gestational age.[24] However, it is unlikely that this scenario applies to all CMN.

It is presumed that both genetic and environmental factors may be operative in the histogenesis of CMN; however, only very limited information is currently available on this subject.

FAMILIAL AGGREGATION

Small CMN have been reported to aggregate in families,[25] and there is evidence for a similar phenomenon for larger varieties of CMN.[9] A clear-cut mode of inheritance, however, has not been established.

ASSOCIATIONS

CMN, especially larger or giant forms, have been associated with a number of developmental deformities such as elephantiasis of the extremities, anatomic asymmetry, hypertrophy of cranial bones, scoliosis, spina bifida, and club foot.[7,9,26,27] An association with neurofibromatosis has been suggested because of phenotypic similarity,[9] but the relationship has not been proved.[27]

CLINICAL FEATURES

The clinical characteristics of CMN are related to size and age (see Tables 5-2, 5-3 and 5-4).[1,2,4–9,17,26] Small congenital nevi less than 1.5 cm in greatest diameter may be indistinguishable from common acquired nevi, and documentation at birth may be the only means of confirming a congenital origin.[5] In general, CMN in the range of 1.5 to 10 or 20 cm in diameter are well-circumscribed, elongate or oval lesions that are usually only slightly elevated.[1] Many CMN may be relatively flat and tan or light brown in infancy and may resemble a café-au-lait macule. However, most CMN of this size exhibit a relatively uniform brown or dark brown color with increasing age of the child.[1] Some CMN also exhibit a mottled but relatively homogeneous coloration with shades of red-brown that have an almost mahogany appearance. Dark brown speckling also may be found in some nevi. Coarse, terminal hair follicles are found on a regular basis.

TABLE 5-5
Frequency Distribution of Nevus Depth versus Size of CMN in Infants under 1 Year of Age

	Frequency, %			
	Small	*Medium*	*Large*	*Total*
Junctional	2 1.8	0 0.0	0 0.0	2 1.8
Superficial	7 6.4	2 1.8	0 0.0	9 8.2
Deep dermal	13 11.8	29 26.4	6 5.4	48 43.6
Subcutaneous	2 1.8	35 31.8	14 12.7	51 46.4
TOTAL	24 21.8	66 60.0	20 18.2	110 100.0

Note: Chi-squared analysis suggests significant association between nevus cell depth and size of the lesion ($p < 0.0001$).

Intermediate- or medium-sized CMN measuring up to 10 or 20 cm in longest diameter frequently have a well-defined, round, oval, or elongate morphology and an orderly distribution of pigment.[1] Most of these nevi are brown, but they range in color from tan to dark brown or black. A speckled or mottled appearance is also common.

Giant CMN occupy a large area of the cutaneous surface, and hence the term *garment* or *bathing trunk nevus* accurately depicts this appearance.[1,7,9] Such CMN often involve a large portion of the dorsal surface of the individual. The surface topography of giant nevi shows considerable variation. These nevi are most often raised and exhibit a variably papular, lumpy, rugose, or even verrucous surface. The skin surface may be shiny or contain numerous terminal hairs. Soft-tissue hypertrophy may mimic changes found in neurofibromatosis. The color is most often a dark brown or black, but considerable variegation of pigment is often noted. Giant CMN are also remarkable for scattered, smaller satellite nevi on the skin surface beyond the garment nevus.[7,26]

All sizes of CMN have been noted to develop hypo- or depigmented halos and loss of pigmentation either within the nevus or on normal skin and to undergo variable degrees of regression.[28]

HISTOPATHOLOGY

The histologic characteristics observed in CMN are related to the size of the nevus primarily and to a lesser degree to the age of the individual.[2,5,6,18,21,29] Although it has been suggested that the histologic pattern of a CMN changes with age,[2,13,30] there is now evidence that the depth of nevus cell involvement throughout the dermis and subcutis is established early and remains for the most part unchanged.[31–33] However, the superficial (intraepidermal and superficial dermal) components of a CMN may mature in some instances. It is believed that immature disordered patterns such as pagetoid spread, large irregular nests, and cytologic atypia do diminish (or mature) with time.[29,30] However, the latter conclusion must be made with some circumspection because of the rather prominent morphologic heterogeneity throughout many CMN.[29]

Histopathologic Features of Congenital Nevi in the First Year of Life

A study of 110 unselected CMN of all sizes from infants less than 1 year of age was conducted recently at Children's Hospital Boston.[29] As shown in Table 5-5, 90 percent of CMN involved the deeper half of the dermis, and 47 percent involved the subcutaneous fat (Fig. 5-1). There was also a striking correlation between nevus size and nevus depth (chi-squared, $p < 0.0001$). Thus 62 percent of small CMN, 97 percent of medium-sized CMN, and 100 percent of large CMN extended into the lower half of the reticular dermis or subcutis. The only junctional nevi were small CMN (8 percent of small CMN). Only 9 CMN (7 were small CMN) involved the superficial reticular dermis only. These findings indicate that the depth of nevus involvement that is characteristic of CMN is established very early in life and correlates with the size of CMN.

The pattern of dermal involvement also tended to correlate with overall nevus size. The predominant dermal pattern was a diffuse, interstitial infiltration of the reticular dermis by nevus cells in 61 percent of CMN (see Fig. 5-1B). The latter pattern correlated with larger CMN. Smaller CMN tended to exhibit a patchy periadnexal/

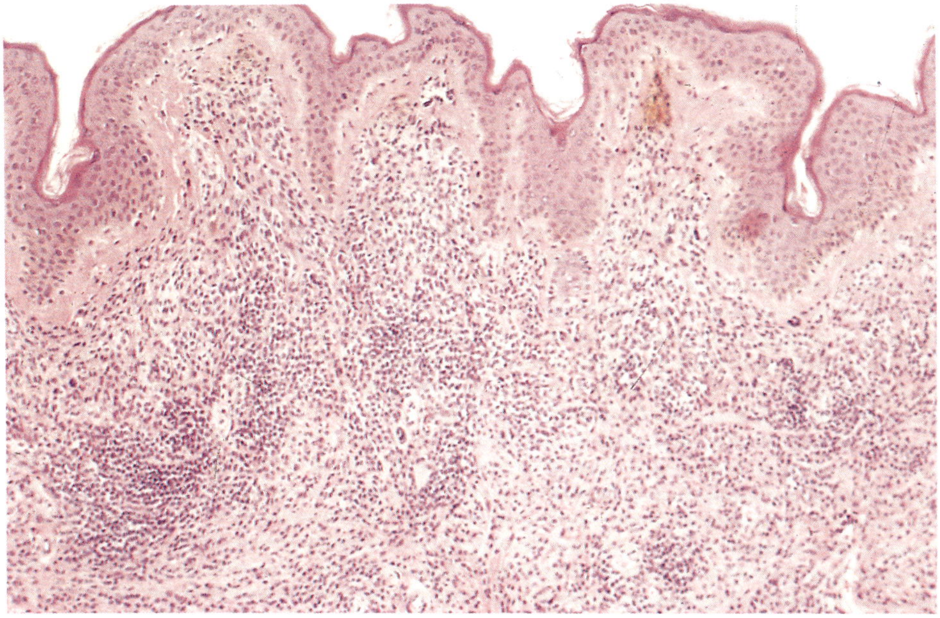

A

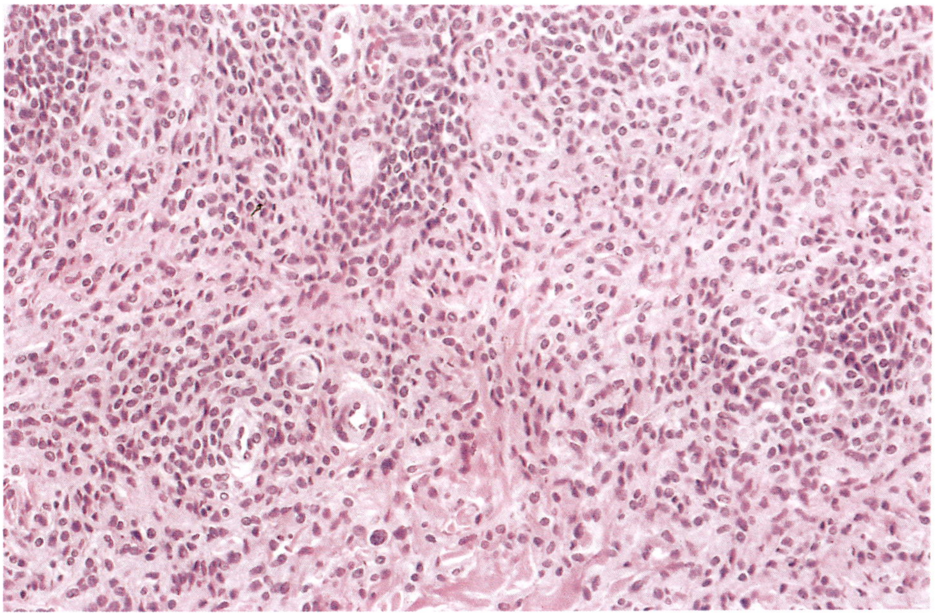

B

FIGURE 5-1

Large congenital nevus. (A) Nevus cells diffusely infiltrate dermis (H&E, × 100). (B) Maturation with descent of nevus cells in reticular dermis. Cellularity decreases from top to bottom as nevus cells are dispersed among collagen bundles at bottom of field (H&E, × 200). (C) Diffuse permeation of collagen of reticular dermis by nevus cells (H&E, × 200). (D) Nevus cells involve fibrous trabeculae of subcutaneous fat (H&E, × 40). (E) Higher magnification of part D showing diffuse infiltration of fibrous trabeculae (H&E, × 200).

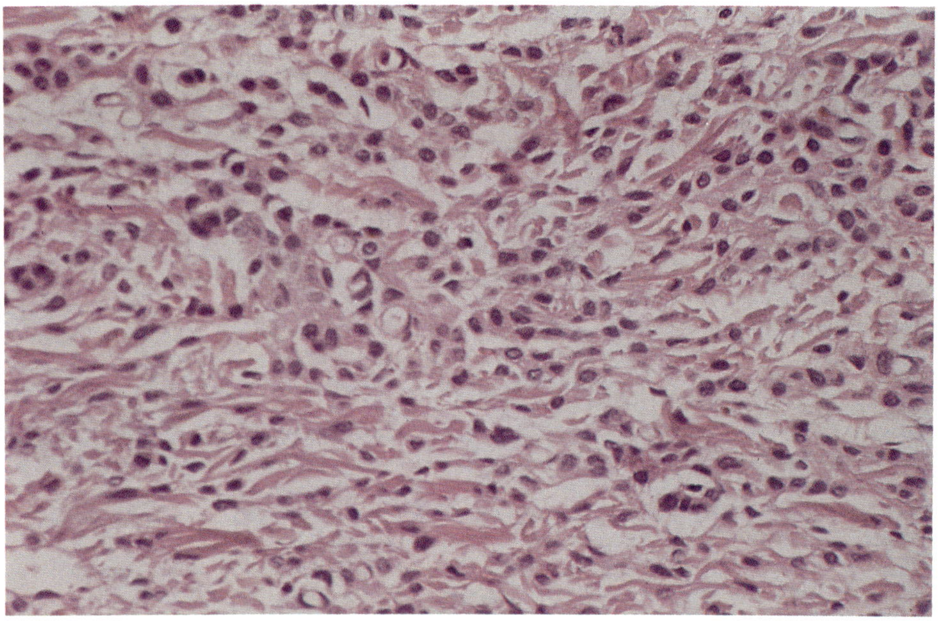

C

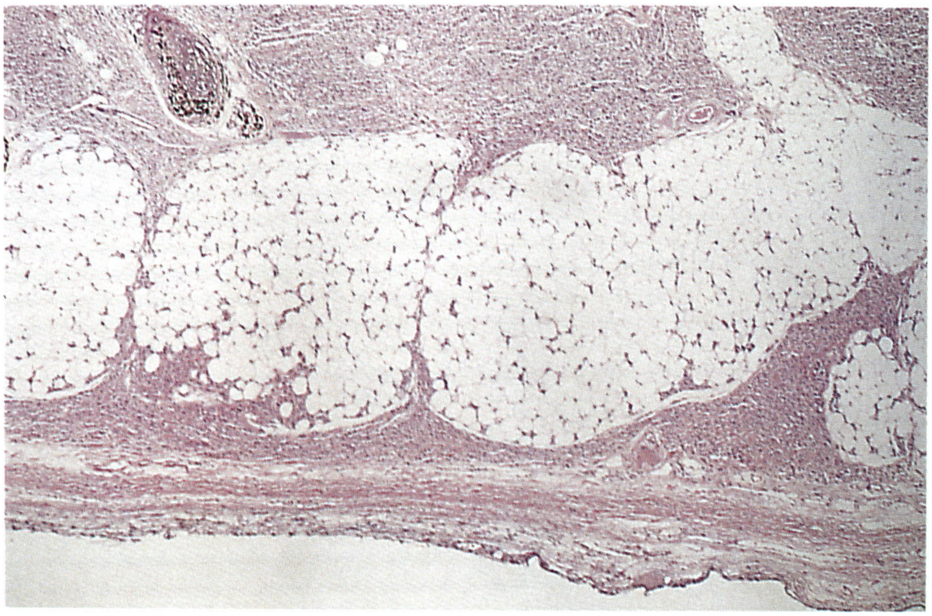

D

FIGURE 5-1 *(Continued)*

perivascular pattern (Fig. 5-2). There was a rather striking affinity of nevus cells for eccrine ducts, particularly just after birth (Fig. 5-3A).

Cytologic atypia has been reported to be somewhat more common and prominent in the CMN of neonates and infants,[30] even though its biologic significance has been questioned. In the preceding study, 29 percent of CMN showed cytologic atypia of the intraepidermal component (Table 5-6), but this was only minimal or slight in almost all the cases.[29] The presence of cytologic atypia did not correlate with CMN size, anatomic site, or other gross morphologic features. Melanoma was not observed in any CMN. These findings indicate that cytologic atypia is probably not as common as was believed and that melanoma is exceedingly rare if it occurs at all in this age group (see below).

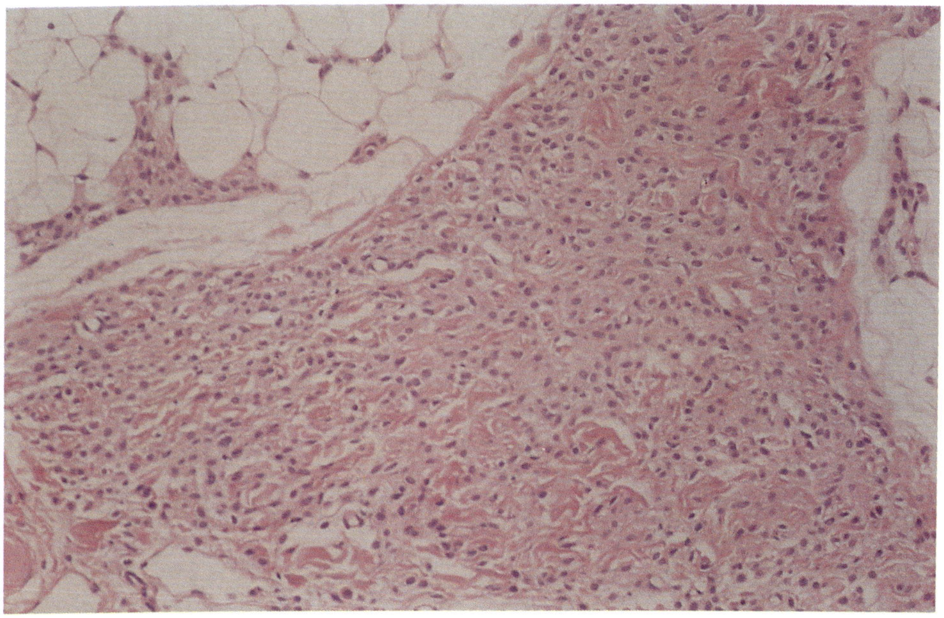

E

FIGURE 5-1 *(Continued)*

Histopathology Features of Relatively Small CMN

Recent evidence indicates that small CMN display considerable heterogeneity of their histologic features.[2,4,5] Some may be entirely junctional and some may be indistinguishable from acquired nevi[2,29,34] (Fig. 5-4). Many small nevi, particularly those measuring less than 1.5 cm in diameter, also demonstrate what has been termed a superficial pattern[6,29] (Fig. 5-2A and C). The latter characterization refers to junctional nests of nevus cells alone or a compound or entirely dermal pattern with aggregates of nevus cells extending to no greater depth than the upper half of the reticular dermis. Such a pattern also may be seen in a significant percentage of acquired nevi. Up to 28 percent of acquired nevi also may exhibit nevus cells extending into the lower two-thirds of the reticular dermis.[5]

Thus many relatively small CMN show the superficial pattern mentioned above and often do not involve the lower third of the reticular dermis as originally reported by Mark and colleagues.[1,5,6] According to Mark et al.,[1] the latter finding was considered to be characteristic of a congenital onset regardless of nevus size.[1] In contradistinction to acquired nevi, small CMN are commonly notable for the following patterns of (usually superficial) dermal involvement: 1) formation of a diffuse plaque of nevus cells filling the papillary dermis, 2) close association of nevus cells with or within appendageal and neurovascular structures of the superficial reticular dermis (and sometimes deeper), and 3) nevus cells being disposed among, "fanning out" between, or splaying collagen bundles of the reticular dermis as single cells, files, and cords of cells (two cells in tandem) (see Figs. 5-1C and 5-2F). CMN also show a typical pattern of maturation of nevus cells from superficial to deep dermis. Near the epidermal surface, nevus cells tend to be aggregated in nests and may exhibit epithelioid cell features.[1,29] (see Fig. 5-4B). With increasing depth, the nevus cells often demonstrate greater separation (i.e., splaying) and slightly diminished cellular and nuclear sizes (see Fig. 5-1B). Extension of nevus cells into the subcutaneous fat is usually a feature observed in larger varieties of congenital nevi but occasionally occurs in small CMN.[1,29] (Fig. 5-1D).

With increasing sizes of CMN, there is greater tendency for deep dermal, appendageal, and neurovascular involvement[5,6,21,29] (Tables 5-7 and 5-8). However, even some congenital nevi less than 1.5 cm in diameter tend to exhibit involvement of eccrine and follicular units at the mid-reticular dermis level or deeper much more commonly than acquired nevi.[32]

Histopathologic Features of Larger CMN

Giant CMN, most medium-sized CMN, and a percentage of nevi less than 10 cm in diameter tend to exhibit distinctive features[5-8,21,29] (see Tables 5-3, 5-4, 5-7, and 5-8). Probably the most characteristic feature shared by these larger varieties of congenital nevi is the pattern of diffuse proliferation of nevus cells throughout the reticular dermis with frequent extension into the subcutaneous

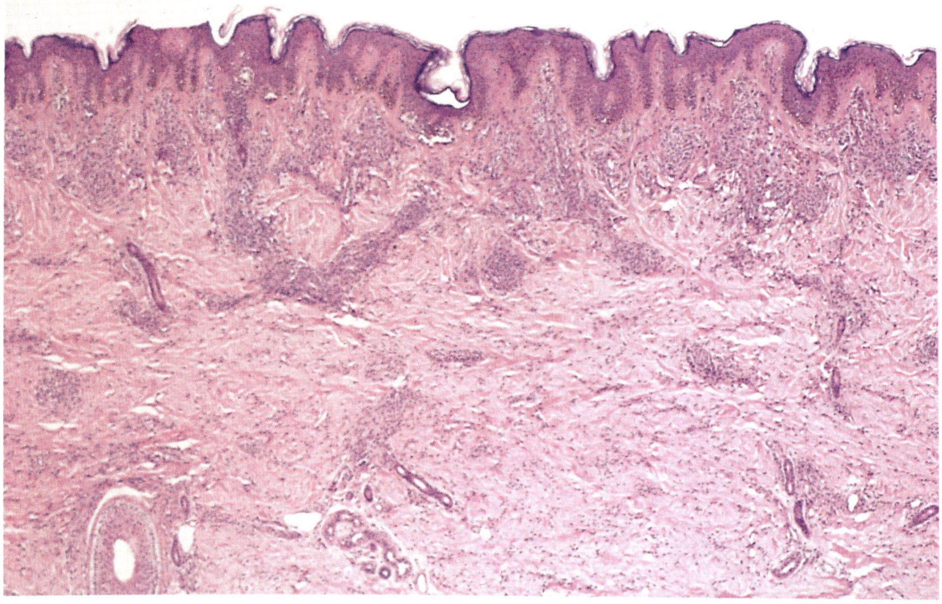

A

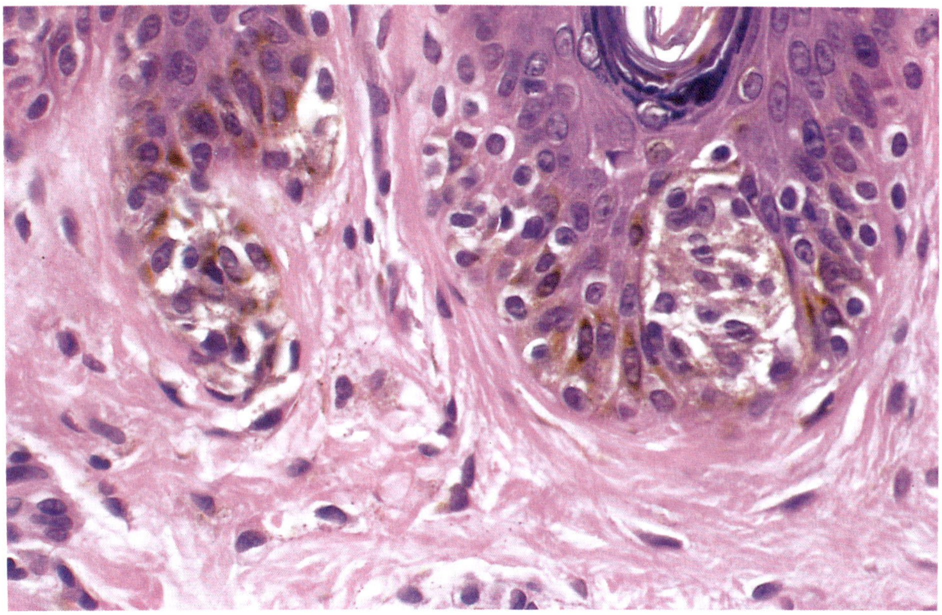

B

FIGURE 5-2

Small congenital nevus. (A) There are aggregates of nevus cells in papillary dermis and distributed throughout reticular dermis in association with blood vessels and adnexal structures (H&E, × 40). (B) Junctional nests are indistinguishable from those in an acquired nevus (H&E, × 400). (C) Discreet nests of nevus cells in reticular dermis simulate inflammatory infiltrates as in a gyrate erythema (H&E, × 100). (D) Perivascular and interstitial disposition of nevus cells in reticular dermis (H&E, × 200). (E) Nevus cells show perivascular cuffing typical of congenital nevi (H&E, × 400). (F) Splaying of nevus cells among collagen bundles as single cells and files of cells (H&E, × 200).

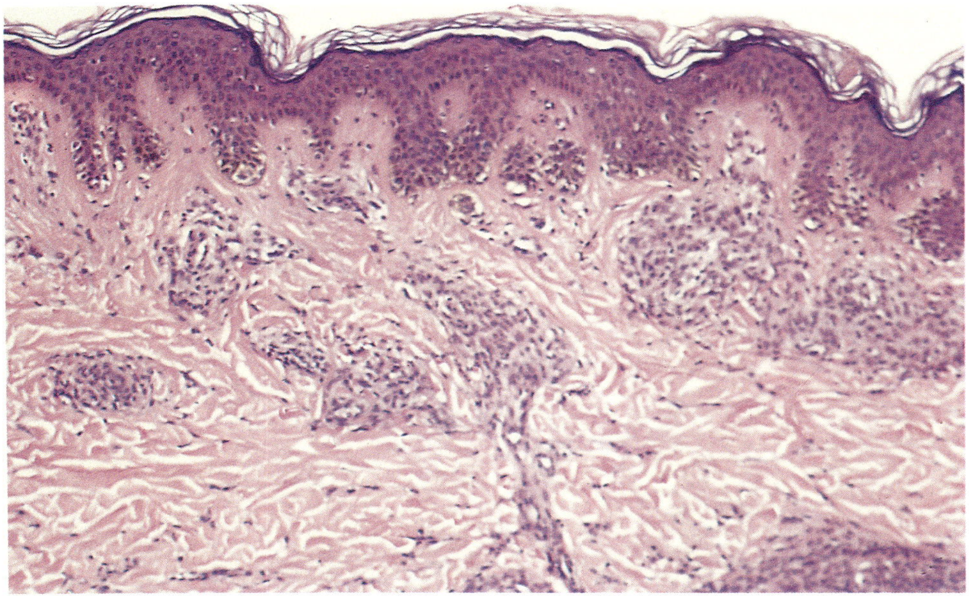

C

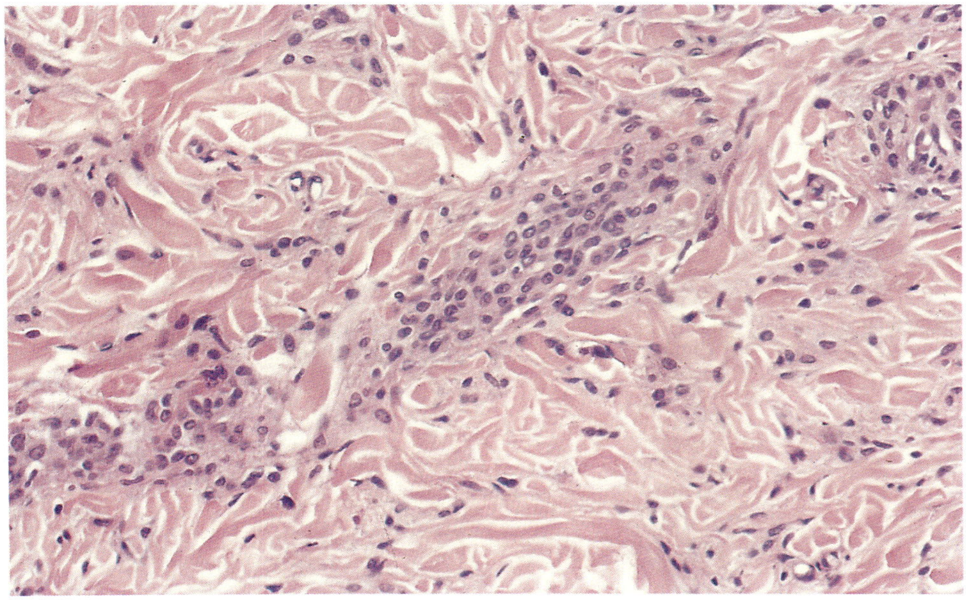

D

FIGURE 5-2 *(Continued)*

fat.[1,6,7,21,29] There is usually a grenz zone separating the epidermis from the dermal infiltration of nevus cells.[21,35] (see Fig. 5-1A). The nevus cells tend to infiltrate collagen in an orderly and uniform pattern. The nevus cells also often extend along the fibrous trabeculae of the subcutaneous fat (see Fig. 5-1E). In some instances, there is infiltration of fat lobules.[1,29] Aggregates of nevus cells also tend to cuff or be present within follicular epithelium, sebaceous glands, eccrine ducts and glands, the perineurium of nerve twigs, and the walls of vascular structures[1,4,5,29] (see Figs. 5-2C–E and Fig. 5-3). The rather striking perivascular and periadnexal cuffing of nevus cells in some congenital nevi may closely resemble an inflammatory process such as a gyrate erythema (see Fig. 5-2C). Such a presentation may be designated as an "inflammatory" pattern of congenital nevi. The nevus cells

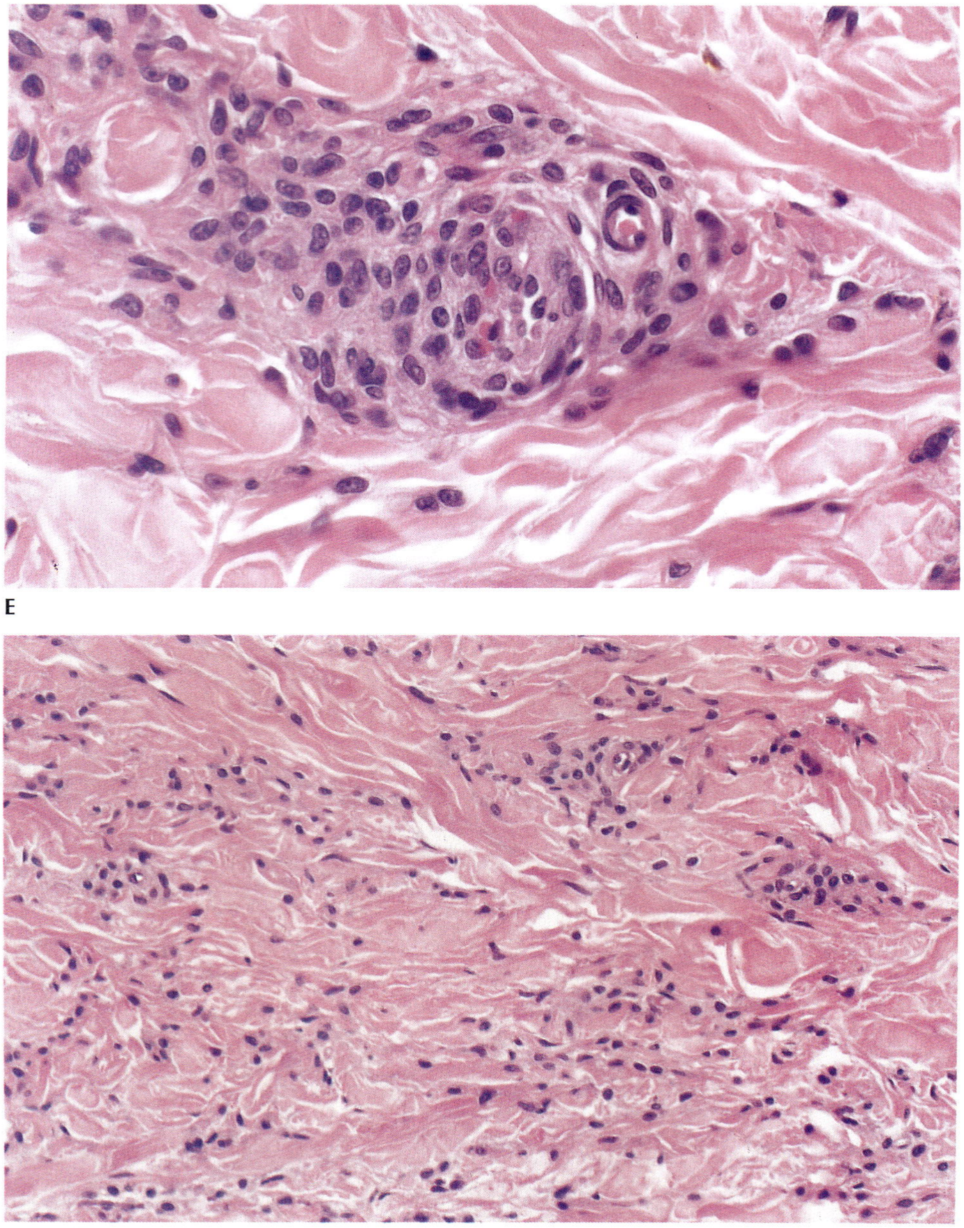

E

F

FIGURE 5-2 *(Continued)*

usually exhibit small uniform nuclei comparable with those in common acquired nevi. Occasional junctional nests of nevus cells are also observed. Foci of hypercellularity are also noted to a variable extent within the dermal population of cells[29] (Fig. 5-5). Both hair follicles and appendageal smooth-muscle bundles may be enlarged.[5,29]

A subset of large/giant CMN is also characterized by spindle cell or neuroidal differentiation resembling the histologic pattern of a neurofibroma (neuroid CMN).[7,27] In the latter instance, the constituent cells have a wavy configuration and are embedded in a delicate stroma. Neural differentiation resembling neural tubules or pseudomeissnerian structures is also a typical histologic feature[1,7,27] (Fig. 5-6). Such nevi may be associated with congenital anomalies such as club foot and spina bifida.[27]

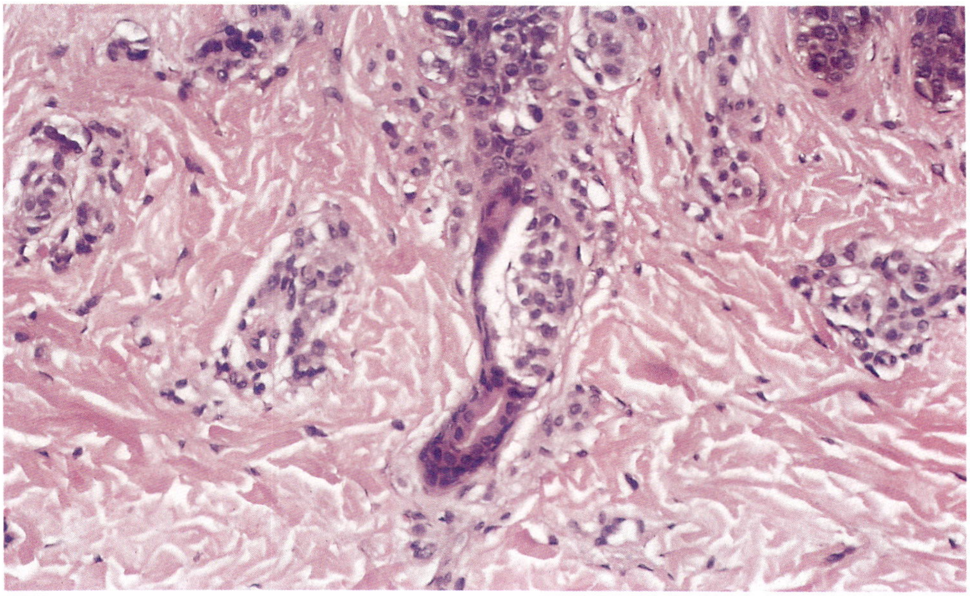

A

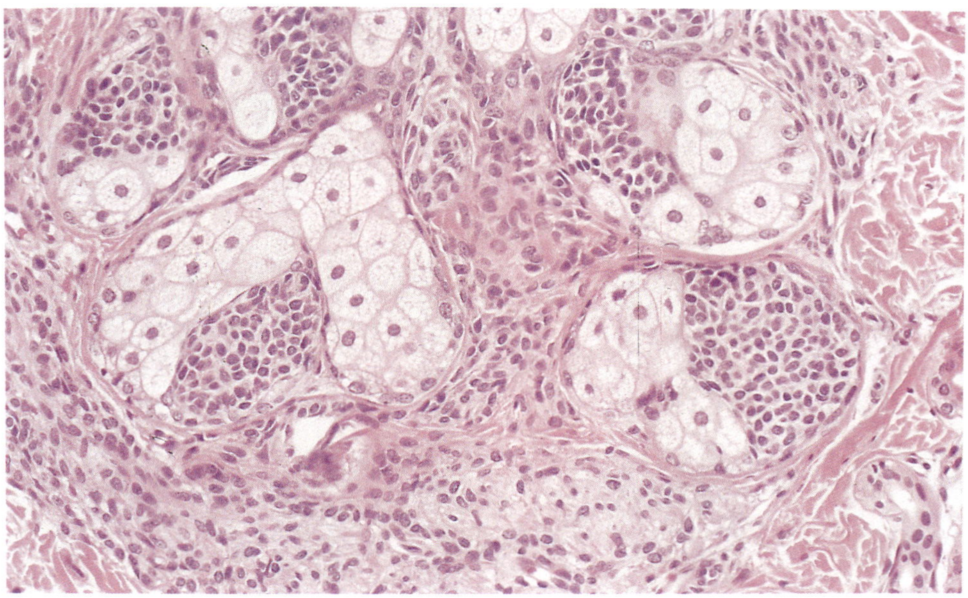

B

FIGURE 5-3

Congenital nevus. (A) Nest of nevus cells within eccrine sweat duct (H&E, × 200). (B) Nests of nevus cells within sebaceous lobules (H&E, × 200). (C) High magnification of part B (H&E, × 400).

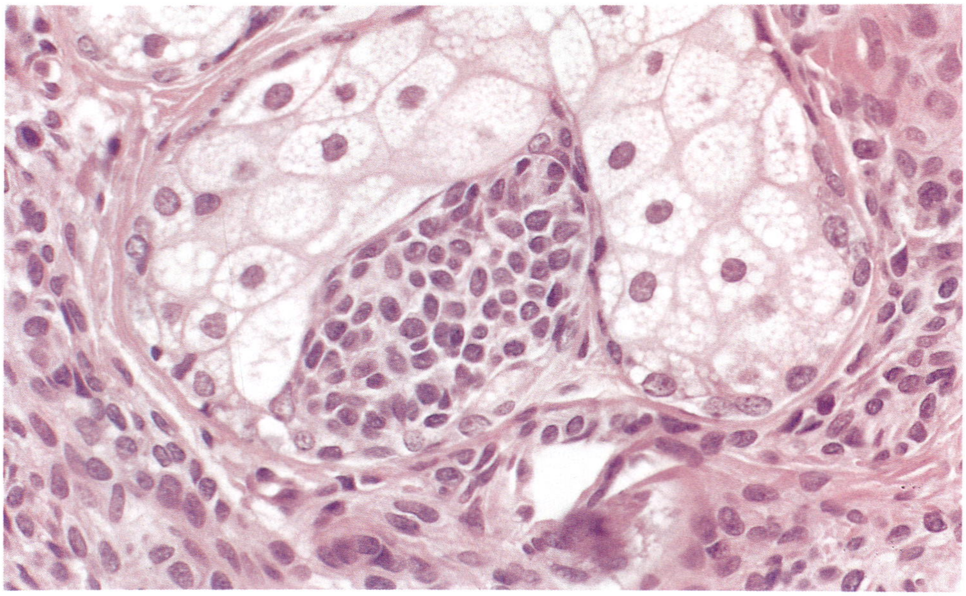

FIGURE 5-3 *(Continued)*

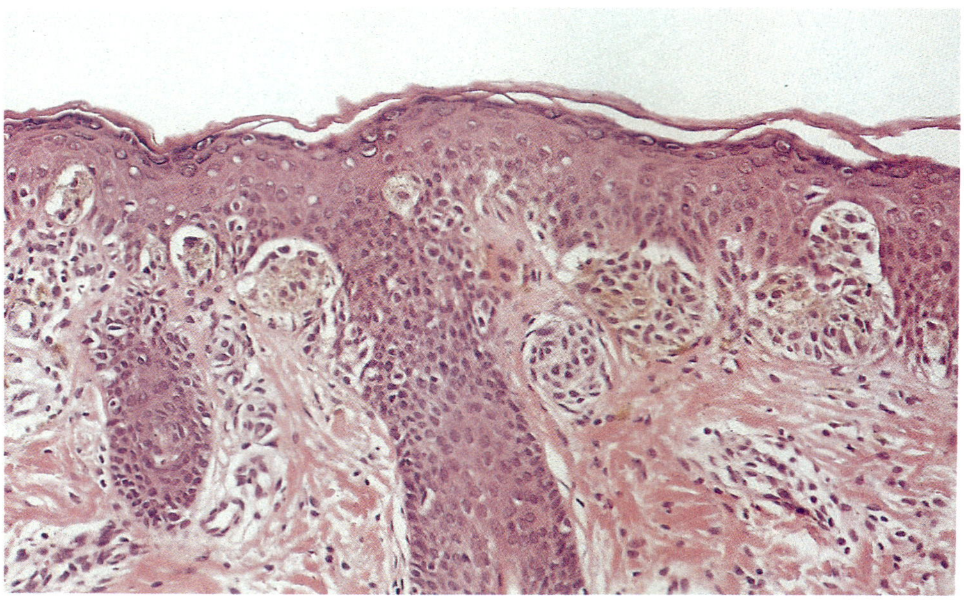

FIGURE 5-4
Small congenital nevus. This lesion shows a prominent junctional component with only limited involvement of the papillary dermis (H&E, × 200).

TABLE 5-6
Frequency Distribution of Atypia versus Size of CMN in Infants under 1 Year of Age

	Frequency, %			
	Small	*Medium*	*Large*	*Total*
No atypia	16 14.6	36 32.7	16 14.6	68 61.8
Atypia	8 7.3	30 27.3	4 9.5	42 38.2
TOTAL	24 21.9	66 60.0	20 18.2	110 100.0

Note: According to chi-squared analysis, atypia was not significantly associated with size of the congenital nevus ($p > 0.1$).

TABLE 5-7
Distribution of Nevus Cell Involvement in Acquired and Congenital Nevi by Size

		Congenital		
	Acquired	*< 1.5 cm*	*1.5–19.9 cm*	*Giant*
Junctional nesting	+ +	+ +	+ +	+ +
Papillary dermis	+ +	+ +	+ +	+ +
Upper reticular dermis, interstitial	+	+ +	+ +	+ +
Upper reticular dermis, appendageal and/or neurovascular	±	+ +	+ +	+ +
Lower reticular dermis, interstitial	−	±	+ +	+ +
Lower reticular dermis, appendageal and/or neurovascular	−	±	+ +	+ +
Subcutaneous	−	±	+ +	+ +

Key: + +, frequent; +, common; ±, may occur; −, usually not present.

TABLE 5-8
Histologic Patterns of Congenital Melanocytic Nevi

Acquired nevus pattern	Mostly small CMN
Patchy periadnexal, perivascular pattern	Small to large CMN
Diffuse infiltration of reticular dermis, subcutis	Mostly large/giant CMN
Neuroid pattern, resembling neurofibroma	Mostly large/giant CMN
Spindle and epithelioid cell nevus pattern	Mostly large/giant CMN
Blue nevus pattern (both ordinary and cellular blue nevus)	Mostly large/giant CMN

Large CMN also may show a variety of other patterns suggesting that they are indeed hamartomas of neural crest differentiation.[8] Such nevi may contain heterologous elements such as cartilage, bone, adipose tissue, vascular malformation, hemangioma, lymphangioma, mastocytoma, and schwannoma.[1,7–9,27] Foci resembling blue nevus, cellular blue nevus, and spindle and epithelioid cell nevus are noted occasionally. The latter histologic picture thus may qualify as a combined nevus if found in the context of an otherwise typical CMN.

Epidermal changes

The epidermal changes in CMN are not distinctive and vary from almost no change to florid papillomatous or polypoid configurations.[1,5,7,35] Lentiginous epidermal and melanocytic hyperplasia are possibly more common in CMN than in acquired nevi.

DISTINCTION OF RELATIVELY SMALL CMN FROM ACQUIRED NEVI

The distinction of small or any type of CMN from acquired nevi is only important if small CMN are proved to have greater risk for the development of melanoma than

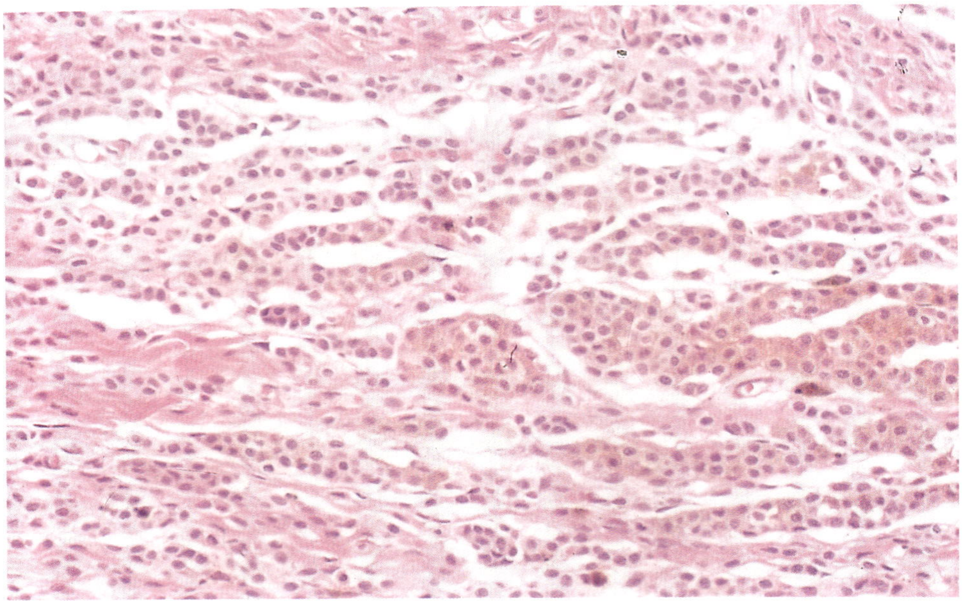

FIGURE 5-5
Large congenital nevus. Area of increased cellularity in reticular dermis. Such foci are common in large CMN (H&E, × 200).

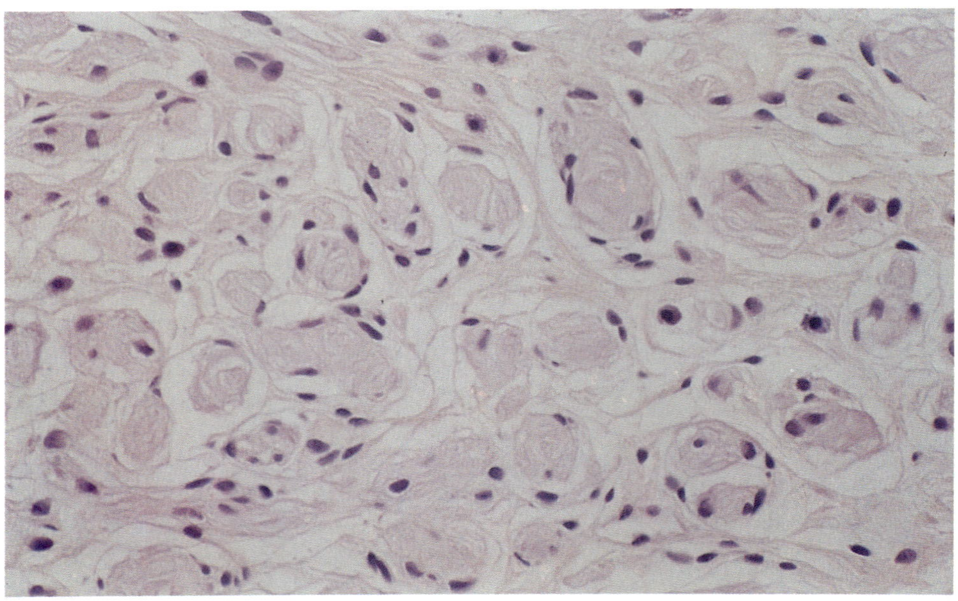

FIGURE 5-6
Large congenital nevus. There is prominent neurotization of nevus cells in dermis. The nevus cells form structures resembling Meissner-Wagner corpuscles (H&E, × 400).

acquired nevi.[5] At present, there is no conclusive proof that there is a significant difference in melanoma risk between the latter two types of nevi. However, some authors do believe that there is sufficient circumstantial evidence for a difference in melanoma risk.[19,20]

As has been mentioned already, because of the histologic overlap between small CMN and acquired nevi, there are no features with 100 percent specificity and 100 percent sensitivity for recognition of CMN.[5] Thus some CMN will be indistinguishable from common acquired nevi (see Table 5-7). Nonetheless, the presence of nevus cells in the lower half of the reticular dermis, in an appendageal/neurovascular pattern, or both will enable one to detect a majority of small CMN.[5,35] It should be emphasized that absence of the latter features does not preclude a congenital origin.[5,35]

CONGENITAL NEVI WITH ATYPICAL FEATURES

Architectural Disorder and/or Cytologic Atypia

As with other types of melanocytic nevi, all varieties of congenital nevi may exhibit varying degrees of architectural and cytologic atypia of both the intraepidermal and dermal components[8,29] (Table 5-9). Perhaps one of the most common findings in congenital nevi is the presence of lentiginous melanocytic proliferation associated with or without some variation in junctional nesting pattern and generally low-grade cytologic atypia of the intraepidermal melanocytes.[29] The latter changes are comparable with those seen in typical acquired dysplastic nevi, and thus such nevi might be designated as *dysplastic* congenital nevi.

TABLE 5-9

Atypical Variants of Congenital Nevi and Atypical Proliferations Arising in Congenital Nevi

Intraepidermal proliferations
- "Dysplastic" congenital nevus
  - Lentiginous melanocytic proliferation
  - Variation in junctional nesting
  - Slight to severe nuclear atypia
- Congenital nevus with pagetoid spread
  - Variant in children with little or no cytologic atypia
  - Simulant of superficial spreading melanoma

Dermal proliferations
- Atypical cellular proliferations
  - Mainly spindle cells
  - Mainly epithelioid cells
  - Mainly small cells
  - Blend with surrounding congenital nevus (maturation),
  - Variable degrees of cytologic atypia
- Tumors composed of the preceding cell types and associated with indeterminate biologic behavior

Intraepidermal Pagetoid Spread of Melanocytes

Another common finding, particularly in congenital nevi in individuals under the age of 10 and especially in the first year of life, is the pattern of upward migration of intraepidermal melanocytes[29,30,36–38] (Fig. 5-7A). Although the latter changes may be alarming, the proliferation is usually orderly and often confined to the lower half of the epidermis, and the cytologic atypia is absent or low-grade.[29] It should be emphasized that one may encounter a spectrum of atypicality within the intraepidermal component ranging from little or no atypia to frank melanoma in situ (see Fig. 5-7B).

Dermal Nodular Proliferations

Large/giant CMN may give rise to intradermal nodular melanocytic proliferations[8,29,36–38] (Figs. 5-8 to 5-12 and Tables 5-9 and 5-10). Such proliferations may occur in the superficial or deep reticular dermis and are characterized by the formation of cellular nodules. The constituent cells in these nodules may be epithelioid, spindled, or small cell in nature.[8,29,36–38] The degree of melaninization may range from little or none to heavy. Varying degrees of cytologic atypia, mitotic activity, and occasionally necrosis may be observed. Most of these cellular aggregates tend to blend with the surrounding background nevus (see Fig. 5-8B). The vast majority of such proliferations, particularly in the neonatal period, are biologically benign despite atypical histologic features (see Figs. 5-8 to 5-10). Nonetheless, all patients should receive close follow-up for evidence of recurrence. Small round cell tumors should be evaluated especially carefully for malignancy (see Figs. 5-8 and 5-10). Many of these nodular proliferations are composed of enlarged epithelioid (see Fig. 5-9) or spindle cells containing an increased cellular content of granular melanin. Usually the melanin does not have the finely divided ("dusty") character observed in melanoma cells. The nuclei in these cells also tend to show an overall uniformity and an evenly dispersed chromatin pattern compared with the more striking pleomorphism and clumped chromatin of melanoma cells[29] (see Fig. 5-9).

MELANOMA DEVELOPING IN CONGENITAL NEVI

Conventional melanoma originating from an intraepidermal site is observed most commonly in relatively small CMN[21,36] (Fig. 5-13 and Table 5-11). Such melanomas are usually of the superficial spreading or nodular type. However, such melanomas are uncommonly observed in

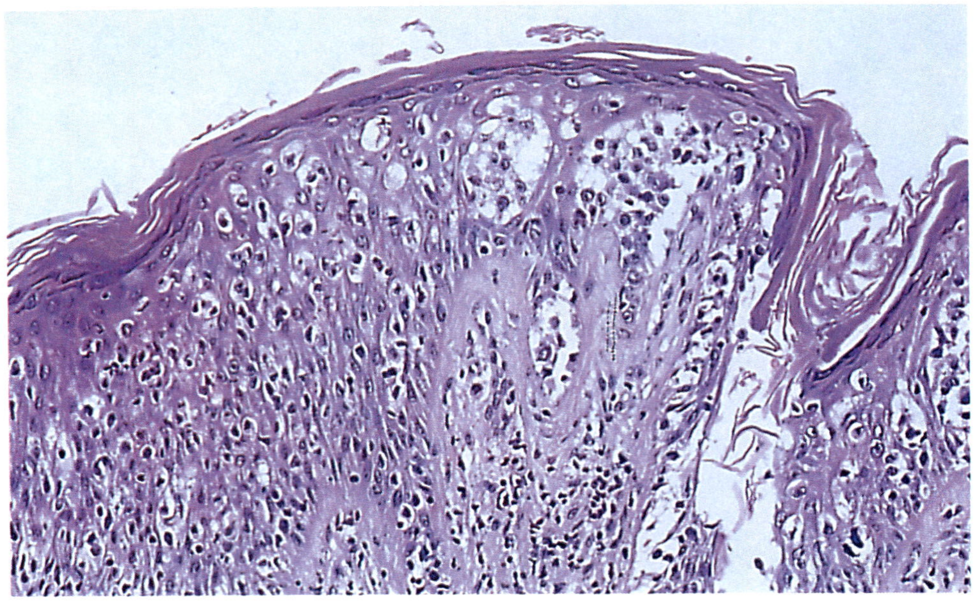

A

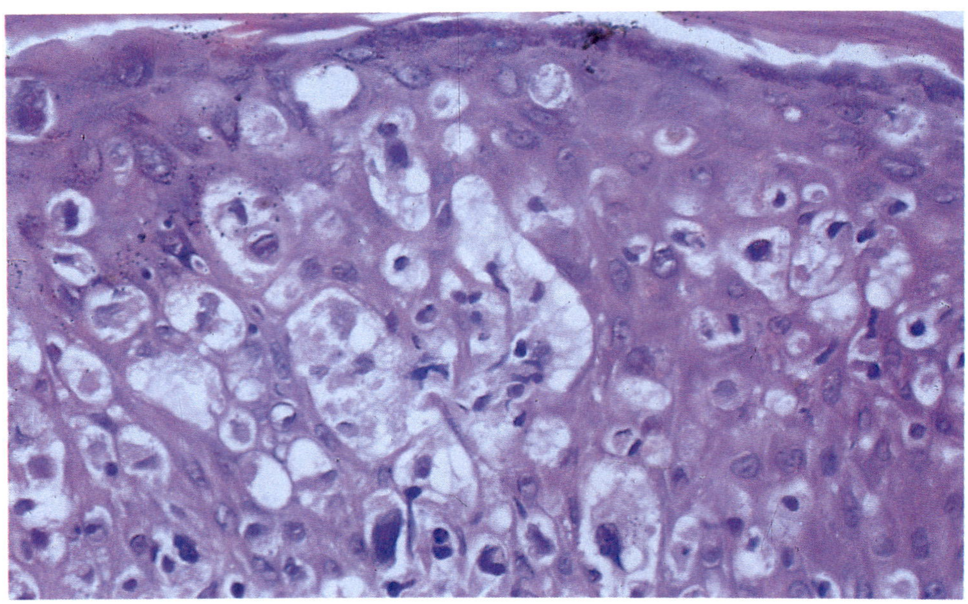

B

FIGURE 5-7

Congenital nevus with intraepidermal pagetoid spread. (A) The epidermis overlying a small congenital nevus shows extensive pagetoid spread (H&E, × 100). (B) Atypical epithelioid melanocytes scattered throughout epidermis. The findings qualify as melanoma in situ (H&E, × 400).

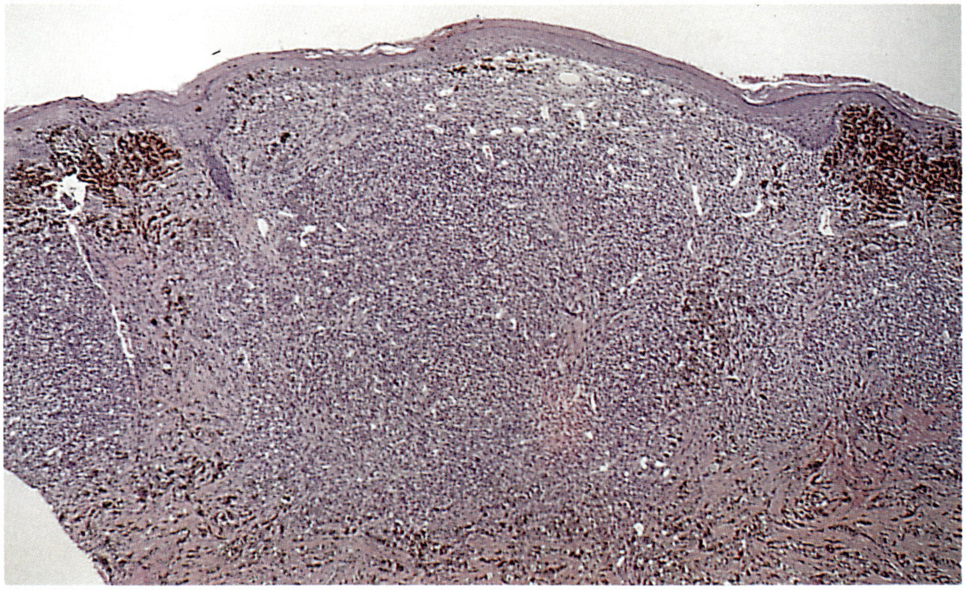

A

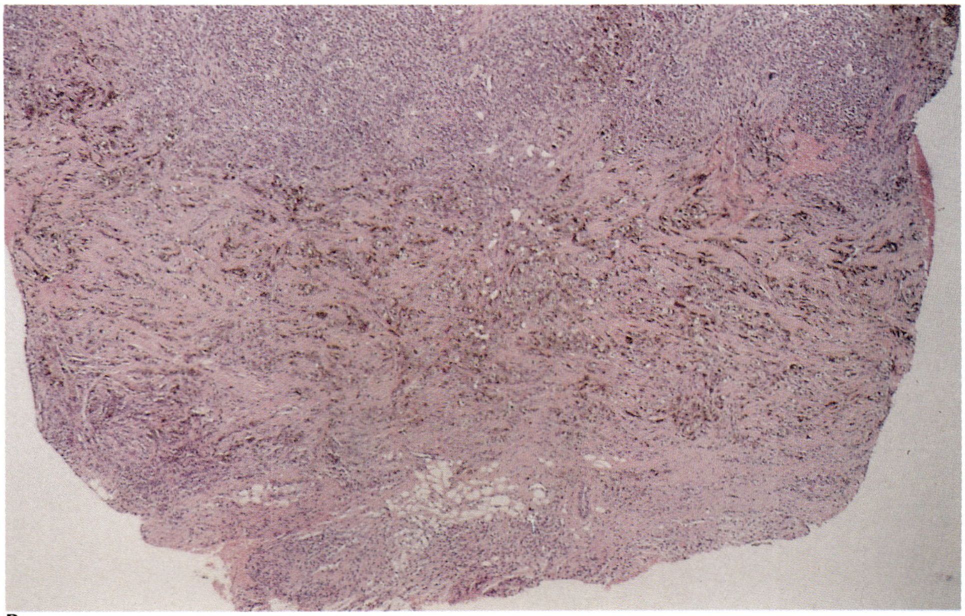

B

FIGURE 5-8

Superficial dermal atypical nodular proliferation in medium-sized congenital nevus of newborn. (A) Large compact cellular nodule in superficial and middle dermis resulting in elevated surface (H&E, × 40). (B) Deep reticular dermis shows maturation of nevus from part A. The nevus cells are dispersed among collagen bundles in an orderly pattern (H&E, × 40). (C) Compact cellular nodule composed of relatively small monotonous cells (H&E, × 100). (D) Higher magnification of part C shows cohesive nodule of cells exhibiting low-grade atypia. Such a proliferation is often misdiagnosed as melanoma. The patient has had no evidence of recurrence on follow-up (H&E, × 400).

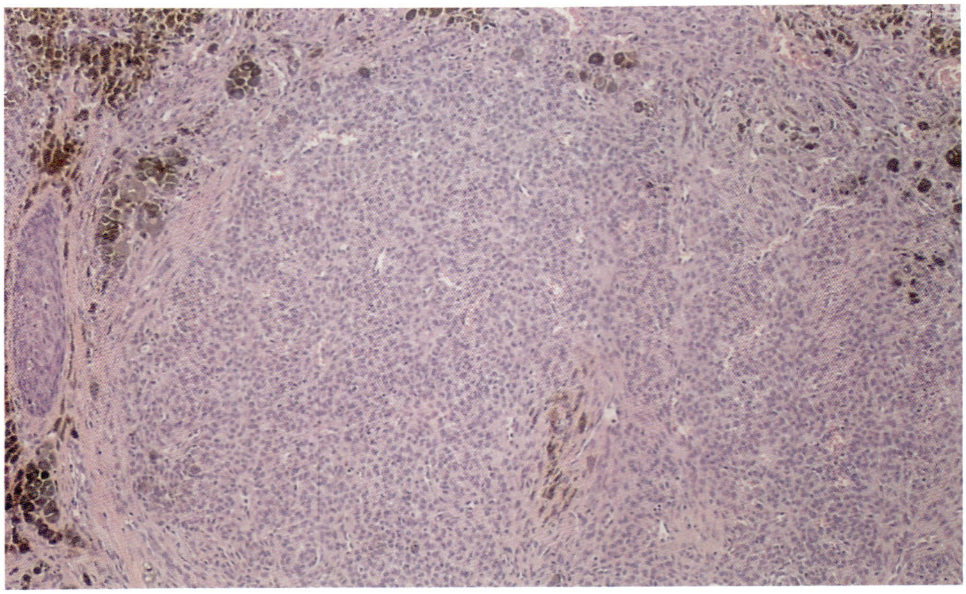

C

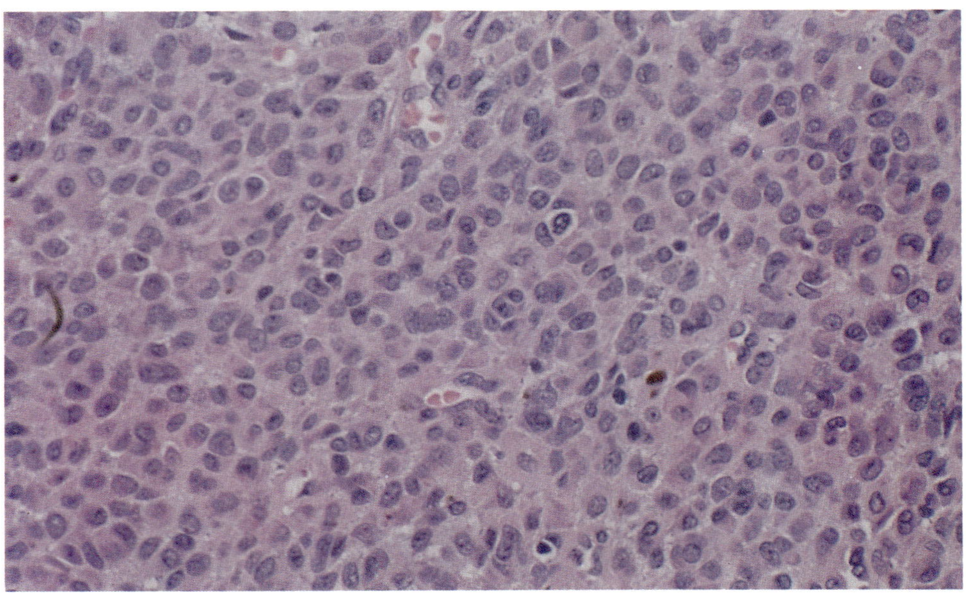

D

FIGURE 5-8 *(Continued)*

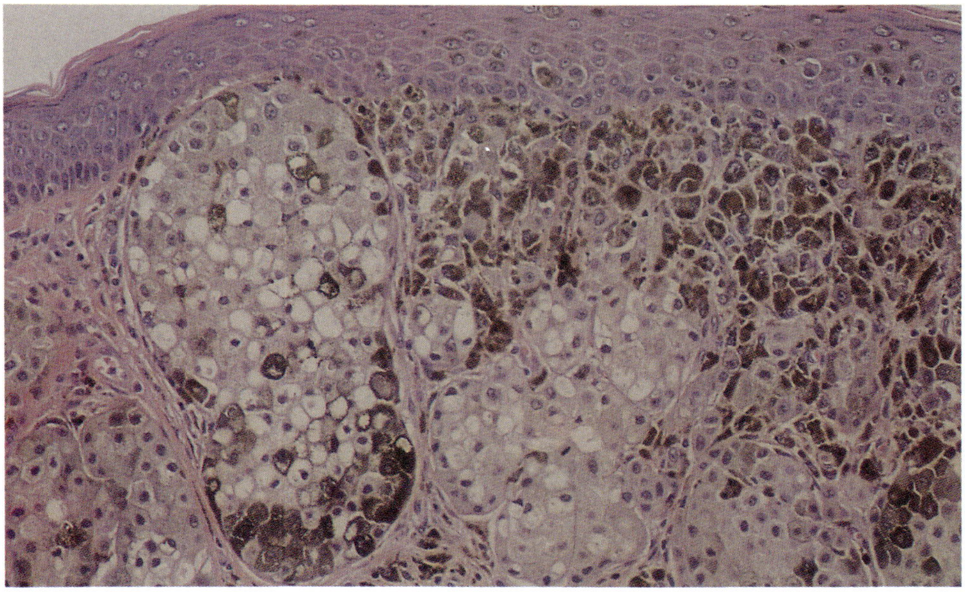

A

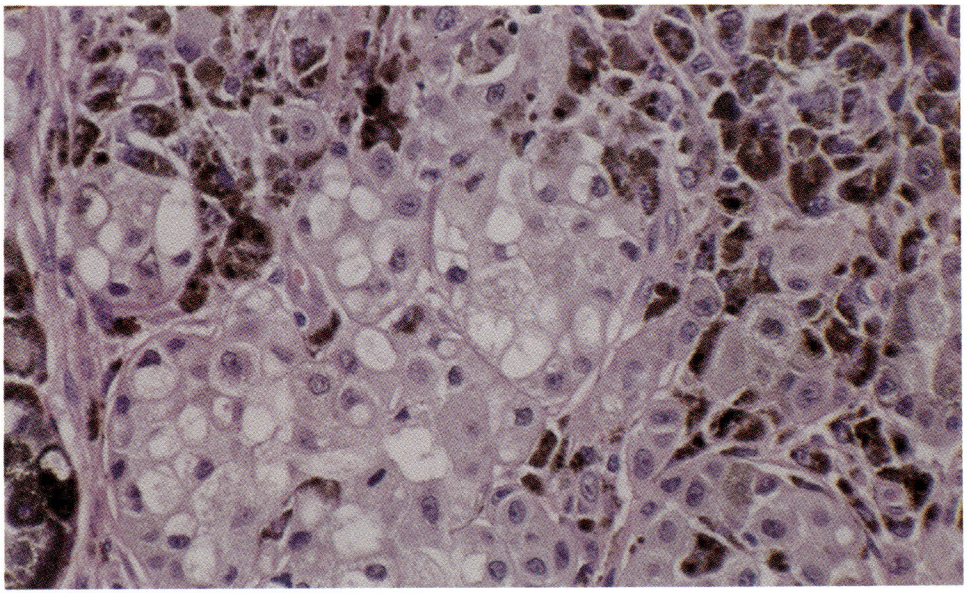

B

FIGURE 5-9

Atypical nodular proliferation in congenital nevus of newborn. (A) Superficial nodule contains atypical epithelioid cells simulating melanoma. The nevus exhibited maturation with descent into the dermis. No evidence of recurrence has been observed in this patient (H&E, × 200). (B) Higher magnification of part A showing epithelioid cells with some pleomorphism of nuclei. Many nuclei have fairly uniformly dispersed chromatin (H&E, × 400).

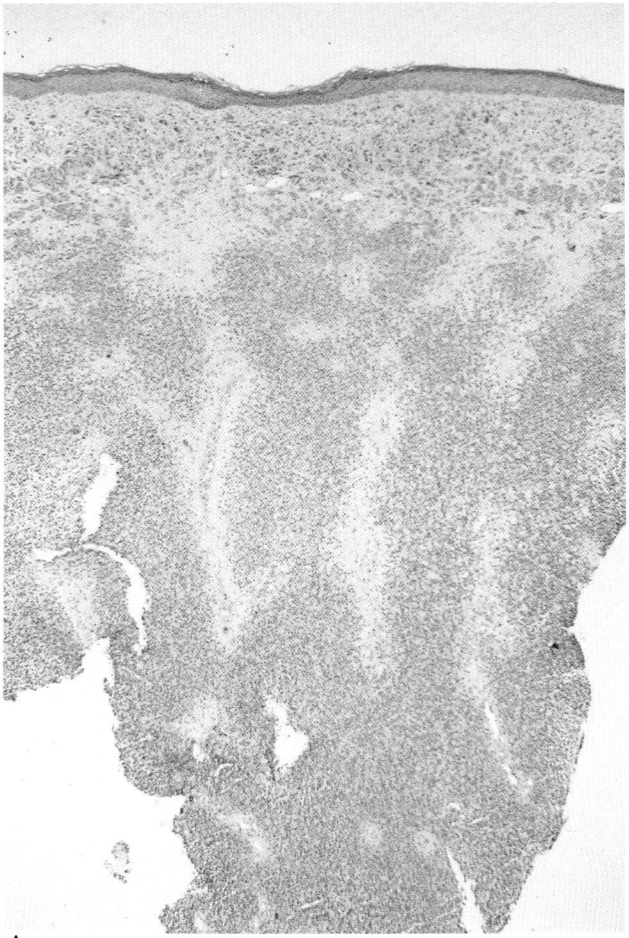

A

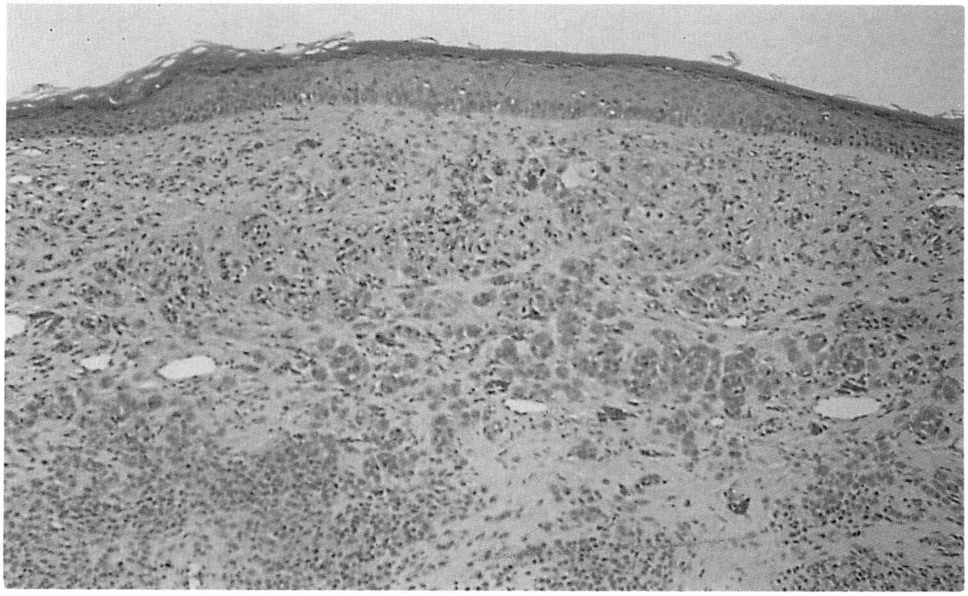

B

FIGURE 5-10

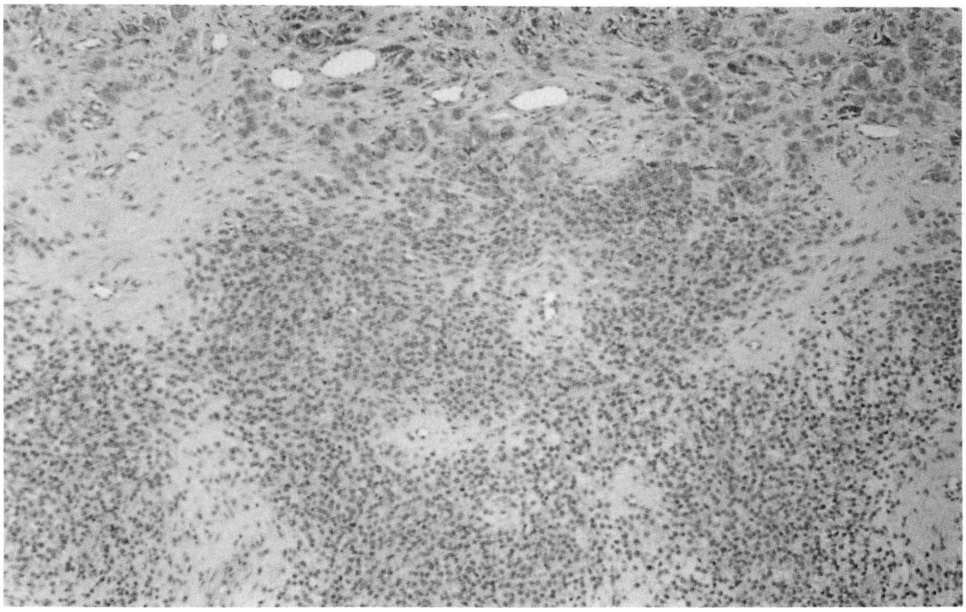

C

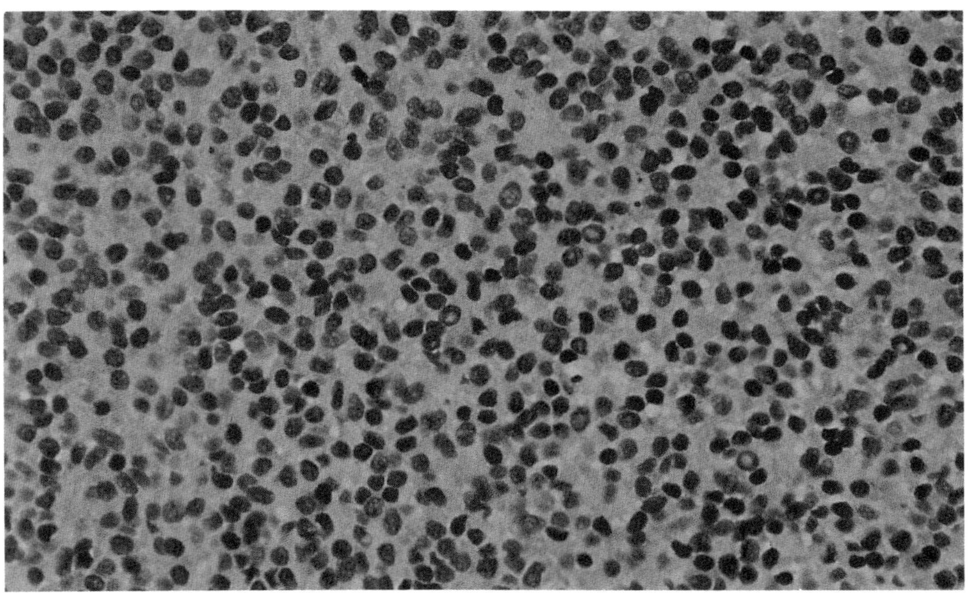

D

FIGURE 5-10 *(Continued)*

Atypical nodular proliferation in giant congenital nevus of newborn. (A) Highly cellular aggregates of relatively small cells fill most of dermis but there is maturation from superficial to deep (H&E, × 40). (B) Superficial dermis contains epithelioid-appearing cells (H&E, × 100). (C) Maturation from superficial epithelioid cells to smaller cells at the bottom of the field (H&E, × 100). (D) High magnification of part C showing aggregate of relatively monomorphous small cells. There was regression of this lesion (H&E, × 400).

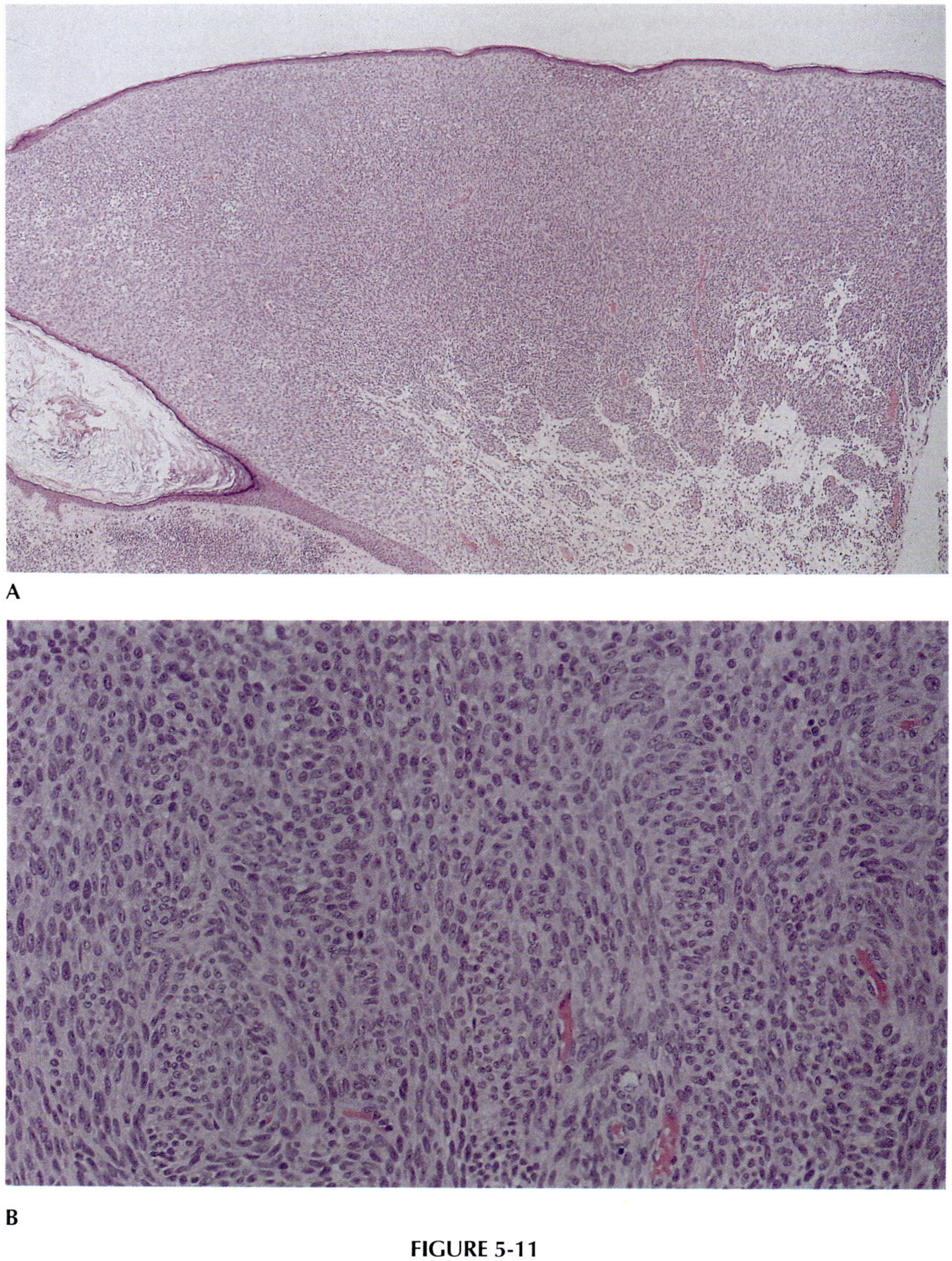

FIGURE 5-11

Atypical nodular proliferation in congenital nevus. (A) The papillary dermis is expanded by nodular aggregates of relatively small cells (H&E, × 100). (B) Higher magnification of (A) (H&E, × 200). (C) The proliferation simulates nevoid or verrucous melanoma (H&E, × 400).

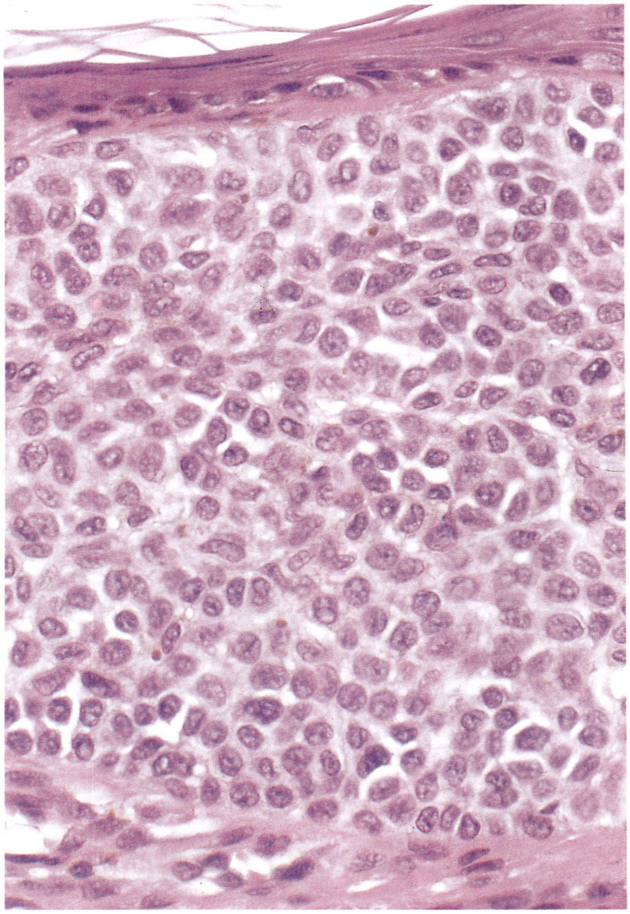

C

FIGURE 5-11 *(Continued)*

TABLE 5-10

Intraepidermal and Dermal Proliferations Developing in Large/Giant Congenital Nevi

Benign	*Indeterminate/Malignant*
1. Epithelioid cell Intraepidermal Pagetoid spread in nevi	Pagetoid melanoma (superficial spreading type)
Dermal Expansile nodule of epithelioid cells	Melanoma, epithelioid cell type
Epithelioid schwannoma	Malignant epithelioid schwannoma
2. Pigmented spindle cell Dermal Expansile nodule of spindle cells	Melanoma, pigmented spindle cell type
3. Spindle cell with schwannian/perineurial differentiation Dermal Neurofibroma-like tumor Schwannoma	Malignant peripheral nerve sheath tumor
4. Small round cell Dermal Expansile nodule of small cells	Small cell melanoma ("lymphoblastic" type)
5. Specific mesenchymal ("ectomesenchymal") differentiation Cartilage Lipoma Hemangioma	Rhabdomyosarcoma
6. Neuronal elements Ganglioneuroma	Ganglioneuroblastoma
7. Unclassified or undifferentiated neoplasms	Undifferentiated sarcoma

Source: Adapted from Hendrickson and Ross.[34]

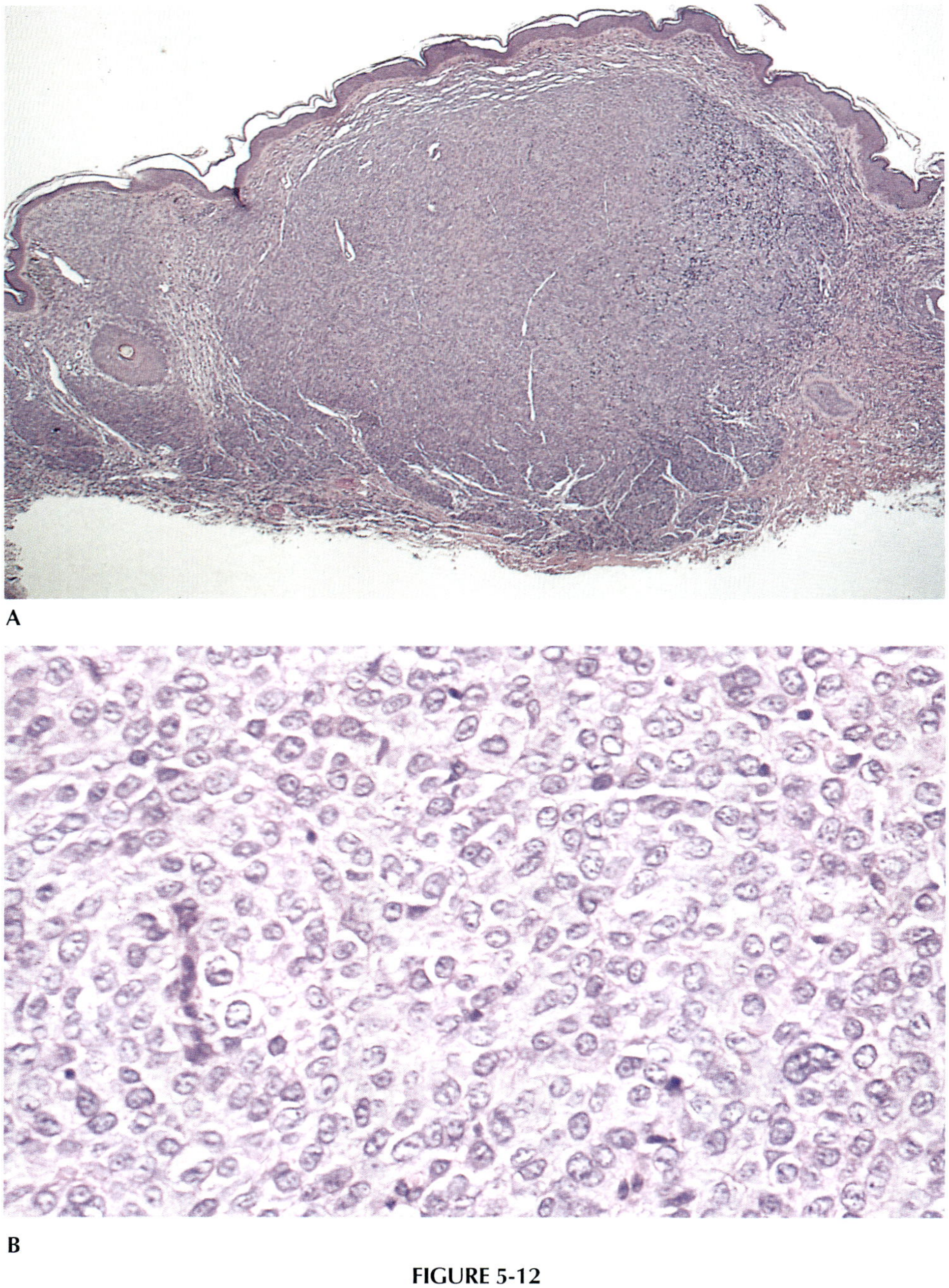

FIGURE 5-12

Atypical nodular proliferation in congenital nevus. (A) Compact nodule in superficial dermis (H&E, × 40). (B) Higher magnification of part A showing monotypic cells with relatively little cytoplasm. This proliferation simulates nevoid melanoma. Careful monitoring of patients with such lesions is needed (H&E, × 400).

large/giant CMN.[36,37] The great majority of melanomas developing in the latter setting are dermal and composed of epithelioid cells, spindle cells, or small round cells resembling malignant lymphoma[7,8,36–38] (Fig. 5-14 and Table 5-12). Some melanomas may have the characteristics of malignant blue nevus or malignant epithelioid schwannoma.[36,39] Such tumors usually manifest cohesive cellular nodules distinctly different from the surrounding nevus, substantial nuclear pleomorphism, necrotic cells, mitotic activity, and striking cellularity.[36–38] Interpretation of such tumors may be exceedingly difficult, and it may not always be possible to arrive at a final diagnosis of benign or malignant tumor. As already mentioned, melanoma in newborns and infants under 1 year of age is rare and must always be

TABLE 5-11
Précis: Melanoma Originating in Relatively Small Congenital Nevi (< 10 cm)

Clinical features	
	Onset after puberty
	Peak ages—20–30 and 50–60 years
	Melanoma often develops at periphery of CMN
	CMN relatively flat
Histopathology	
	Virtually all melanomas have intraepidermal origin
	Superficial spreading and nodular melanomas most common types
	CMN mostly involve upper two-thirds or half of dermis

TABLE 5-12
Précis: Melanoma Originating in Large/Giant Congenital Nevi

Clinical features	
	Onset most commonly in first decade (~60%) but at any age
	Median age 5 years
	Mean age 8.6 years
	True biologic melanoma rare or almost nonexistent under 1 year of age
	Development of or enlarging cutaneous nodule
	Darkening or lightening of skin
Histopathology	
	Majority originate in dermis
	Expansile tumors composed of epithelioid cells, spindle cells, or small round cells

seriouslyquestioned.[37,38] Furthermore, the vast majority of epithelioid and spindle cell nodular proliferations developing in CMN, particularly in young individuals, are benign or not aggressive[29,37,38] (see Figs. 5-8 to 5-12). Thus the pathologist should be cautious in rendering a diagnosis of melanoma in the latter circumstances. A prudent approach is to ensure complete surgical removal of such nodular lesions and to monitor the patient carefully for recurrence or metastasis. On the other hand, many of the true biologic forms of melanoma arising in giant CMN are of the small cell type[7,8,36–38] (see Fig. 5-14). The cells forming such melanomas are disposed in sheets in a delicate myxoid stroma.[8,36] The cells are closely crowded, have minimal cytoplasm, and contain small round or slightly oval nuclei with dense, uniformly dispersed chromatin. The cells take on the appearance of lymphoblastic lymphoma or comparable "blastic" tumors (see Fig. 5-14B). Mitotic figures and nuclear debris are also commonly observed.

OTHER MESENCHYMAL TUMORS

As delineated by Hendrickson and Ross,[36] giant CMN may exhibit specific mesenchymal differentiation and rarely give rise to hamartomatous mesenchymal tumors containing cartilage, vascular channels, and other elements.[36] Rarely, liposarcoma, rhabdomyosarcoma, ganglioneuroblastoma, and other primitive sarcomas have been reported to arise in giant congenital nevi.[8,36,40]

LEPTOMENINGEAL MELANOCYTOSIS (NEUROCUTANEOUS MELANOSIS)

CMN, not necessarily large or giant, involving the scalp, neck, or posterior midline may be associated with melanocytic proliferations localized to the cranial and/or spinal leptomeninges[7–19] (Table 5-13). Histologically, aggregates of melanocytes are present in the basal subarachnoid cisterns. The latter lesion may be asymptomatic or result in hydrocephalus, either communicating or noncommunicating type, seizures, mental retardation, other neurologic signs, and leptomeningeal melanoma. Meningeal biopsy may be necessary to confirm a diagnosis of leptomeningeal melanocytosis.

FOCAL MELANOCYTIC AGGREGATES IN SKIN, PLACENTA, AND LYMPH NODES ASSOCIATED WITH LARGE/GIANT CONGENITAL NEVI

There have been occasional reports of melanocytic lesions or satellites identified in the skin (Fig. 5-15), placenta, and lymph nodes of patients with large/giant CMN.[41–44] Explanations for these peculiar lesions have included arrested or aberrant migration of neural crest elements during embryogenesis and benign metastases from the large CMN. There is evidence supporting both hypotheses. Further investigation is needed to establish the pathogenesis of these lesions.

TABLE 5-13
Précis: Leptomeningeal Melanocytosis Associated with Congenital Melanocytic Nevi (Neurocutaneous Melanosis)

Cranial or spinal leptomeningeal involvement
Scalp, neck, or posterior midline CMN
Hydrocephalus, communicating or noncommunicating type
Seizures
Neurologic signs
Mental retardation
Meningeal melanoma

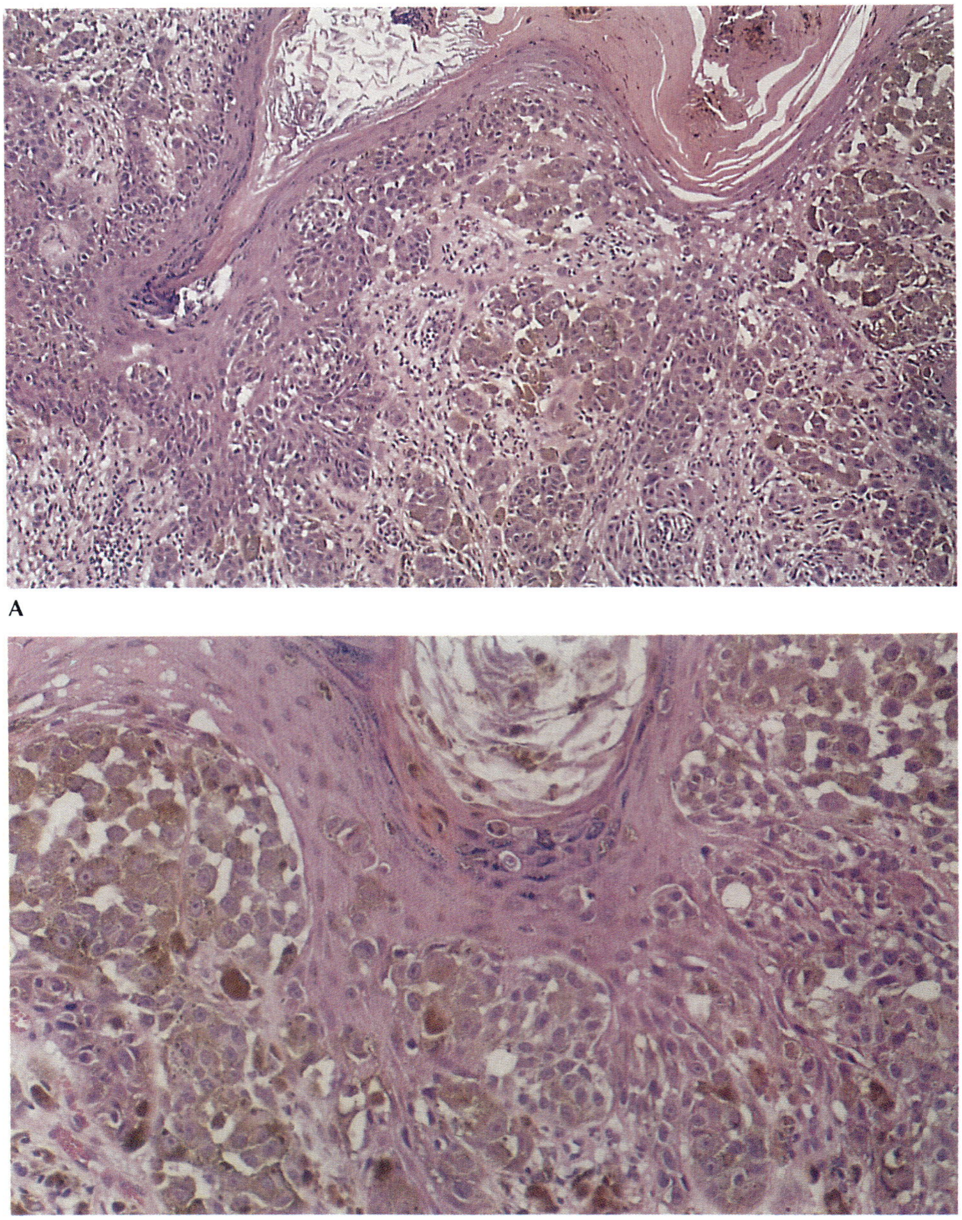

A

B

FIGURE 5-13

Melanoma arising from intraepidermal component of small congenital nevus. (A) The lesion exhibits pagetoid spread and invasion of dermis (H&E, × 100). (B) High magnification of part A showing large intraepidermal nests of melanoma cells with pagetoid spread (H&E, × 200).

DIFFERENTIAL DIAGNOSIS

The differential diagnosis for small CMN less than 1.5 cm in diameter is primarily that of acquired melanocytic nevi and dysplastic nevi. Since there are no specific features for small CMN histologically, the distinction from acquired nevi often rests on documentation at birth. Acquired dysplastic nevi are superficial proliferations that often involve the papillary dermis resulting in a compound nevus (see Chap. 9).

One particular problem associated with CMN is the presence of prominent upward migration of melanocytic cells throughout the epidermis in congenital nevi of

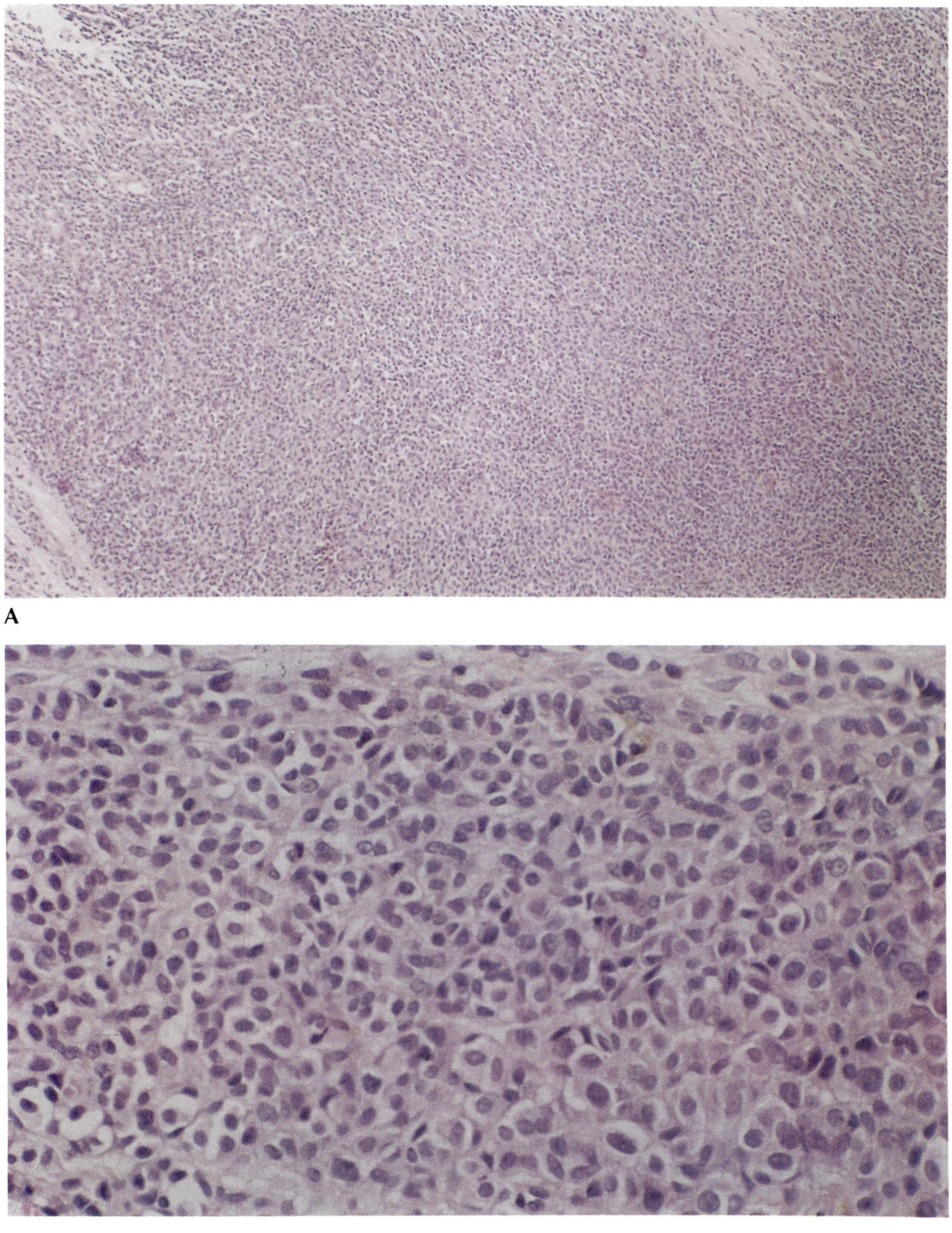

FIGURE 5-14

Small cell melanoma arising in dermal component of congenital nevus. (A) Diffuse sheet of small cells in deep dermis (H&E, × 100). (B) Uniform population of cells resembling lymphoma. The patient died of metastases (H&E, × 400).

children and particularly neonates. These proliferations suggest melanoma in situ or even invasive melanoma (see Fig. 5-7). However, in general, the pattern within the epidermis has an orderly character, and many of the cells do not reach the granular layer. Furthermore, careful examination will reveal low-grade or no cytologic atypia of these cells. In our experience and in the experience of others, virtually all these proliferations are benign.

Another diagnostic difficulty is the distinction of tumoral dermal nodules in large CMN from melanoma. Relatively small nodules generally measuring less than 1 cm in greatest diameter are common in giant CMN. These

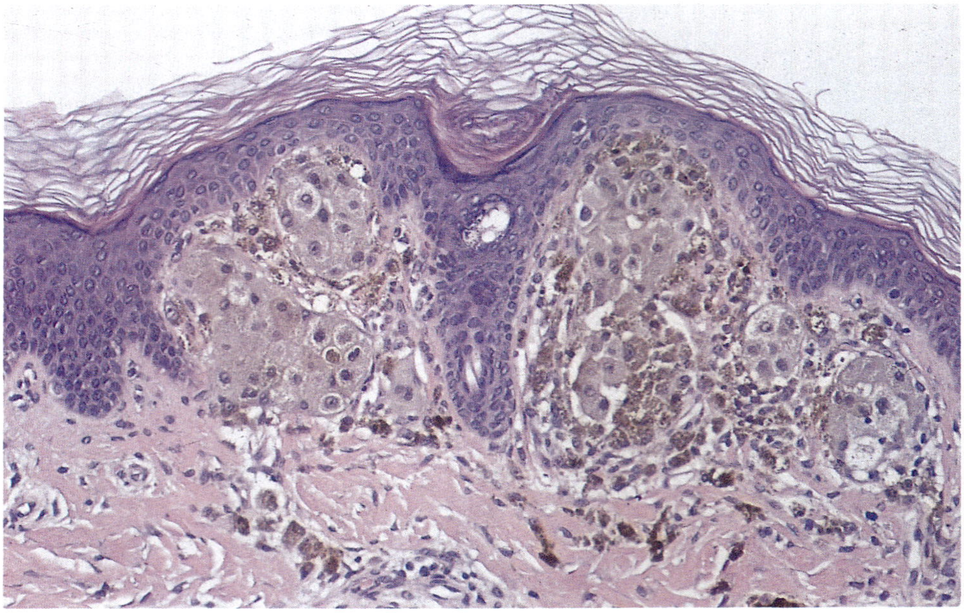

A

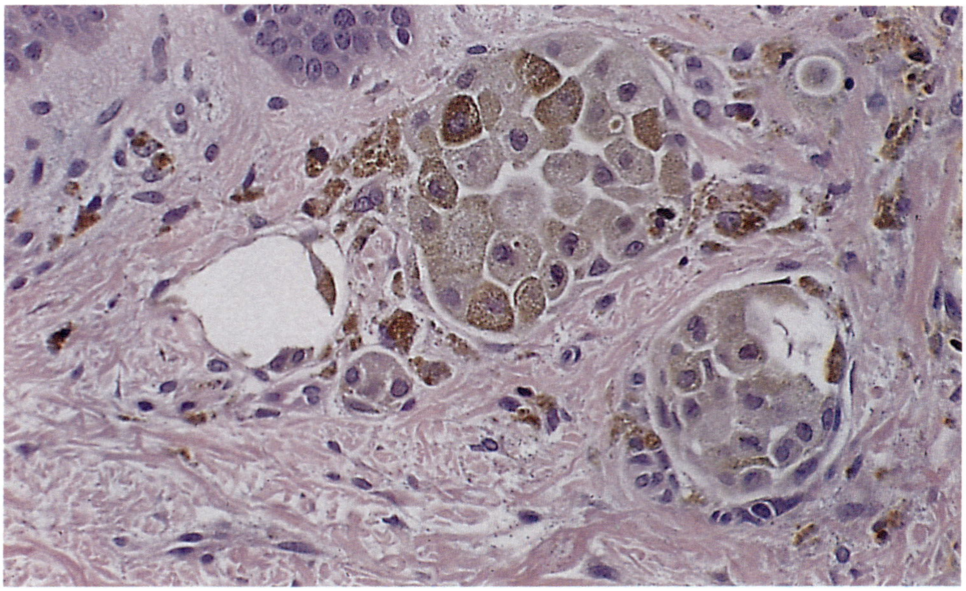

B

FIGURE 5-15

Cutaneous satellite lesion in newborn with medium-sized congenital nevus and atypical nodular proliferation. (A) Well-circumscribed nodular aggregate of atypical epithelioid cells in papillary dermis suggesting metastasis (H&E, × 200). (B) Another satellite lesion in papillary dermis suggesting lymphatic invasion. Such lesions are possibly explained by benign metastases or aberrant migration of neural crest–derived cells (H&E, × 400).

TABLE 5-14
Variants of Congenital Melanoma and Summary of Patients Reported

	No. of Patients	Sex	Location of Melanoma	Outcome
Transplacental metastatic melanoma from maternal source	3	M	Widespread visceral metastases	3 infants dead (within 1 year) 3 mothers dead (from metastatic melanoma)
De novo melanoma	8	7M, 1F	Head and neck 3 Trunk 2 Extremities 3	2 dead (4 to 7 months) 6 alive (follow-up 1 to 18 years)
Melanoma arising in large/giant congenital nevus	12	6M, 6F	Trunk 10 Genitalia 1 Head 1	5 dead 6 alive 1 unknown

nodules exhibit compact cellularity, and the constituent cells are usually larger and exhibit variable degrees of cytologic atypia (see Figs. 5-8 to 5-12). The distinction from melanoma relates to the gradual blending of the cellular nodule with the surrounding nevus cells in the dermis. The presence of an abrupt margin between the tumor nodule and the surrounding nevus is abnormal and suggests melanoma. The presence of necrotic cells, significant cytologic atypia, and easily found mitotic activity are also features suggesting melanoma. Age is a significant factor to be considered in the evaluation of these proliferations. A diagnosis of melanoma should be made with extreme caution in individuals under the age of 1 year.[29,37,38]

RISK FACTORS FOR THE DEVELOPMENT OF MELANOMA IN CMN

Potential risk factors for the development of melanoma in CMN have not been systematically studied. Such variables might include overall size or surface area (perhaps correlating with total number of nevus cells present), evidence of hypopigmentation or regression, intraepidermal or dermal melanocytic proliferations with architectural disorder and cytologic atypia, and other variables such as DNA aneuploidy and the expression of cell surface antigens.[45–47] Atypical melanocytic proliferations would seem to correlate with increased melanoma risk but have not been sufficiently investigated as markers of elevated melanoma risk. Abnormal DNA content has been reported in CMN and to have a higher prevalence in large/giant CMN versus small CMN.[45–47] However, whether DNA aneuploidy is associated with elevated melanoma risk in CMN has not been established. The expression of two or more cell surface (progression-associated melanoma) antigens in CMN has been correlated with progression to melanoma in a series of 36 CMN.[47]

CONGENITAL MELANOMA

The presence of malignant melanoma at birth is exceedingly rare and may be classified into three varieties[48–50] (Table 5-14). The first type, of which only three cases have been reported (reviewed in Trozak et al.[49]), is characterized by maternal melanoma metastatic to the fetus.[51] Neonates usually present at birth with widespread visceral metastases and are dead of disease within days to months. The placenta usually shows gross and histopathologic evidence of metastatic melanoma in such cases. Primary congenital melanoma is also vanishingly rare and may develop de novo or in association with a giant congenital nevus. Only eight cases of de novo congenital melanoma have been reported[49,52–59] (see Table 5-14). Among this small group of patients, only two succumbed to the melanoma. Congenital melanoma developing in giant congenital nevi also has been described in a small number of patients[26,50,60–66] (see Table 5-14). Only five such patients have died from disseminated melanoma.

Because of the small number of primary congenital melanomas reported and only very limited descriptions of their histopathologic features or none at all, it is not possible to make any definitive statements about primary congenital melanoma. However, it should be emphasized that because of the extreme rarity of these lesions, a diagnosis of congenital or neonatal melanoma must be viewed with considerable skepticism.[29] Virtually all such lesions are biologically benign. Examination of these highly atypical tumors with reference to karyotype, expression of cell surface antigens, growth in soft agar, and other parameters has shown that they have the properties of an immature proliferative but benign tumor.[37,64] DNA image analysis of a similar congenital tumor associated with a CMN has failed to show any evidence of abnormal DNA content (Schmidt BS, Barnhill RL, unpublished observations, 1992).

TABLE 5-15
Précis: Melanoma in Individuals less than 20 Years of Age

Clinical features	
Males = females	
Mean age 16 years	
Very few cases under age 10 years/puberty	
Distribution similar to adults	
Head and neck	21.8%
Extremities	39.7%
Trunk	37.2%
Clinical characteristics similar to adult patients	
Histopathology	
Similar to adult melanomas	
Lentigo maligna	1.5%
Superficial spreading	67.2%
Nodular	23.4%
Acral lentiginous	7.8%
Ulceration	14.1%
Tumor thickness mean 1.76 mm (range 0.32 to 5.22 mm)	
Differential diagnosis	
Spitz nevus	
Other melanocytic nevi	
Prognosis	
Similar to adults	
Five-year actuarial survival 76%	

Source: Reintgen et al.[74]

CHILDHOOD MELANOMA

The incidence of melanoma increases with age but is exceptionally rare in prepubertal individuals (estimated incidence approximately 0.4 percent among all melanomas)[67,68] and uncommon under the age of 20 years (incidence approximately 2 percent).[69] With the realization that many cases of childhood melanoma in the past had been considered spindle and epithelioid cell (Spitz) nevi, it has become evident that malignant melanoma is much less common and has no better prognosis in children compared with adults.[48,70–74] Analysis of melanomas in individuals under the age of 20 years shows fairly similar clinical and histologic features compared with melanomas in adults[69,74] (Table 5-15). It should be noted, however, that there are too few cases of melanoma reported in prepubescent children to make any definitive statements about melanomas in this age group. It will be necessary to obtain such information from multiple centers or through a central registry.

REFERENCES

1. Mark GJ, Mihm MC, Liteplo MG, et al: Congenital melanocytic nevi of the small and garment type. *Hum Pathol* 4:395–418, 1973.
2. Walton RG, Jacobs AH, Cox AJ: Pigmented lesions in newborn infants. *Br J Dermatol* 95:389–396, 1976.
3. Cramer SF: The melanocytic differentiation pathway in congenital melanocytic nevi: Theoretical considerations. *Pediatr Pathol* 8:253–265, 1988.
4. Stenn KS, Arons M, Hurwitz S: Patterns of congenital nevocellular nevi. *J Am Acad Dermatol* 9:388–393, 1983.
5. Rhodes AR, Silberman RA, Harrist TJ, Melski JW: A histologic comparison of congenital and acquired nevomelanocytic nevi. *Arch Dermatol* 121:1266–1273, 1985.
6. Everett MA: Histopathology of congenital pigmented nevi. *Am J Dermatopathol* 11:11–12, 1989.
7. Reed WB, Becker SW Sr, Becker SW Jr, Nickel WR: Giant pigmented nevi, melanoma, and leptomeningeal melanocytosis. *Arch Dermatol* 91:100–118, 1965.
8. Reed RJ: Giant congenital nevi: A conceptualization of patterns. *J Invest Dermatol* 100 (Suppl):300S–312S, 1993.
9. Rhodes AR: Neoplasms, benign neoplasias, hyperplasias, and dysplasia of melanocytes. In Fitzpatrick TB, Eisen AZ, Wolff K, Freedberg IM, Austen KF (eds): *Dermatology in General Medicine* (ed 4). New York, McGraw-Hill, 1993, pp 1026–1037.
10. Pers AFM: Naevus pigmentosus giganticus: Indikationer for operative Behandling. *Ungeskrift Laeger* 125:613–619, 1963.
11. Lorentzen M, Pers M, Bretteville-Jensen G: The incidence of malignant transformation in giant pigmented nevi. *Scand J Plast Reconstr Surg* 71:163–167, 1977.
12. Lanier VC Jr, Pickrell KL, Georgiade NG: Congenital giant nevi: Clinical and pathologic considerations. *Plast Reconstr Surg* 58:48–54, 1976.
13. Greeley PW, Middleton AG, Curtin JW: Incidence of malignancy in giant pigmented nevi. *Plast Reconstr Surg* 36:26–37, 1965.
14. Pilney FT, Broadbent TR, Woolf RM: Giant pigmented nevus of the face: Surgical management. *Plast Reconstr Surg* 40:469–474, 1967.
15. Kopf AW, Bart RS, Hennessey P: Congenital nevocytic nevi and malignant melanoma. *J Am Acad Dermatol* 1:123–130, 1979.
16. NIH Consensus Conference: Precursor to malignant melanoma. *JAMA* 251:1864–1866, 1984.
17. Kaplan EN: The risk of malignancy in large congenital nevi. *Plast Reconstr Surg* 53:421–428, 1974.
18. Rhodes AR, Wood WC, Sober AJ, Mihm MC Jr: Nonepidermal origin of malignant melanoma associated with a giant congenital nevocellular nevus. *Plast Reconstr Surg* 67:782–790, 1981.
19. Rhodes AR, Sober AJ, Day CL, et al: The malignant potential of small congenital nevocellular nevi: An estimate of association based on a histologic study of 234 primary cutaneous melanomas. *J Am Acad Dermatol* 6:230–241, 1982.
20. Rhodes AR, Melski JW: Small congenital nevocellular nevi and the risk of cutaneous melanoma. *J Pediatr* 100:219–224, 1982.
21. Illig L, Weidner F, Hundeiker M, et al: Congenital nevi less than or equal to 10 cm as precursors to melanoma: 52 cases, a review, and a new conception. *Arch Dermatol* 121:1274–1281, 1985.
22. Castilla EE, da Graca Dutra M, Orioli-Parreiras IM: Epidemiology of congenital pigmented naevi: I. Incidence rates and relative frequencies. *Br J Dermatol* 104:307–315, 1981.

23. Kroon S, Clemmensen OJ, Hastrup N: Incidence of congenital melanocytic nevi in newborn babies in Denmark. *J Am Acad Dermatol* 17:422–426, 1987.
24. Hamming N: Anatomy and embryology of the eyelids: A review with special reference to the development of divided nevi. *Pediatr Dermatol* 1:51–58, 1983.
25. Rhodes AR, Slifman NR, Korf BR: Familial aggregation of small congenital nevomelanocytic nevi. *Am J Med Genet* 22:315–326, 1985.
26. Pack GT, Davis J: Nevus giganticus pigmentosus with malignant transformation. *Surgery* 49:347–354, 1961.
27. Solomon L, Eng AM, Bené M, Loeffel D: Giant congenital neuroid melanocytic nevus. *Arch Dermatol* 116:318–320, 1980.
28. Albert VA, Barnhill RL, Sober AJ: Leukoderma in association with giant congenital nevi: Report of 2 cases. *Dermatology* 185:140–142, 1992.
29. Fleischli M, Barnhill RL: Histologic features of congenital melanocytic nevi less than a year of age (abstract). *J Cutan Pathol* 20:541, 1993.
30. Silvers DN, Helwig EB: Melanocytic nevi in neonates. *J Am Acad Dermatol* 4:166–175, 1981.
31. Zitelli JA, Grant MG, Abell E, Boyd JB: Histologic patterns of congenital nevocytic nevi and implications for treatment. *J Am Acad Dermatol* 11:402–409, 1984.
32. Nickoloff BJ, Walton R, Pregerson-Rodan K, et al: Immunohistologic patterns of congenital nevocellular nevi. *Arch Dermatol* 122:1263–1268, 1986.
33. Rhodes AR: Congenital nevomelanocytic nevi: Histologic patterns in the first year of life and evolution during childhood. *Arch Dermatol* 122:1257–1262, 1986.
34. Clemmensen OJ, Kroon S: The histology of "congenital features" in early acquired melanocytic nevi. *J Am Acad Dermatol* 19:742–746, 1988.
35. Walsh MY, MacKie RM: Histologic features of value in differentiating small congenital melanocytic nevi from acquired naevi. *Histopathology* 12:145–154, 1988.
36. Hendrickson MR, Ross JC: Neoplasms arising in congenital giant nevi: Morphologic study of seven cases and a review of the literature. *Am J Surg Pathol* 5:109–135, 1981.
37. Mancianti ML, Clark WH, Hayes FA, Herlyn M: Malignant melanoma simulants arising in congenital melanocytic nevi do not show experimental evidence for a malignant phenotype. *Am J Pathol* 136:817–829, 1990.
38. Clark WH Jr, Elder DE, Guerry D IV: Dysplastic nevi and malignant melanoma. In Farmer ER, Hood AF (eds): *Pathology of the Skin.* Norwalk, Conn, Appleton and Lange, 1990, pp 684–756.
39. Weidner N, Flanders DJ, Jochimsen PR, Stamler FW: Neurosarcomatous malignant melanoma arising in a neuroid giant congenital melanocytic nevus. *Arch Dermatol* 121:1302–1306, 1985.
40. Zúniga SR, Las Heras J, Benvenisto S: Rhabdomyosarcoma arising in a congenital nevus associated with neurocutaneous melanosis in an neonate. *J Pediatr Surg* 22:1036–1038, 1987.
41. Demian SDE, Donnelly WH, Frias JL, Monif GRG: Placental lesions in congenital giant pigmented nevi. *Am J Clin Pathol* 61:438–442, 1974.
42. Sotelo-Avila C, Graham M, Hanby DE, Rudolph AJ: Nevus cell aggregates in the placenta: A histochemical and electron microscopic study. *Am J Clin Pathol* 89:395–400, 1988.
43. Jauniaux E, de Meeus M-C, Verellen G, et al: Giant congenital melanocytic nevus with placental involvement: Long-term follow-up of a case and review of the literature. *Pediatr Pathol* 13:717–721, 1993.
44. Hara K: Melanocytic lesions in lymph nodes associated with congenital naevus. *Histopathology* 23:445–451, 1993.
45. Stenziger W, Suter L, Schumann J: DNA aneuploidy in congenital melanocytic nevi: Suggestive evidence for premalignant changes. *J Invest Dermatol* 82:569–572, 1984.
46. Newton JA, Camplejohn RS, McGibbon DH: The flow cytometry of melanocytic skin lesions. *Br J Cancer* 58:606–610, 1988.
47. Steijlen PM, Hamm H, van Erp PEJ, et al: Immunohistologic evidence for the malignant potential of congenital melanocytic nevi. *J Invest Dermatol* 92:366–370, 1989.
48. Skov-Jensen T, Hastrup J, Lambrethsen E: Malignant melanoma in children. *Cancer* 19:620–626, 1966.
49. Trozak DJ, Rowland WD, Hu F: Metastatic malignant melanoma in prepubertal children. *Pediatrics* 55:191–204, 1975.
50. Roth ME, Grant-Kels JM, Kuhn K, et al: Melanoma in children. *J Am Acad Dermatol* 22:265–274, 1990.
51. Potter JF, Schoeneman M: Metastasis of maternal cancer to the placenta and fetus. *Cancer* 25:380–388, 1970.
52. Coe HE: Malignant pigmented mole in an infant. *Northwest Med* 24:181, 1925.
53. Lyall D: Malignant melanoma in infancy. *JAMA* 202:1153, 1967.
54. Oldhoff J, Koudstall J: Congenital papillomatous malignant melanoma of the skin. *Cancer* 21:1193–1197, 1968.
55. Conn A, Nicolescu F, Popescu G: Malignant melanoma developing in intrauterine life. *Rom Med Rev* 15:41–42, 1971.
56. Voinov EA, Semskov VS, Maleskina LA: Case of congenital skin melanoma. *Arkh Patol* 35:78–80, 1973.
57. Stromberg BV: Malignant melanoma in children. *J Pediatr Surg* 14:465–467, 1979.
58. Hayes FA, Green AA: Malignant melanoma in childhood: Clinical course and response to chemotherapy. *J Clin Oncol* 2:1229–1234, 1984.
59. Prose NS, Laude TA, Heilman ER, Coren C: Congenital malignant melanoma. *Pediatrics* 79:967–970, 1987.
60. Fish J, Smith EB, Canby JP: Malignant melanoma in childhood. *Pediatr Surg* 59:309–315, 1966.
61. Sweet LK, Connerty HV: Congenital melanoma: Report of a case in which antenatal metastasis occurred. *Am J Dis Child* 62:1029–1040, 1941.
62. Borges AF, Lineberger AS: Malignant melanoma without metastasis in a giant nevus. *Ann Plast Surg* 12:454–460, 1984.
63. Schneiderman H, Wu AY-Y, Campbell WA, et al: Congenital melanoma with multiple prenatal metastases. *Cancer* 60:1371–1377, 1987.
64. Angelucci D, Natali PG, Amerio PL, et al: Rapid perinatal growth mimicking malignant transformation in a giant congenital melanocytic nevus. *Hum Pathol* 22:297–301, 1991.
65. Baader W, Kropp R, Tapper D: Congenital malignant melanoma. *Plast Reconstr Surg* 90:53–56, 1992.

66. Workman ML, Kaye VN, Anderson PM, Cunningham BL: Malignant melanoma with evidence of maturation arising from a giant congenital nevocellular nevus. *Ann Plast Surg* 28:381–385, 1992.
67. Mahre E: Malignant melanomas in children. *Arch Pathol Microbiol Scand* 59:184–193, 1963.
68. Boddie AW, Smith L, McBride CM: Malignant melanoma in children and young adults. *South Med J* 71:1074–1078, 1978.
69. Bader JL, Li FP, Olmstead PM, et al: Childhood malignant melanoma: Incidence and etiology. *Am J Pediatr Hematol Oncol* 7:341–345, 1985.
70. Malec E, Lagerlöf B: Malignant melanoma of the skin in children registered in the Swedish Cancer Registry during 1959–1971. *Scand J Plast Reconstr Surg* 11:125–129, 1977.
71. Pratt CB, Palmer MK, Thatcher N, Crowther D: Malignant melanoma in children and adolescents. *Cancer* 47:392–397, 1981.
72. Moss ALH, Briggs JC: Cutaneous malignant melanoma in the young. *Br J Plast Surg* 39:537–541, 1986.
73. Partoft S, Østerlind A, Hou-Jensen K, Drzewiecki KT: Malignant melanoma of the skin in children (0 to 14 years of age) in Denmark, 1943–1982. *Scand J Plast Reconstr Surg* 23:55–58, 1989.
74. Reintgen DS, Vollmer R, Seigler HF: Juvenile malignant melanoma. *Surg Gynecol Obstet* 168:249–253, 1989.

6

Spitz Nevi and Variants

SPITZ NEVUS

Synonyms: Spitz's nevus, Spitz tumor, spindle and epithelioid cell nevus of large spindle and/or epithelioid cells, spindle cell nevus, juvenile melanoma, benign juvenile melanoma

The spindle and epithelioid cell nevus, commonly referred to as *Spitz nevus,* is a melanocytic, usually acquired nevus with a distinct histopathologic appearance. The characteristics that set this nevus apart from other nevi are the presence of large epithelioid and/or spindle cells in varying proportions. The lesion is frequently misdiagnosed as malignant melanoma.

Terminology

Examples of melanocytic tumors resembling malignant melanoma on gross and microscopic appearance but behaving clinically in a benign manner were first described by Darier and Civatte[1] in 1910 and Miescher[2] in 1933. The discrepancy between histologic features that were at that time thought to represent melanoma and the benign clinical behavior was noted especially in children. This led Pack and Anglem[3] to develop the concept of "prepubertal melanoma." They used this term for melanocytic tumors, which histologically mimicked melanoma but failed to metastasize. Spitz's major contribution was to establish histologic criteria to distinguish such lesions, which she termed *juvenile melanoma,* from true metastasizing melanoma.[4] In her original series of childhood melanomas, the presence of giant cells was highlighted as the single most distinctive feature favoring the diagnosis of a juvenile tumor.

Subsequently, it became apparent that lesions clinically and histologically similar to those described by Spitz occurred also in adults, although less frequently.[5,6] The concept of a distinct type of benign melanocytic tumor which was different from other known nevi emerged. The original term used by Spitz, *juvenile melanoma,* and its modification by Kopf and Andrade,[7] *benign juvenile melanoma,* were ultimately abandoned because the term *melanoma* indicated malignancy and the lesion also could be found in adults.[6] A number of alternative terms have been proposed to name this lesion. Helwig[8] suggested *spindle and epithelioid cell nevus.* This name emphasizes the distinct cell types of this nevus and is widely accepted. The term *nevus of large spindle and/or epithelioid cells*[9] has been proposed as a more precise name, since the spectrum of cytologic appearances of this nevus includes not only an admixture of both cell types but also exclusively spindle or epithelioid cells. However, this term appears too long and cumbersome for routine diagnostic use. The term *Spitz nevus* seems reasonable because of its simplicity. This nondescriptive term allows one to include a spectrum of similar albeit variable histomorphology and does not carry misleading connotations.

Since the early descriptions of Spitz nevi, it has become apparent that variants exist which share certain features with Spitz nevi but are distinct enough to justify a separate terminology. Of these, desmoplastic Spitz nevus and pigmented spindle cell nevus are included in this chapter.

The term *spitzoid* or *spitzian* is often used when lesions resemble Spitz nevi in one way or another but lack sufficient other features needed for diagnosis as Spitz nevus.

Spitzoid features have been described in melanomas as well as in congenital and dysplastic nevi.

Epidemiology

Spitz nevi are relatively uncommon. Epidemiologic data regarding their incidence, age distribution, sex preference, and geographic or ethnic predilection are scarce. Their annual incidence in Queensland, Australia, was estimated to be 1.4 cases per 100,000 people compared with 25.4 cases per 100,000 people for cutaneous melanoma.[10] Most cases are diagnosed in children or adolescents. In a series of 262 patients with Spitz nevi in 1960, 85 percent were infants and children.[11] In later series reported in the 1970s, the proportion of adult patients over 20 years of age was larger, reaching 20 to 30 percent of the cases.[9,10,12] However, in these later series, there is probably a referral bias leading to an overrepresentation of adult patients.[13] Although most Spitz nevi are acquired, congenital Spitz nevi occur[14,15] and may account for as many as 7 percent of cases. Spitz nevi are uncommon but do occur in individuals beyond the ages of 40 to 50 years.[12]

There is no obvious sexual predilection, although most reports indicate a slight female preponderance, especially in young adults.[13] It has been suggested that the female preponderance of Spitz nevi in this age group may reflect the greater likelihood of their removal for cosmetic purposes.[9] Most published cases of Spitz nevi have been described primarily in Caucasians.[13] Spitz nevi are thought to be rare in blacks and Asians.[9,13]

Familial aggregation of Spitz nevi has been reported in identical twin boys,[7] but the role of genetic factors has not been investigated systematically. It is believed that the great majority of Spitz nevi are sporadic with unknown etiology.

Clinical Features

Anatomic Site. Spitz nevus may occur anywhere on the body. However, there is a predilection for the face, especially the cheeks, and the lower extremities.[6,11,16] In a large series of solitary Spitz nevi,[17] 30 percent of 652 lesions were located on the lower extremities, 26 percent on the head, and 25 percent on the upper extremities. Most series report a female preponderance for lesions from the lower extremities.[13]

Appearance and Presentation. Spitz nevi may present in a number of different ways. The most common form, typically observed in children, is that of a solitary, asymptomatic, red/pink or flesh-colored, hairless, dome-shaped nodule.[13,18] Some lesions may be tan, brown, or even black in color. Pigmentation tends to be seen more often in adolescents and adults.[16,19] The surface appearance is usually smooth but may be verrucous. Pedunculated and polypoid forms have been described,[7] and telangiectasia may be noted.[7] Scale-crust, erosion, and ulceration are uncommon and, when present, generally reflect exogenous trauma.[10] While in children the nodules tend to be slightly soft, in adults they are more often firm.[9,18] Borders are usually sharp but may be irregular. In one series, 73 percent of cases had lesions measuring less than 0.6 cm, and in 94 percent the lesions were less than 1 cm in size,[10] although sizes up to 3 cm have been reported rarely.[11] Some Spitz nevi are pruritic and tender.[13] The duration of solitary Spitz nevus is usually less than 9 months[13] but may vary from 1 month to more than 20 years.

Biologic Course. The natural history of Spitz nevi has not been clearly delineated. As previously mentioned, a small percentage of these lesions are present at birth, and some acquired ones are long-standing. Although there has been speculation that these lesions involute as do conventional nevi[20] or possibly evolve to conventional nevi, these outcomes have not been documented. In most instances, there is a clinical history of recent onset or change. The vast majority of lesions with characteristics of Spitz nevi are benign. However, because of the histologic resemblance of Spitz nevi to some melanomas, the presence of atypical variants, and occasional metastases from such lesions, there is some justification for the belief that uncommonly or rarely melanoma may develop in association with Spitz nevi. The exact nature and classification of these lesions await definitive study. An aggressive variant termed *malignant Spitz nevus* has been reported to result in regional lymph node metastases (see below).[21]

Multiple Spitz Nevi

Multiple Spitz nevi have been reported to occur either in a grouped (agminate) or disseminated pattern.[22–25] The disseminated type is characterized by numerous (up to hundreds) Spitz tumors all over the body, typically sparing the palms, soles, and mucous membranes. Only a few cases have been reported to date, primarily affecting adults. In a review of 33 cases from the literature, 11 instances were reported in which multiple agminate Spitz nevi arose within a congenital circumscribed area of hyperpigmentation, most often described as a café-au-lait macule.[25] Multiple agminate Spitz nevi affected women nearly twice as often as men, tended to occur on average earlier in life (76 percent younger than 6 years of age) than solitary Spitz nevi, and showed a predilection for the face (50 percent of the cases), most often the cheeks. Some congenital forms have been reported.[15] Agminate Spitz nevi have been reported to follow trauma such as previous excision of a solitary Spitz nevus, sunburn, and radiation therapy.[26]

Clinical Differential Diagnoses

As the variety of presentations suggests, the clinical features of Spitz nevus are usually not distinctive enough to allow a correct diagnosis on clinical grounds alone. Weedon[13] reports that a correct clinical diagnosis is made in only about 20 percent of childhood cases and in less than 10 percent of adult lesions. The most frequent clinical diagnosis is that of a common acquired melanocytic nevus. In about 10 percent of cases, malignant melanoma is suspected. Other lesions, which may be mimicked by Spitz nevi on gross appearance and have been mentioned in the differential diagnoses of various series, include pyogenic granuloma, juvenile xanthogranuloma, dermatofibroma, verruca vulgaris, insect-bite granuloma, molluscum contagiosum, neurofibroma, adnexal tumors, and mastocytoma.[13]

Histopathology

Spitz nevi may be junctional, compound, or intradermal (Figs. 6-1 to 6-7). The majority (about two-thirds or more) are compound lesions (see Fig. 6-1). Between 5 and 10 percent of the cases are junctional[13,27] (see Fig. 6-7). Intradermal Spitz nevi account for approximately 12 to 20 percent of the lesions and are seen mainly in adults[13,27,28] (see Fig. 6-2).

The most distinctive histologic feature of Spitz nevus and an absolute prerequisite for its diagnosis is the presence of large epithelioid and/or spindle-shaped melanocytes or an admixture thereof[13] (see Fig. 6-3). A number of other features in addition to cell type, however, need to be assessed before a final diagnosis of Spitz nevus can be rendered.[9,10,13] Some of these features, such as symmetry or sharp lateral demarcation, bear more weight than others, such as retraction spaces or perivascular distribution of lymphocytic infiltrates. These features are summarized in Table 6-1.

Spindle and/or Epithelioid Cell Type. Spindle cell melanocytes in Spitz nevi are elongated, fusiform, and often plump (see Figs. 6-3B and 6-4A and C). Occasional tapered cytoplasmic processes resembling dendrites may be observed. They possess centrally located nuclei that are comparable in size with or even larger than nuclei of keratinocytes (see Fig. 6-4C). Nuclear contours are typically smooth and regular. The chromatin pattern is usually finely dispersed or slightly vesicular. Typically, a distinct, single, centrally located, round eosinophilic or amphophilic nucleolus is present. The cytoplasm is usually well developed with recognizable cytoplasmic borders. In most cases, the cytoplasm appears eosinophilic but may be bluish.

At the dermoepidermal junction, the spindle cells are arranged in fascicles or elongated nests, characteristically in vertical orientation to the epidermal surface and often adjacent to elongated rete ridges (see Fig. 6-3A). In some instances, the spindle cells have whorled or concentric arrangements within nests. Both the overall size of the nests and the size of the individual melanocytes within them are variable and tend to decrease in the deeper parts of the lesion. Melanocytes may be tightly packed or loosely aggregated within their nests and fascicles. In the dermis, the spindle cell melanocytes of Spitz nevi are also arranged in fascicles but may be more angulated in their orientation to the epidermal surface (Fig. 6-4B and C).

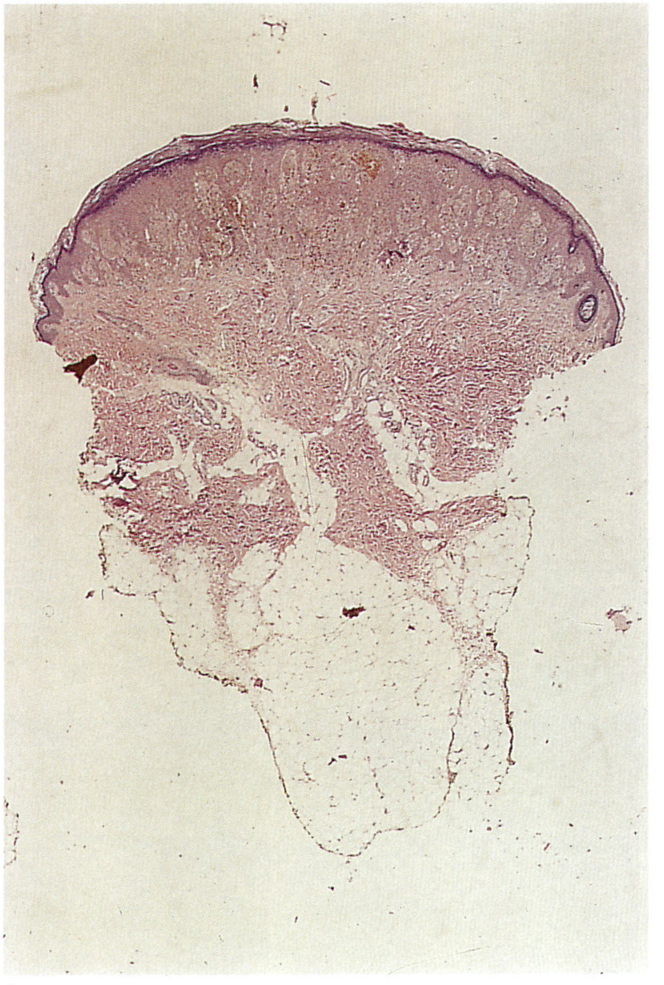

A

FIGURE 6-1

Spitz nevus (pigmented spindle and epithelioid cell nevus). (A) Note small size, dome-shaped morphology, striking symmetry, and sharp lateral demarcation (H&E, × 10). (B) Higher magnification of part A, again illustrates overall symmetry of lesion. There is moderate epidermal hyperplasia with a smooth surface topography (H&E, × 20). (C) Sharp lateral demarcation of nevus (H&E, × 100).

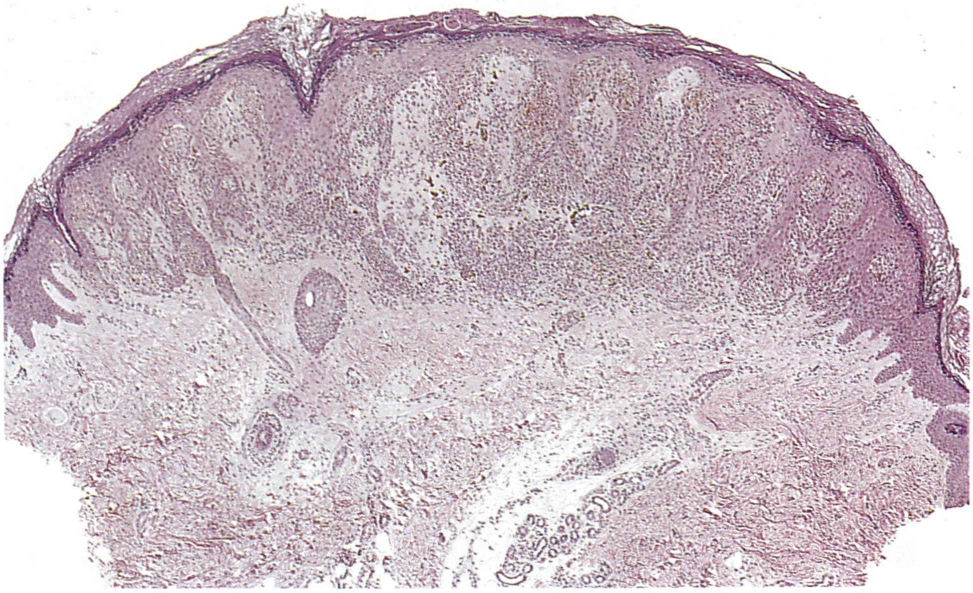

B

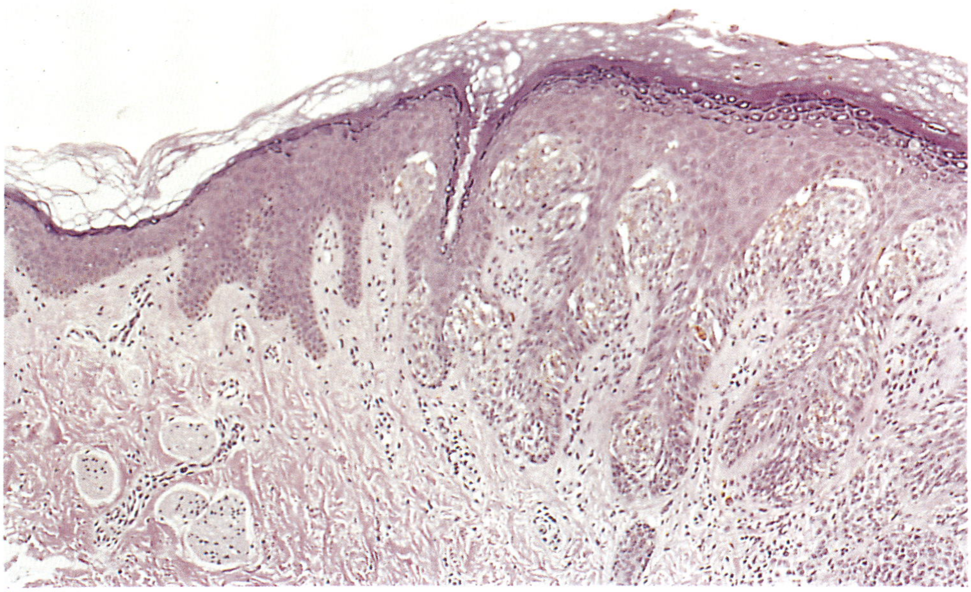

C

FIGURE 6-1 *(Continued)*

Their plumper appearance, their nuclear features, and their arrangement in vertically streaming fascicles make spindle cell melanocytes of Spitz nevi quite distinct from spindle cells of other nevi, such as the slender dendritic cells of blue nevi or the melanocytes with schwannian features (type C melanocytes) of common acquired nevi.

Epithelioid melanocytes in Spitz nevi are large, round, oval, polygonal, rhomboidal, or polyangular cells with distinct cellular borders (see Fig. 6-5A). Their nuclei are enlarged, round, oval, and sometimes irregularly shaped or lobulated. The nuclei have similar chromatin patterns as the spindle cell forms and also frequently show one large, centrally placed nucleolus. In some cases, the cytoplasmic and/or nuclear contours may become very irregular, leading to a pleomorphic appearance. This is particularly pronounced when large multinucleated forms are

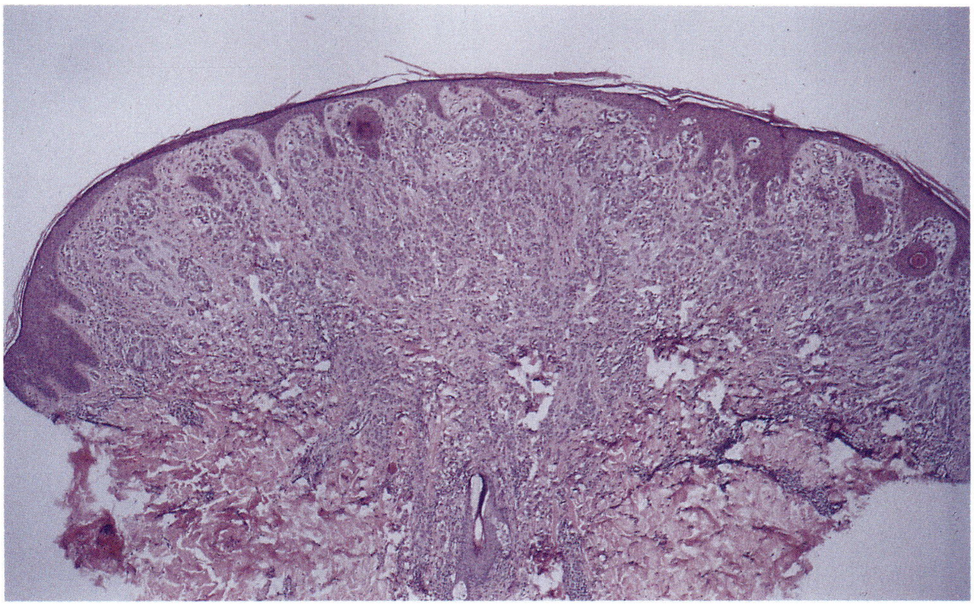

FIGURE 6-2
Spitz nevus, mainly dermal type. The lesion is notable for its dome-shaped profile, symmetry, and inverted wedgelike extension into the dermis (H&E, × 40).

present (see Fig. 6-3C). Such pleomorphism may be more striking than in melanoma but usually affects only a minority of cells. Multinucleated cells are often seen when epithelioid forms constitute the predominant cell type of a Spitz nevus. The cytoplasm of epithelioid cells is usually abundant with a homogeneous eosinophilic or bluish, sometimes ground-glass appearance. Melanin is typically absent or scarce.

The two cell types may be admixed in varying proportions, but either may occur alone. Regardless of the proportion of spindle or epithelioid cells, one of the most characteristic features of Spitz nevus is the uniformity of the cells and nuclei. From side to side in horizontal zones, the cells tend to show a strikingly uniform appearance and size. However, from top to bottom, despite maintaining a monotonous appearance, the cells and nuclei usually diminish in size (see "Maturation" below). In all age groups, Spitz nevi with predominant spindle cell morphology are the most common type, and they are especially prevalent in adults.[26] Spitz nevi of the epithelioid cell type are observed mainly in childhood. In one study, 89 percent of the tumors contained predominantly spindle cells and 11 percent primarily epithelioid cells.[10] Compound epithelioid-type Spitz nevi usually show small junctional nests, often consisting of only a few cells. In contrast, large junctional nests are often observed in predominantly spindle cell Spitz nevi.

While the presence of spindle and/or epithelioid cells is a prerequisite for the diagnosis of Spitz nevus, they must appear in an appropriate architectural arrangement before a final diagnosis of Spitz nevus can be made. The major architectural criteria are symmetry and sharp lateral demarcation. These criteria, which are thought to reflect ordered growth and favor benignancy, are not unique to Spitz nevi but also apply to the evaluation of other melanocytic nevi.

Symmetry. Symmetry is a feature assessed on scanning magnification (see Figs. 6-1A and 6-2). Symmetry in Spitz nevi is a symmetry from *side to side;* i.e., the halves of the lesion around a central vertical axis are similar to one another. Common architectural appearances on histologic sections that convey symmetry are those of a semicircle with the epidermal surface as convexity or a trapezoid whose width decreases from epidermal top to bottom in the dermis (see Fig. 6-2). The presence of symmetry is an important feature distinguishing Spitz nevus from melanoma, where uneven lateral and/or deep growth is common.

Sharp Lateral Demarcation. Sharp lateral demarcation is a characteristic feature of the junctional component of Spitz nevi (see Figs. 6-1A and B and 6-2). The impression of sharp demarcation is conveyed by the presence of nests rather than single cells at the lateral borders and by an abrupt transition from an epidermis with a

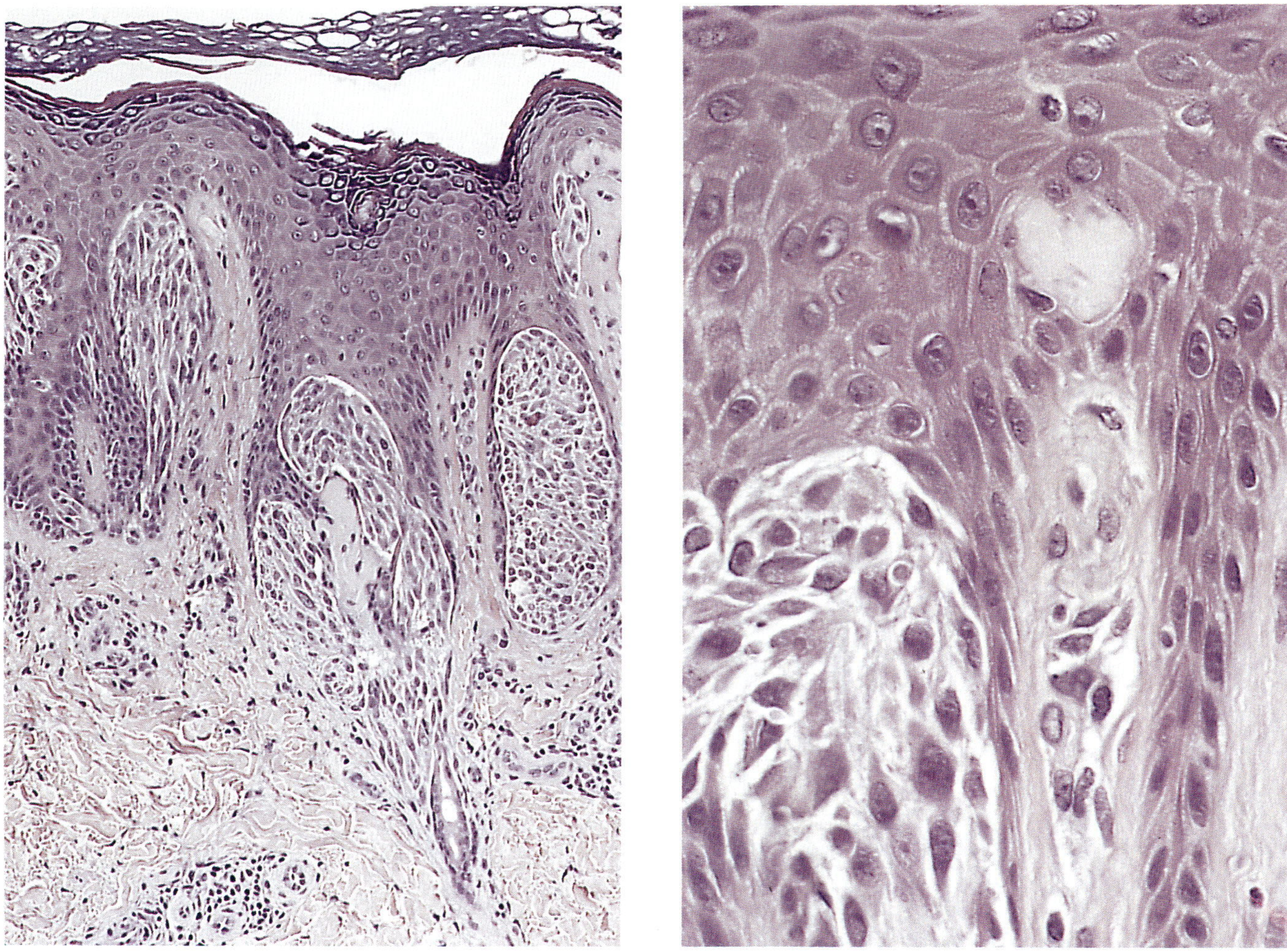

A B

FIGURE 6-3

Spitz nevus. (A) There are large intraepidermal nests of large spindle and epithelioid cells. Note "raining down" pattern (H&E, × 100). (B) Higher magnification showing junctional nest of spindle cells and epithelioid cells. Within epidermis above dermal papilla is a coalescent aggregate of eosinophilic globules (Kamino bodies) (H&E, × 400). (C) Nevus giant cells along dermoepidermal junction (H&E, × 400).

high density of nested or single melanocytes to an adjacent area of epidermis devoid of melanocytic proliferation (see Fig. 6-1C). The lateral borders become poorly circumscribed when there is lateral intraepidermal melanocytic growth that gradually diminishes without an abrupt termination. Also, marked variation in the position of nevus nests at the periphery with intervening "skip areas" devoid of nests and lentiginous junctional growth at the periphery that extends beyond the lateral borders of the dermal component (lateral extension or "shoulder phenomenon") contribute to a loss of lateral demarcation at the dermoepidermal junction.

Zonation. Zonation in Spitz nevi is conveyed by the appearance of layers of differing morphology from top to bottom. Several features can give the appearance of zonation. Epithelioid giant cells, if present in a Spitz nevus, typically form a superficial cell layer at the dermoepidermal junction and are rarely seen deeper, thereby contributing to a zonal structure.[13] The cytologic features of the spindle and/or epithelioid cells may change from above downwards, leading to a gradient in cell size and shape such as from large plump cells at the top to smaller or slender cells at the bottom (see Fig. 6-5B). This phenomenon of cytologic alteration or involution, in which the melanocytes of Spitz nevi progressively

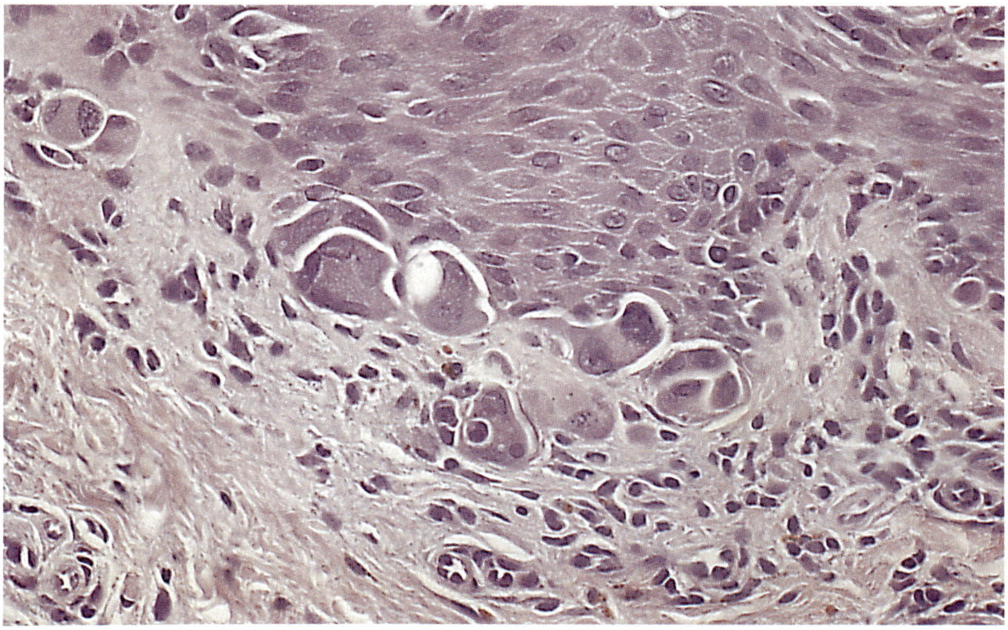

C

FIGURE 6-3 *(Continued)*

TABLE 6-1
Précis: Spitz Nevus

Clinical features
- Configuration: papule or nodule, often dome-shaped
- Size: small (usually < 1 cm)
- Profile: smooth surface topography
- Color: pink/red; darker forms occur
- Age: majority in children and adolescents
- Location: face and extremities most common
- Number: usually solitary; rare multiple forms occur
- Symptoms: commonly asymptomatic, rarely pruritic
- History of growth: months, usually less than a year

Histopathology
- Cytologic features
  - Spindle and/or epithelioid cell type*
  - Overall monomorphous population of cells*
  - Occasional striking pleomorphism in a minority of cells
- Architectural features
  - Symmetry*
  - Sharp lateral demarcation*
  - Zonation in depth (e.g., maturation)*
  - Orderly nondisruptive infiltration of collagen by Spitz nevus cells*

Other helpful diagnostic features
- Absent or rare, but not atypical, mitoses in deep parts*
- Giant nevus cells
- Irregular contours of growth at deep margin*
- Kamino bodies
- Paucity or absence of single-cell upward spread
- Junctional clefts
- Loss of cohesion between cells (retraction spaces)
- Perivascular or diffuse inflammatory infiltrate
- Superficial distribution of pigmentation
- Telangiectasia and edema
- Epidermal hyperplasia

*Most helpful features.

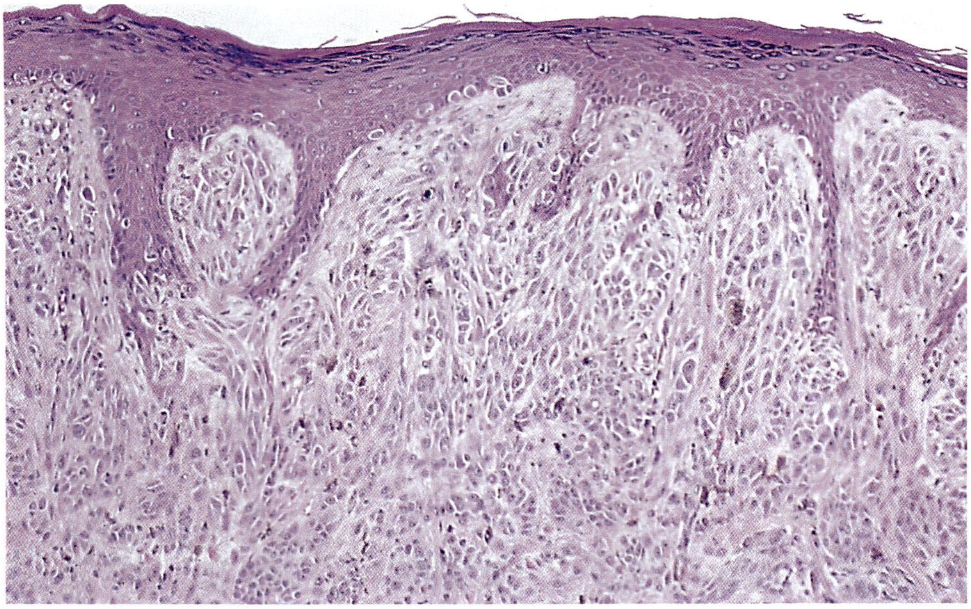

A

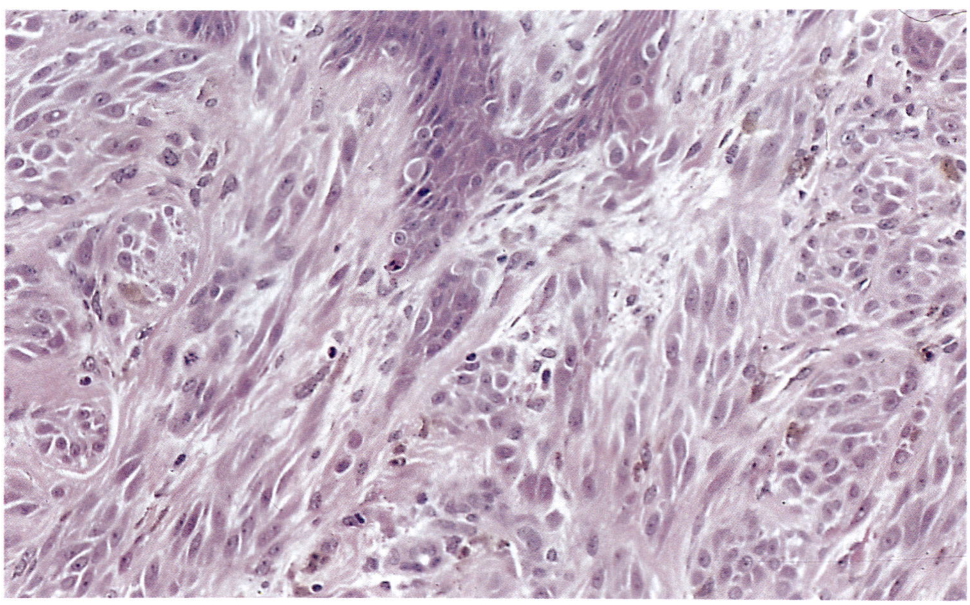

B

FIGURE 6-4

Spitz nevus. (A) Diffuse sheet of spindle cells in upper dermis (H&E, × 100). (B) Fascicles of large spindle cells with abundant cytoplasm (H&E, × 200). (C) Note striking uniformity of spindle cells. The cells have abundant pink cytoplasm. Also note uniformity of nuclei. The chromatin is evenly dispersed, and one or two nucleoli are present (H&E, × 400).

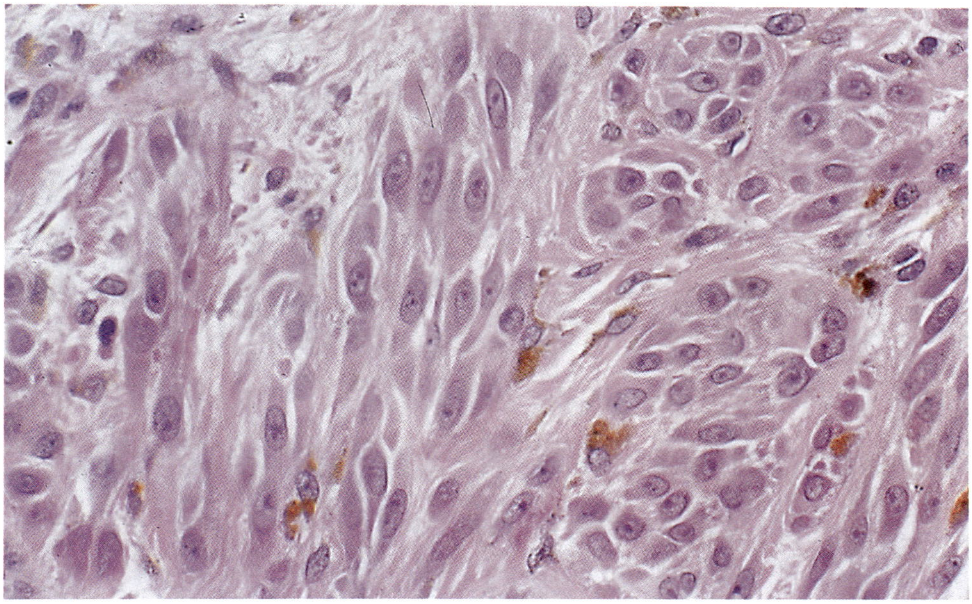

C

FIGURE 6-4 *(Continued)*

come to resemble melanocytes of conventional nevi in deeper parts of the lesions, also has been termed *maturation.*[13]The frequency of maturation in Spitz nevi varies considerably among published accounts. Kernen and Ackerman[6] found maturation in only 4 of their 27 cases. In Weedon and Little's review[10] of 211 cases, maturation was present in 25 percent. Of 41 compound and intradermal Spitz nevi, 31 showed maturation in a recent report by Binder and coworkers.[27] Architectural features also may show a gradient, such as the transition from larger nests at the dermoepidermal junction to smaller nests near the deep margin of the nevus. With this transition from top to bottom, the cellular elements exhibit a nondisruptive insinuation among collagen bundles without induction of new stroma (see Fig. 6-5B). Finally, the distribution of pigment may be zonal. If melanin is present in Spitz nevi, it is largely confined to cells immediately subjacent to the epidermis in the majority of cases.[13] In contrast to zonation in Spitz nevi, melanoma characteristically displays a more disorderly and disruptive growth pattern.

Although maturation is thought to reflect growth control and is an important feature favoring benignity, it does not necessarily equate with benignity. Features suggesting maturation also have been reported in melanomas (pseudomaturation).

Irregular Contours of Growth at Deep Margin. Spitz nevi typically display a single-cell or single-file infiltrative growth pattern at their base.[13] However, the deep parts of the nevus still appear to merge with, but not distort, the normal dermal architecture. Although melanocytes stretch finger-like into the dermis, they seem to separate and ease apart, but not destroy, dermal collagen bundles[27] (see Fig. 6-5B). The impression of merging may be emphasized by a gradual decrease in the size of dermal fascicles or nests of melanocytes, ultimately to single cells. The orderly cellular infiltration at the deep margin of Spitz nevi is one of the most important histologic features distinguishing Spitz nevi from melanoma and cannot be overemphasized. On the other hand, the presence of compact nodules with pushing margins raises suspicion for melanoma.

Absent or Rare Mitoses in Deep Parts

Mitoses are a variable finding in Spitz nevi. Binder and colleagues[27] reported mitoses in 7 of 43 Spitz nevi, while according to Weedon,[13] they may be found in more than half the cases. In an individual lesion, they may be numerous, rare, or absent. Mitoses occur most commonly in the upper portion of the lesion and are usually bipolar. Al though an occasional mitosis in the deeper parts of the lesion or a rare atypical mitosis may be observed in benign Spitz nevi, they should nonetheless prompt careful evaluation of the lesion for melanoma. In an architecturally minimally altered lesion, the presence of mitoses indeeply located melanocytes, in particular the finding of an atypical mitosis, may be diagnostically the most important clue to recognize the lesion as atypical and to suspect melanoma.

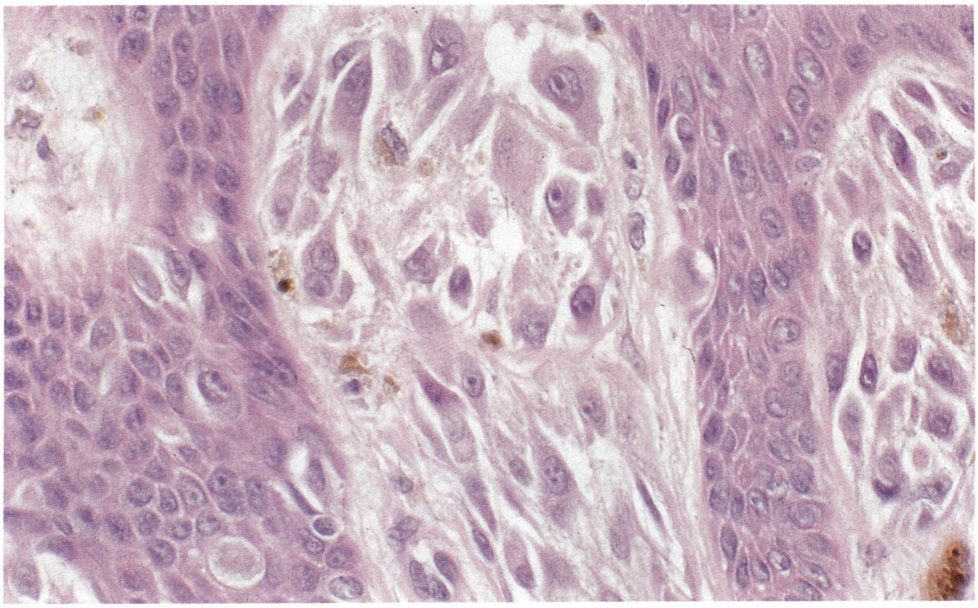

A

FIGURE 6-5

Spitz nevus. (A) Large epithelioid cells and spindle cells in papillary dermis. Note angular contours of cells; some are triangular, rhomboidal, and polygonal in morphology. The cytoplasm is pink with a ground glass appearance. Many nuclei contain prominent nucleoli (H&E, × 400). (B) Maturation of Spitz nevus. Note diminution in cell and nuclear sizes. The cells disperse among collagen on entering the reticular dermis from above. There is no disruption of collagen or induction of stroma (H&E, × 100).

Giant Nevus Cells. The presence of giant nevus cells was emphasized by Spitz in her original report.[4] They are found in at least 50 percent of cases.[13] Giant cells may be multinucleate or contain only one nucleus. They are typically located near the dermoepidermal junction (see Fig. 6-3C) and are rarely found in the deep parts of a Spitz nevus.

Kamino Bodies. Kamino and colleagues[29] reported the presence of eosinophilic amorphous globules, either singly or in aggregates, at the dermoepidermal junction in 60 percent of their 293 Spitz nevi (see Fig. 6-3B). These globules constitute a useful histologic feature of Spitz nevi but are not diagnostic since they are also found with some regularity in malignant melanoma. In Kamino's original report, only 2 percent of malignant melanoma were found to have eosinophilic globules. Arbuckle and Weedon[30] found them in 86 percent of Spitz nevi, 12 percent of malignant melanomas and 8 percent of benign compound nevi in their examination of 50 cases of each entity. They studied 10 sections from each case and reported that Kamino bodies were found in only 15 percent of Spitz nevi if only a single section was examined.[13]

Eosinophilic globules in Spitz nevi often coalesce to form irregular masses, while in melanomas, if present, they are usually smaller and rarely coalesce.[13] Coalescence is typically seen at the dermoepidermal junction in lesions with numerous and highly cellular junctional nests. Individual small pink bodies, probably representing apoptotic melanocytes, tend to be located in the spinous cell layer and may be the only form of pink globules in lesions with rare junctional nests and more prominent intraepidermal single cell growth pattern. Kamino et al.[29] had noted that the eosinophilic globules stained positively with periodic acid–Schiff (PAS) and trichrome stains in Spitz nevi but not in malignant melanoma. However, others have not been able to confirm this finding and questioned the reliability of these staining methods for distinguishing melanomas from Spitz nevi.[13]

Ultrastructurally, Kamino bodies are composed of amorphous masses and bundles of filaments.[30] Immunohistochemically, they contain basement membrane components, including collagen types IV and VII, as well as laminin.[31,32] Degenerate material derived from melanocytes and keratinocytes also may be present.[29]

Paucity or Absence of Single-Cell Upward Spread. Pagetoid spread of single melanocytes is frequently found at all levels of the epidermis in malignant melanoma. This process can occur in Spitz nevus, however, but usually to a lesser extent (see Fig. 6-7). In one recent study of 43 Spitz nevi, scattered suprabasal melanocytes were seen in 16

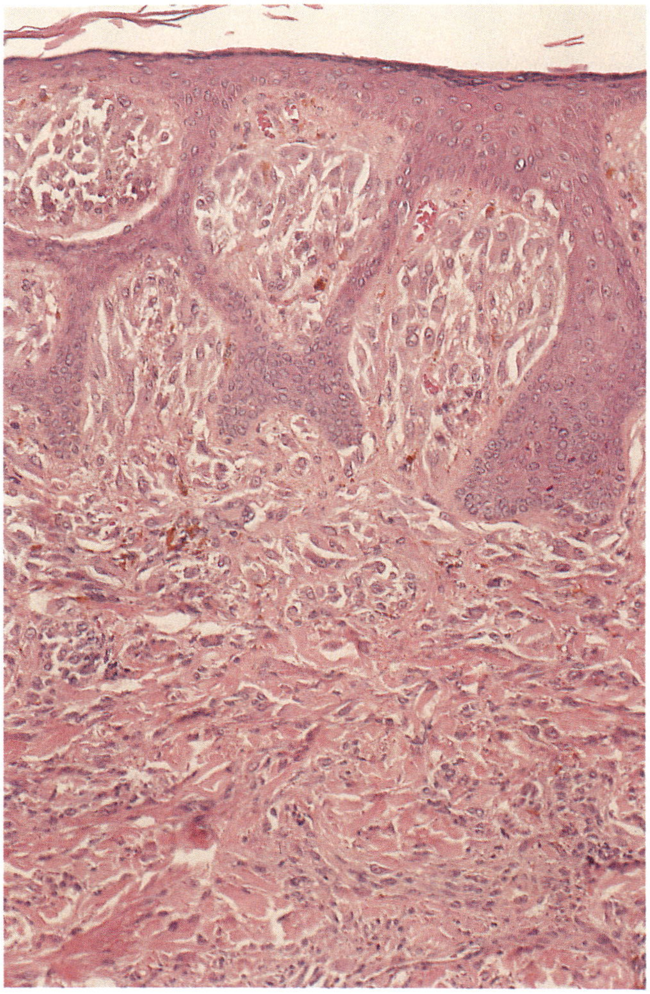

B

FIGURE 6-5 *(Continued)*

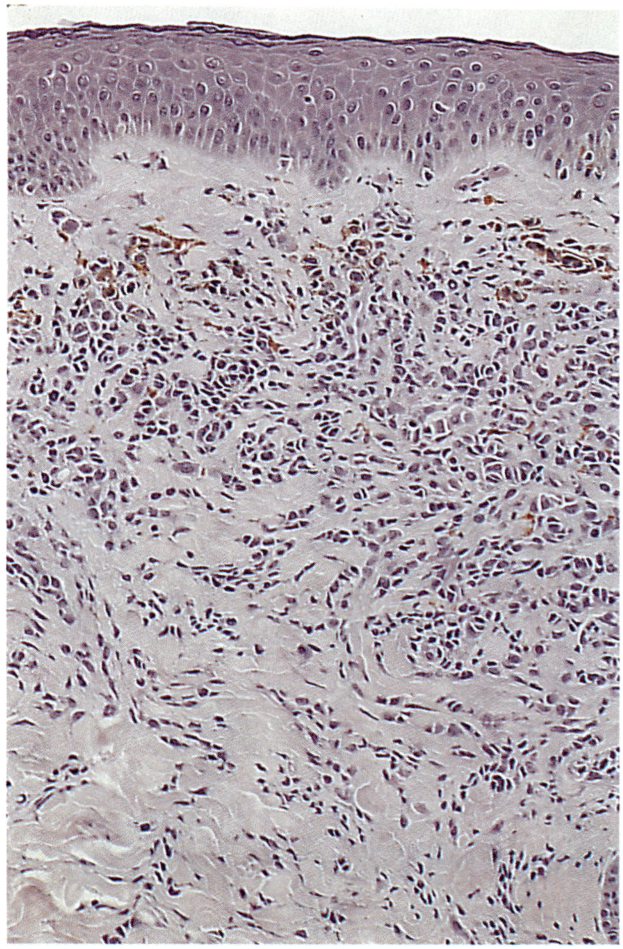

A

FIGURE 6-6

Spitz nevus. (A) The lesion shows maturation from top to bottom. The overall cellularity is reduced near the base of the lesion. The cells infiltrate the collagen as cords of cells and individual cells. The stroma is slightly sclerotic (H&E, × 100). (B) Higher magnification of part A (H&E, × 100). (B) Higher magnification of part A (H&E, × 200).

percent.[27] When upward migration of melanocytes is present in Spitz nevus, it often takes the form of nests of two or more cells extending toward the stratum corneum.[13] Such transepidermal elimination of nests is especially common in childhood lesions but may be found at any age. Pagetoid spread of melanocytes or transepidermal elimination of nests in Spitz nevus is characteristically limited to the epidermis overlying the junctional and/or dermal nevus component. If upward migration is found peripheral to the central part of the nevus, the lesion should be scrutinized carefully to rule out melanoma.[13]

Junctional Cleavage. At the dermoepidermal junction, the fascicles of spindle cells in Spitz nevi, typically following the course of elongated rete ridges, are often separated by a cleftlike retraction space from the adjacent epidermis, a result of tissue shrinkage during processing[13] (see Fig. 6-1C). This feature is present in about half the cases of Spitz nevi but is probably less common in malignant melanomas. Because it seems a useful feature that can help in the differential diagnosis from melanoma, the phenomenon of junctional cleavage has been called a "meaningful artifact."

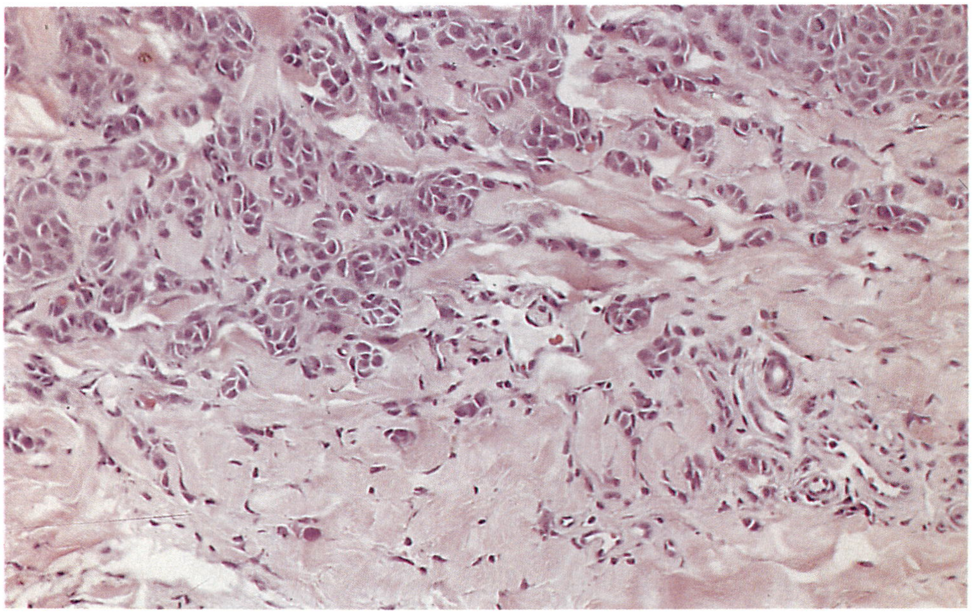

B

FIGURE 6-6 *(Continued)*

phenomenon of junctional cleavage has been called a "meaningful artifact."

Loss of Cohesion. Loss of cohesion may be seen within fascicles or nests of melanocytes, which is reflected by the presence of spaces between individual cells. This allows a loosely packed appearance of melanocytes within the confines of a nest. Loss of cellular cohesion tends to be more pronounced in epithelial cell nests than in spindle cell aggregates.[13]

Adnexal Involvement. Spitz nevi and their variants have a striking propensity to involve hair follicles and eccrine ducts. In most instances, intraepidermal fascicles of cells track along the adventitial sheaths of appendageal structures into the papillary dermis and often into the reticular dermis. Knowledge of the prevalence of this morphologic feature in Spitz nevi and their variants is important because such a finding might otherwise raise undue concern about melanoma.

Perivascular or Diffuse Inflammatory Infiltrate. The distribution of the inflammatory infiltrate in Spitz nevi can be a helpful diagnostic feature. It tends to be perivascular but also may be diffuse in some Spitz nevi. On the other hand, in melanomas, the inflammatory infiltrate is often at the base and not uncommonly associated with tumor regression.[13]

Other Features. A number of other features have been suggested as helpful in the distinction of Spitz nevi from malignant melanoma, such as the type or distribution of pigment, epidermal hyperplasia, edema, and telangiectasia.[13,26,33] As part of the overall constellation of findings, these features may be helpful. However, their diagnostic usefulness is limited. Although they appear more common in Spitz nevi, they are observed frequently enough in melanoma to preclude their diagnostic value.

PIGMENTATION. Spitz nevi are usually only lightly pigmented or amelanotic. Pigment is prominent in only about 10 percent of cases.[13] When it is present, it is typically superficial, especially near the dermoepidermal junction. While the texture of the pigment is typically fine and dusty in melanomas, it is said to be coarser in Spitz nevi.

EPIDERMAL HYPERPLASIA. Epidermal hyperplasia is a common finding in Spitz nevi (see Fig. 6-1B). In one study, acanthosis was seen in 58 percent of Spitz nevi and pseudoepitheliomatous hyperplasia in 74 percent of cases.[27]

TELANGIECTASIA AND EDEMA. A zone of telangiectatic fibrous tissue, typically in the superficial dermis, partly or completely separating the epidermis from the upper melanocytes is observed in about 50 percent of Spitz nevi. Edema is less common and prominent in only about 10 percent of Spitz nevi.[13]

Spitz Nevus with Architectural Disorder and Cytologic Atypia (Atypical Spitz Nevus)

Spitz nevi with atypical features are encountered not uncommonly, yet standardized criteria for recognizing or categorizing such lesions are not available. Architectural

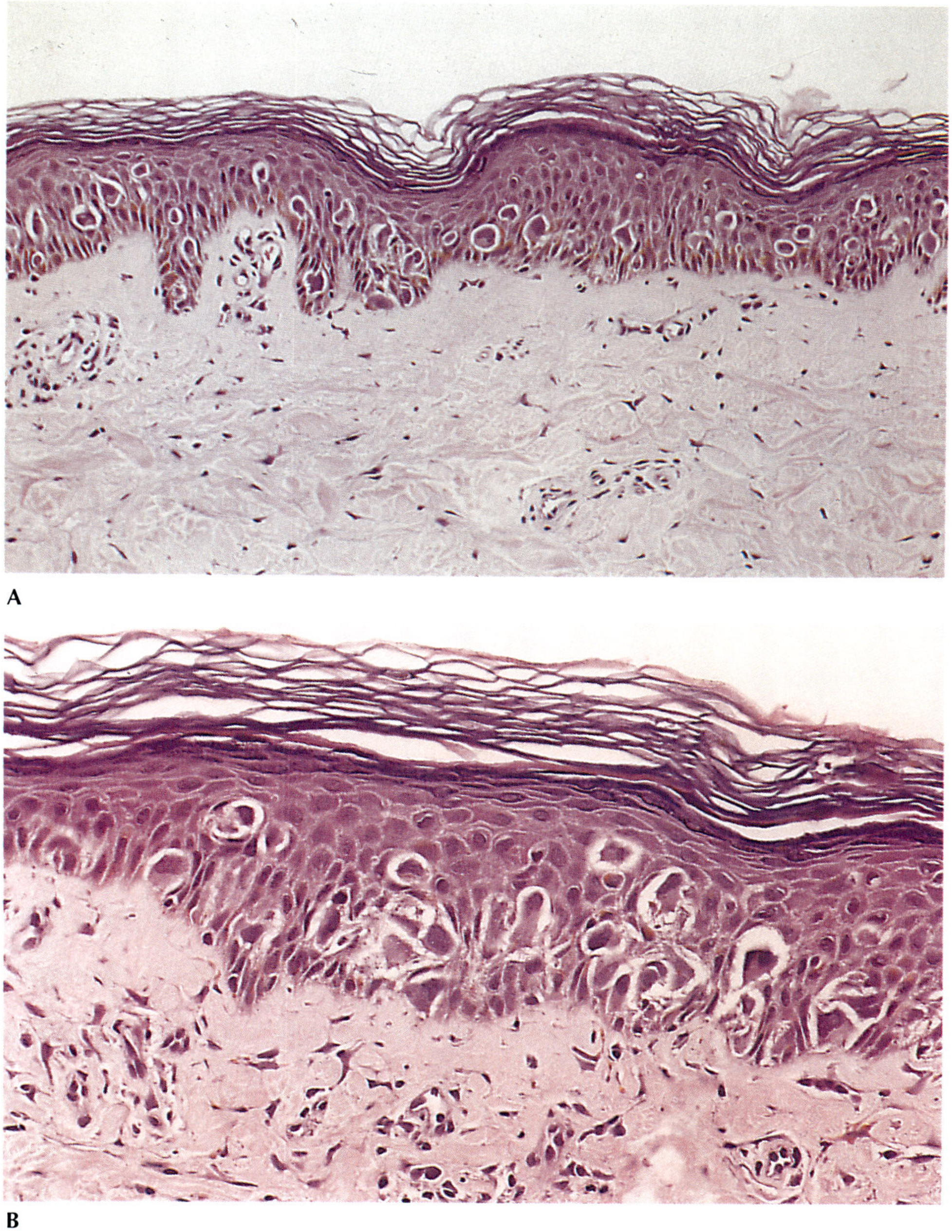

A

B

FIGURE 6-7

Spitz nevus with intraepidermal pagetoid spread (A) Pagetoid spread suggests melanoma in situ (H&E, × 100). (B) Note characteristic cytologic details of Spitz nevus cells. The cells are polyangular and contain abundant ground-glass cytoplasm, and the nuclei have dispersed chromatin (H&E, × 200).

and cytologic criteria for diagnosing and grading atypical nevi and melanocytic proliferations are discussed in Chapter 9. In general, atypical features may be subdivided into those involving primarily the epidermis (conventional melanocytic dysplasia) or the dermis/subcutis. The latter two subcategories of features may occur together to varying extents or separately.

Atypical Features of the Intraepidermal Component. As discussed in Chapter 9, Spitz nevi (and pigmented spindle cell nevi) may show morphologic features of conventional dysplastic nevi and thus may be considered to have architectural disorder and/or cytologic atypia (melanocytic dysplasia) (Table 6-2). The essential criteria for diagnosis are (1) disordered architectural patterns of the intraepidermal component, i.e., lentiginous melanocytic proliferation and/or significant variation in junctional nesting (variations in size, shape, orientation, spacing of junctional nests; horizontal confluence and bridging of nests; diminished cellular cohesion of nests) and (2) unequivocal cytologic atypia of melanocytes (Fig. 6-8). The features of such Spitz nevi are outlined in Table 6-2.

TABLE 6-2
Spitz Nevus/Pigmented Spindle Cell Nevus with Architectural Disorder and Cytologic Atypia

I. Intraepidermal variant
  A. Architectural disorder
    1. Disordered intraepidermal melanocytic proliferation*
      a. Lentiginous or single-cell pattern*
      b. Disordered junctional nesting*
        (1) Variation in size, shape, orientation, spacing, cellular cohesion of nests
        (2) Horizontal confluence and bridging of nests
      c. Pagetoid spread
    2. Asymmetry
    3. Poor circumscription
    4. Lateral extension of intraepidermal component ("shoulder phenomenon")
  B. Cytologic atypia*
    1. Nuclear pleomorphism
    2. Variation in nuclear chromatin patterns
    3. Nuclear enlargement
    4. Variation in nucleoli
  C. Host response
    1. Patchy to bandlike mononuclear infiltrates in papillary dermis
    2. Fibroplasia
II. Dermal variant
  A. Architectural disorder*
    1. Expansile nodules
    2. Increased cellularity
    3. Loss of cellular cohesion
    4. Asymmetry
    5. Deep extension
    6. Lack of maturation or orderly infiltration of collagen
    7. Ulceration
    8. Necrosis
  B. Cytologic atypia (as above)
  C. Mitotic activity
    1. Numerous mitoses
    2. Mitoses at base of lesion
    3. Atypical mitoses
  D. Host response
    1. Prominent mononuclear cell infiltrates
    2. Formation of tumor stroma

*Essential criteria for diagnosis.

Intraepidermal or Mainly Intraepidermal Spitz Nevi with Prominent Pagetoid Spread. A distinctive variant of Spitz nevus that has received little attention in previously published series is the mainly intraepidermal or junctional subtype with a prominent pagetoid pattern. This variant may occur anywhere but is encountered most commonly on the lower extremities of young women. The most important reason for recognizing this lesion is its frequent misdiagnosis as in situ/radial-growth-phase melanoma. The clinical findings are often unremarkable. Most lesions measure less than 5 or 6 mm and are diagnosed as a nevus or atypical nevus.

Scanning magnification usually discloses a mainly intraepidermal proliferation of enlarged epithelioid cells usually devoid of melanin (see Fig. 6-7A). The proliferation commonly has an overall symmetry from side to side and is often fairly well demarcated. However, some lesions have ill-defined margins. Many of these lesions show a combination of both a single-cell and nested proliferation of epithelioid melanocytes. The single-cell proliferative pattern is often both basilar and pagetoid and commonly varies within the lesion (see Fig. 6-7B). Typical junctional nests of epithelioid cells with associated clefting are also usually present and may be quite small in size. Nests of cells or single Spitz nevus cells may or may not be present in the papillary dermis. Often the degree of pagetoid spread is focal or limited; however, it may be prominent in some lesions, raising the possibility of melanoma in situ (see Fig. 6-7B).

Atypical Features of the Dermal Component. As outlined in the second part of Table 6-2, certain Spitz nevi may demonstrate prominent atypicality of the dermal component. These various features include the presence of compact cellular nodules, increased cellularity, diminished cellular cohesion, asymmetry, deep extension into the lower-most dermis or subcutis, deep bulbous or pushing growth pattern, lack of maturation or orderly infiltration of collagen, cytologic atypia, mitotic activity especially

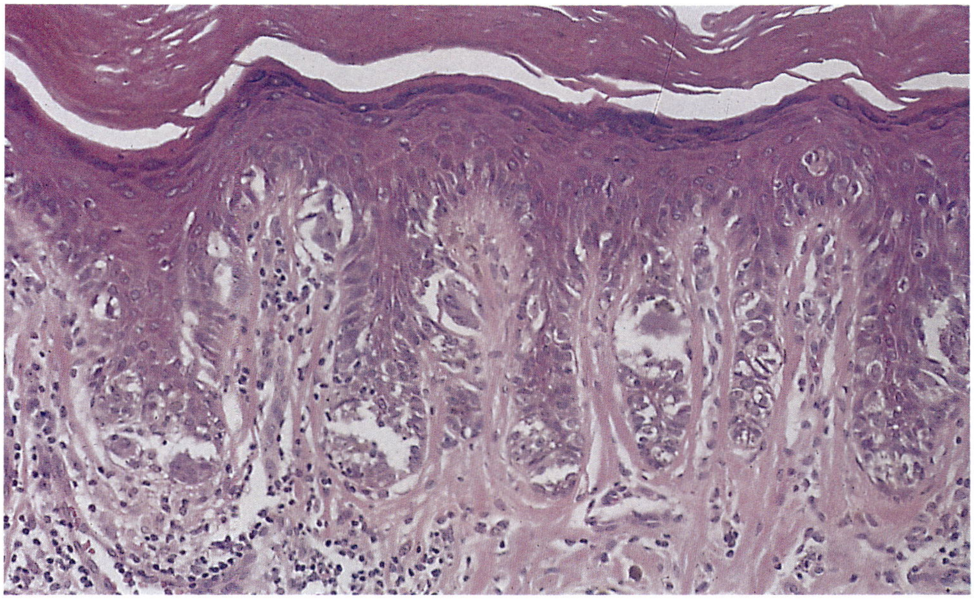

A

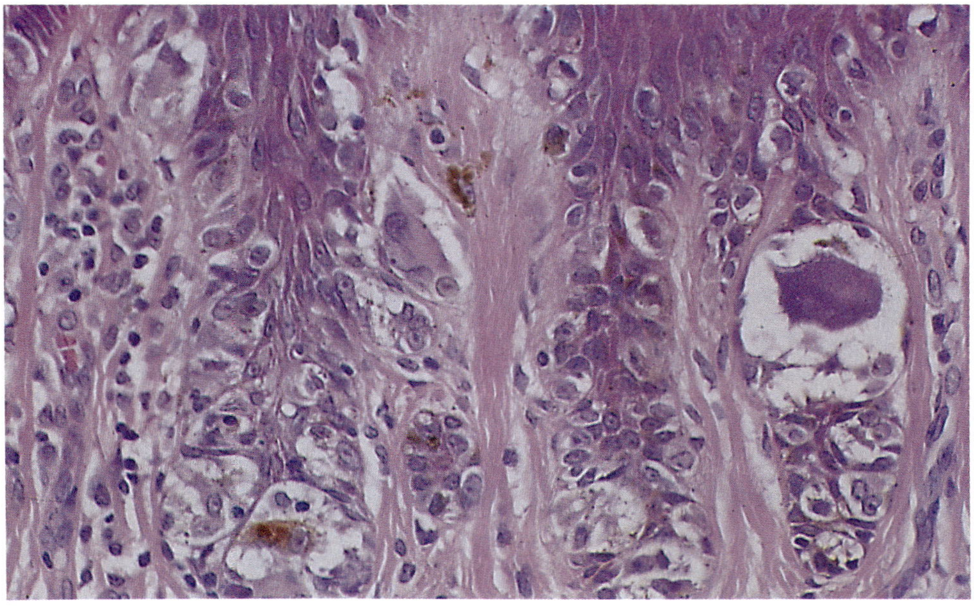

B

FIGURE 6-8

Spitz nevus with architectural disorder and cytologic atypia. (A) The lesion demonstrates architectural disorder, as indicated by lentiginous melanocytic proliferation and variation in junctional nesting pattern (H&E, × 200). (B) Higher magnification shows disordered and atypical intraepidermal melanocytes. The cells also exhibit the features of Spitz nevus cells: abundant ground-glass cytoplasm, angulated contours, and characteristic multinucleate giant cells (H&E, × 400). (C) Disordered nesting of enlarged epithelioid cells. These cells again show features of Spitz nevus cells but in addition display nuclear atypia (H&E, × 400). (D) This field demonstrates horizontal confluence of enlarged fusiform cells typical of Spitz nevus. The cells have a monotonous appearance and contain nuclei with evenly dispersed chromatin. (H&E, × 400).

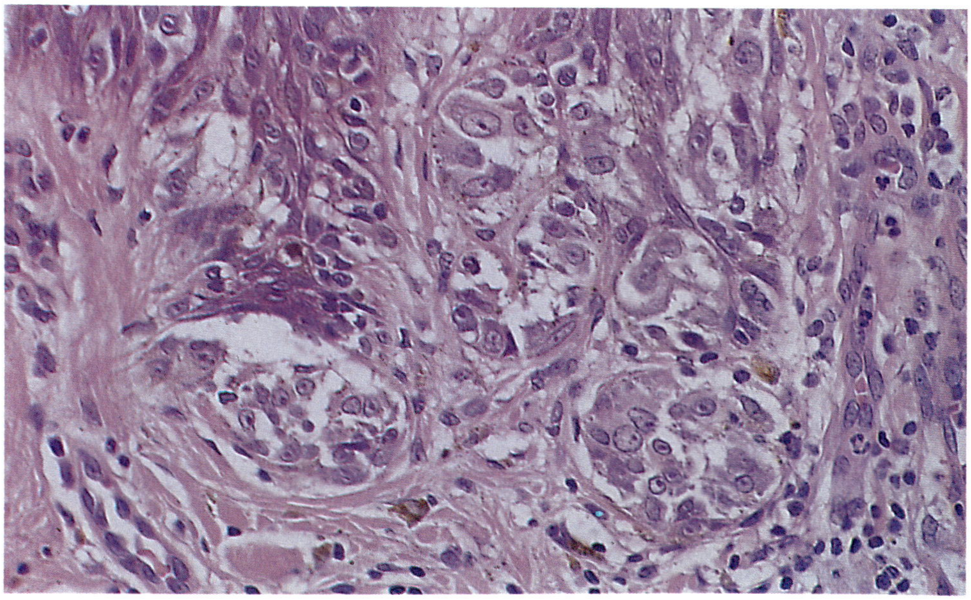

C

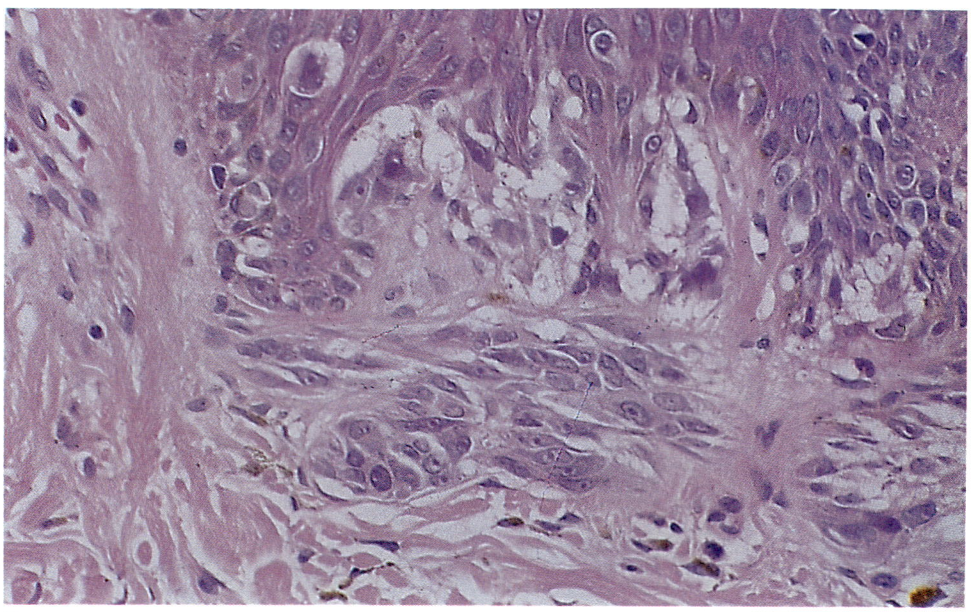

D

FIGURE 6-8 *(Continued)*

deep, and mononuclear infiltrates (Fig. 6-9). Because of the rarity of such lesions and the lack of sufficient follow-up in many instances, the significance of these various features has not been elucidated. There is little question that the presence of these various features in any given lesion is highly worrisome for melanoma and that as these features increase in number and severity the likelihood of melanoma increases.

Smith and colleagues[50] reported a series of 32 such lesions designated as "malignant Spitz nevus." These tumors developed in relatively young individuals (41 percent ≤ age 14 years and 82 percent ≤ 29 years of age) and were located on the head and neck and extremities. Regional lymph node metastases occurred in 6 individuals, but on limited follow-up (mean 6 years) of these 6 patients and 24 additional patients, all were disease-free. Thus it is apparent that there is insufficient information currently available to know the biologic potential of many such Spitz tumors with atypicality of the dermal component.

In evaluating such lesions, a number of factors should be weighed in the final interpretation. Clinical factors such as the age of the patient, location of the tumor, clinical appearance, history of recent change in long-standing stable lesions, size greater than 1 cm, and family history of melanoma should be considered carefully. The older the patient, especially individuals beyond the age of 30 years, the much greater is the likelihood of malignancy. As a general rule, one's threshold for diagnosing melanoma in such lesions should correlate inversely with the age of the patient, i.e., a high threshold for very young individuals and a lower threshold for elderly individuals. However, it should be stressed that there are many exceptions. The location of atypical tumors on sites less commonly involved by Spitz nevus, such as the back, is also another such factor suggesting careful scrutiny of the lesion for melanoma. After weighing these various factors and a clear-cut diagnosis of melanoma cannot be made, a practical approach is to communicate this situation to the clinician and patient. We advise that such atypical tumors be completely excised with surgical margins of approximately 1 cm and that the patient be monitored carefully as if he or she has melanoma, i.e., regular examinations for evidence of recurrence or metastasis. We do not believe that lymph node dissections should be performed unless palpable and persistent lymphadenopathy is present. It must be stressed that all such lesions should be managed on an individual basis.

Differential Diagnosis

A number of melanocytic and nonmelanocytic lesions share morphologic features with Spitz nevi and their atypical variants. The intraepidermal or junctional variants of Spitz nevi must first of all be discriminated from in situ or early invasive melanoma. These intraepidermal Spitz nevi often show relatively small size, symmetry, evidence of growth control, and sharp circumscription compared with melanoma. Of particular importance are the cytologic characteristics of the epithelioid cells; they tend to be fairly monotypic with abundant pinkish cytoplasm that has a ground-glass appearance rather than the granular cytoplasm often observed in melanoma cells. The nuclei of Spitz nevus cells are also fairly uniform with evenly dispersed chromatin versus the pleomorphism of melanoma cells.

Compound and dermal Spitz nevi and their atypical variants also must be discriminated from melanoma. The features outlined above and listed in Tables 6-1 and 6-3 provide criteria for this distinction, which can be made confidently for cases of typical Spitz nevi or typical melanoma (Table 6-4). However, in a number of cases, the lesions are atypical, and some of the features associated with benignancy are missing. The absence or incomplete development of major diagnostic features, such as symmetry or sharply demarcated lateral borders, is of concern and should prompt a careful search for features of melanoma. Even if symmetry and sharp lateral demarcation are observed, the presence of extensive pagetoid spread, the lack of maturation in depth, and the presence of prominent cellularity of the dermal component, nuclear pleomorphism of more than a small proportion of cells, cohesive cellular nodules in the dermis, or deeply located (albeit rare) mitoses are worrisome.

Detailed knowledge of diagnostic criteria and their relative weight is critical in the histologic assessment of such atypical lesions. When an atypical lesion is present, we consider it appropriate to indicate in a comment whether the lesion shows only slight atypicality or its features approach melanoma. Depending on the severity of the atypia, we state that the diagnosis of malignant melanoma cannot be excluded completely. A diagnosis of malignancy should not be made unless there is sufficient histologic evidence so that overtreatment and undue psychological burden for the patient can be avoided.

As discussed above and in Chapter 9, atypical forms of Spitz nevi may show many features of dysplastic nevi and in a general sense may be "dysplastic." Distinction from dysplastic nevi is based primarily on the presence of the characteristic cell types of Spitz nevi.

Aside from melanoma and dysplastic nevi, Spitz nevus needs to be distinguished from its variants desmoplastic nevus, pigmented spindle cell nevus, and as other melanocytic nevi with features shared by Spitz nevi. The characteristics of these nevi are discussed in the respective paragraphs and chapters of this book.

A number of nonmelanocytic, primarily histiocytic lesions also may simulate Spitz nevus and need to be considered in the differential diagnosis. Juvenile xanthogranuloma lacks a junctional component and typically has Touton giant cells.[34] In a lesion with rare or no giant cells, the finding of histiocytes with foamy cytoplasm or the presence of eosinophils is helpful. In contrast to Spitz nevi, the cells in juvenile xanthogranuloma are typically not immunoreactive with S-100 protein. Spitz nevi differ from cellular neurothekeoma[35] by the presence of junctional nests, maturation, or melanin pigment and by the feature of individual cells infiltrating the dermis at the base of the lesion. The stroma in cellular neurothekeoma

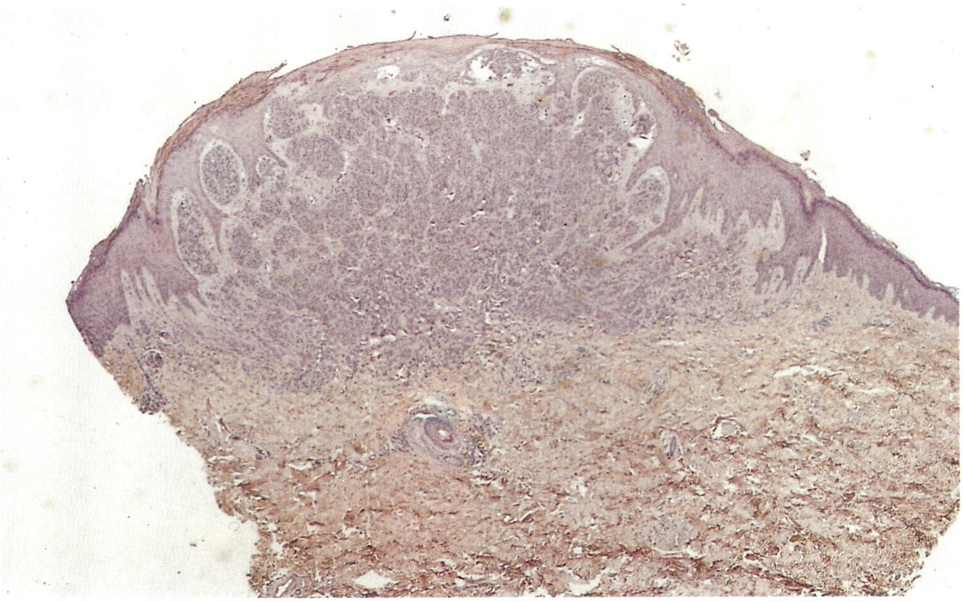

A

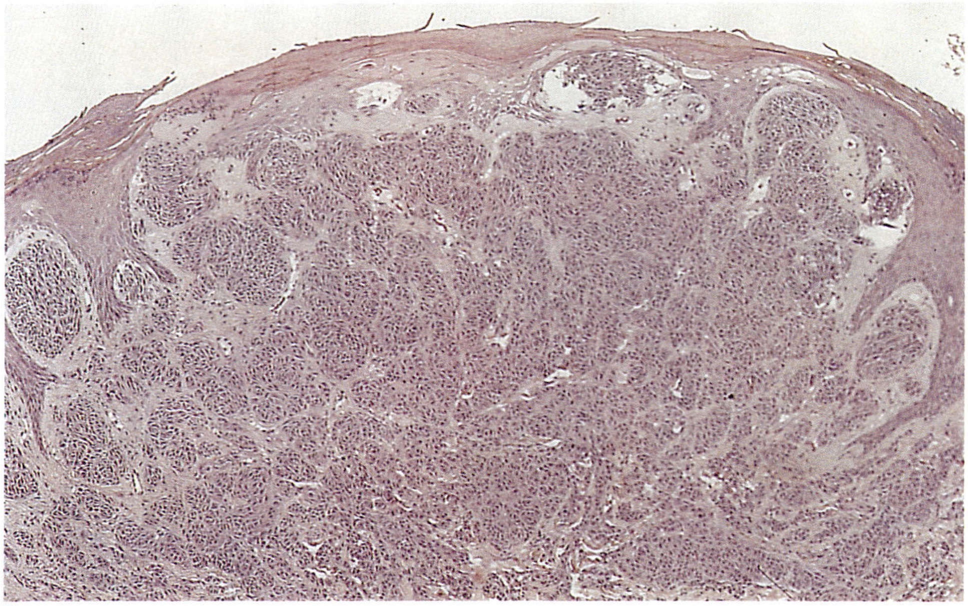

B

FIGURE 6-9

Atypical Spitz nevus. (A) The lesion is dome-shaped and fairly symmetric but is characterized by an expansile cellular nodule with only slight maturation. These are the atypical features (H&E, × 20). (B) The nodule is characterized by a monotonous cellular appearance which is acceptable from side to side but not from top to bottom (H&E, × 40). (C) Dyscohesion of junctional nest. The cells have the cellular attributes of Spitz nevus cells; they are monotonous, angular, and have abundant pink cytoplasm (H&E, × 100). (D) Nests of epithelioid cells at base of lesion. Two mitotic figures are present in this field (H&E, × 200).

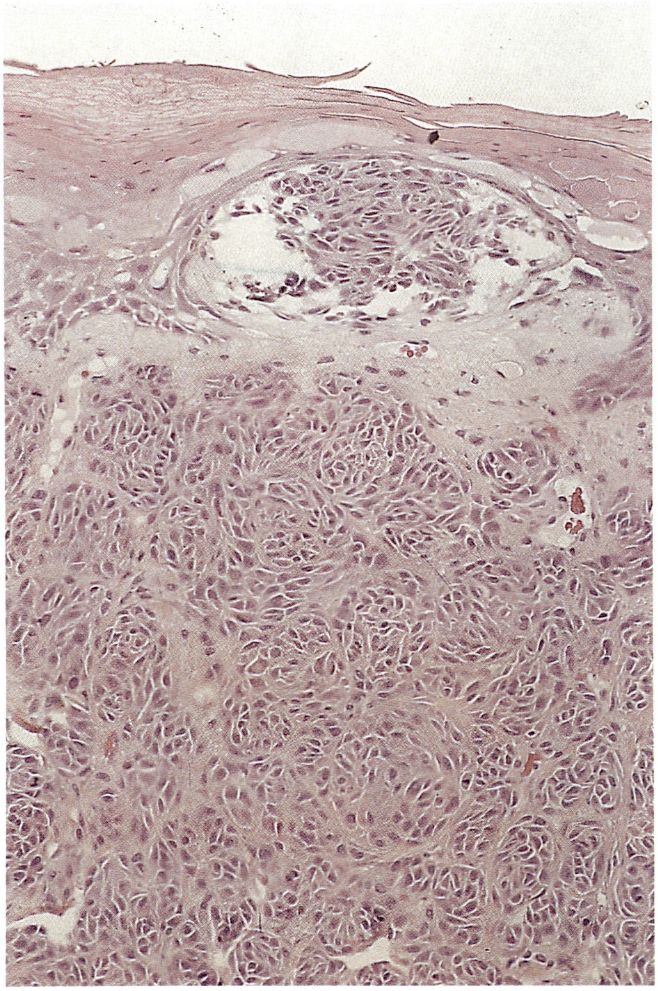

C

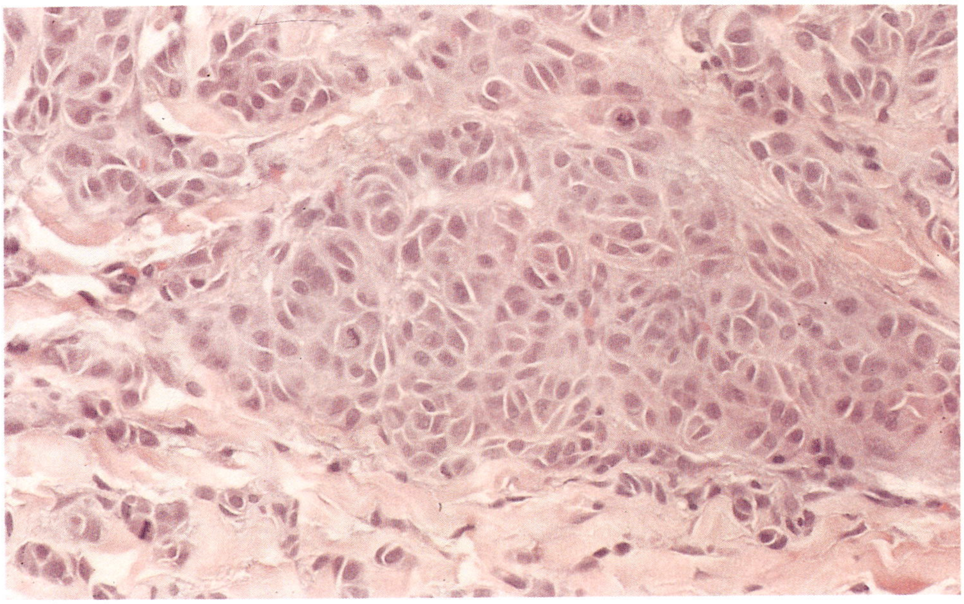

D

FIGURE 6-9 *(Continued)*

TABLE 6-3
Comparison of Spitz Nevus, Atypical Spitz Nevus, and Melanoma

	Spitz Nevus	*Spitz Nevus with Architectural Disorder and Cytologic Atypia*	*Melanoma*
Size	Usually < 1 cm	Often > 1 cm	Usually > 1 cm
Symmetry	Symmetric	Often asymmetric	Asymmetric
Lateral borders	Sharply demarcated	Often poorly defined	Often poorly defined
Lateral extension	Uncommon	Common	Common
Lentiginous melanocytic proliferation	Uncommon	Variable	Common
Irregular nesting	Uncommon	Common	Frequent
Upward migration	Common in children, nests > single cells	Variable, prominent on occasion	Frequent, usually as single cells
Ulceration	Uncommon	Variable	Common
Kamino bodies	Common	Common	Less common
Cell type	Monomorphous	Monomorphous	Pleomorphic
Deep extension	Uncommon	Common	Variable
Expansile nodules	Uncommon	Common	Frequent
Maturation/zonation	Common	Uncommon	Uncommon
Deep border	Orderly infiltrating pattern	Often rounded, "pushing"	Irregular or "pushing"
Cellularity	Variable	Prominent	Prominent
Cytologic atypia	Uncommon	Common	Prominent
Cellular cohesion	Diminished	Diminished	Variable
Mitoses, deep	Uncommon	Common	Frequent
Atypical mitoses	Uncommon	Variable	Common
Mononuclear infiltrates	Perivascular	Patchy	Bandlike, patchy

is usually slightly myxoid. Epithelioid cell histiocytoma[36] is another recently described lesion that can mimic Spitz nevus. It occurs primarily as a solitary nodule in adulthood (mean age of 42 years), most commonly on the lower limbs. It lacks a junctional component, often has an epidermal collarette, and is composed of a proliferation of large epithelioid cells with polygonal or triangular outlines which do not show a gradient in size from above downward to the base. Epithelioid histiocytomas usually show prominent vascularity with clustering of epithelioid cells around blood vessels. A small number of cells may be S-100 protein- positive, but the majority are not. However, staining for factor XIIIa is common, for which melanocytes in Spitz nevi are said to be negative. Reticulohistiocytoma of the skin is characterized by the presence of giant cells with abundant ground-glass eosinophilic cytoplasm.[34] These cells often have large hyperchromatic nuclei. They are usually more densely aggregated than melanocytes in Spitz nevi and may have an accompanying mixed inflammatory infiltrate of lymphocytes, plasma cells, and eosinophils. The cytoplasm of the giant cells is positive for periodic acid–Schiff stain and resistant to diastase. If no intraepidermal melanocytes can be found, then melanin stains and immunoreactivity for S-100 protein may be of help. Melanin stains are negative, and the cells in reticulohistiocytoma lack immunoreactivity for S-100 protein.

Rarely, exclusively intraepidermal/junctional Spitz nevi may mimic *Paget's disease* or *Bowen's disease*, both of which can be distinguished from Spitz nevus by immunoreactivity for cytokeratins.[37]

Metastasizing Spitz Nevus. Melanocytic lesions classified as Spitz nevi have been reported to spread to regional lymph nodes.[5,7,21,38,39] The concept of localized, presumably "benign" metastases has been proposed to explain this rare phenomenon. However, these metastasizing melanocytic lesions, albeit resembling in many ways Spitz nevi, tended to be unusually large and deep or showed other uncommon features.[21,26] It is therefore possible to consider an alternative explanation and to view these tumors as unusual melanomas with spitzoid features

TABLE 6-4
Differential Diagnosis of Spitz Nevus

Melanocytic lesions
- Malignant melanoma, in particular nodular melanoma
- Dysplastic nevi with features of Spitz nevus
- Variants of nevi with spindle and/or epithelioid cells
  - Pigmented spindle cell nevus
  - Desmoplastic Spitz nevus
  - Plexiform spindle cell nevus/deep penetrating nevus
  - Cellular blue nevus
  - Various "combined" nevi

Non-melanocytic lesions
- Paget's disease
- Bowen's disease
- Dermatofibroma
- Epithelioid histiocytoma
- Reticulohistiocytoma
- Cellular neurothekeoma

which may have a less aggressive potential for spread beyond regional lymph nodes. The data available do not allow clear-cut conclusions on this issue.

Invasion of lymphatic spaces, which has been demonstrated in 7 of 49 Spitz nevi in children, may be a histologic curiosity and is not in itself a predictor of metastasis (even if benign). No evidence of metastasis was found during a follow-up period of up to 14 years.[40]

Special Techniques

The diagnosis of Spitz nevus still rests on light microscopic morphologic features. A number of additional techniques have been used in an attempt to facilitate the distinction between Spitz nevus and malignant melanoma. Ultrastructurally, a distinct type of cell was reported to be characteristic of Spitz nevus. This cell was described as containing a large number of premelanosomes, oriented around the Golgi complex, without melanin synthesis.[41] However, the applicability of electron microscopy to the routine diagnostic workup of Spitz nevi appears limited. A difference in the numbers of AgNORs between Spitz nevi and melanomas has been suggested.[42] However, there was overlap in the results, which questions the usefulness of this technique to resolve diagnostic dilemmas. Rode et al.[43] compared the intensity of staining of Spitz nevi and melanoma with antibodies for S-100 protein and neuron-specific enolase. The staining intensity for both markers appeared lower in Spitz nevi. In the same study, nuclear DNA content was examined.[43] The cells in Spitz nevi showed a normal diploid pattern in the majority of cases. Several investigators using a variety of techniques to determine DNA ploidy were unable to discriminate between Spitz nevi and malignant melanoma.[44,45]

DESMOPLASTIC SPITZ NEVUS

Synonyms: sclerosing Spitz nevus, desmoplastic nevus.

Clinical Features

Although the desmoplastic Spitz nevus is considered by many to be an unusual variant of Spitz nevus,[46,47] some authors maintain that this lesion is a distinct entity.[48] Desmoplastic Spitz nevus typically presents as a firm, dome-shaped papule or nodule, measuring up to 1 cm in greatest diameter and is most often located on the extremities.[9,46,47] In many instances, the lesion is flesh-colored and suggests a dermatofibroma. This variant of Spitz nevus primarily affects adults, with a peak incidence in the third decade. However, it also may be encountered in children. Usually, the patient gives a history that the lesion has been present for months or even years.

Histologic Features

The desmoplastic Spitz nevus is characterized by a poorly circumscribed growth of large polygonal or elongated melanocytes in a collagen-rich stromal background[9,46,47] (Fig. 6-10, Table 6-5). It is usually a wholly intradermal

TABLE 6-5
Précis: Desmoplastic Spitz Nevus

Clinical features
- Firm papule or nodule
- Adults (peak incidence in third decade)
- Most commonly located on extremities

Histopathology
- Spindle and/or epithelioid cells
- Predominantly intradermal location of melanocytes
- Sometimes junctional component
- Dermal stroma with increased collagen
- Usually circumscribed, but with ill-defined borders
- Often vaguely wedge-shaped
- Usually diffuse distribution of cells with low cell density
- Typically small nests and single melanocytes
- Maturation often present
- Mitoses absent or rare
- Multinucleate giant cells not uncommon (usually superficial)
- Melanin usually sparse or absent

Differential diagnosis
- Desmoplastic melanoma
- Sclerosing blue nevus
- Dermatofibroma

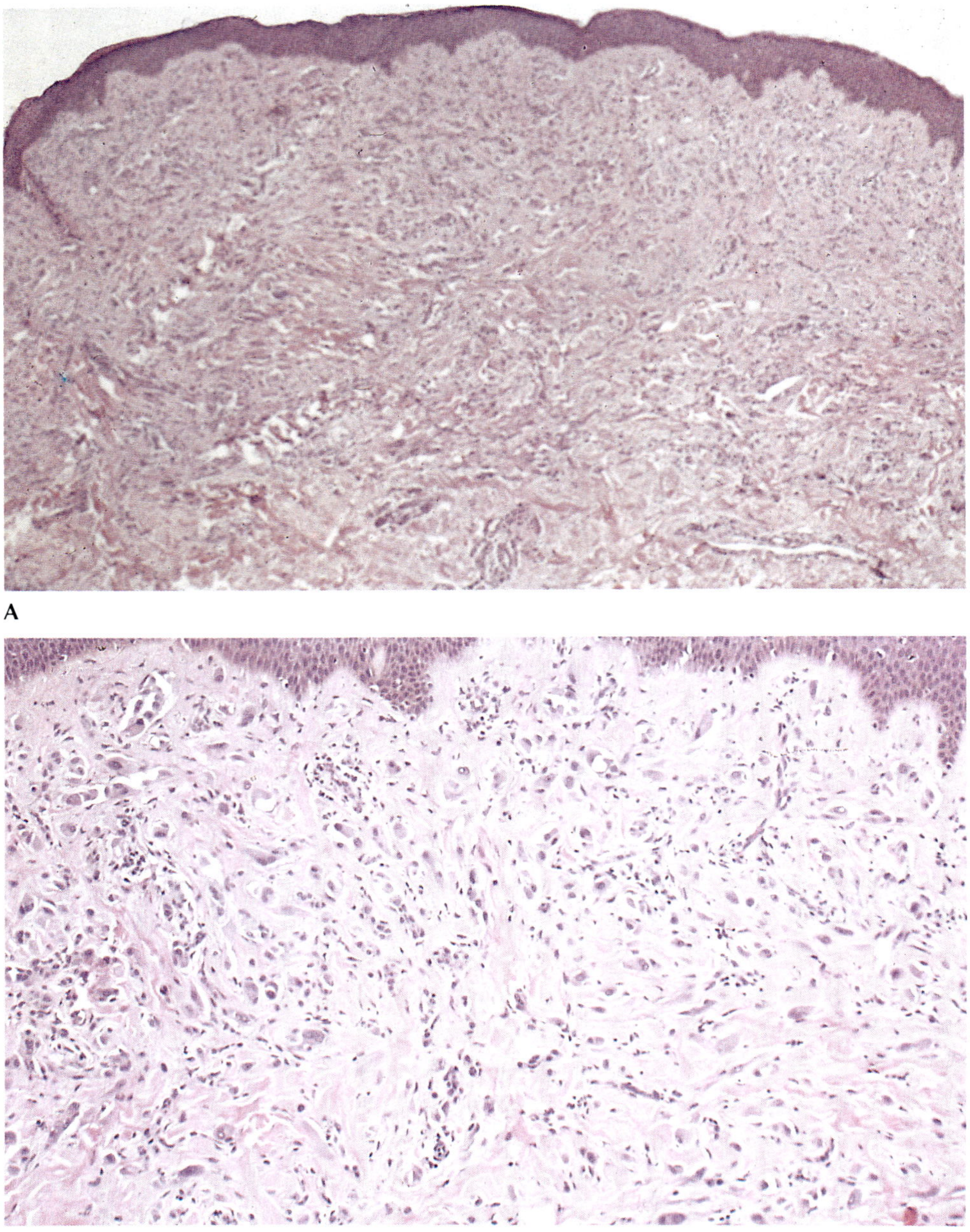

B

FIGURE 6-10

Desmoplastic Spitz nevus. (A) The lesion is entirely intradermal and characterized by a nondescript appearance at this magnification. Nonetheless, the tumor exhibits symmetry and an orderly pattern (H&E, × 40). (B) Nests, cords, and individual cells dispersed in sclerotic dermis (H&E, × 200). (C) Typical epithelioid cells of Spitz nevus scattered throughout sclerotic dermis. Note pink homogeneous quality of collagen. The Spitz nevus cells infiltrate the collagen without disruption (H&E, × 400).

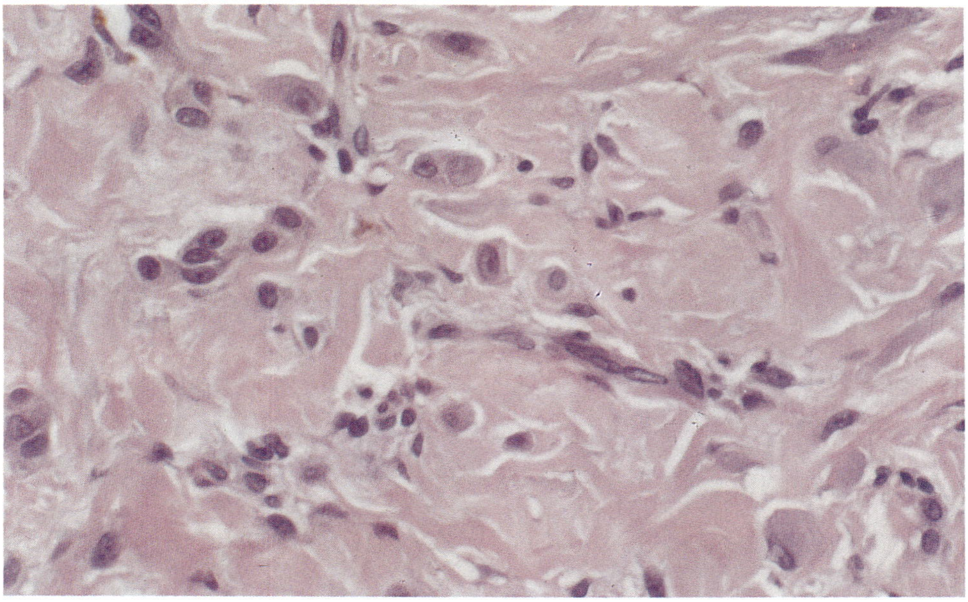

C

FIGURE 6-10 *(Continued)*

lesion, although minor junctional components may be present (see Fig. 6-10A). It should be noted that the desmoplastic changes in Spitz nevi may comprise the entire lesion or any portion of it. In the superficial dermis, melanocytes may be grouped in nests or aggregates, while in the deeper parts of the lesions, they tend to infiltrate singly between typically thickened collagen bundles (see Fig. 6-10B). The latter phenomenon is maturation, as in other Spitz nevi. Scattered multinucleated giant cells or large pleomorphic forms may be present. Cytologically, the melanocytes of desmoplastic Spitz nevi are characterized by nuclei that are often hyperchromatic with clumped or finely dispersed chromatin (see Fig. 6-10C). Nucleoli are commonly inconspicuous but may be prominent, especially in larger cells. The size of the nuclei tends to diminish as melanocytes approach the base of the lesion, which is usually ill-defined. Mitoses are rare (usually <1 per 20 high-power fields).[26] A lymphohistiocytic infiltrate may be present but is generally sparse.

Differential Diagnosis

The major differential diagnostic problem with desmoplastic Spitz nevus is its distinction from desmoplastic melanoma. A number of features help to distinguish desmoplastic Spitz nevus from desmoplastic melanoma (Table 6-6). The desmoplastic Spitz nevus may present in a similar fashion to desmoplastic melanoma, i.e., an indurated amelanotic or slightly pigmented nodule. However, in other respects, the desmoplastic Spitz nevus is strikingly different from desmoplastic melanoma. There is a predilection for the extremities of young individuals versus the head and neck of elderly persons in desmoplastic melanoma. Histologically, desmoplastic Spitz nevi tend to be small, well-circumscribed, superficial lesions, whereas desmoplastic melanomas are often larger, poorly demarcated, and characterized by deep involvement of the dermis or subcutis. The desmoplastic variant of Spitz nevus also shows maturation, i.e., isolation of individually smaller cells with increasing depth versus little or no such transition in desmoplastic melanoma. As outlined above,

TABLE 6-6
Desmoplastic Spitz Nevus versus Desmoplastic Melanoma

	Desmoplastic Spitz Nevus	*Desmoplastic Melanoma*
Preferred site	Extremities	Head and neck
Preferred age group	Early adulthood	Late adulthood
Melanocytic atypia		
Intraepidermal	Rare	Common
Dermal	Not uncommon, but usually slight	Common, often more than slight
Mitoses	Rare	Variable
Necrosis	Absent	Occasional
Maturation	Common	Uncommon

the cell types in the two processes tend to be rather different. Desmoplastic Spitz nevi contain typical large epithelioid or fusiform cells, whereas desmoplastic melanoma is notable for pleomorphic spindle cells often with hyperchromatic nuclei.

A benign melanocytic lesion that may be confused with this variant of Spitz nevus is blue nevus. Although blue nevi may have pronounced sclerosing features, it is usually a more ill-defined melanocytic lesion than desmoplastic Spitz nevus and is composed of a more slender and more diffusely pigmented melanocytic population than the plumper cells of Spitz nevi.

Nonmelanocytic dermal spindle cell lesions that may share morphologic features of desmoplastic Spitz nevus are dermatofibroma, reticulohistiocytoma, and epithelioid cell histiocytoma (see above).

PIGMENTED SPINDLE CELL NEVUS

Synonyms: pigmented spindle cell nevus of Reed, pigmented spindle cell tumor

Clinical Features

The pigmented spindle cell nevus (PSCN) is a distinctive clinicopathologic entity important to recognize because of its frequent confusion with melanoma. PSCN usually presents as a symmetric, sharply circumscribed, dark brown or black papule or nodule.[46,49–51] It is typically a small lesion, often measuring less than 0.6 cm in diameter. Hypopigmented halos surrounding the lesion have been described[49] but are rare. PSCN is preferentially located on the extremities, especially the thigh, and less often on the trunk or arm. The lesion is uncommon in the head and neck region. It appears to affect women slightly more than men.[46,50] The peak incidence of the lesion is in the third decade, but it may occur in children as well as in late adult life. Occasional PSCN are congenital. There is usually a history of recent onset.

Histopathology

The architectural profile of PSCN at scanning magnification tends to be rather characteristic and is quite helpful in their recognition. These lesions are usually relatively small, strikingly well circumscribed, and remarkable for a slightly elevated, flat-topped plaquelike appearance of the epidermis (Fig. 6-11). The epidermis is often of fairly uniform thickness throughout or may diminish in thickness at the margins. However, some variants of PSCN may show elongation of epidermal rete ridges, but this is not the usual case. Although the PSCN may be junctional or compound, many are almost entirely intraepidermal. If dermal involvement occurs, the spindle cell elements are usually confined to the papillary dermis.

The PSCN is also remarkable for the presence of uniform, delicate, spindle cells present in tightly packed fascicles in its most typical presentation (see Fig. 6-11B). These fascicles of cells tend to have a fairly uniform and symmetric spacing and size within the epidermis. The fascicles are often vertically oriented (Fig. 6-12A) but also may form concentric arrangements (Fig. 6-12B) and be horizontally disposed.

The nests or fascicles vary in size and density. They are often closely apposed to each other and may be fused. They tend to be centered at or near the dermoepidermal junction and sometimes fill the majority of junctional space of the lesion. The predominant cellular growth pattern is within nests or fascicles. However, some PSCN, particularly in children, may show florid upward migration of single melanocytes closely simulating melanoma in situ (see Fig. 6-11D). Epithelioid cells may be present but only as a minor cell population.[50] The fusiform cells are often slightly more slender than the spindle cells of "classic" Spitz nevus (see Fig. 6-12B). Their nuclei are equal in size or smaller than the nuclei of adjacent keratinocytes.[52] A decrease in nuclear size from top to bottom may or may not be present, but many PSCN are not sufficiently thick for such an assessment to be meaningful. The nuclear shape is typically oval and regular. The chromatin pattern is usually finely stippled. Nucleoli may be inconspicuous or prominent.[52] A particularly important feature that is very useful in the recognition of PSCN is the uniformity of nuclei. Nuclear pleomorphism or anisochromasia is rare and, if present, needs to be viewed as an atypical feature.

Also in contrast to ordinary Spitz nevus, melanocytes of PSCN contain variable amounts of granular melanin. Heavy pigmentation also may involve the adjacent keratinocytes, cornified layer, and papillary dermis, giving the lesion a very dark color on gross appearance.[46]

It must be stated clearly that there is a histologic continuum of Spitz nevus and PSCN (Table 6-7). One will encounter many nevi showing varying degrees of transition between these two poles of the spectrum. For example, some nevi may exhibit slender spindle cells typical of PSCN yet at the same time contain somewhat larger fusiform cells that are less heavily melaninized. The latter cells would be more suggestive of Spitz nevus (Table 6-8).

The PSCN grows in an expansile fashion. The lateral intraepidermal growth is usually sharply demarcated with an abrupt transition from closely apposed nests to uninvolved epidermis. However, occasional lateral lentiginous proliferation of single melanocytes can be present and does not preclude the diagnosis of PSCN (see below).

In contrast to the infiltrative-appearing, often wedge-shaped deep portion of a Spitz nevus, the base of PSCN is

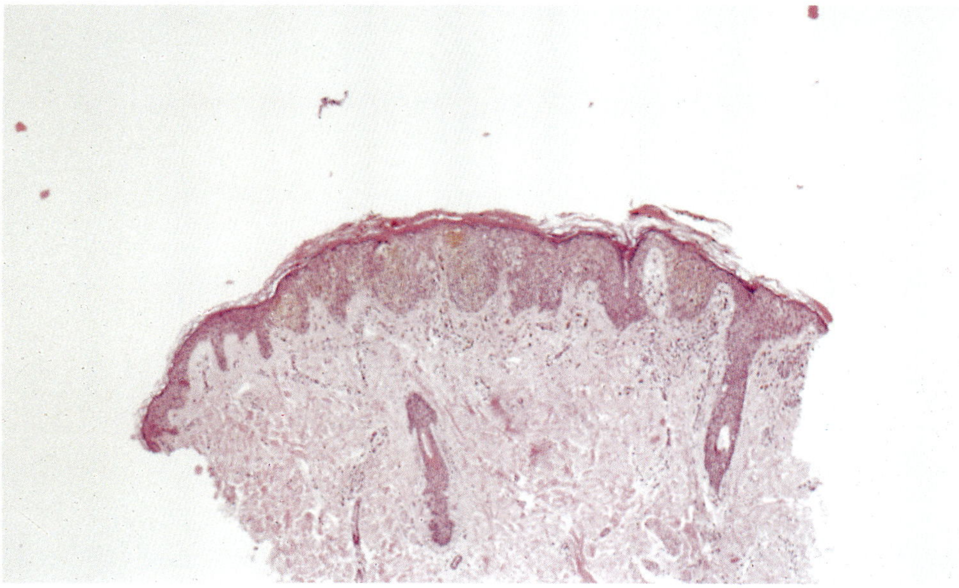

A

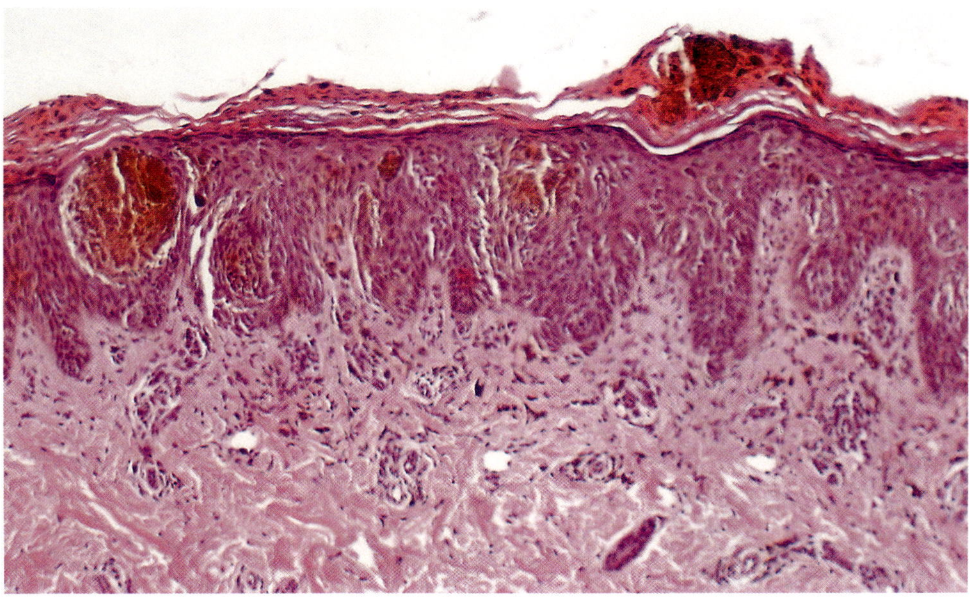

B

FIGURE 6-11

Pigmented spindle cell nevus. (A) The lesion is small, symmetric, and well-circumscribed (H&E, × 40). (B) Scattered intraepidermal nests of spindle cells, some heavily pigmented (H&E, × 100). (C) Fascicles of spindle cells are vertically disposed and seem to be part of the thickened epidermis (H&E, × 200). (D) Prominent pagetoid spread simulating melanoma in situ. Nonetheless, the lesion has all the features of a benign process noted in part A (H&E, × 400).

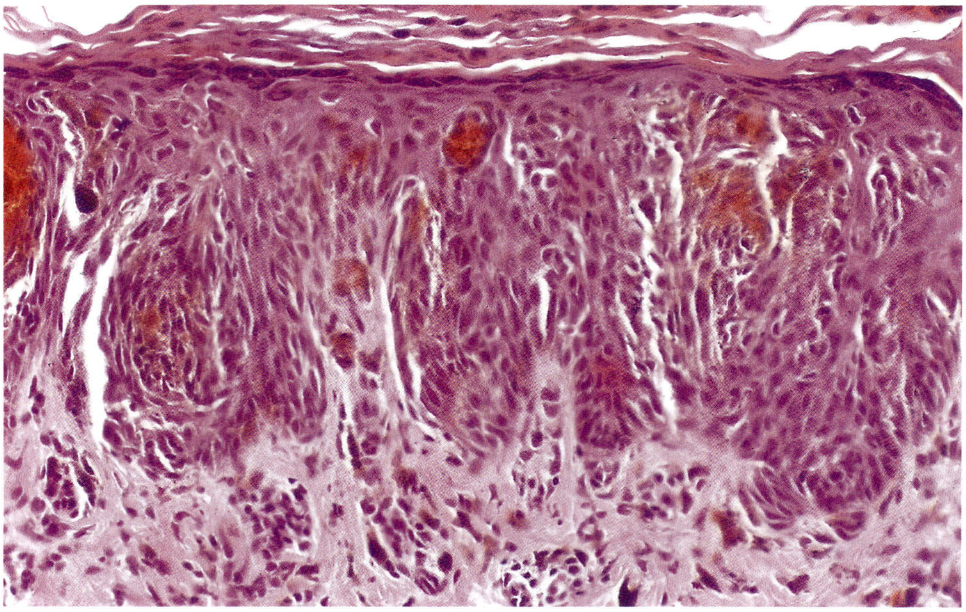

C

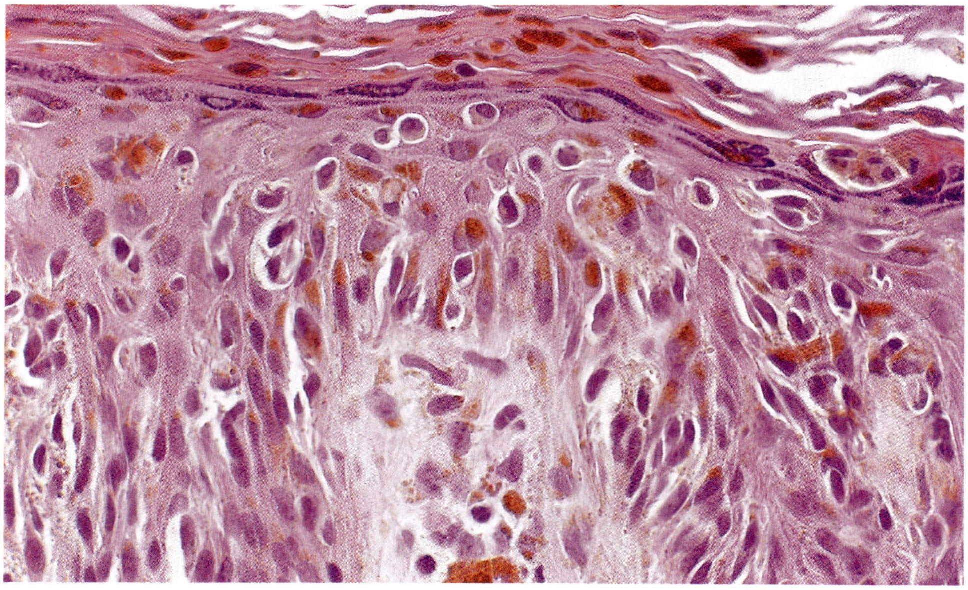

D

FIGURE 6-11 *(Continued)*

typically broad with pushing borders if papillary dermal involvement is present (see Fig. 6-12A). Compact rounded nests of relatively small cuboidal nevus cells often characterize the dermal component of PSCN. These cells often contain less pigment than intraepidermal spindle cells. The expansile nature of the papillary dermal nests may prompt scrutiny to rule out melanoma. However, the cytologic characteristics of such cells are usually unremarkable, and one can observe a maturation from the intraepidermal cells to the lower-most nevus cells at the base of the lesion. Extension into the reticular dermis is much less frequent than in Spitz nevus.[26]

As in Spitz nevus, shrinkage during tissue processing may lead to prominent clefts between fascicles of spindle cells from the adjacent epidermis. The same process leads also to retraction spaces separating melanocytes from each

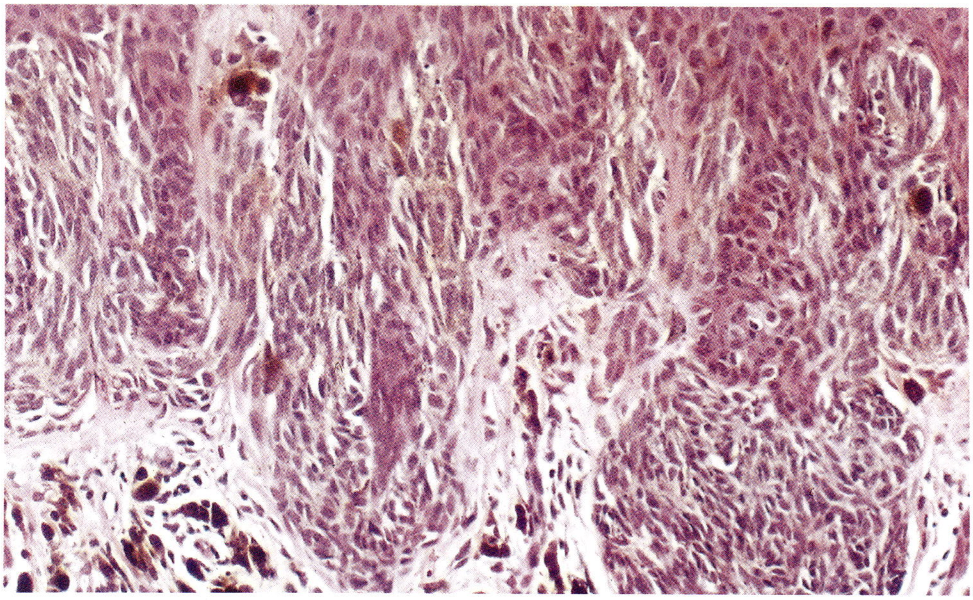

A

FIGURE 6-12
Pigmented spindle cell nevus. (A) Vertically oriented fascicles of spindle cells and compact nest of cells in papillary dermis (H&E, × 200). (B) Uniform spindle cells in concentric whorl (H&E, × 400).

other and giving them a loosely aggregated appearance. As already mentioned, upward single-cell extension of melanocytes toward the stratum corneum and transepidermal elimination of nests are not uncommon.[53] However, lateral pagetoid melanocytic spread raises the suspicion for melanoma.

A rather characteristic feature of PSCN, also shared with Spitz nevus, is the proclivity of fascicles of spindle cells to track along skin appendages. One typically observes fascicles extending from the intraepidermal component to involve eccrine ducts or hair follicles, often following these structures into the reticular dermis. These nests or fascicles tend to be compact and commonly fusiform in shape. This striking feature may suggest lentigo maligna, and the entire lesion should be carefully evaluated with this in mind.

Kamino bodies are seen less commonly than in Spitz nevus, but they can be found in the majority of cases if serial step sections are examined.[54] A patchy lymphocytic infiltrate with an admixture of melanophages is usually present at the base of the lesion, a feature that may cause confusion with melanoma.

Pigmented Spindle Cell Nevus with Architectural Disorder and Cytologic Atypia. The same discussion applies to the atypical variants of PSCN as previously elaborated for atypical forms of Spitz nevus (see Table 6-2). However, most atypical variants of PSCN are primarily intraepidermal. Substantial overlap may occur with conventional dysplastic nevi (Fig. 6-13).

Differential Diagnosis

Pigmented spindle cell nevus and its atypical variants must be distinguished from the radial growth phases of lentigo maligna and superficial spreading melanoma and from dysplastic nevus. Important features that distinguish PSCN from melanoma are listed in Table 6-9.

PSCN (particularly atypical forms) and lentigo maligna may show considerable similarity on occasion. Both are typically composed of pigmented spindle cells that may be arranged in junctional nests and may involve skin appendages to a striking degree. It is unusual for PSCN to occur on sun-exposed skin of the head and neck of older individuals, but this occasionally happens. Discrimination of the two is based on the usual small size, sharp circumscription, predominantly nested pattern, and uniformity of cell type in PSCN. Lentigo maligna, on the other hand, tends to be broader, poorly circumscribed, and usually typified by a mainly basilar single-cell proliferation of pleomorphic melanocytes. Rare lesions may show such striking overlap that distinction may not be possible. In such circumstances, we recommend that such lesions be excised completely with a cuff of normal tissue and that the patients be monitored carefully for aggressive behavior.

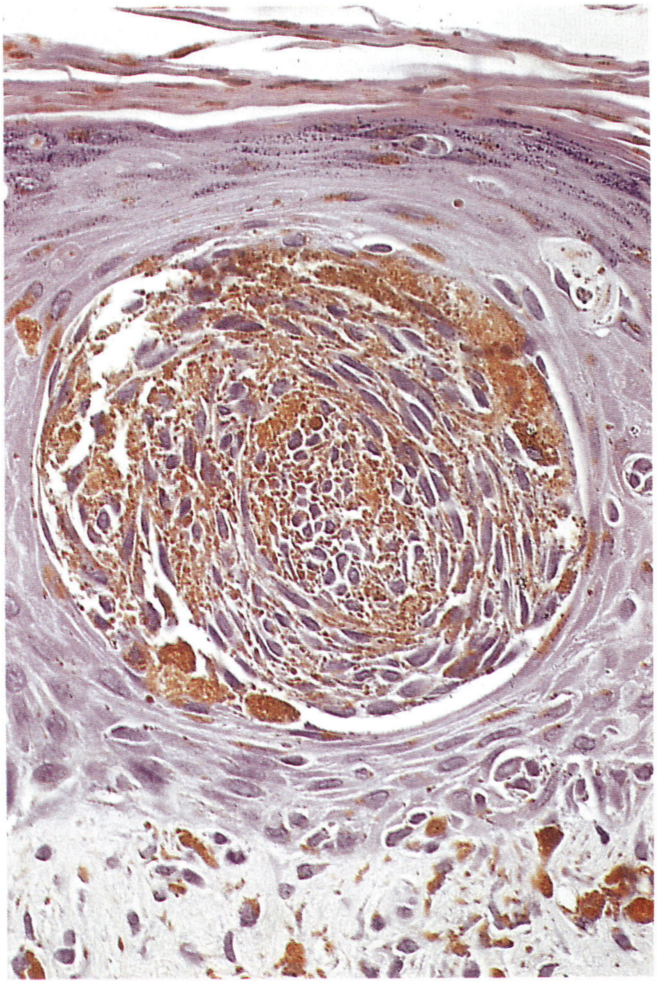

B

FIGURE 6-12 *(Continued)*

TABLE 6-7
Précis: Pigmented Spindle Cell Nevus

Clinical features
- Peak incidence in third decade
- Most often located on extremities (especially thigh)
- Women ≥ men
- Small (usually smaller than 0.6 cm)
- Symmetric
- Pigmented (usually evenly, often heavily)
- Sharply circumscribed
- Papule or nodule
- History of recent onset

Histopathology
- Junctional or compound nevus
- Predominantly spindle cells, but occasional epithelioid cells
- Spindle cells more slender and delicate than in Spitz nevi
- Uniform population of cells from side to side
- Symmetric configuration
- Predominance of junctional nests or fascicles
- Typically ovoid nests with fusiform cells oriented vertically
- Often confluence of nests leading to irregular shapes
- Sharp lateral borders, occasional lentiginous lateral spread
- Usually abundant coarse melanin
- Uniform nuclear features
- Decrease in cell size from top to bottom ("maturation")
- Mitoses not uncommon in intraepidermal component
- Absent or rare dermal mitoses

Differential diagnosis
- Lentigo maligna melanoma
- Superficial spreading (pagetoid) melanoma
- Dysplastic nevus

TABLE 6-8
*Comparison of Spitz Nevus and Pigmented Spindle Cell Nevus**

	Spitz Nevus	*Pigmented Spindle Cell Nevus*
Surface topography	Dome-shaped	Plaque-like or gently elevated
Epidermal hyperplasia	Prominent, often almost pseudoepitheliomatous	Platelike
Pagetoid spread	Variable, may be prominent	Common
Dermal architecture	Inverted wedge often	Rounded nests of cells usually confined to papillary dermis
Cell type	Enlarged epithelioid cells, spindle cells	Slender spindle cells, occasional transitional Spitzlike spindle cells, epithelioid cells uncommon
Melanin content	Often minimal, prominent on occasion	Spindle cells contain granular melanin; epidermis and papillary dermis contain substantial melanin deposits

*This table lists features noted at the poles of a morphologic continuum.

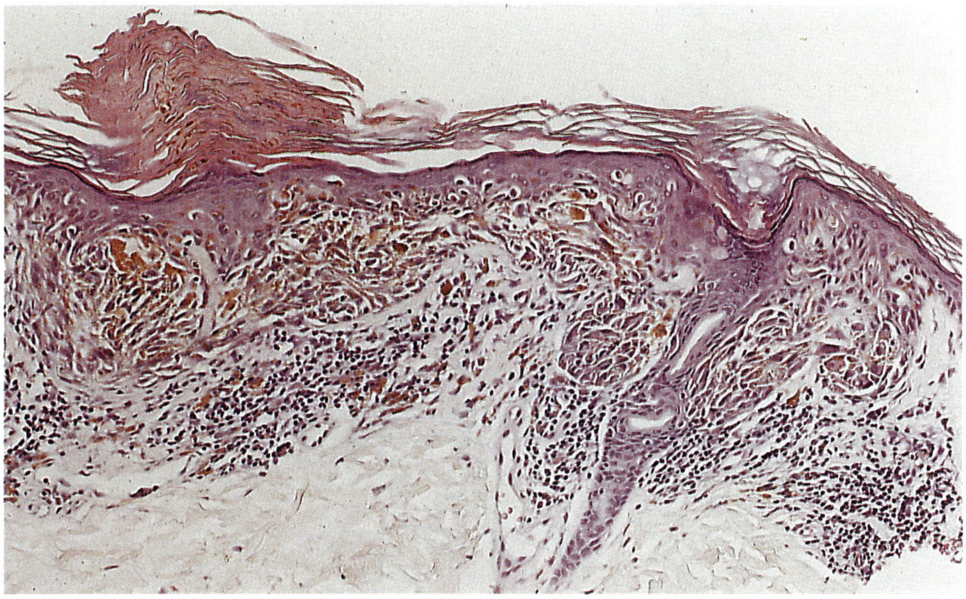

A

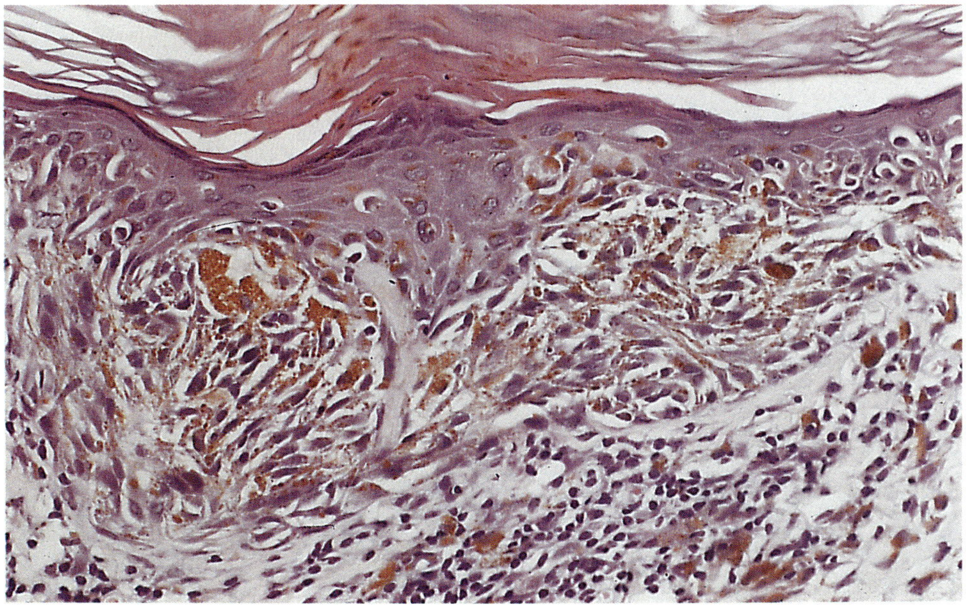

B

FIGURE 6-13

Pigmented spindle cell nevus with architectural disorder and cytologic atypia. (A) Note confluence of nests along dermal epidermal junction, an abnormal architectural feature resembling conventional dysplastic nevus (H&E, × 100). (B) Higher magnification showing horizontal confluence. The nevus is recognizable as a pigmented spindle cell nevus because the cells are fusiform and contain melanin. Kamino bodies are also present in this field (H&E, × 200).

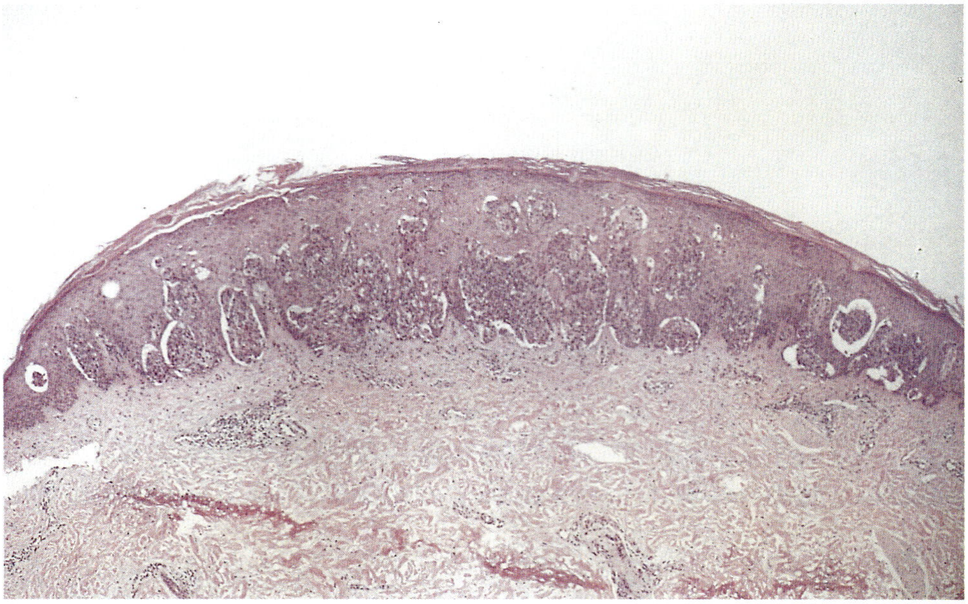

A

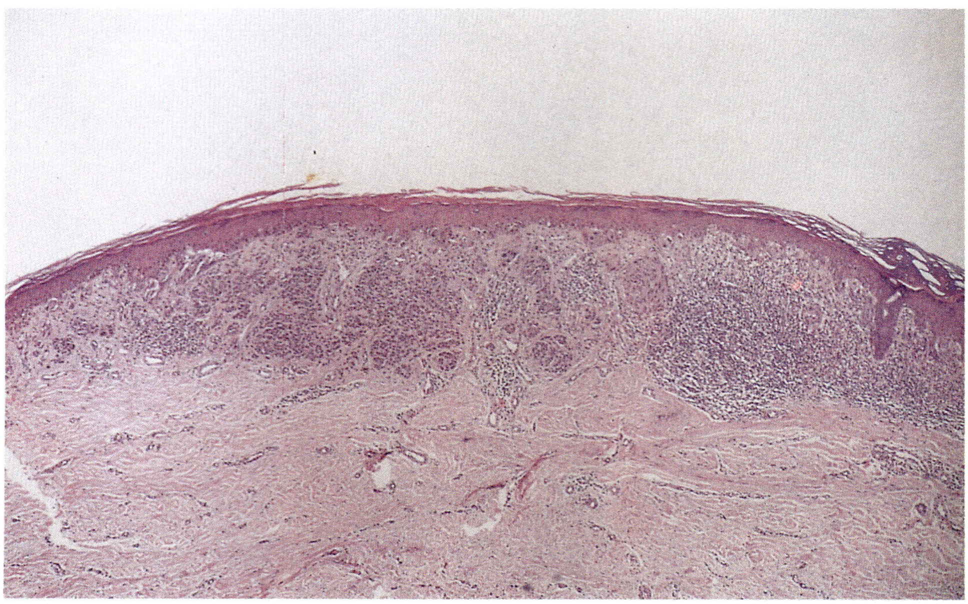

B

FIGURE 6-14

Recurrent Spitz nevus. (A) Original lesion extended to margin of excision. Note striking symmetry and orderly arrangement of cells in the initial lesion (H&E, × 40). (B) Recurrent lesion resected over one year later. This lesion is larger in size, shows a larger dermal component, and variation in the arrangement of dermal nests (H&E, × 40). (C) Higher magnification of (B). Note variability in size and shape of both junctional and dermal nests of melanocytes. There is a cohesive nest of enlarged spindle cells in the right side of the field. Despite this architectural disturbance, the typical cytologic features of Spitz nevus cells can be recognized (H&E, × 200).

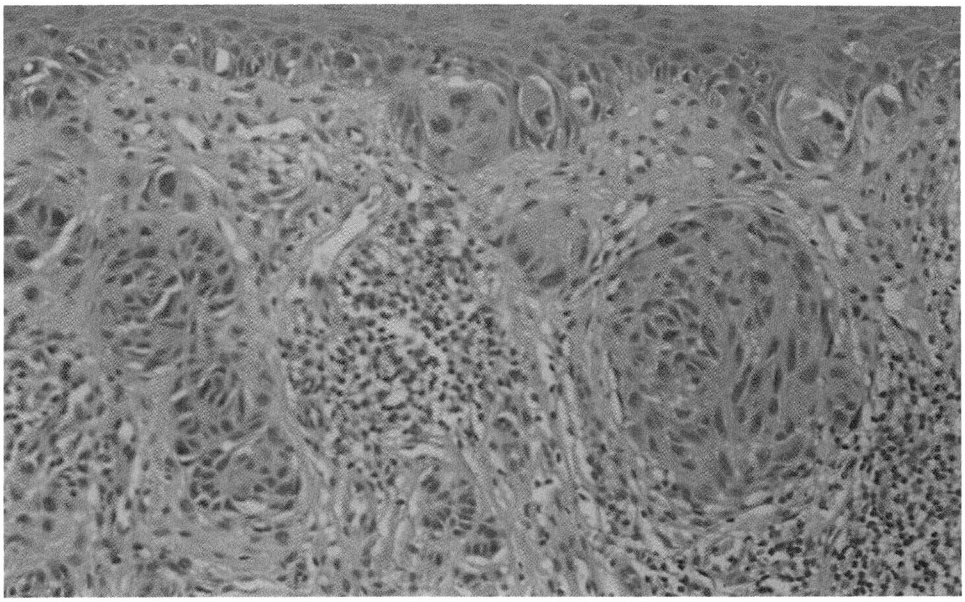

C

FIGURE 6-14 *(Continued)*

TABLE 6-9
Pigmented Spindle Cell Nevus and Atypical Variants versus Lentigo Maligna and Superficial Spreading Melanoma

	PSCN	*Atypical PSCN*	*Lentigo Maligna*	*Superficial Spreading Melanoma*
Symmetry	+	±	−	−
Sharp lateral borders	+	±	−	−
Cytologic uniformity	+	±	−	−
Regularity of nests	+	±	−	−
Maturation	+	±	−	−
Prominent vertical orientation of spindle cells	+	+	±	−
Involvement of appendages	+	+	+	±
Prominent coarse pigmentation	+	+	+	−

PSCN and atypical variants of PSCN are often confused with the radial growth phase of superficial spreading melanoma because of prominent pagetoid spread. This is one of the most commonly encountered problems in the pathology of melanocytic lesions. As discussed above, one must rely on clinical factors, i.e., young age, anatomic site (e.g., the extremities), as well as the overall morphologic appearance. PSCN are typically small, well-demarcated, symmetric, and orderly. Even with striking pagetoid spread in some lesions, the latter features argue strongly in favor of a benign process, especially if present in a young individual and on a site such as the thigh. However, atypical forms of PSCN are extremely challenging, and all the clinical and histologic features must be weighed carefully in the final interpretation. In many instances, a clear-cut diagnosis of melanoma cannot be made based on the constellation of findings. In such a situation, we often diagnose such lesions as pigmented spindle cell nevus (or melanocytic proliferation) with architectural disorder and cytologic atypia and recommend careful follow-up of the patient for recurrence. In our experience, recurrence of such lesions appears to be extremely rare.

The same features characteristic of PSCN, such as cytologic uniformity and nuclear regularity, as well as its tendency to contain vertically disposed melanocytes ("raining down") to the epidermal surface, help to distinguish PSCN from dysplastic nevus, in which the melanocytes are oriented more parallel to the epidermal surface and show more cytologic variability and atypia. Dysplastic nevi are generally less cellular and often display a pronounced lentiginous melanocytic proliferation with elongation of the rete ridges and associated papillary dermal fibrosis, which are not typical features of PSCN. However, some atypical forms of PSCN show substantial overlap with conventional dysplastic nevi and are in effect "dysplastic" PSCN. Discrimination of the two lesions thus may not be reproducible. Such lesions may be designated as PSCN with architectural disorder and cytologic atypia or dysplastic nevus with features of PSCN.

TABLE 6-10
Precís: Recurrent Spitz Nevus

Clinical features
- Mean age 14 years (range 3 to 34 years)
- Locations: head, extremities common
- Scar-like plaque or nodule, suggesting keloid
- Pink nodule suggesting Spitz nevus
- Often larger than original lesion

Histopathology
- Original lesions have positive margins
- Often larger than original lesion
- Asymmetry more common
- Dermal involvement more prominent than in original lesion, extension into deep reticular dermis or even subcutis
- Epithelioid cells more prevalent than in initial specimens
- Greater nuclear pleomorphism and hyperchromatism compared to original lesion
- Maturation usually present
- Mitoses not increased

Differential diagnosis
- Melanoma
- Spitz nevus with architectural disorder and cytologic atypia
- Desmoplastic Spitz nevus

RECURRENT SPITZ NEVUS

Judging from the number of cases reported and the experience of most dermatopathologists, recurrence of Spitz nevus is extremely rare.[55-57] This is probably a realistic impression since Spitz nevus itself is uncommon. Because of its rarity and the likelihood of referral bias, reliable data on the prevalence of recurrent Spitz nevi are difficult to obtain. Another caveat that must be considered is the actual diagnosis of the original lesion when recurrence does occur, i.e., could the original lesion have been an atypical variant of Spitz nevus or even melanoma? In any event, the prevalence of recurrent Spitz nevus must be rare (probably under 5 to 10 percent of all Spitz nevi). For example, in the series of 49 Spitz nevi reported by Kaye and Dehner,[57] there were no recurrences even among 24 lesions extending to the margins of excision.

Well-documented reports of recurrent Spitz nevus are limited, but in the series described by Stern,[56] there is useful information available. Stern reported 16 patients with recurrent Spitz nevi among which the original lesion was available for histopathologic examination in 13 cases.

Clinical Features

The average age at recurrence was 14 years with a range of 3 to 34 years according to Stern.[56] Males predominated over females (10M:6F), and the most common site was the head. Shave biopsy was the most common procedure performed. The mean time to recurrence was 13 months (range 2 months to 3 years). The most common clinical presentation of recurrence was a scar-like lesion suggesting a keloid or less likely a raised pink nodule typical of Spitz nevus.

Histopathology

Examination of the original specimens as described by Stern[56] will usually disclose features typical of Spitz nevus (Fig. 6-14A). However, virtually all of the initial lesions extend to the margins of the specimen. Rather characteristic findings noted in most recurrent Spitz nevi are the tendency of the lesion to be larger in overall size, to involve the dermis to a much greater extent (Fig. 6-14B), to show a predominance of epithelioid cells (as opposed to spindle cells in the original lesion), to possibly exhibit greater architectural disorder (Fig. 6-14C) and nuclear pleomorphism and hyperchromatism (as compared to the original lesion), and to show fibrosis of the surrounding stroma. Stern observed a striking propensity of recurrent Spitz nevi to involve the deep reticular dermis and even superficial subcutaneous fat.[56] Mitotic figures were not increased in recurrent lesions compared to the initial nevi.

Differential Diagnosis

The recurrent Spitz nevus must be distinguished from melanoma, atypical forms of primary Spitz nevus, and desmoplastic Spitz nevus. As with the conventional recurrent melanocytic nevus, it is necessary that the original biopsy be examined to establish a diagnosis of Spitz nevus and to determine if the initial lesion extended to the surgical margins. As has been mentioned previously, almost all recurrent Spitz nevi are associated with positive margins in the original lesion. Examination of the original specimen also is necessary to exclude melanoma since recurrent Spitz nevi may exhibit histologic features suggesting melanoma to a greater extent than the initial lesion. Clinical presentation also should figure into the discrimination of recurrent Spitz nevus from melanoma, i.e., younger age, location, and so on (see previous discussions for typical Spitz nevus). Although recurrent Spitz nevus may display unusual histologic features, careful examination should disclose in most instances maturation, typical cytologic characteristics of Spitz nevus, and absence of mitotic figures at the base of the lesion.[55,56]

As discussed previously for atypical Spitz nevi, some recurrent Spitz nevi may be particularly difficult to distinguish from melanoma. Because of the rarity of recurrent Spitz nevus and the lack of data on long-term follow-up, we advise a similar management strategy as that outlined for markedly atypical Spitz nevi (see previous discussion). The possibility of aggressive behavior should be discussed with the clinician and patient. Such lesions should have adequate reexcision and the patient followed carefully on a periodic basis for potential recurrence.

As noted by Stern,[56] recurrent Spitz nevus may be indistinguishable from desmoplastic Spitz nevus without knowledge of the clinical recurrence.

Clinical Course

Insufficient information is available on the clinical outcome of patients with recurrent Spitz nevi.[55,56] Long-term follow-up is needed to definitively exclude unusual presentations of melanoma. Second recurrences of Spitz nevi have been described, but these recurrences have also been related to previously positive margins.[56] Metastases have not been reported to our knowledge.[55–57]

REFERENCES

1. Darier J, Civatte A: Naevus ou naevo-carcinoma chez un nourisson. *Bull Soc Franc Derm Syph* 21:61–63, 1910.
2. Miescher G: Faszikulaerer Typus des Pigementzellennaevus. In Jadassohn, J (ed): *Handbuck der Haut unde Geschlechtskrankheiten,* Vol. 12. Berlin, Springer-Verlag, 1933,12 pp 1034–1036.
3. Pack G, Anglem T: Tumors of soft somatic tissues in infancy and childhood. *J Pediatr* 15:372–400, 1939.
4. Spitz S: Melanomas of childhood. *Am J Pathol* 24:591–609, 1948.
5. Allen A, Spitz S: Malignant melanoma: A clinicopathological analysis of the criteria for diagnosis and prognosis. *Cancer* 6:1–45, 1953.
6. Kernen J, Ackerman L: Spindle cell nevi and epithelioid cell nevi (so-called juvenile melanomas) in children and adults: A clinicopathological study of 27 cases. *Cancer* 13:612–625, 1960.
7. Kopf A, Andrade R. Benign juvenile melanoma. In Kopf A, Andrade R (eds): *Yearbook of Dermatology, 1965–1966.* Chicago, Year Book Medical Publishers, 1966, pp 7–52.
8. Helwig E: Seminar on skin neoplasms and dermatoses. In *Proceedings of the Twentieth Seminar of the American Society of Clinical Pathologists, Sept. 11, 1954.* American Society of Clinical Pathologists, 1955, pp 63–67.
9. Paniago-Pereira C, Maize J, Ackerman A: Nevus of large spindle and/or epithelioid cells (Spitz's nevus). *Arch Dermatol* 114:1811–1823, 1978.
10. Weedon D, Little J: Spindle and epithelioid cell nevi in children and adults: A review of 211 cases of the Spitz nevus. *Cancer* 40:217–225, 1977.
11. Allen A: Juvenile melanomas of children and adults and melanocarcinomas of children. *Arch Dermatol* 82:325–335, 1960.
12. Coskey R, Mehregan A: Spindle cell nevi in adults and children. *Arch Dermatol* 108:535–536, 1973.
13. Weedon D: The Spitz nevus. *Clin Oncol* 3:493–507, 1984.
14. McWorther H, Woolner L: Pigmented nevi, juvenile melanomas, and malignant melanomas in children. *Cancer* 7:564–585, 1954.
15. Palazzo J, Duray P: Congenital agminated Spitz nevi: Immunoreactivity with a melanoma-associated monoclonal antibody. *J Cutan Pathol* 15:166–170, 1988.
16. Peters M, Goellner J: Spitz nevi and malignant melanomas of childhood and adolescence. *Histopathology* 10:1289–1302, 1986.
17. Gartmann H, Ganser M: Der Spitz-Naevus. Spindelzellen und/oder Epithelienzellennaevus. Eine klinische Analyse von 652 Tumoren. *Z Hautkr* 60:22–28, 1985.
18. Rhodes A: Neoplasms: Benign neoplasias, hyperplasias, and dysplasias of melanocytes. In Fitzpatrick TB, Eisen AZ, Wolff K, Freedberg IM, Austen KF, (eds): *Dermatology in General Medicine* (ed 4). New York, McGraw-Hill, 1993, pp 996–1077.
19. Echevarria R, Ackerman LV: Spindle and epithelioid nevi in the adult: Clinicopathologic report of 26 cases. *Cancer* 20:175–189, 1967.
20. Allen A: Juvenile melanomas and malignant melanomas. *Surg Gynecol Obstet* 104:735–754, 1957.
21. Smith K, Skelton H, Lupton G, Graham J: Spindle cell and epithelioid cell nevi with atypia and metastasis (malignant Spitz nevus). *Am J Surg Pathol* 13:931–939, 1989.
22. Lancer H, Muhlbauer J, Sober A: Multiple agminated spindle cell nevi: Unique clinical presentation and review. *J Am Acad Dermatol* 8:707–711, 1983.
23. Wallace H: Eruptive juvenile melanomata. *Br J Dermatol* 91(Suppl 10):37–38, 1974.
24. Weimar V, Zuehlke R: Multiple agminate spindle and epithelioid cell nevi in an adult. *Arch Dermatol* 114:1383–1384, 1978.
25. Hamm H, Happle R, Broecker E: Multiple agminate Spitz nevi: Review of the literature and report of a case with distinctive immunohistological features. *Br J Dermatol* 117: 511–522, 1987.
26. Mooi W, Krausz T: Spitz naevus, desmoplastic Spitz naevus and pigmented spindle cell naevus. In Mooi W, Krausz T (eds): *Biopsy: Pathology of Melanocytic Disorders.* London, Chapman and Hall, 1992, pp 156–185.
27. Binder S, Asnog C, Paul E, Cochran A: The histology and differential diagnosis of Spitz nevus. *Semin Diagn Pathol* 10:36–46, 1993.
28. Merot Y, Frenk E: Spitz nevus (large spindle and/or epithelioid cell nevus): Age-related involvement of the suprabasal epidermis. *Virchows Arch [A]* 415:97–101, 1989.
29. Kamino H, Misheloff E, Ackerman A, et al: Eosinophilic globules in Spitz's nevi: New findings and a diagnostic sign. *Am J Surg Pathol* 1:319–324, 1979.
30. Arbuckle S, Weedon D: Eosinophilic globules in the Spitz nevus. *J Am Acad Dermatol* 7:324–327, 1982.
31. Havenith M, van Zandvoort E, Cleutjens J, Bosman F: Basement membrane deposition in benign and malignant nevomelanocytic lesions: An immunohistochemical study with antibodies to type IV collagen and laminin. *Histopathology* 15:137–146, 1989.
32. Schmoeckel C: How consistent are dermatopathologists in reading early malignant melanoma and lesions "precursor" to them? An international survey. *Am J Dermatopathol* 6(Suppl):13–24, 1984.

33. Elder D, Murphy G: Spindle and epithelioid cell nevus (Spitz nevus): Atlas of tumor pathology. In Elder D, Murphy G (eds): *Melanocytic Tumors of the Skin.* Washington, Armed Forces Institute of Pathology, 1990, pp 40–57.
34. Peters M: Histiocytic and Langerhans cell reactions. In Farmer ER, Hood AF (eds): *Pathology of the Skin.* Norwalk, Conn, Appleton and Lange, 1990, pp 249–272.
35. Barnhill RL, Mihm MC: Cellular neurothekeoma: A distinctive variant of neurothekeoma mimicking nevomelanocytic tumors. *Am J Surg Pathol* 14:113–120, 1990.
36. Wilson-Jones E, Cerio R, Smith N: Epithelioid cell histiocytoma: A new entity. *Br J Dermatol* 120:185–195, 1989.
37. Guldhammer B, Norgaard T: The differential diagnosis of intraepidermal malignant lesions using immunohistochemistry. *Am J Dermatopathol* 8:295–301, 1986.
38. Reed R: Malignant Spitz nevus. Case presented at the Clinicopathology Conference, American Academy of Pathology Meeting, New York, December 1980.
39. Delacretaz J: Melanoma juvenile (melanome de Spitz) a evolution maligne. *Dermatologica* 139:79–83, 1969.
40. Howat A, Variend S: Lymphatic invasion of Spitz nevi. *Am J Surg Pathol* 9:125–128, 1985.
41. Ainsworth A, Folberg R, Reed R, Clark W: Melanocytic nevi, melanocytomas, melanocytic dysplasias, and uncommon forms of melanoma. In Clark WH Jr, Goldman LT, Mastrangelo MJ (eds): *Human Malignant Melanoma.* New York, Grune and Stratton, 1979, pp 167–208.
42. Howat A, Giri D, Cotton D, Slater D: Nuclear organizer regions in Spitz nevi and malignant melanomas. *Cancer* 63:474–478, 1989.
43. Rode J, Williams R, Jarvis L, et al: S-100 protein, neuron-specific enolase, and nuclear DNA content in Spitz nevus. *J Pathol* 161:41–45, 1990.
44. Winokur T, Palazzo J, Johnson W, Duray P: Evaluation of DNA ploidy in dysplastic and Spitz nevi by flow cytometry. *J Cutan Pathol* 17:342–347, 1990.
45. LeBoit P, Fletcher H: A comparative study of Spitz nevus and nodular melanoma using image analysis cytometry. *J Invest Dermatol* 88:753–757, 1987.
46. Reed R, Ichinose H, Clark W, Mihm MC: Common and uncommon melanocytic nevi and borderline melanomas. *Semin Oncol* 2:119–147, 1975.
47. Barr R, Morales R, Graham J: Desmoplastic nevus. A distinct histologic variant of mixed spindle and epithelioid cell nevus. *Cancer* 46:557–564, 1980.
48. MacKie RM, Doherty VR: The desmoplastic melanocytic naevus: A distinct histological entity. *Histopathology* 20:207–211, 1992.
49. Gartmann H: Der pigmentierte Spindelzellentumor. *Z Hautkr* 56:862–876, 1981.
50. Smith N: The pigmented spindle cell tumor of Reed: An underdiagnosed lesion. *Semin Diagn Pathol* 4:75–87, 1987.
51. Barnhill RL, Mihm MC: Pigmented spindle cell nevus and its variants: Distinction from melanoma. *Br J Dermatol* 121:717–726, 1989.
52. Sagebiel R, Chinn E, Egbert B: Pigmented spindle cell nevus: Clinical and histologic review of 90 cases. *Am J Surg Pathol* 8:645–653, 1984.
53. Sau P, Graham J, Helwig E: Pigmented spindle cell nevus. *Arch Dermatol* 120:1615, 1984.
54. Wistuba I, Gonzalez S: Eosinophilic globules in pigmented spindle cell nevus. *Am J Dermatopathol* 12:268–271, 1990.
55. Omura EF, Kheir SM: Recurrent Spitz's nevus. *Am J Dermatopathol* 6:207–212, 1984.
56. Stern J: Recurrent Spitz's nevi: A clinicopathologic investigation. *Am J Dermatopathol* 7(Suppl):49–50, 1985.
57. Kaye VN, Dehner LP: Spindle and epithelioid cell nevus (Spitz nevus): Natural history following biopsy. *Arch Dermatol* 126:1581–1583, 1990.

7

Dermal Melanocytoses, Blue Nevi, and Related Conditions

The subject of this chapter includes blue nevi and related proliferations of melanocytes, usually dendritic or spindled, primarily involving the reticular dermis.[1-74] The nomenclature for this group of lesions is somewhat confusing and inconsistent. Some of this confusion is related to clinical description ("blue nevus") for some entities and histologic characterization for others ("cellular" blue nevus). Inconsistency results from histologic overlap with other melanocytic lesions such as spindle and epithelioid cell nevi or pigmented peripheral nerve sheath tumors[75-78] (see Chap. 8).

The classification of lesions within this general category is based on assessing a number of features: clinical appearance; anatomic site of lesion; localization in the reticular dermis, subcutis, etc; the extent to which the lesion is made up of dendritic versus spindle-shaped melanocytes; degree of cellularity of lesion; degree of fibrosis (sclerosis); degree of melanization and accumulation of melanophages; overall architecture—fibrous nodule, cellular nodule or nests, plexiform configuration; presence of other nevus components—junctional, compound elements; and degree of cytologic atypia and mitotic activity[5,29,39,40,43] (Fig. 7-1).

The bluish appearance of these various lesions is related primarily to depth of melanin in the dermis and the Tyndall phenomenon. The longer wavelengths of visible light penetrate the reticular dermis and are absorbed by the melanin. However, the shorter wavelengths, representing the bluish part of the color spectrum, do not penetrate so deeply and are reflected back from the superficial dermis and epidermis. The result is that the lesion appears blue to the observer.

HISTOGENESIS

The dermal melanocytoses and blue nevi are thought to result from the dermal arrest and accumulation of cells migrating from the neural crest.[30,67] In contrast to ordinary nevi, it is believed that these migratory cells never reach the epidermis. Based on the affinity of many of these lesions for hair follicles, an origin from hair follicles is possible. The immediate origin of the cells comprising the dermal melanocytoses and blue nevi has been postulated to be either (1) melanocytes or (2) melanogenic Schwann cells.[68,69] Recent ultrastructural studies have shown a remarkable similarity between blue nevus cells and schwannoma cells.[71-73] Both cell types are reported to exhibit basal lamina, desmosome-like junctional structures, and compound melanosomes.[68,70] Based on the latter studies, a schwannian origin of blue nevus has been proposed. However, some authorities have not confirmed the presence of an external lamina in association with blue nevus cells of the skin, a finding arguing against schwannian differentiation.[74] Blue nevus cells also can be distinguished from Schwann cells because only the former cells contain premelanosomes, and melanosomes,[68] whereas Schwann cells do not. In addition, the compound melanosomes observed in pigmented Schwann cells are most likely derived from phagocytosis rather than synthesis of melanin.[74] It also has been shown recently that the monoclonal antibody HMB-45 reacts with blue nevus cells but not with Schwann cells,[67] unless they contain melanin, as in pigmented schwannoma. Taking into account all these observations, Sun and colleagues[67] have proposed that blue nevi, rather than being purely melanocytic or schwannian,

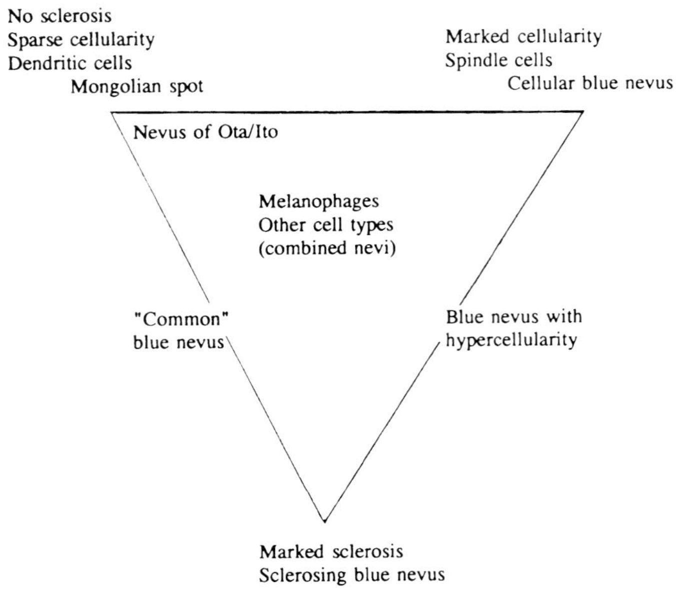

FIGURE 7-1
Histologic spectrum of blue nevus and related conditions. The particular disorder is defined by the degree of dermal sclerosis (none to marked), the degree of cellularity (sparse to marked), and the cell types present (mainly dendritic cells, mainly spindle cells, other cell types, and melanophages).

originate from a progenitor cell with features of both melanocytes and Schwann cells. Nonetheless, the general consensus at present is that cutaneous blue nevi are derived from melanocytes rather than Schwann cells.

DERMAL MELANOCYTOSES

Mongolian spot
Nevus of Ota
Nevus fuscocaeruleus zygomaticus (acquired nevus of Ota-like macules, Sun's nevus)
Acquired dermal melanocytosis of the face and extremities
Nevus of Ito
Dermal melanocyte hamartoma

These six entities are related because they are all essentially bluish macular lesions that histologically demonstrate scattered dendritic melanocytes in the reticular dermis with little or no stromal alteration[1–25] (Table 7-1).

Mongolian spot

Clinical Features. Mongolian spots are oval or round, often poorly defined macules varying in color from slight gray to blue-black or dark brown[1,2,4,5] (see Table 7-1). There is no change in the skin texture. The lesions most often affect the lumbosacral region but may be seen in other (ectopic or aberrant) locations. The size of Mongolian spots varies from less than 1 cm to over 10 cm. These lesions are present at birth but usually regress spontaneously by 3 to 4 years of age. However, some lesions may persist until the second decade or even into adulthood. Mongolian spots have been observed in over 90 percent of black and Native American newborns, 81 percent of Asians, 70 percent of Hispanics, and 10 percent of Caucasians.[4] The development of malignant melanoma in a typical Mongolian spot has not been reported.

Histopathology. The Mongolian spot is characterized by widely spaced dendritic melanocytes localized to the lower half or two-thirds of the reticular dermis.[5] The dermis is unaltered, and melanophages are usually not present. The melanocytes are generally bipolar with their axes oriented parallel to the skin surface and situated in low density between individual collagen bundles. The individual cells have slender, lengthy cytoplasmic processes (dendrites) that contain finely divided melanin granules. The nuclei are often obscured by melanin but, when visible, have clumped chromatin patterns.

Differential Diagnosis. Mongolian spots are distinguished from other dermal dendritic lesions by location (sacral area), disappearance in infancy, and sparse number of dermal melanocytes without melanophages or fibrosis. Persistent ectopic "Mongolian spots" may be difficult to discriminate from nevus of Ota and nevus of Ito.

TABLE 7-1
Differential Features of Dermal Melanocytoses

Feature	*Mongolian Spot*	*Nevus of Ota*	*Nevus of Ito*	*Blue Nevus*
Onset	Birth or soon after	Birth or soon after	Birth or soon after	Birth or later in life
Size	5 cm or larger	5 cm or larger	5 cm or larger	0.2–1.5 cm
Color	Gray-tan, slate blue	Brown, slate blue	Brown, slate blue	Bluish black
Surface	Macular	Macular, rarely discrete papules	Macular, rarely discrete papules	Papular
Hair	Normal for site	Normal for site	Normal for site	Normal for site
Distribution	Midline	Unilateral	Unilateral	Unilateral
Number	Single, can be multiple	Single	Single	Single, rarely multiple
Site	Lumbosacral	First and second division trigeminal nerve	Shoulder and upper arm	Extensors of extremities: dorsa of hands and feet, buttocks, face
Racial incidence	Asians and dark-skinned races	Asians and dark-skinned races	Asians and dark-skinned races	More common in dark-skinned races
Familial incidence	Common	Rare	Rare	None
Sex	No difference	80% in females	80% in females	60% in females
Age of appearance	At birth	60% at birth	60% at birth	At or just after birth
Spontaneous fate	Usually disappears during first few years of life	Persist, rarely disappear	Persist, rarely disappear	Persist
Tendency to malignancy	Never reported	Rare	Rare	Rare
Histologic features	Scattered dermal melanocytes in lower half of dermis in low concentrations	Moderate number of dermal melanocytes in upper dermis	Moderate number of dermal melanocytes in upper dermis	Common form has high concentration of dermal melanocytes in middle and lower third of dermis; melanophages usually present; cellular form also contains bundles of spindle-shaped cells
Ultrastructure	Fully developed melanocytes with only mature melanosomes; virtually no premelanosomes	Fully developed melanocytes with only mature melanosomes; virtually no premelanosomes	Fully developed melanocytes with only mature melanosomes; virtually no premelanosomes	Fully developed melanocytes with only mature melanosomes; virtually no premelanosomes

It is likely that some previously reported examples of ectopic Mongolian spots are in fact nevus of Ota or nevus of Ito.

Nevus of Ota (Nevus Fuscocaeruleus Ophthalmomaxillaris)

Clinical Features. This hamartomatous or nevoid condition usually presents at birth or in childhood as a unilateral speckled bluish macule involving the periorbital region, forehead, temple, cheek, or nose.[5–15] The areas correspond to the distribution of the first two branches of the trigeminal nerve. Examination also may disclose involvement of the sclera, conjunctiva, cornea, retina, or oral and nasal mucosa. Brownish lentigo-like lesions and bluish papules or nodules are occasionally associated with nevus of Ota. About 13 percent of cases are bilateral. The natural history of nevus of Ota is persistence with slight extension of the process.

The development of malignant melanoma in association with nevus of Ota has only been recorded in a few instances.[16,17] However, patients with involvement of the eye also have been observed to develop melanoma of the choroid, iris, orbit, and brain.

Nevus Fuscocaeruleus Zygomaticus (Acquired Nevus of Ota-Like Macules, Sun's Nevus)

Clinical Features. The development of bilateral bluish macules in the zygomatic areas of the face has been reported primarily in Chinese and Japanese women.[18,19] The affected individuals have ranged in age from 19 to 69 years. In contrast to typical nevus of Ota, there is no involvement of either the eye or oral mucosa by the melanocytosis.

Acquired Dermal Melanocytosis of the Face and Extremities

Clinical Features. This particular disorder is associated with bilateral bluish or brownish discoloration of the face, somewhat similar to nevus of Ota, but also associated with involvement of the extensor surfaces of the upper extremities and possibly the palms.[20] This particular entity is associated with onset in adults in a similar fashion to the acquired bilateral nevus zygomaticus.

Nevus of Ito (Nevus Fuscocaeruleus Acromiodeltoideus)

Clinical Features. The nevus of Ito is closely related to nevus of Ota but is distinguished by its unilateral distribution involving the supraclavicular, scapular, or deltoid regions.[8] Similar to nevus of Ota, this lesion has a mottled appearance with bluish or brownish macules. Onset is noted at birth or later in childhood. The nevus of Ito may occur in association with nevus of Ota. The development of malignant melanoma in nevus of Ito has been recorded.[21]

Dermal Melanocyte Hamartoma

Clinical Features. The term *dermal melanocyte hamartoma* has been used to describe a small number of developmental abnormalities usually present at birth and exhibiting extensive involvement of the skin.[22–25] In one particular instance, there was almost complete involvement of the skin. Other reported cases include extensive involvement of a lower extremity and segmental coalescence of bluish macules.

Histopathology. The histologic changes of the last five entities described above are very similar for the bluish macules.[8,9,12] Scattered dermal melanocytes with prominent dendritic processes are noted in the upper dermis without alteration of the dermal stroma (Fig.7-2A). There may be involvement of the papillary dermis, and in some instances, there is aggregation of these cells about sebaceous glands, eccrine ducts, blood vessels, and cutaneous nerves. Uncommonly, there may be extension of these cells into the subcutaneous fat. As in Mongolian spot, the cells contain prominent deposits of fine melanin granules (See Fig. 7-2B). Melanophages, in general, are uncommon. The density of melanocytes is greater than in Mongolian spot.

Based on the examination of 450 cases of Ota's nevus, Hirayama and Suzuki[12] have recently reported a new histopathologic classification of this entity. The classification is related to the location of melanocytes in the dermis: (1) superficial type (melanocytes present in the superficial dermis), (2) deep type, (3) diffuse type (melanocytes scattered throughout entire dermis), (4) superficial dominant type, and (5) deep dominant type. These authors also noted that cheek lesions tended to have a superficial pattern, whereas all other sites were typified by diffuse, deep, or deep dominant patterns.[12]

The brownish macules demonstrate dermal melanocytes located very close to the epidermis. In these areas, slight basilar melanocytic hyperplasia and basal layer hypermelanosis also may be present.[8]

The slightly raised or papular lesions that may be seen in these lesions demonstrate an even greater concentration of dendritic melanocytes, resembling the findings seen in blue nevus.

Differential Diagnosis. In general, the dermal melanocytoses discussed above are distinguished from blue nevi by the absence of or only limited collagenization or deformation of the dermis by cellular aggregates and a predominately single-cell disposition of dendritic melanocytes. On the other hand, blue nevi tend to distort the fabric of the dermis by the presence of increased fibrous tissue, cellular accumulation, or both. It must be pointed out that there is some degree of histologic overlap or merging of the dermal melanocytoses and blue nevi. Final categorization of a particular lesion must take into account clinical features such as size, surface topography (macular versus papular surface), and location. Classification of some lesions may be somewhat arbitrary (nevus of Ito versus patch-like blue nevus); in some instances, a descriptive diagnosis may be preferred, such as dermal melanocytosis.

BLUE NEVUS

Historically, the classification of blue nevus has included two variants based on clinical and histologic findings.[5,27–49] The first type of blue nevus, generally known as the *common blue nevus,* is the most frequent subtype, primarily involving the dorsal aspects of the hands and feet, having a relatively small diameter (<1 cm), and characterized primarily by the presence of dendritic melanocytes with variable fibrosis histologically. The less prevalent, larger variant, the *cellular blue nevus,* has been defined primarily by nests of relatively amelanotic spindle cells in addition

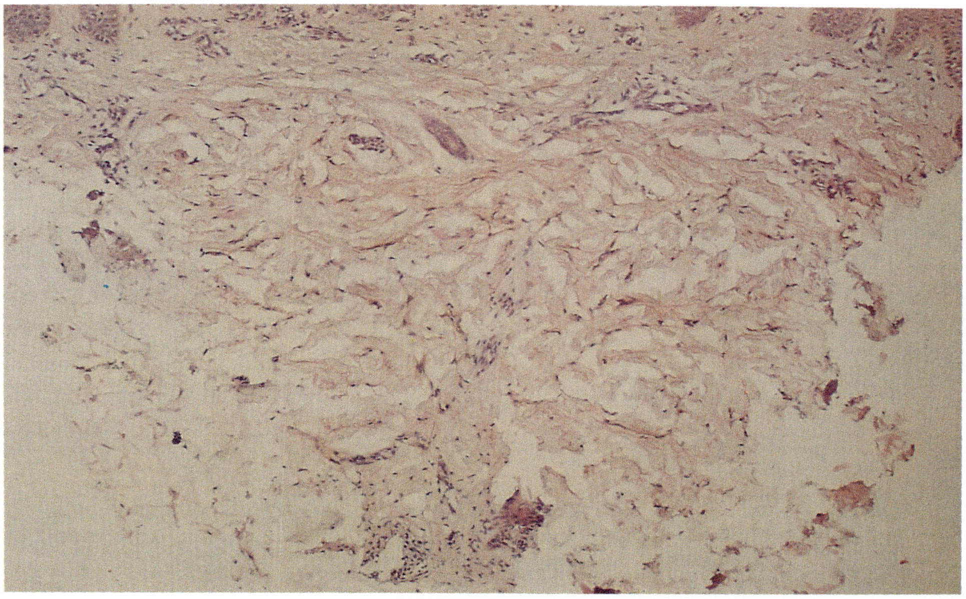

A

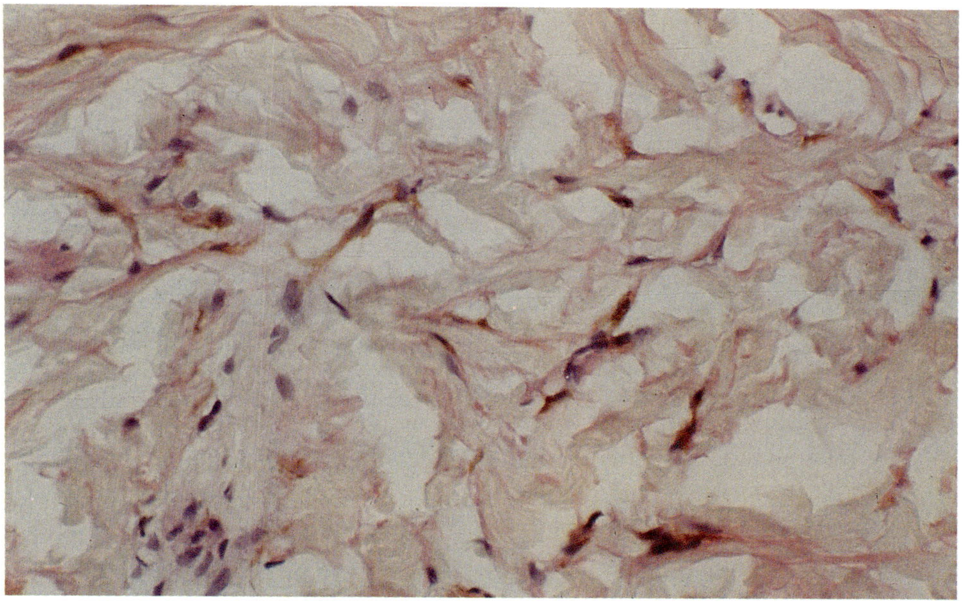

B

FIGURE 7-2

Nevus of Ito. (A) A punch biopsy shows a largely unaffected dermis. There are increased numbers of pigmented dendritic cells in the mid-reticular dermis scattered among collagen bundles. Neither fascicles of cells nor fibrosis is present, as would be observed in blue nevus (H&E, × 100). (B) Higher magnification showing scattered dendritic melanocytes with delicate cytoplasmic processes containing melanin (H&E, × 400).

TABLE 7-2
Précis: Ordinary (common) Blue Nevus

Clinical features
- Onset birth or later
- Women > men
- Located on face, dorsum of wrist or foot, buttock
- 2–10 mm or larger
- Well circumscribed
- Symmetric
- Dome-shaped often
- Uniform blue, blue-gray, blue-black
- No alteration of skin markings
- Regular borders

Histopathology
- Symmetry
- Alteration of dermis by variable admixture of dendritic melanocytes (usually heavily melaninized), melanophages, and fibrosis
- Dendritic cells often in bundles
- Periadnexal aggregation of dendritic cells often
- Infiltration of smooth muscle, nerves

Differential diagnosis
- Other dermal melanocytoses
- Desmoplastic melanoma
- Regressed melanoma

to the dendritic melanocytic component. However, examination of sufficient numbers of blue nevi reveal that there is indeed a spectrum of histologic changes rather than necessarily two well-defined subtypes of blue nevus. The histologic changes that may be seen in the spectrum of blue nevi include variable number and density of dendritic melanocytes, number of melanophages, degree of fibrosis, and variable number and disposition of spindle cells. The spindle cell component may consist of individually disposed spindle cells, spindle cells arranged in fascicles, and finally, arrangement of spindle cells in compact nests, as seen in the classic cellular blue nevus. Finally, some blue nevi contain cellular elements from other nevi such as ordinary nevi or spindle and epithelioid cell nevi and have been designated *combined nevi*[35] (see Chap. 8). Thus the final histologic characterization of a blue nevus must encompass the varying proportions of the histologic features mentioned, as well as other concerns such as degree of cytologic atypia. The clinical characteristics of some blue nevi also may warrant attention, such as a plaquelike or agminated configuration.[5,36,59–65] The following classification of blue nevi therefore is based on the predominant histologic changes.

Ordinary (common) Blue Nevus (Dendritic-Fibrotic Type)

Clinical Features. The most common form of blue nevus usually presents as a well-demarcated, slightly raised or dome-shaped, bluish papule[5,27–29,40] (Table 7-2). The color is usually a uniform slate gray, blue-black, or black. The borders are generally regular, and these nevi usually measure less than 1 cm in diameter. They are located primarily on the dorsal aspects of the hands and feet and they involve the face and scalp as well. Onset is generally in childhood but may occur later in life. Melanoma has only rarely been reported to originate from this type of blue nevus.[37]

Histopathology. This form of blue nevus is characterized by an aggregation of dendritic melanocytes, generally in the upper dermis, with formation of a space-occupying mass that deforms the dermis[5,29,40] (Fig. 7.3A and Table 7-2). In many instances, compact cellular bundles of dendritic melanocytes are horizontally-disposed with an overall elongated or lens-shaped configuration. The lesion may occur anywhere in the reticular dermis and even in the papillary dermis. In general, there are fascicles of dendritic cells with frequent aggregation about appendages and neurovascular bundles (see Fig. 7-3B). The cells are generally bipolar or stellate and are characterized by lengthy dendritic processes (Fig. 7-3B and 7-4). Most cells contain a dense accumulation of relatively fine melanin granules. The nuclei are ovoid with uniform chromatin patterns. Melanophages are usually present and may be the principal cell type in some cases. These cells are distinguished from the blue nevus cells by the lack of dendrites, the polygonal morphology of the cell, and the presence of coarser melanin granules. Variable degrees of fibrosis are also present (see Fig. 7-3B).

Differential Diagnosis. This type of blue nevus shares the common dendritic cell type noted in the dermal melanocytoses already discussed. The blue nevus differs from the preceding entities by showing a greater concentration of dendritic melanocytes that results in a deformation of the reticular dermis and is accompanied by varying degrees of fibrosis and melanophage accumulation. However, the papular and nodular lesions within nevus of Ota or nevus of Ito are indistinguishable from this variant of blue nevus.[8] The differential diagnosis also might include primary or metastatic melanoma, possibly with some degree of regression. In general, however, blue nevi can be distinguished from melanoma by their small size, overall symmetry, lack of cytologic atypia, and absence of mitotic activity and necrosis. On occasion, a tattoo may suggest blue nevus because of dark pigment within macrophages of the dermis. However, in contrast to a blue nevus, tattoos are usually characterized by intense black pigment (other colors may be present) versus the brown granules of melanin, perivascular arrangement of pigment-containing macrophages, and usual absence of dendritic melanocytes and fibrosis.

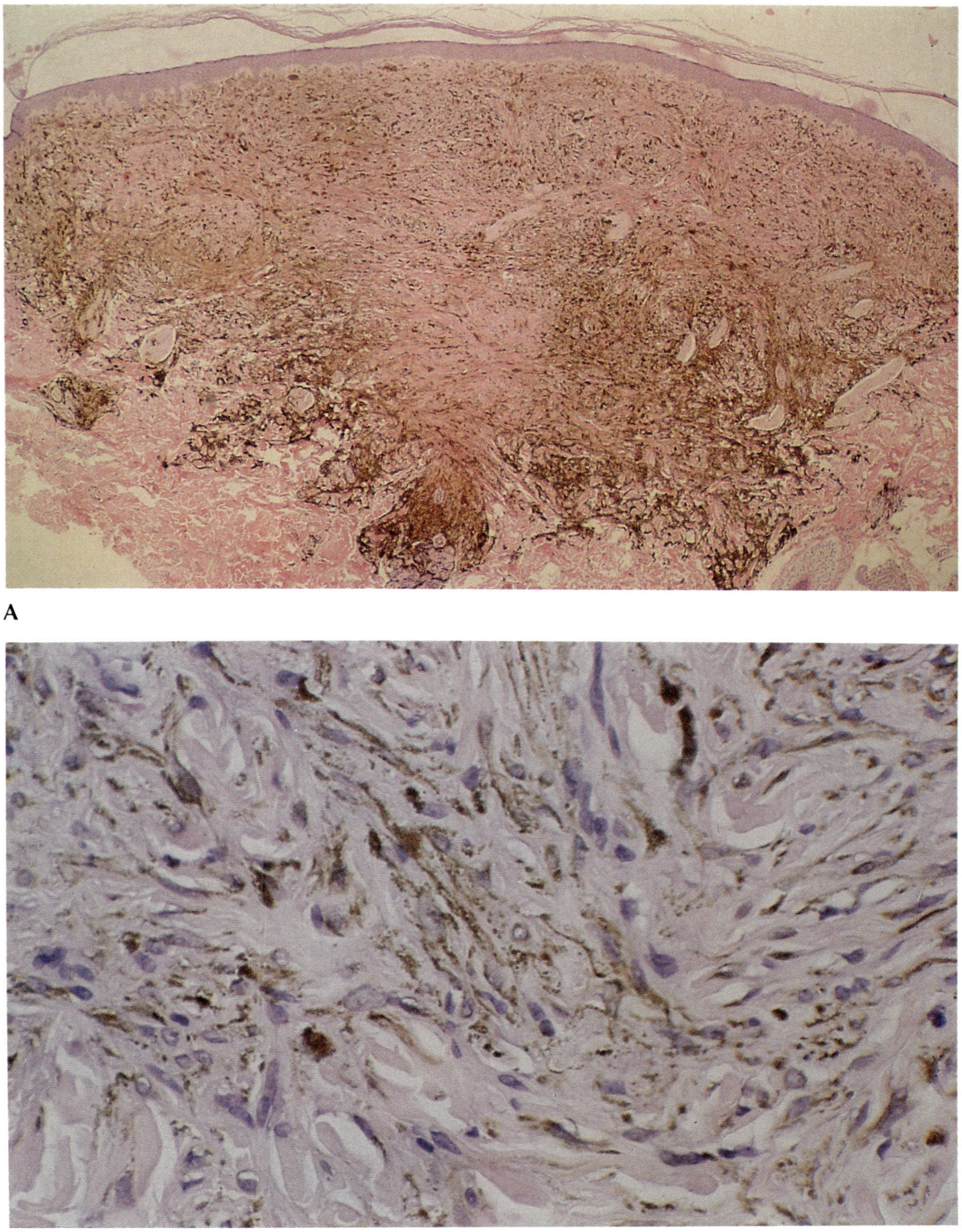

A

B

FIGURE 7-3

Blue nevus, ordinary type. (A) The lesion is slightly raised and has an inverted wedge configuration in the reticular dermis. The nevus is composed of numerous pigmented dendritic cells in a slightly fibrotic matrix (H&E, × 40). (B) The dendrites are easily identified by their melanin content (H&E, × 400).

Sclerosing Blue Nevus

This variant of blue nevus is distinguished from the other types based on a prominent fibrous or sclerotic stroma.

Histopathology. This variant of blue nevus is characterized by the formation of a symmetric and fairly well circumscribed fibrous nodule occupying the dermis (Figs. 7-5 and 7-6). The fibrous component is conspicuous relative to the cellular elements. The cellular elements generally consist of a relatively sparse number of dendritic melanocytes, variable numbers of melanophages, and occasional relatively small numbers of spindle cells (see Fig. 7-6). This variant may represent the later stages in the

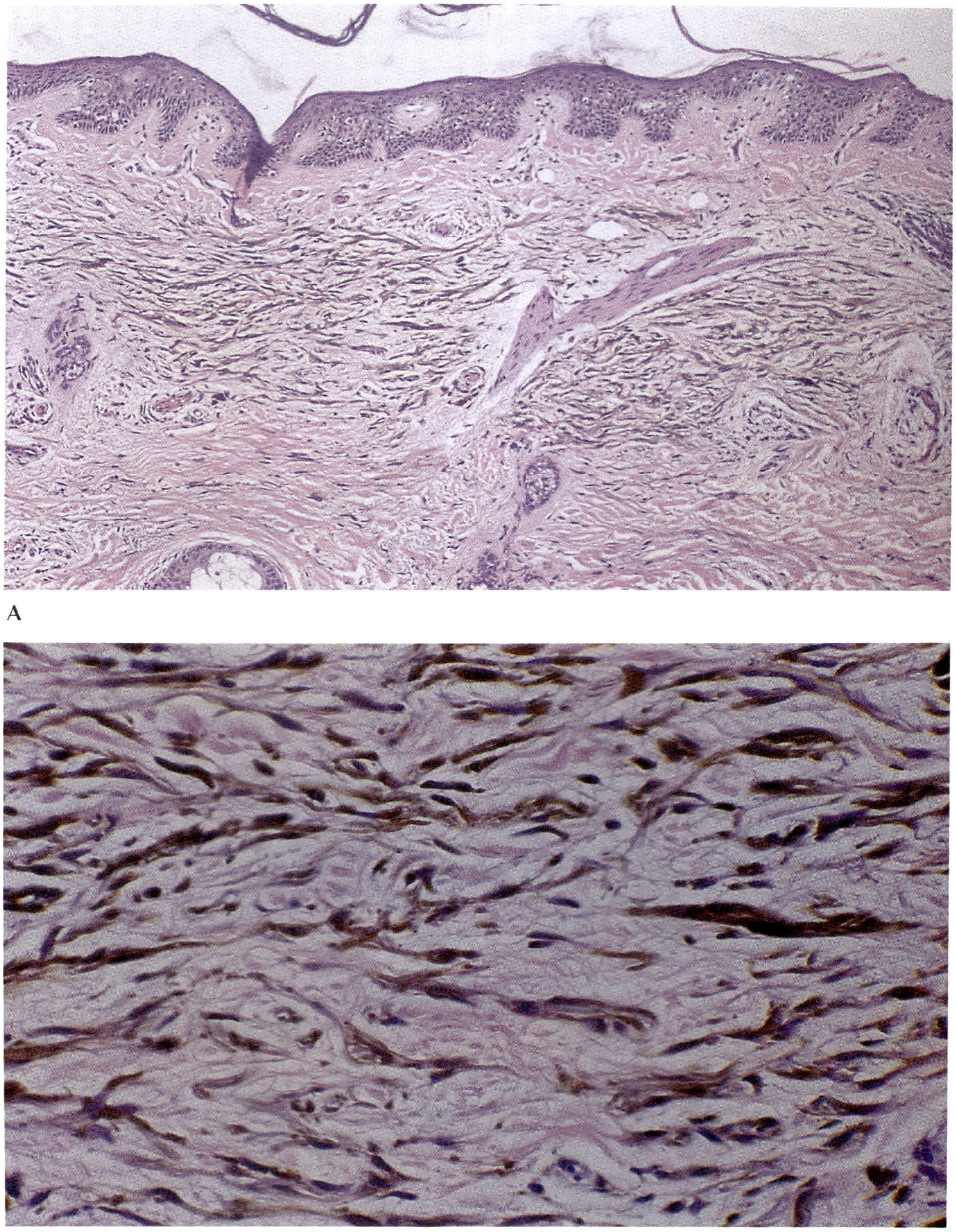

FIGURE 7-4

Blue nevus. (A) The lesion is composed mainly of dendritic, horizontally disposed melanocytes in the upper dermis (H&E, × 100). (B) High magnification of part A (H & E, × 400).

natural history of some blue nevi, although this has not been confirmed definitely.

Differential Diagnosis. Entities to be distinguished from sclerosing blue nevus include dermatofibroma, particularly the hemosiderotic variant, sclerosing Spitz nevus, and desmoplastic melanoma (Table 7-3) (see also Chap. 10). The type of dermatofibroma associated with prominent deposits of hemosiderin can closely mimic blue nevus. However, the typical epidermal changes resembling seborrheic keratosis are usually found with dermatofibroma, as well as the typical infiltrating pattern of cells in dermatofibroma. Close inspection of the pigment granules in dermatofibroma usually will reveal the golden refractile character of hemosiderin. If necessary, special

TABLE 7-3
Comparison of Sclerosing Blue Nevus and Desmoplastic-Neurotropic Melanoma

Sclerosing Blue Nevus	*Desmoplastic Melanoma*
Clinical Features	
Common	Rare
Age mean 38.6 years	Age mean 60 years
Women > men	Men ≥ women
Dorsal hands, feet, face	Head and neck, sun-exposed skin
Blue, blue-black	Flesh-colored papule or nodule, may have tan or brown component
Histopathology	
Usually no intraepidermal component	About 85% have intraepidermal component, often lentigo maligna
Symmetry	Asymmetry often
Well-demarcated fibrous nodule with rounded contours in dermis	Fibrous nodule often extending into deep reticular dermis or subcutis
Orderly arrangement of dendritic cells	Fascicles of cells oriented in all directions
Melanin often present	Melanin often absent
Little or no cytologic atypia	Often enlarged hyperchromatic spindle-shaped nuclei
Infiltration of cutaneous nerves (orderly)	Perineurial and endoneurial invasion
Usually no mitoses	Usually at least 1 or 2 mitoses/mm^2
Usually no mucin	Mucinous stroma on occasion
Immunohistochemistry	
S-100 protein +	S-100 protein +
HMB-45 +	HMB-45 − (in most cases)

stains for iron and melanin can be useful in distinguishing these two entities. The desmoplastic or sclerosing form of Spitz nevus is usually easily separated from blue nevus because there is usually no pigment in the Spitz variant and the cell type is usually epithelioid. Desmoplastic melanoma is distinguished from sclerosing blue nevus by the presence of an atypical lentiginous melanocytic proliferation, the presence of fascicles of markedly atypical spindle cells, and the minimal pigment present in desmoplastic melanoma (see Table 7-3). However, the distinction of early desmoplastic melanoma from sclerosing blue nevus occasionally may be quite difficult. Diagnosis must be based on weighing the degree of cellularity, the degree of cytologic atypia, the presence of necrotic cells, mitotic activity, and clinical presentation.

Blue Nevus, Spindle Cell Variant

This variant of blue nevus is distinguished histologically by the relative prominence of spindle cell elements relative to dendritic cells and fibrous tissue.

Histopathology. In addition to the presence of variable numbers of dendritic melanocytes, melanophages, and fibrosis, this variant of blue nevus is characterized by conspicuous numbers of spindle cells that infiltrate the stroma singly or in fascicles[5,43] (Fig. 7-7). In some instances, these lesions may have a plexiform configuration; i.e., there may be fairly discreet cellular foci of spindle cells extending into the deep reticular dermis or subcutaneous fat. Cytologically, the spindle cells are characterized by oval or elongate nuclei with relatively dispersed uniform chromatin patterns. Occasional small nucleoli may be observed. Mitotic figures are rare and should be cause for concern.

Differential Diagnosis. As with the preceding entity, the differential diagnosis is primarily that of spindle and epithelioid cell nevi and desmoplastic melanoma. In general, distinction from spindle and epithelioid cell nevi is based on the presence of dendritic melanocytes and fibrosis in blue nevi. As discussed earlier, the discrimination of blue nevi from desmoplastic melanoma is based on the presence or absence of an epidermal component; i.e., lentiginous melanocytic dysplasia frequently noted in desmoplastic melanoma but not in blue nevi, overall symmetry with desmoplastic melanoma generally showing more disordered growth than a blue nevus, presence of

TABLE 7-4
Précis: Cellular Blue Nevus

Clinical features	
Onset	birth, childhood, adolescence
Age	mean 33 (range 6–85) years
Site	buttocks, sacrococcygeal area, forearm/wrist, leg/ankle/foot, scalp, face
Gray-blue to blue-black papule, nodule	
Usually well circumscribed	
Regular borders	
Size	0.3–3 cm
Histopathology	
Symmetry	
Localization to reticular dermis	
Often deep extension with bulging, nodular configuration, rounded, well-demarcated inferior margin	
Heterogeneity of patterns	
Biphasic pattern most common	
Melanin-laden dendritic melanocytes and fibrosis and	
Bundles of amelanotic fusiform cells	
Alveolar pattern	
Fascicles or nests of fusiform cells compartmentalized by fibrous trabeculae	
Fascicular pattern	
Fascicles of spindle cells often with clear cytoplasm and prominent schwannian differentiation	
Atypical cellular blue nevus	
Marked cytologic atypia	
Enlarged bizarre cells	
Multinucleate cells	
Lacunae containing melanophages	
Cystic degeneration in central part of nevus with loose edematous stroma	
Few or no mitotic figures	
Necrosis absent or uncommon	
Differential diagnosis	
Malignant blue nevus	
Metastatic melanoma	
Clear cell sarcoma	

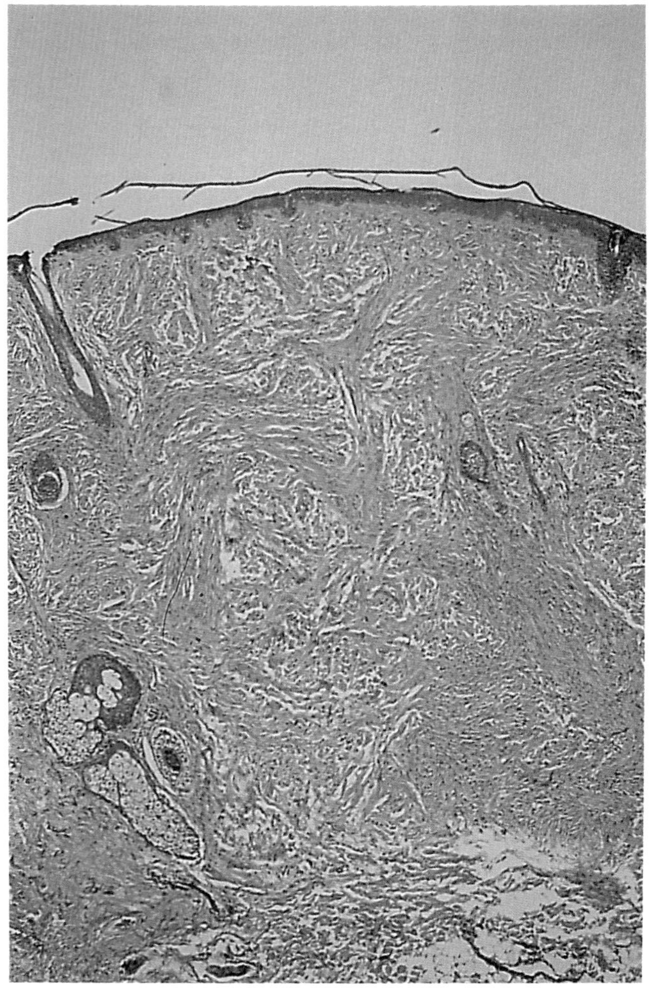

A

FIGURE 7-5
Blue nevus. (A) The lesion contains almost no pigment and consists of a symmetric fibrotic nodule (H&E, × 40). (B) Oval and fusiform cells disposed in fibrotic dermis. There is a resemblance to dermatofibroma (H&E, × 200).

cytologic atypia in desmoplastic melanoma as manifested by pleomorphic and hyperchromatic spindle cells, mitotic activity with atypical mitotic figures in desmoplastic melanoma but not in blue nevus, and a presence of necrotic cells in desmoplastic melanoma but not in blue nevus.

"Compound" Blue Nevus

This is a histologic variant of blue nevus defined by intraepidermal proliferation of dendritic melanocytes.[38]

Clinical Features. Only six cases have been reported.[38] The mean age was 31 years (range 11 to 51 years), and the most common site was the trunk. The lesions measured 2 to 4 mm in diameter and were described as blue-gray, blue-black, or black.

Histopathology. The unique feature of these lesions is the presence of basilar epidermal proliferation of heavily pigmented dendritic melanocytes.[38] Junctional nests are not present. The papillary and upper reticular dermis contains a fairly well circumscribed aggregate of spindle and dendritic melanocytes, usually heavily melanized with numerous melanophages.

Differential Diagnosis. The compound blue nevus must be distinguished from a combined blue nevus, pigmented spindle cell nevus, variant of deep penetrating/plexiform nevus, melanoma, and regressed melanoma.

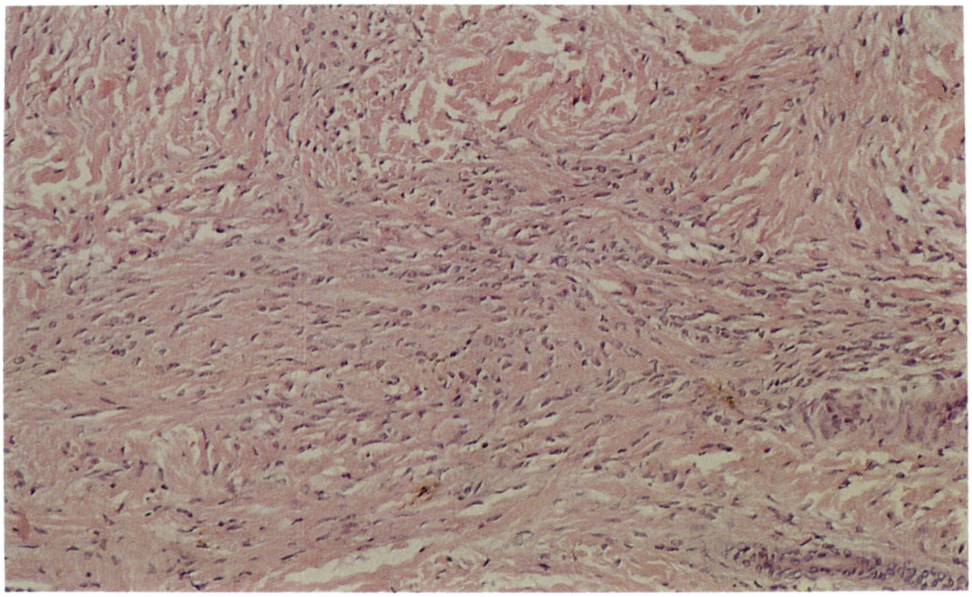

B

FIGURE 7-5 *(Continued)*

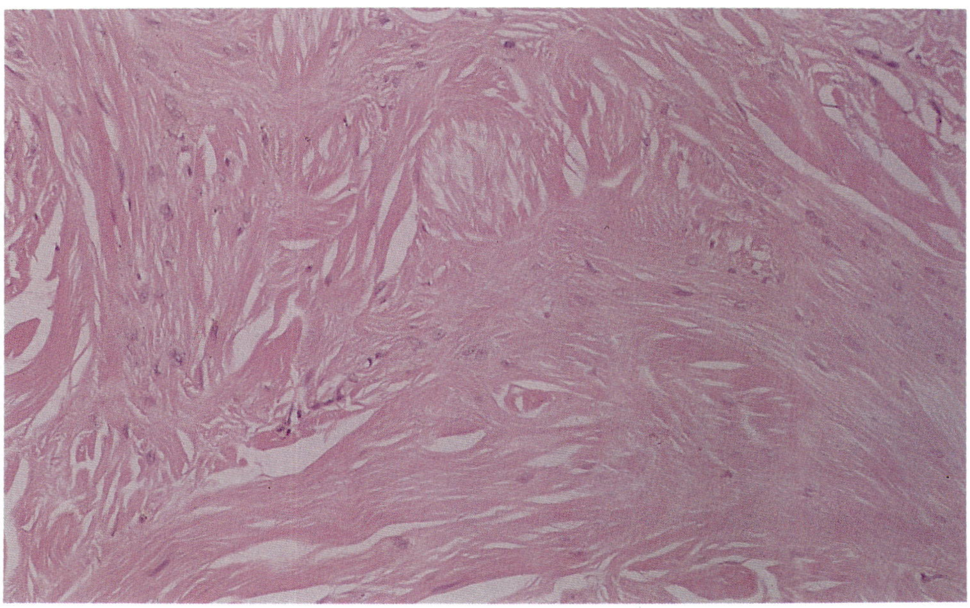

FIGURE 7-6

Blue nevus, sclerotic type. Note markedly hyalinized collagen and dearth of cells (H&E, × 200).

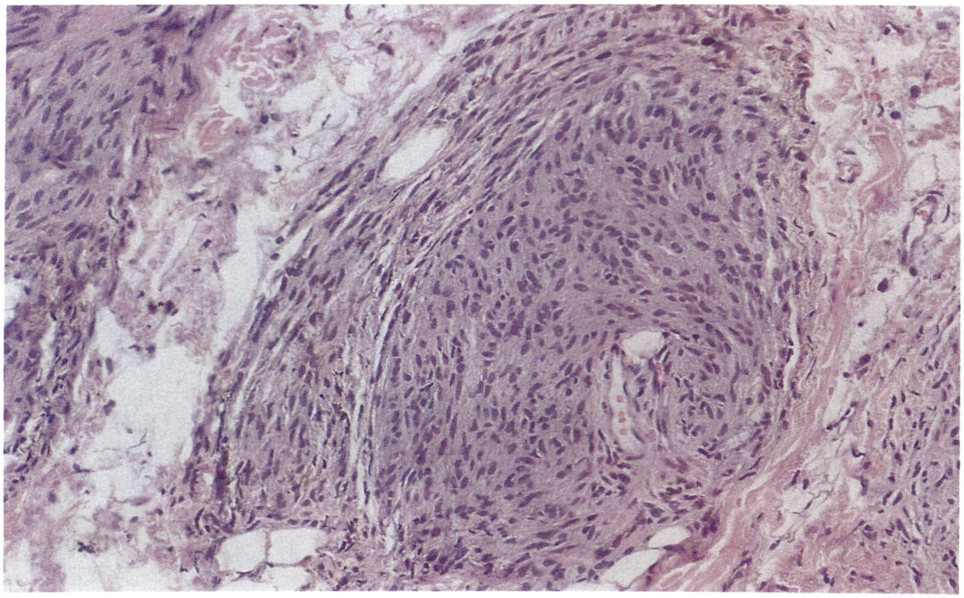

FIGURE 7-7
Blue nevus, spindle cell variant. Circumscribed cellular focus in deep dermis resembles palisaded encapsulated neuroma (H&E, × 200).

Cellular Blue Nevus

Clinical Features. The cellular blue nevus (CBN) is less common than the typical dendritic and fibrotic variant.[5,28,39-43,49] CBN are generally 1 to 2 cm in diameter with a blue, blue-black, or black coloration and most commonly involve the buttocks, sacral area, or scalp (Table 7-4). They are generally diagnosed between the ages of 10 and 40 years and are usually asymptomatic. Frequently, the natural history is that of persistence, but rarely these lesions may undergo transformation to malignant blue nevus. Incomplete excision of CBN is rarely associated with recurrence.

Histopathology. As already mentioned, it is clear that there is a continuum from ordinary blue nevi to cellular blue nevi. Blue nevi are thus characterized by varying proportions of pigmented dendritic cells, oval, elongate, fusiform cells arranged in various configurations and exhibiting varying degrees of melaninization, melanophages, and fibrosis[39-43,49] (Figs. 7-8 and 7-9A and Table 7-4). Size, depth, and architecture also figure into this spectrum. No criteria have been established as to what proportion of a blue nevus should consist of fusiform cells in order to qualify as a cellular blue nevus. The heterogeneity of CBN is further discussed in Chapter 8.

The following criteria are proposed for diagnosis of CBN: The lesion should occupy the reticular dermis, at least a third to a half of the lesion should contain oval to fusiform cells, and the overall architecture should be multilobular or plexiform with deep extension, occasionally into subcutaneous fat.

Architecture of CBN. In general, CBN occupy a major portion of, if not the entire reticular dermis and are notable for a rounded, well-demarcated lobular configuration[39-43,49] (see Fig. 7-9A). The lesion may show a single lobular mass with a well-defined horizontal inferior margin that parallels or bulges into the subcutaneous fat, or alternatively, there may be two or more lobules or digitate bulbous projections that extend into the deep reticular dermis or subcutaneous fat; these bulbous structures also may display a plexiform spatial arrangement (see Figs. 7-8A and 7-9B).

Composition of CBN. CBN are remarkable for their heterogeneity, and it is apparent that the morphologic limits of CBN have not been clearly defined. For example, the distinction from common blue nevi, some pigmented peripheral nerve sheath tumors, and other unusual melanocytic nevi may be problematic (see Chap. 8). Essential for the diagnosis are cellular foci of round, oval, elongate, or fusiform cells that constitute at least a third to a half, if not most of the tumor (see Fig. 7-8C and 7-9C). These cells are arranged in a number of patterns and vary considerably as to melanin content. As opposed to the frequent diffuse distribution of melanin-laden dendritic melanocytes in the ordinary type of blue nevus, the fusiform cells of CBN

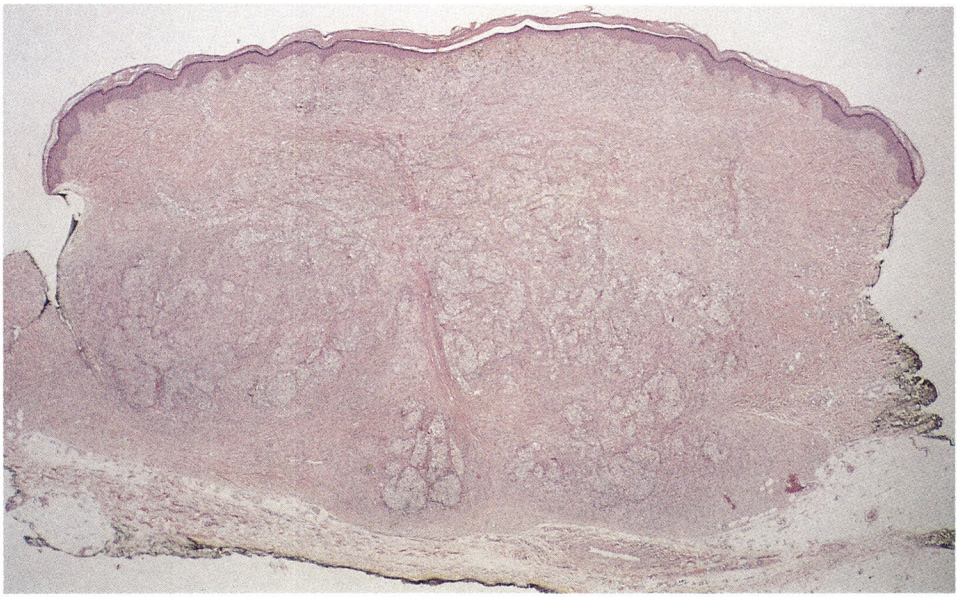

A

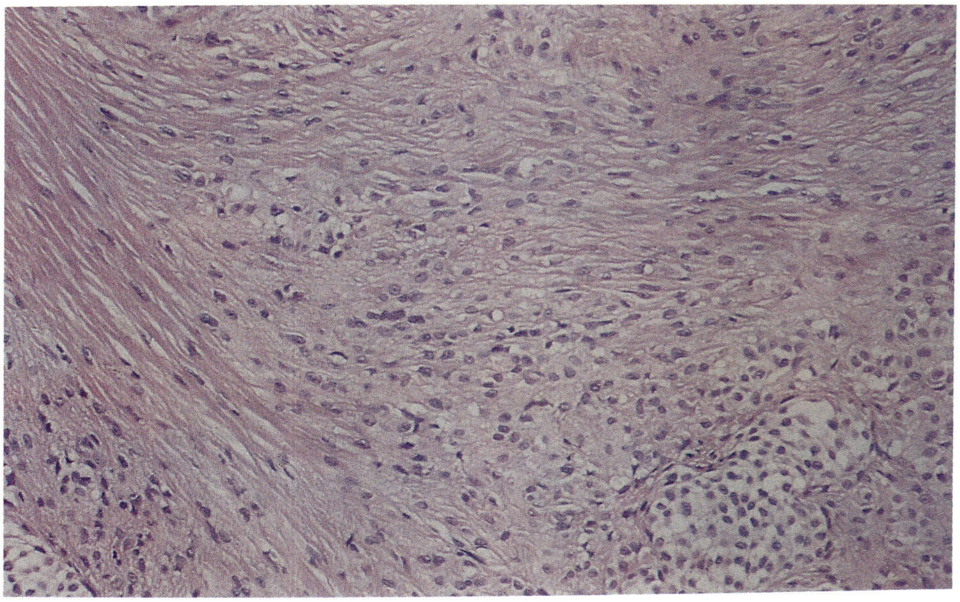

B

FIGURE 7-8

Blue nevus, cellular variant. (A) This lesion occupies the entire dermis and displays a well-demarcated, slightly rounded deep margin (H&E, × 20). (B) Fibrotic area containing scattered cells and little if any melanin (H&E, × 100). (C) Discreet nests of round, oval, and slightly elongate cells with clear cytoplasm (H&E, × 400).

are usually arranged in variably organized nests or bundles (see Figs. 7-9 D–F). These bundles may or may not be encapsulated by fibrous tissue. In some instances, there are fascicles of fusiform cells oriented randomly in all directions without evidence of compartmentalization. However, a common pattern is that of compact, highly cellular nests or fascicles separated by fibrous trabeculae. There may be linear or concentric arrangements of cells within these nests. Often pigmented dendritic melanocytes and melanophages are present in the peripheral fibrous tissue surrounding the cellular fascicles (see Fig. 7-9E). The sizes of fascicles or nests may vary considerably. There may be large lobules of fusiform cells constituting much of the tumor without any intervening fibrous tissue. The presence of well-defined, rounded nests of cells has been described as the "alveolar" pattern in CBN.[43,49]

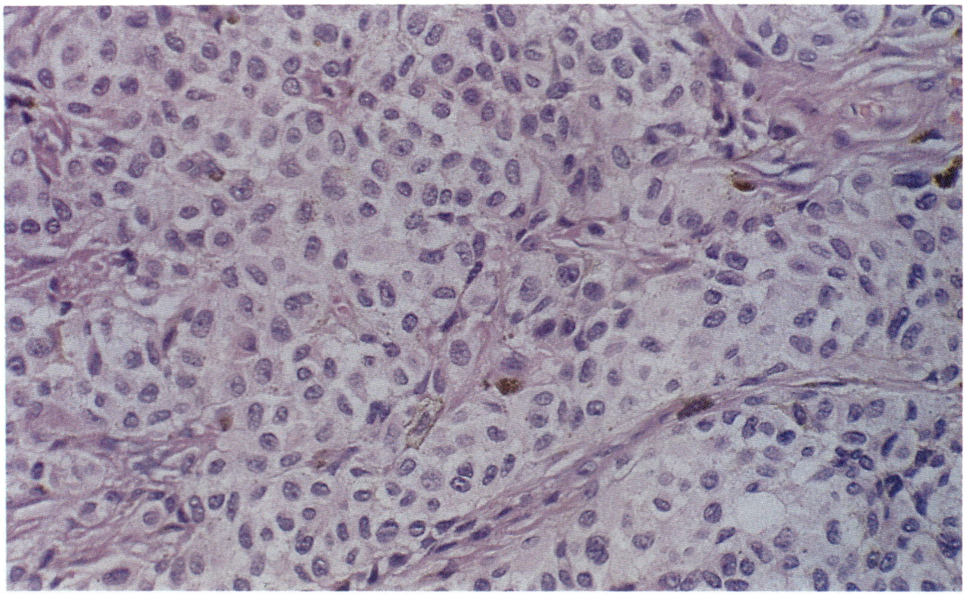

C

FIGURE 7-8 *(Continued)*

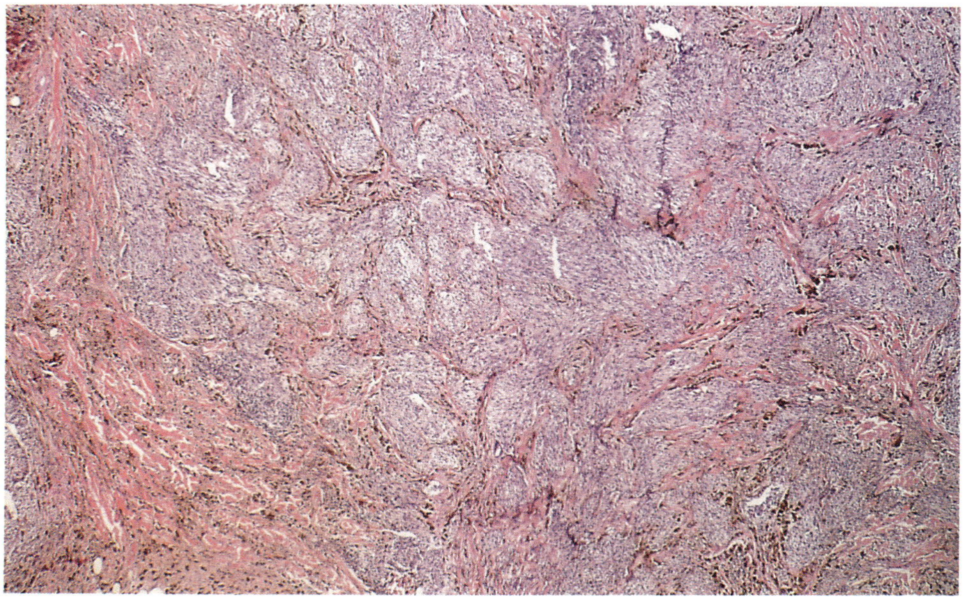

A

FIGURE 7-9

Cellular blue nevus. (A) Pale-staining central area corresponds to nests and fascicles of fusiform cells. Fibrosis and pigment are at the periphery of this area (H&E, × 40). (B) Characteristic bulbous configuration of cellular blue nevus extending into subcutis (H&E, × 20). (C) Well-defined compact nests of fusiform cells bounded by fibrous tissue (H&E, × 100). (D) Fascicles of fusiform cells with slightly eosinophilic or clear cytoplasm (H&E, × 200). (E) Melanophages are present in fibrous trabeculae separating the cellular fascicles (H&E, × 400). (F) Higher magnification of part E. Fusiform cells have vacuolated cytoplasm and elongate nuclei. The nuclei have dispersed chromatin and occasional nucleoli are present. There is a striking resemblance to clear cell sarcoma (melanoma of soft parts) (H&E, × 600).

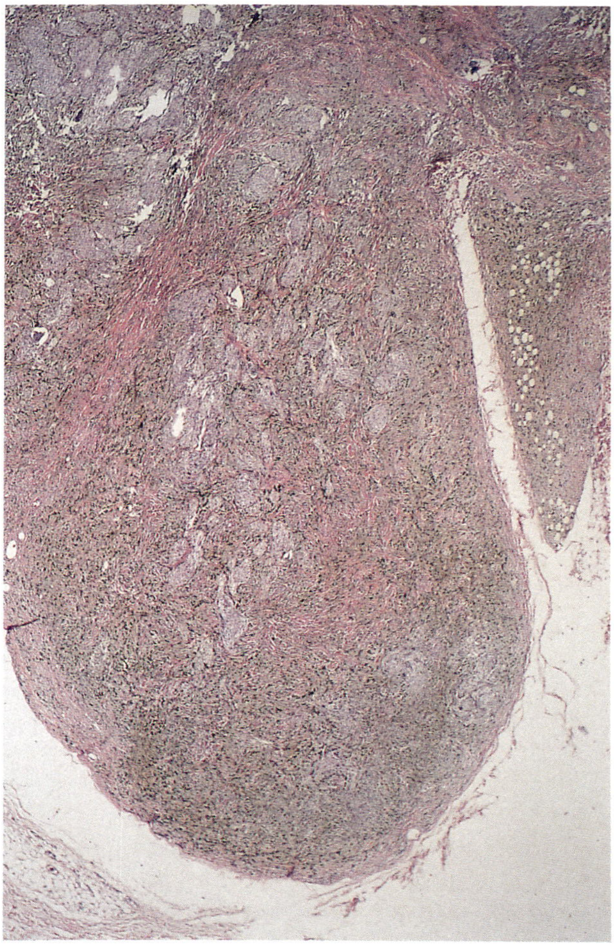

B

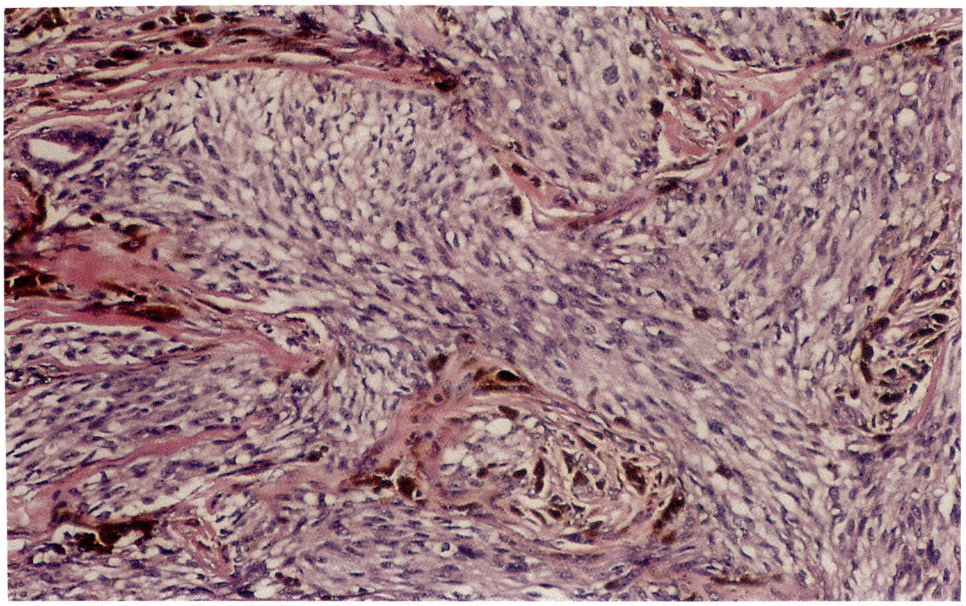

C

FIGURE 7-9 *(Continued)*

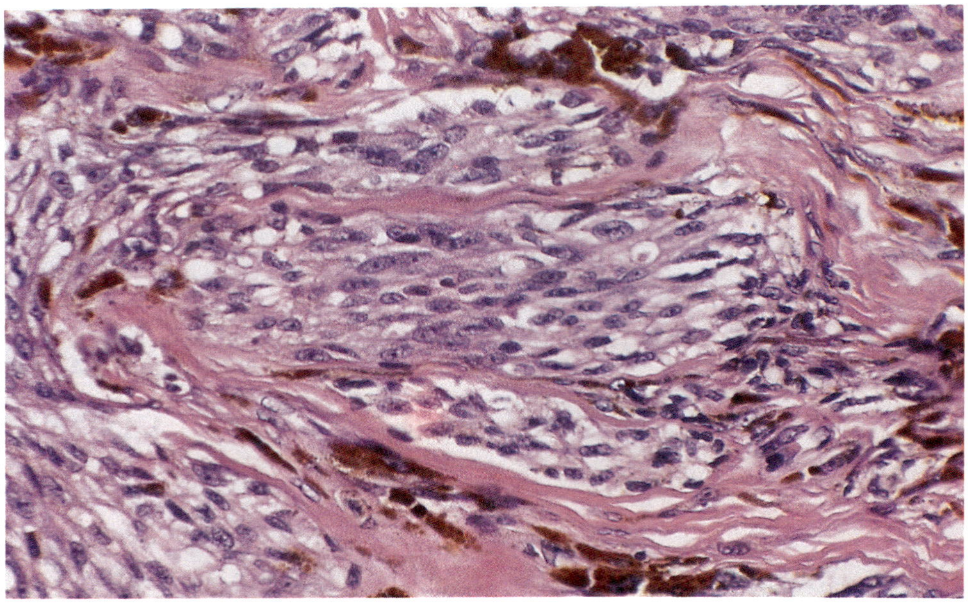

D

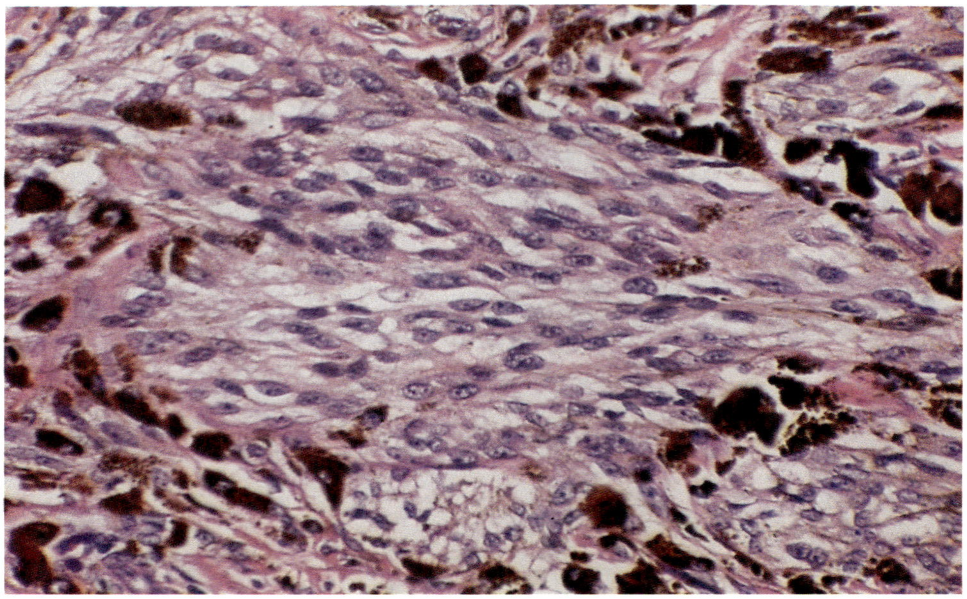

E

FIGURE 7-9 *(Continued)*

In some CBN, fascicles of spindle cells may have striking schwannian differentiation and may merge with and infiltrate cutaneous nerves.[49]

The cells comprising the "cellular" foci in CBN are most often fusiform or spindle-shaped but also may be round or oval (see Figs. 7-8C and 7-9F). These cells are usually somewhat enlarged but may be relatively small on occasion. The cell's boundaries are often ill-defined, and the cytoplasm is usually either clear, vacuolated, slightly eosinophilic, or bluish. In many CBN, the fusiform cells do not contain readily apparent melanin by conventional microscopy. Because of the paucity or absence of melanin, these cellular foci appear pale or clear on scanning magnification, in contrast to the often heavily pigmented areas containing dendritic melanocytes, melanophages, and sclerosis. The latter pale areas are quite helpful in

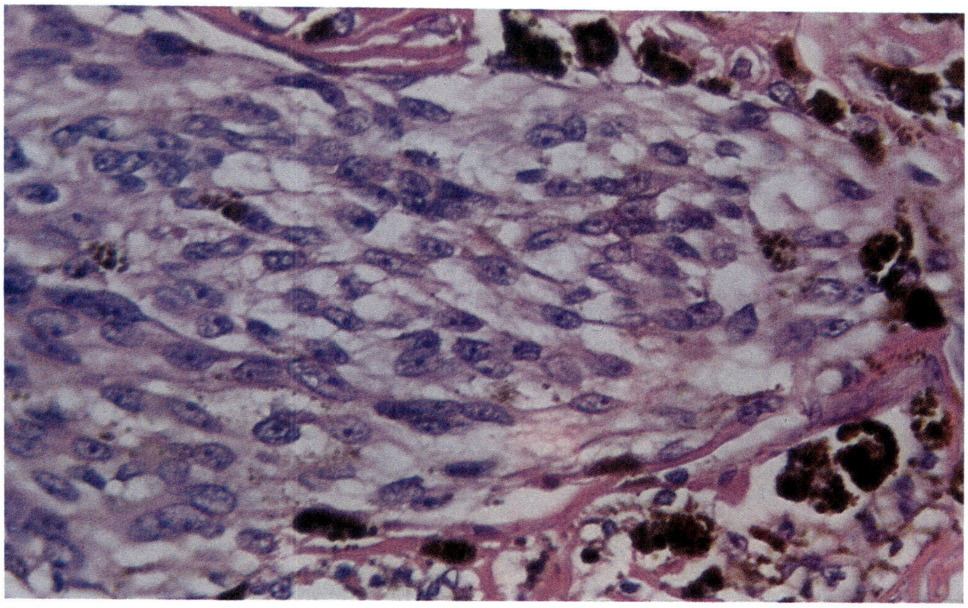

F

FIGURE 7-9 *(Continued)*

recognizing CBN. However, the degree of melaninization may vary from barely visible fine granular melanin to heavy pigmentation obscuring cytologic detail. Usually, the dendritic melanocytes and melanophages contain the heaviest deposition of melanin. However, the latter cells are usually located in peripheral fibrous trabeculae or in areas of sclerosis.

The nuclei of these cells are usually round, oval, or fusiform and commonly are somewhat enlarged (Fig. 7-9F). The chromatin tends to be evenly dispersed, and one or more small nucleoli are often observed. Minimal or low-grade nuclear pleomorphism is noted in many CBN. However, this should not be pronounced. Similarly, occasional mitoses are described in many CBN. As a general rule, if 2 or more mitoses are present per square millimeter, the lesion should be evaluated carefully for other corroborating evidence of malignancy.

Multinucleate giant cells are noted occasionally in the cellular areas and may be numerous in some CBN. Such giant cells also may occur in areas of cystic degeneration[49] (see below).

Occasional CBN are composed of discreet nests of amelanotic round or oval cells analogous to the usual fusiform cells (see Fig. 7-8C). Such nests are separated in the typical fashion by fibrous trabeculae that usually contain some dendritic melanocytes and melanophages. Recognition of other features of CBN such as a lobular, well-demarcated configuration and clinical features are necessary for diagnosis as CBN. Such presentations point out the heterogeneity of CBN, relationships to other melanocytic nevi, and problems of proper nosology (see Chap. 8).

Other Morphologic Features of CBN. Perhaps two-thirds or so of CBN have a so-called biphasic pattern, and this refers to a component of common blue nevus, i.e., areas containing pigmented dendritic melanocytes, variable sclerosis, and melanophages.[43–49] These areas are often in the superficial dermis overlying or at the periphery of cellular lobules. These areas are indistinguishable from ordinary blue nevi and provide evidence that all blue nevi are indeed a continuum.

A rather characteristic feature of CBN is the presence of cystic degeneration ("encystification"), which is often centrally located[42,49,50] (Fig. 7-10). The latter changes are probably indistinguishable from those occurring in ancient schwannoma and may have an ischemic or traumatic basis. These degenerative changes are typified by edema, myxoid stromal alteration, some degree of diminished cellularity, and scattered melanophages. Alterations of blood vessels also tend to be a prominent feature. Commonly, ectatic blood vessels show hyalinization of their walls and thrombosis, features suggesting a component of ischemia. Both ordinary blue nevi and CBN are immunoreactive with S-100 protein and HMB-45.[67]

Atypical Cellular Blue Nevus

There are variants of CBN that may be extremely difficult to distinguish from malignant blue nevus (melanoma).[49,54]

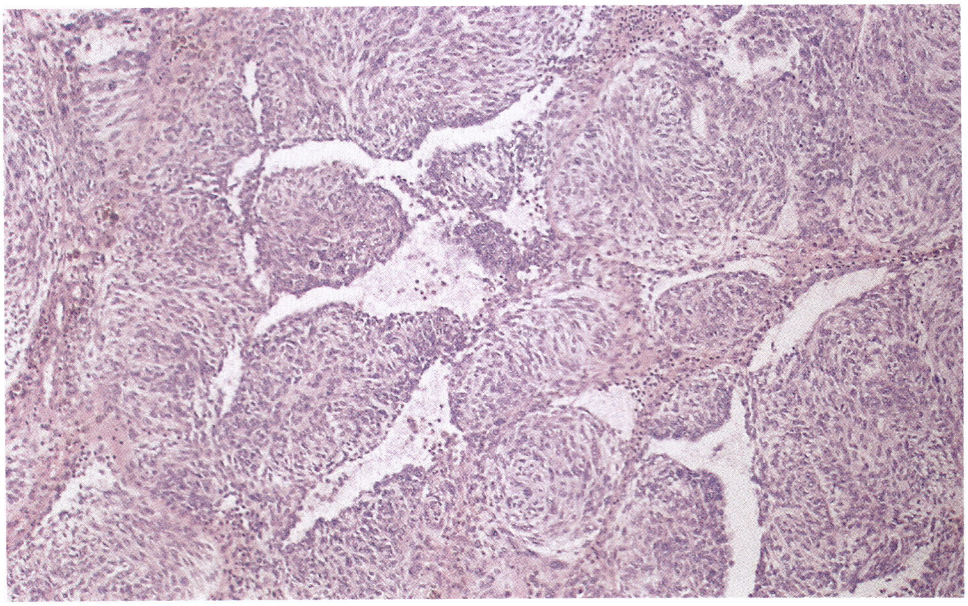

A

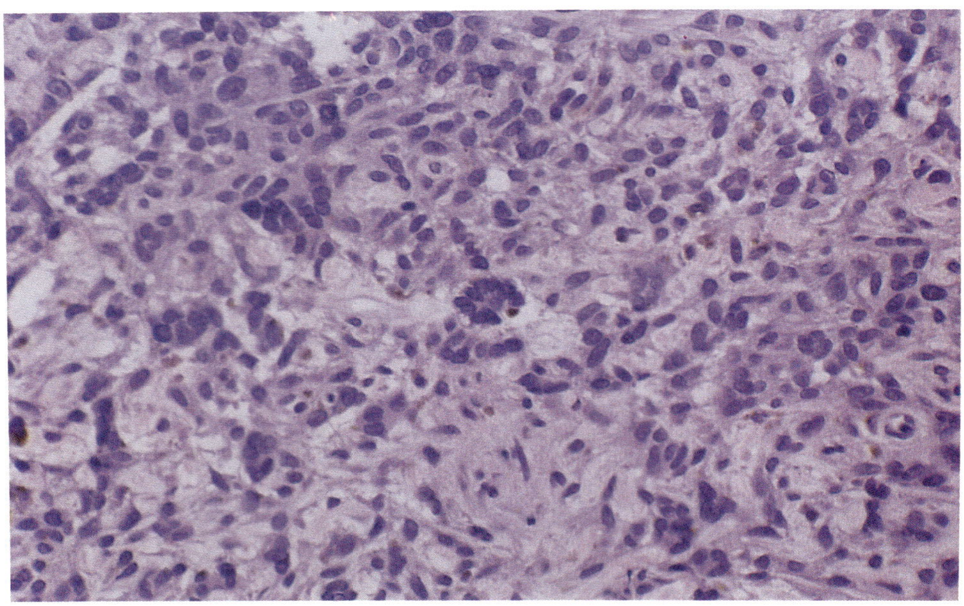

B

FIGURE 7-10

Cellular blue nevus with central cytic degeneration. (A) Nests of cells are separated by edema and myxoid stroma (H&E, × 100). (B) The cells exhibit pleomorphism and occasional multinucleate giant cells are present (H&E, × 400).

The clinical history associated with such lesions is usually that of recent change or enlargement.

Histopathology. Atypical variants of CBN are generally characterized by large size, deep extension, and large expansile nests of spindle cells.[49,54] These large tumoral aggregates of cells display greater cellularity than what is seen normally in typical CBN. There is also greater cellular pleomorphism with hyperchromatism and variation of nuclear characteristics. Nucleoli may be prominent as well. There also may be greater mitotic activity in such lesions. The distinction from melanoma may be quite difficult. Such discrimination is based on determining that a

TABLE 7-5
omparison of Cellular Blue Nevus and Malignant Blue Nevus

Cellular Blue Nevus	*Malignant Blue Nevus*
Clinical Features	
Mean age 32.6 (7–60) years	Mean age 48.8 (30–75) years
Women > men	Men > women
Buttocks, sacrococcygeal area, extremities	Scalp
Size 1.8 cm (1–2 cm)	Size 2.5 cm (1.3–4 cm)
Blue, blue-gray, blue-black nodule	Blue, blue-black nodule
Histopathology	
Component of ordinary blue nevus in 60%	Blue nevus component, cellular 92%
Symmetry	Asymmetry
Lobular or multilobular	Lobular or multilobular
Cytologic atypia, Low-grade or absent	Substantial cytologic atypia
Mitoses < 1–2/10 HPF	Mitoses 1–2/10 HPF
Usually no atypical mitoses	Atypical mitoses
Necrosis uncommon	Necrosis in 33%
	Pronounced heterogeneity in most tumors

majority of the cells have a fairly uniform appearance, that necrosis is absent or not prominent, and that atypical mitotic figures are not present. Otherwise, a diagnosis of malignant melanoma must be weighed carefully.

Differential Diagnosis. The differential diagnosis of CBN (and atypical CBN) includes malignant blue nevus (MBN) (malignant melanoma arising in association with cellular blue nevus),[52,53] well-differentiated forms of malignant melanoma, metastatic melanoma, and clear cell sarcoma (see Chap. 10). MBN is an extremely rare entity, and thus this diagnosis should only be made after careful evaluation (Table 7-5). The clinical history of a long-standing blue nevus with subsequent change or finding an associated benign blue nevus remnant (usually CBN) is extremely important for the diagnosis of MBN. Without the latter criterion, MBN cannot be distinguished from conventional melanoma, whether primary or metastatic. The MBN is discriminated from CBN by greater degrees of cytologic atypia, greater mitotic activity with atypical forms, and necrosis. It is important to emphasize that there may be considerable heterogeneity within MBN, and the diagnosis has been missed because of this histologic variation.[52,53] The presence of a concomitant conventional blue nevus element favors a diagnosis of CBN. It cannot be overemphasized that although MBN is vanishingly rare, atypical CBN should be completely excised and the patients monitored very carefully for recurrence. Metastases from such lesions have been observed after the passage of several years. Thus, because of the unusual nature of these lesions, their rarity, and the lack of long-term follow-up, the biologic potential of atypical forms of CBN is largely unknown and requires further study.

Clear cell sarcoma may have a very similar appearance to CBN (see Fig. 7-9F) but has greater cytologic atypia, mitotic activity, and generally involves deep soft tissue of the extremities (see Chap. 10).

Lymph Node Involvement by Cellular Blue Nevus

For some time it has been recognized that foci of CBN may be encountered on occasion in regional lymph nodes.[55,56] These regional lymph nodes have almost always been axillary or inguinal lymph nodes proximal to a CBN on an extremity. These nodal foci of CBN most commonly have involved the subcapsular peripheral sinuses and parenchyma of the lymph nodes, which are sites involved by metastatic cancer, but also the lymph node capsule. Because of the nodal localization of these cellular aggregates, explanations for this phenomenon have included benign metastases and aberrant histogenesis of CBN in lymph nodes.[55,56] It is possible that both hypotheses may be operative.

The most important point regarding this phenomenon is that it is recognized and not misdiagnosed as metastatic melanoma or MBN. Similarly, it is important that a cutaneous lesion, if present, is not misdiagnosed as MBN simply because of the lymph node involvement. This is not to say that the distinction between CBN and MBN is not difficult or that MBN with metastasis does not exist. Thus it is incumbent on the pathologist to be certain that there

TABLE 7-6
Précis: Plaque-Type Blue Nevus

- Clinical features
  - Congenital or later onset
  - Site anywhere
  - Size 1–17 cm
  - Plaque, either confluent or, composed of numerous macules and papules
  - Blue-gray to blue-black
  - May increase in size
- Histopathology
  - Features of ordinary to cellular blue nevus
- Differential diagnosis
  - Melanoma

are sufficient changes for malignancy in such a circumstance, i.e., pronounced cytologic atypia, necrosis, mitotic activity, etc., before rendering a diagnosis of metastatic melanoma (or metastatic MBN) and primary MBN.

Patchlike Blue Nevus

Clinical Features. This lesion is a macular area of blue-gray pigmentation varying in size from 1 to several centimeters, clinically resembling a Mongolian spot.[57,58]

Histopathology . In contrast to Mongolian spots, the patchlike blue nevus contains a greater number of dendritic melanocytes in the dermis.

Plaque-Type Blue Nevus

Clinical Features. This is a variant of blue nevus that is often congenital and characterized by a palpable area of blue-gray pigmentation measuring 1 to several centimeters or more in diameter.[5,59–64] The plaque is either a single lesion or composed of multiple but distinct papules. There is probably a close relationship between eruptive or agminated blue nevi, patchlike blue nevus, pilar neurocristic hamartoma and plaque-type blue nevus.[65]

Histopathology. The histologic features are similar to those of ordinary blue nevi, but there may be predominant periappendageal aggregation of dendritic melanocytes. There also may be foci of hypercellularity, i.e., compact bundles of spindle cells.

Pilar Neurocristic Hamartoma

Clinical Features. This rare hamartomatous process is characterized by multiple perifollicular papules occupying an area of skin measuring several centimeters in diameter.[65] Individual papules have been reported to vary in color from tan to blue or black. There is some similarity to patchlike and plaquelike blue nevi in humans and equine melanotic disease.

Histopathology. This lesion is notable for prominent perifollicular accumulation of dendritic melanocytes that show extension to nearby eccrine ducts. The intervening reticular dermis contains scattered pigmented dendritic cells resembling Mongolian spots.

Target Blue Nevus

This is an uncommon type of blue nevus important to recognize because of its possible clinical confusion with melanoma.[66]

Clinical Features. The two cases reported to date have occurred on the dorsal aspect of the foot of young adult males.[66] The lesions have been about 1 cm in greatest diameter and dome-shaped and showed a target appearance. Each lesion was characterized by a central dark blue nodule surrounded by a flesh-colored annulus and more peripheral blue-black macular annulus. Both patients reported that their lesions had changed in color during the preceding year.

Histopathology. On scanning magnification, one can detect a zonal alteration in the number of pigment-containing cells corresponding to the target-like clinical appearance.[66] The dark central nodule has the features of a typical blue nevus, i.e., a fibrotic tumor containing pigmented dendritic cells and fusiform cells. The flesh-colored annulus, although exhibiting dermal sclerosis, is remarkable for significantly reduced numbers of pigment-containing cells. However, the most peripheral zone of the lesion has, in contrast, significant numbers of the pigmented dendritic cells.

Differential Diagnosis. The variation in numbers of pigmented dendritic cells in the target blue nevus might suggest an atypical lesion. However, careful inspection will disclose an overall orderly arrangement of the cellular population and fibrosis. In addition, cytologic atypia is generally minimal or absent.

TABLE 7-7
Précis: Target Blue Nevus

Clinical features
Young adults
Approximately 1 cm size
Location dorsal aspect of foot (2 cases)
Dome-shaped nodule
Central gray-black to blue-black area surrounded by flesh-colored annulus and more peripheral macular blue-black annulus
Usual history of recent change
Histopathology
Central nodule contains pigmented dendritic cells, fibrosis, and possibly spindle cells in dermis
Flesh-colored annulus shows fibrosis and reduced number of pigmented dendritic cells
Outer pigmented annulus shows some pigmented dendritic cells
Differential diagnosis
Melanoma with regression

REFERENCES

1. El Bahrawy A: Ueber den Mongolenfleck bei Europaern. *Arch Dermatol Syphilol* 141:171–192, 1922.
2. Larsen NP, Godfrey LS: Sacral pigment spots. *Am J Phys Anthropol* 10:253–274, 1927.
3. Carleton A, Biggs R: Diffuse mesodermal pigmentation with congenital cranial abnormality. *Br J Dermatol* 60:10–13, 1948.
4. Pratt AG: Birthmarks in infants. *Arch Dermatol* 67:302–305, 1953.

5. Dorsey CS, Montgomery H: Blue nevus and its distinction from Mongolian spot and the nevus of Ota. *J Invest Dermatol* 22:225–236, 1954.
6. Ota M, Tanino H: Nevus fusco-caeruleus ophthalmo-maxillaris and melanosis bulbi. *Tokyo Iji Shinshi* 63(3133):1243–1245, 1939.
7. Tanino H: Naevus fusco-caeruleus ophthalmo-maxillaris (Ota). *J Jpn Dermatol* 47:181–203, 1940.
8. Mishima Y, Mevorah B: Nevus Ota and nevus of Ito in American Negroes. *J Invest Dermatol* 36:133–154, 1961.
9. Kopf AW, Weidman AI: Nevus of Ota. *Arch Dermatol* 85:195–208, 1962.
10. Hidano A, Kajima H, Endo Y: Bilateral nevus of Ota associated with nevus of Ito. *Arch Dermatol* 91:357–359, 1965.
11. Hidano A, Kajima H, Ikeda S, et al: Natural history of nevus of Ota. *Arch Dermatol* 95:187–195, 1967.
12. Hirayama T, Suzuki T: A new classification of Ota's nevus based on histopathological features. *Dermatologica* 183:169–172, 1991.
13. Cole HN Jr, Hubler WR, Lund HZ: Persistent, aberrant mongolian spots. *Arch Dermatol Syphilol* 61:244–260, 1950.
14. Hidano A: Persistent Mongolian spot in the adult. *Arch Dermatol* 103:680–681, 1971.
15. Carmichael AJ, Tan CY, Abraham SM: Adult onset Mongolian spot. *Clin Exp Dermatol* 18:72–74, 1993.
16. Kopf AW, Bart RS: Malignant blue (Ota's?) nevus. *J Dermatol Surg Oncol* 8:442–445, 1982.
17. Nödl F, Krüger R: Maligner blauer Nävus bei Nävus Ota. *Hautarzt* 35:421–424, 1984.
18. Hori Y, Kawashima M, Oohara K, Kukita A: Acquired, bilateral nevus of Ota-like macules. *J Am Acad Dermatol* 10:961–964, 1984.
19. Sun C-C, Lu Y-C, Lee EF, Nakagawa H: Naevus fusco-caeruleus zygomaticus. *Br J Dermatol* 117:545–553, 1987.
20. Hidano A, Kaneko K: Acquired dermal melanocytosis of the face and extremities. *Br J Dermatol* 124:96–99, 1991.
21. van Krieken JHJM, Boom BW, Scheffer E: Malignant transformation in a naevus of Ito: A case report. *Histopathology* 12:100–102, 1988. (Brief report)
22. Bashiti HM, Blair JD, Triska RA, Keller L: Generalized dermal melanocytosis. *Arch Dermatol* 117:791–793, 1981.
23. Burkhart CG, Gohara A: Dermal melanocytic hamartoma. *Arch Dermatol* 117:102–104, 1981.
24. Vélez A, Fuente C, Belinchón I, et al: Congenital segmental dermal melanocytosis in an adult. *Arch Dermatol* 128:521–525, 1992.
25. Mevorak B, Frenk E, Delacrétaz J: Dermal melanocytosis. *Dermatologica* 154:107–114, 1977.
26. Levene A: Disseminated dermal melanocytosis terminating in melanoma. *Br J Dermatol* 101:197–205, 1979.
27. Tièche M: Ueber benigne Melanome ('Chromatophorome') der Haut "blaue Naevi." *Virchows Arch [A]* 186:212–229, 1906.
28. Darier J: Le melanome malin mesenchymatieux ou melanosarcome. *Bull Assoc Fr Cancer* 14:221–249, 1925.
29. Montgomery H: The blue nevus (Jadassohn-Tieche): Its distinction from ordinary moles and malignant melanomas. *Am J Cancer* 36:527–539, 1939.
30. Levene A: On the natural history and comparative pathology of the blue naevus. *Ann Roy Coll Surg Engl* 62:327–334, 1980.
31. Bogomoletz W: Blue nevus of oral mucosa. *Br J Dermatol* 80:611–613, 1968.
32. Jao W, Fretzin DF, Christ ML, Prinz LM: Blue nevus of the prostate gland. *Arch Pathol* 91:187–191, 1971.
33. Qizilibash AH: Blue nevus of the uterine cervix. *Am J Clin Pathol* 59:803–806, 1973.
34. Tobon H, Murphy AI: Benign blue nevus of the vagina. *Cancer* 40:3174–3176, 1977.
35. Leopold JG, Richards DB: The interrelationship of blue and common naevi. *J Pathol Bacteriol* 95:37–46, 1968.
36. Shenfield HT, Maize JC: Multiple and agminated blue nevi. *J Dermatol Surg Oncol* 6:725–728, 1980.
37. Modly C, Wood C, Horn T: Metastatic malignant melanoma arising from a common blue nevus in a patient with subacute cutaneous lupus erythematosus. *Dermatologica* 178:171–175, 1989.
38. Kamino H, Tam ST: Compound blue nevus: A variant of blue nevus with an additional junctional dendritic component. A clinical, histopathologic, and immunohistochemical study of six cases. *Arch Dermatol* 126:1330–1333, 1990.
39. Allen AC: A reorientation on the histogenesis and clinical significance of cutaneous nevi and melanomas. *Cancer* 2:28–56, 1949.
40. Lund HZ, Kraus JM: Melanotic tumors of the skin. In *Atlas of Tumor pathology*. Washington, Armed Forces Institute of Pathology, 1962, pp 104–106.
41. Gartmann VH: Neuronaevus blue Masson—cellular blue nevus Allen. *Arch Klin Exp Dermatol* 221:109–121, 1965.
42. Leopold JG, Richards DB: Cellular blue nevi. *J Pathol Bacteriol* 94:247–255, 1967.
43. Rodriguez HA, Ackerman LV: Cellular blue nevus: Clinicopathologic study of forty-five cases. *Cancer* 21:393–405, 1968.
44. Merkow LP, Burt RC, Hayeslip DW, et al: A cellular and malignant blue nevus: A light and electron microscopic study. *Cancer* 24:888–896, 1969.
45. Bird CC, Willis RA: The histogenesis of pigmented neurofibromas. *J Pathol* 97:631–637, 1969.
46. Mishima Y: Cellular blue nevus: Melanogenic activity and malignant transformation. *Arch Dermatol* 101:104–110, 1970.
47. Gartmann H, Müller HD: Über das gemeinsame Vorkommen von blauem Naevus and Naevuszellnaevus. *Z Hautkr* 52:389–398, 1977.
48. Sterchi JM, Muss HB, Weidner N: Cellular blue nevus simulating metastatic melanoma: Report of an unusually large lesion associated with nevus-cell aggregates in regional lymph nodes. *J Surg Oncol* 36:71–75, 1987.
49. Temple-Camp CRE, Saxe N, King H: Benign and malignant cellular blue nevus: A clinicopathological study of 30 cases. *Am J Dermatopathol* 10:289–296, 1988.
50. Michal M, Baumruk K, Skalova A: Myxoid change within cellular blue naevi: A diagnostic pitfall. *Histopathology* 20:527–530, 1992.
51. Hendrickson MR, Ross JC: Neoplasms arising in congenital giant nevi. *Am J Surg Pathol* 5:109–135, 1981.

52. Goldenhersh MA, Savin RC, Barnhill RL, Stenn KS: Malignant blue nevus. *J Am Acad Dermatol* 19:712–722, 1988.
53. Connelly J, Smith JL Jr: Malignant blue nevus. *Cancer* 67:2653–2657, 1991.
54. Avidor I, Kessler E: "Atypical" blue nevus—A benign variant of cellular blue nevus. *Dermatologica* 154:39–44, 1977.
55. Lambert WC, Brodkin RH: Nodal and subcutaneous cellular blue nevi: A pseudometastasizing pseudomelanoma. *Arch Dermatol* 120:367–370, 1984.
56. Lamovec J: Blue nevus of the lymph node capsule: Report of a new case with review of the literature. *Am J Clin Pathol* 81:367–372, 1984.
57. Pariser H, Beerman H: Extensive blue patchlike pigmentation: A morphologic variant of blue nevus? Persistent extrasacral Mongolian blue spot? Diffuse mesodermal pigmentation? *Arch Dermatol Syphilol* 59:396–404, 1949.
58. Radentz WA, Vogel P: Congenital common blue nevus. *Arch Dermatol* 126:124–125, 1990.
59. Upshaw BY, Ghormley RK, Montgomery H: Extensive blue nevus of Jadassohn-Tièche: Report of case. *Surgery* 22:761–765, 1947.
60. Pittman JL, Fisher BK:. Plaque-type blue nevus. *Arch Dermatol* 112:1127–1128, 1976.
61. Hendricks WM: Eruptive blue nevi. *J Am Acad Dermatol* 4:50–53, 1981.
62. Tsoitis G, Kanitakis C, Kapetis E: Naevus bleu multinodulaire en plaque, superficiel et neuroide. *Ann Dermatol Venereol* 110:231–235, 1983.
63. Pfaltz M, Schnyder UW: Verlauf und Ultrastruktur beim plaqueartigen Naevus bleu. *Hautarzt* 40:355–357, 1989.
64. Heymann WR, Yablonsky TM: Congenital appearance of plaque-type blue nevi. *Arch Dermatol* 127:587, 1991.
65. Tuthill RJ, Clark WH Jr, Levene A: Pilar neurocristic hamartoma: Its relationship to blue nevus and equine melanotic disease. *Arch Dermatol* 118:592–596, 1982.
66. Bondi EE, Elder D, Guerry D IV, Clark WH Jr: Target blue nevus. *Arch Dermatol* 119:919–920, 1983.
67. Sun J, Morton TH, Gown AM: Antibody HMB-45 identifies the cells of blue nevi. *Am J Surg Pathol* 14:748–751, 1990.
68. Casadei GP, Grigolato P, Cabibbo E: Blue nevus of the endocervix: A study of five cases. *Tumori* 73:75–79, 1987.
69. Khalil MK, Duguid WP: Neurotropic malignant melanoma of right temple with orbital metastasis: A clinicopathological case report. *Br J Ophthalmol* 71:41–46, 1987.
70. Kjaerheim A, Martinez MG, Montes LF: Blue nevus of the oral cavity. *Oral Surg* 29:718–728, 1970.
71. Lach B, Russell N, Benoit B, Atack D: Cellular blue nevus ("melanocytoma") of the spinal meninges: Electron microscopic and immunohistochemical features. *Neurosurgery* 22:773–780, 1988.
72. Lovas GL, Wysocki GP, Daley TD: The oral blue nevus: Histogenetic implications of its ultrastructural features. *Oral Surg* 55:145–150, 1983.
73. Ro JY, Grignon DJ, Ayla AG, et al: Blue nevus and melanosis of the prostate. *Am J Clin Pathol* 90:530–535, 1988.
74. Ghadially FN: Blue naevus. In *Diagnostic electron microscopy of Tumours.* London: Butterworths, 1980, pp 81, 399–406.
75. Nakai T, Rappaport H: A study of the histogenesis of experimental melanotic tumors resembling cellular blue nevi: The evidence in support of their neurogenic origin. *Am J Pathol* 43:175–199, 1963.
76. Mandybur TI: Melanotic nerve sheath tumors. *J Neurosurg* 41:187–192, 1974.
77. Graham DI, Paterson A, McQueen A, et al: Melanotic tumours (blue naevi) of spinal nerve roots. *J Pathol* 118:839, 1976.
78. Carney JA: Psammomatous melanotic schwannoma. *Am J Surg Pathol* 14:206–222, 1990.

8

Melanocytic Nevi with Phenotypic Heterogeneity

As discussed previously, the developmental biology of melanocytic nevi is poorly understood, and thus explanations for the variance in cell type, melanin content, stroma, and depth currently do not exist. A number of nevi reported in the literature as combined nevus, deep penetrating nevus, plexiform spindle cell nevus, inverted type A nevus, and melanocytic nevus with focal atypical epithelioid cell component (MNFAECC) are notable for unusual histologic features. However, as outlined in Table 8-1, some of these nevi tend to show rather similar clinical and histologic features. The goal of this chapter will be to describe the salient features of the melanocytic lesions named above as they have been reported but also to point out their morphologic similarities and differences where applicable.

THE COMBINED NEVUS

The recognition of two or more fairly distinct populations of melanocytes in melanocytic nevi dates back to the turn of the century[1,2] (Table 8-2). The term *combined nevus* was used initially to describe the combination of ordinary nevus and blue nevus elements[1-5] but was subsequently extended to include components of Spitz nevus and pigmented spindle cell nevus (deep penetrating nevus and plexiform pigmented spindle cell nevus).[6-10] On purely morphologic grounds alone, the combined nevus also encompasses so-called inverted type A nevus and MNFAECC.[11,12]

Clinical Features

The characteristics of the combined nevus are probably related to the predominant cellular population present, e.g., whether blue nevus, Spitz nevus, or other[1-10] (Table 8-3). Most patients have been relatively young, with a mean age of 30.3 years in a recent large series.[10] A predominance of women has been reported consistently in several studies. Most of these nevi measure less than 5 mm in greatest diameter.[8,10]

In nevi with a significant component of blue nevus, the most common sites of involvement are the face, back, and shoulder.[8] Such nevi are often diagnosed as blue nevi because of the predominant dark color. Some of these nevi also may demonstrate a small well-circumscribed blue or blue-black focus, e.g., often 1 to 3 mm in diameter, within an otherwise ordinary flesh-colored, tan, or brown nevus (see MNFAECC below).[8,12]

Nevi with prominent components of Spitz nevus occur commonly on the extremities, as do conventional Spitz nevi.[9] Such nevi are often diagnosed as an unusual nevus, Spitz nevus, dermatofibroma, or possibly melanoma.

Histopathology

Nevi designated as combined may potentially encompass the entire phenotypic repertoire of melanocytic nevi[1-10] (see Table 8-3). It also should be kept in mind that the lesions reported in various studies as combined nevi are most likely a skewed sampling of nevi selected for unusual, atypical, or poorly characterized features.[8-10]

TABLE 8-1
Comparison of Various Histologic Features in Certain Unusual Melanocytic Nevi

		Depth		*Architecture*			*Stroma*	*Cellular Characteristics*					
	Blue Color	*Superficial*	*Deep*	*Inverted Wedge*	*Plexiform*	*Bulbous Contour*	*Sclerosis*	*Epithelioid Cell*	*Pigmented Epithelioid Cell*	*Spindle Cell*	*Pigmented Spindle Cell*	*Dendritic Cell*	*Conventional Nevus Cell*
Spitz nevus	−	++	+	++	±	+	+	++	+	++	+	−	−
Pigmented spindle cell nevus	−	++	−	−	−	−	−	−	+	−	++	−	−
Blue nevus	++	++	++	++	+	+	++	−	−	−	+	++	−
Cellular blue nevus	++	+	++	+	+	++	++	+	+	++	+	+	+
Combined nevus	+	+	+	+	+	+	+	+	+	+	+	+	+
Deep penetrating nevus	++	+	++	++	++	++	+	±	+	+	++	±	−
Plexiform spindle cell nevus	++	+	++	++	++	+	±	±	+	+	++	±	−
Inverted type A nevus	+	+	+	+	±	+	±	+	++	±	+	−	++
Melanocytic nevus with focal atypical epithelioid cell component	+	+	+	±	−	±	±	+	++	+	+	+	+

TABLE 8-2
Summary of Previously Published Accounts of Combined Nevus

Author	*Year*	*Number of Cases*	*Observations*
Tèiche	1906	—	Concept of combined nevus: ordinary plus blue nevus
Dubreuilh and Petges	1912	1	Ordinary and blue nevus
Allen and Spitz	1953	2	Ordinary and blue nevus
Evans	1956	5	Ordinary and blue nevus
Leopold and Richards	1968	20	Ordinary nevus plus common blue or cellular blue nevus
Gartmann and Müller	1977	97	Combinations of ordinary nevus, common blue nevus, cellular blue nevus, and Spitz nevus
Weedon and Little	1977	32	Combinations of Spitz nevus and other nevus cell components, not further specified by authors
Fletcher and Sagebiel	1981	50	Combinations of ordinary nevus, common blue nevus, cellular blue nevus, and Spitz nevus
Rogers et al.	1985	22	Combinations of Spitz nevus, ordinary nevus, and blue nevus
Pulitzer et al.	1991	95	Combinations of ordinary common blue, cellular blue, Spitz, and pigmented spindle cell nevus

TABLE 8-3
Précis: The Combined Nevus

Clinical features
- Any age (3–74 years) but usually < 40 years of age
- Women > men
- Head and neck (especially for blue nevus variants), upper trunk, proximal extremities
- Often component of blue, blue-black
- May have small (1–5-mm) blue, blue-black focus in ordinary nevus
- Size < 6–7 mm in most instances

Histopathology
- Symmetric
- Well circumscribed
- Orderly arrangements of cells
- Two or more of the following:
  1. Ordinary nevus component
  2. Pigmented dendritic melanocytes
  3. Pigmented spindle/epithelioid cells
  4. Amelanotic spindle cells
  5. Spitz nevus cells
- Ordinary nevus component often overlies or is adjacent to other component
- Deep involvement occurs
- Plexiform configuration on occasion

Differential diagnosis
- Cellular blue nevus
- Melanoma

*See Table 8-1.

Furthermore, some of the morphologic combinations reported are based on subjective interpretations that may not necessarily be reproduced by other observers. With these caveats in mind, the common presentations of combined nevus will be described.

One of the most common patterns of combined nevus is that of an ordinary nevus and blue nevus (Figs. 8-1 and 8-2). The ordinary nevus component, as with all combined nevi, may be compound or dermal and often overlies or is adjacent to the blue nevus component (see Fig. 8-1). The blue nevus elements most often consist of heavily pigmented dendritic melanocytes, melanophages, and variable fibrosis. Less commonly, the fusiform cells typical of cellular blue nevus also may be present with or without dendritic cells. The component of blue nevus may extend deeply into the reticular dermis as nests or fascicles, often in a plexiform configuration (see Fig. 8-2). Despite the two or more components, such nevi are usually symmetric, well-circumscribed, orderly and display little or no cellular atypia.

Another common pattern of combined nevus which probably includes inverted type A nevus and MNFAECC is that of an ordinary nevus in combination with discrete foci of pigmented spindle cells and/or pigmented epithelioid cells[11,12] (Fig. 8-3). The latter cells are often enlarged, contain abundant granular melanin, and are disposed in nests or fascicles in the deep portions of or beneath the ordinary nevus, sometimes in a plexiform arrangement. The sizes of the nests or fascicles may vary from being minuscule to large lobular or digitate aggregates. The nuclei are usually slightly enlarged, round, oval, or elongate, and uniform but on occasion show slight to moderate atypia. Melanophages are also frequently associated with these pigmented foci. It should be pointed out that this pattern of combined nevus is also probably morphologically identical to that of deep penetrating nevus and plexiform pigmented spindle cell nevus.[13–16]

Spitz nevi uncommonly are observed in association with ordinary nevus elements[9] (Fig. 8-4). The topographic relationships of these two components include the Spitz nevus component being adjacent to, beneath, or admixed with the common nevus elements.

After the preceding relatively well recognized forms of combined nevus, almost any combination of cell types is possible but rare. Thus one may encounter nevi containing various admixtures of ordinary nevus cells, dendritic melanocytes, Spitz nevus cells, and perhaps other transitional cell types. Atypical features also may be observed, such as melanocytic dysplasia of the intraepidermal component.[6–10]

Inverted Type A Nevus. The morphologic pattern invoked by inverted type A nevus is one probably also encompassed by combined nevus and MNFAECC.[11] The term describes the presence of discrete nests of epithelioid cells, usually pigmented, within the dermal component of an ordinary nevus (see Fig. 8-3). These nests are often deep and may be multifocal. In general, the term has not been accepted into general usage and may not offer any advantages over other terms.

Melanocytic Nevus with Focal Atypical Epithelioid Component. As mentioned earlier, the presence of a focal distinct epithelioid cell component in an ordinary nevus is characteristic of one pattern of combined nevus (see Fig. 8-3). This same morphologic description has been described recently as MNFAECC[12] (Table 8-4). In their study of 73 cases, Ball and Golitz[12] reported that MNFAECC were characterized by the recent appearance of a 1- to 5-mm black macule or papule in a preexisting nevus and a corresponding histologic focus of atypical epithelioid cells. These authors have stressed the importance of distinguishing such a newly developed focus from melanoma. With regard to the pathogenesis of MNFAECC, the authors postulate the development of an abnormal clone of cells, perhaps with a growth advantage over the surrounding ordinary nevus cells. As evidence for their hypothesis, they have shown p53 expression in some of the foci compared with no expression in the background

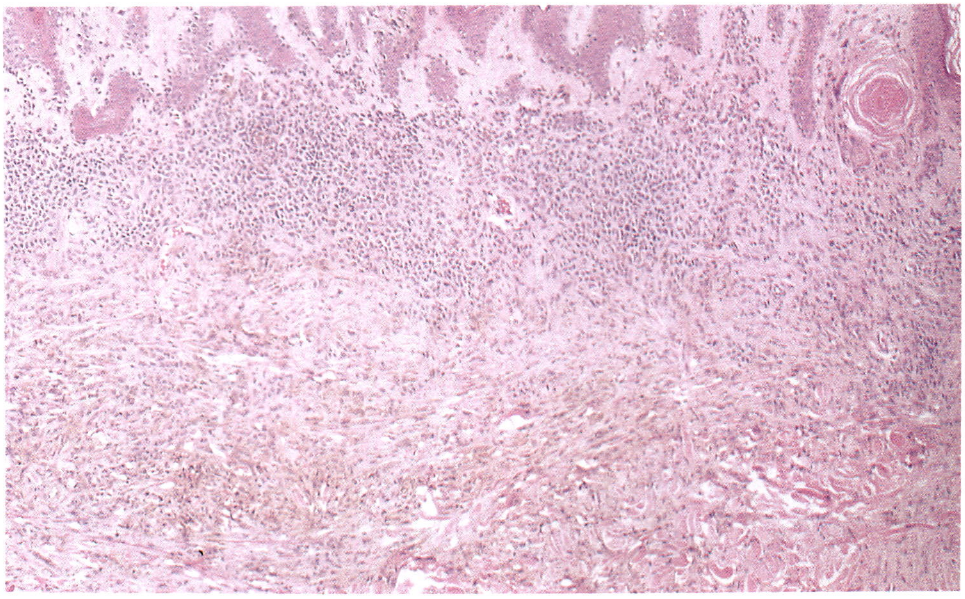

A

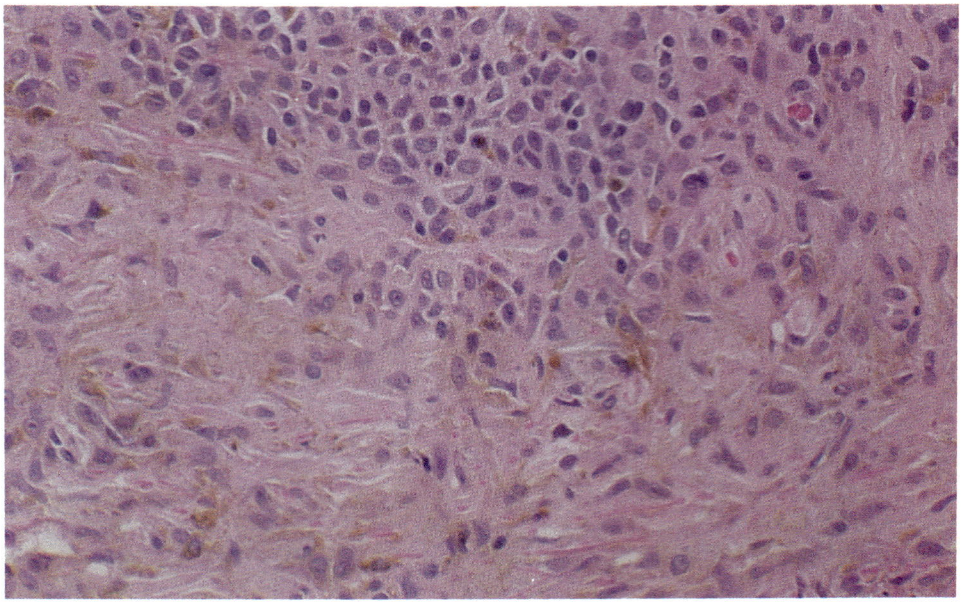

B

FIGURE 8-1

Combined nevus composed of ordinary compound nevus overlying blue nevus. (A) Note well-defined zone of small nevus cells in superficial dermal overlying blue nevus (H&E, × 100). (B) Sheet of small type B nevus cells collides with blue nevus cells. There is slight fibrosis associated with the blue nevus cells (H&E, × 400).

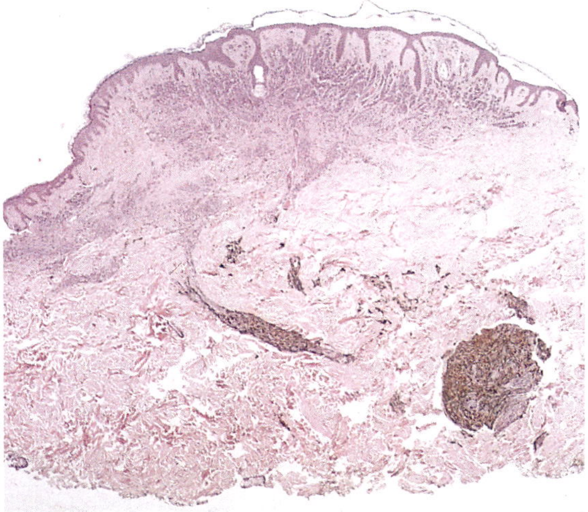

A

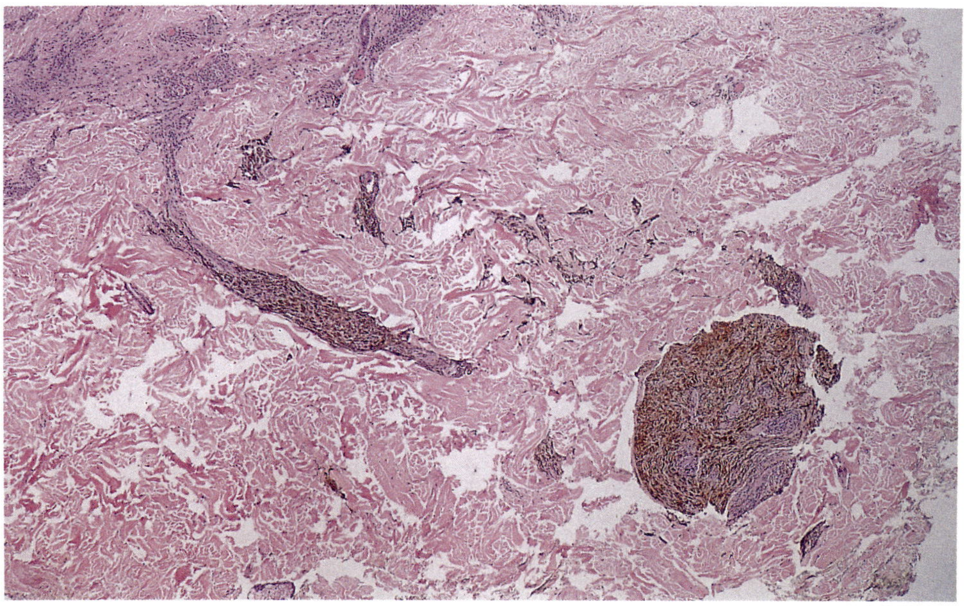

B

FIGURE 8-2

Combined nevus composed of dermal nevus overlying the blue nevus in deep dermis. (A) Note clear separation of the two components (H&E, × 20). (B) Blue nevus has plexiform configuration in deep reticular dermis. The heavily pigmented elements are associated with neurovascular structures (H&E, × 40). (C) Compact nest of pigmented dendritic melanocytes and melanophages associated with cutaneous nerves (H&E, × 200).

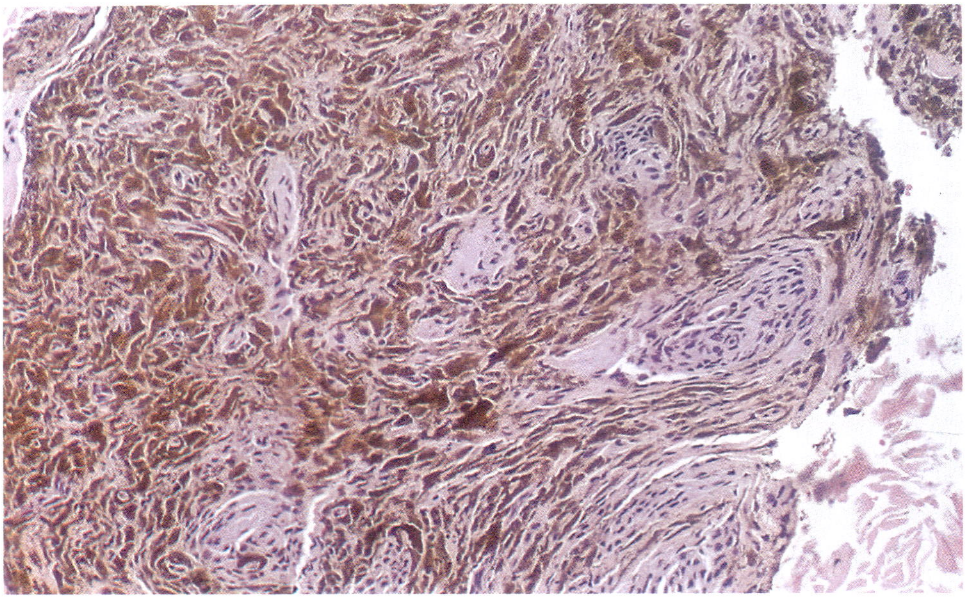

C

FIGURE 8-2 *(Continued)*

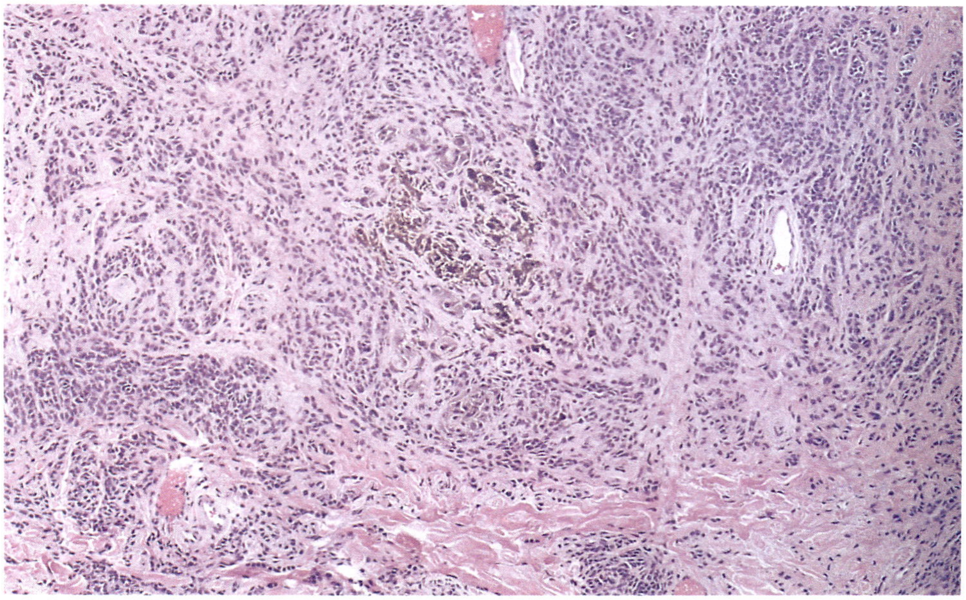

A

FIGURE 8-3

Combined nevus with focal aggregate of pigmented epithelioid cells. (A) Most of the field shows nests and cords of small type B nevus cells. However, there is a small circumscribed aggregate of pigment-containing cells in the center of the field (H&E, × 100). (B) The cells within this aggregate are epithelioid cells and melanophages. These findings also fit the morphologic pattern of inverted type A or clonal nevus (H&E, × 200). (C) The epithelioid cells are enlarged with abundant cytoplasm containing melanin. These cells are also similar to the epithelioid cells of Spitz nevus. The surrounding stroma is slightly sclerotic (H&E, × 400).

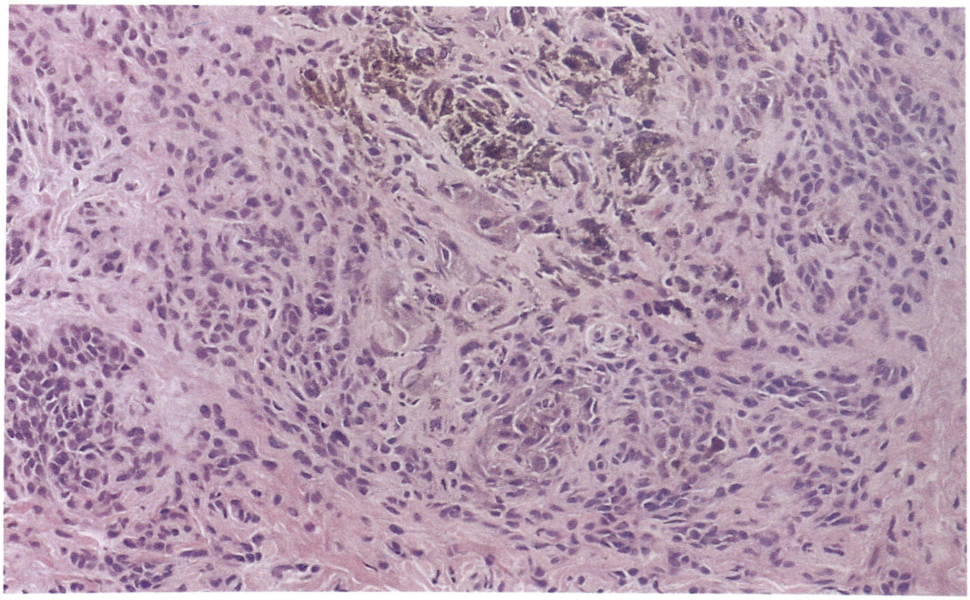

B

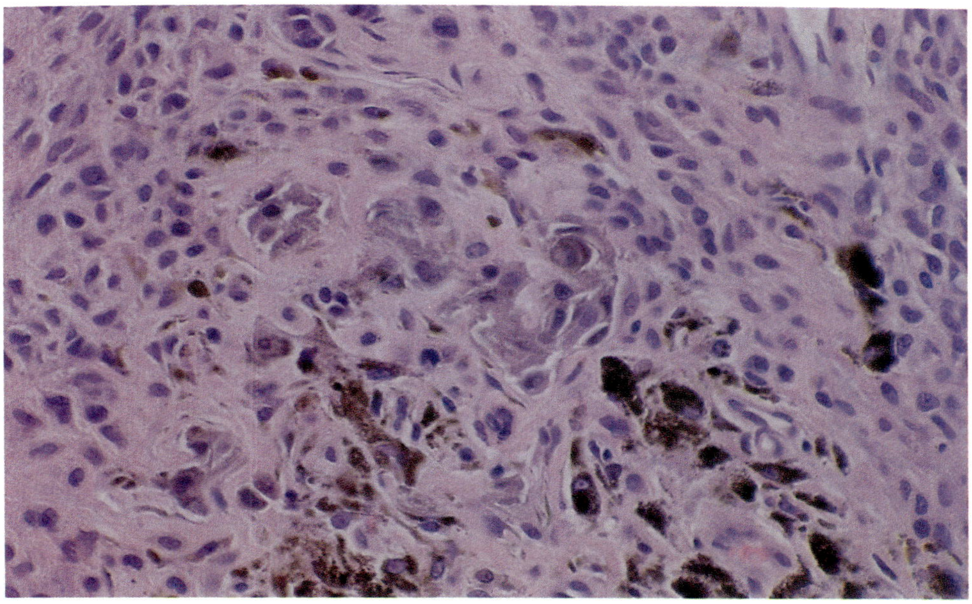

C

FIGURE 8-3 *(Continued)*

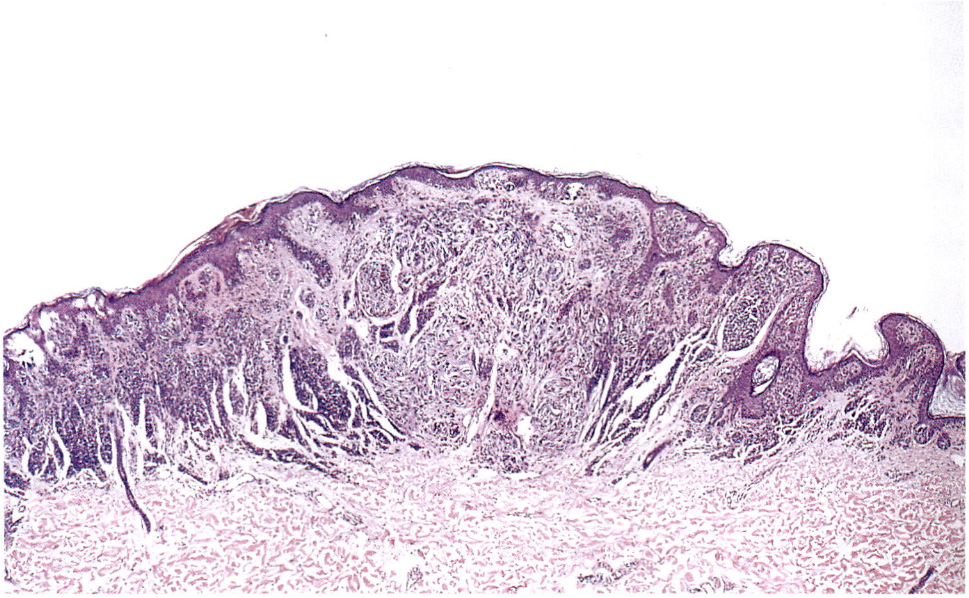

A

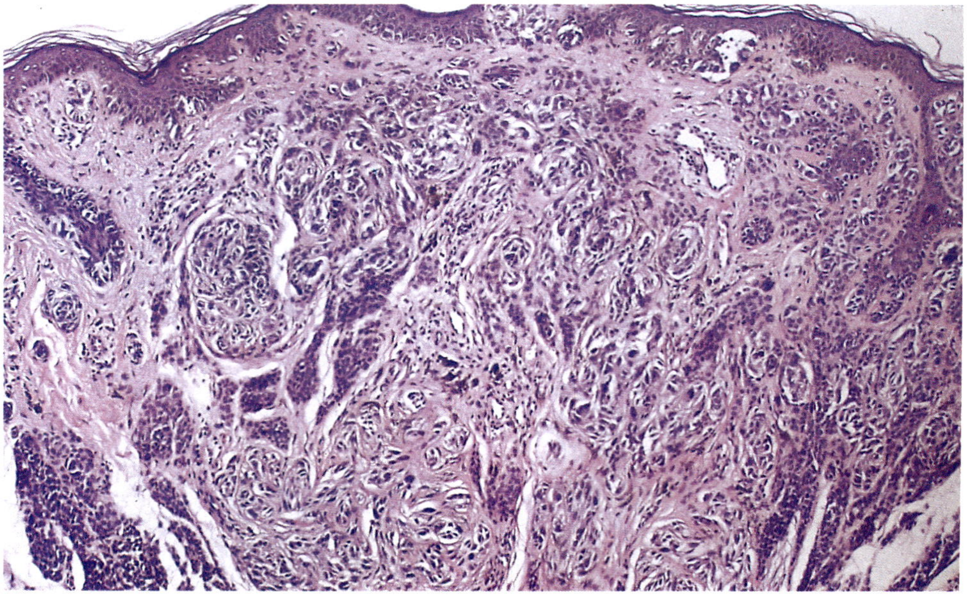

B

FIGURE 8-4

Combined nevus composed of ordinary compound nevus and spindle and epithelioid cell nevus. (A) Dome-shaped lesion with central component of spindle and epithelioid cells surrounded by ordinary compound nevus (H&E, × 40). (B) Central portion of lesion contains spindle and epithelioid cell elements in small nests and fascicles (H&E, × 100). (C) Higher magnification of part B showing bundles of spindled cells and some epithelioid cells. The stroma is slightly fibrotic, and the compartmentalization of the cellular bundles has the appearance of schwannian differentiation (H&E, × 400).

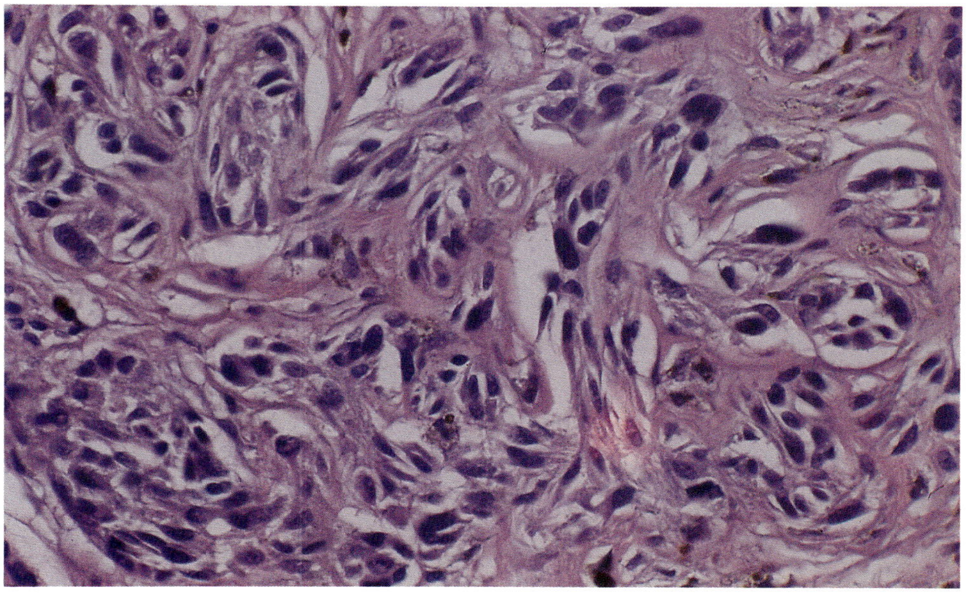

C

FIGURE 8-4 *(Continued)*

nevus. This hypothesis has merit and suggests that focal tumor progression might account for some varieties of combined nevus in which the emergence of a new, altered, or aberrant population of cells has occurred, but this requires further study.

Differential Diagnosis

The differential diagnosis of combined nevus is of course dependent on the particular cellular populations present. However, the histologic change often of most concern to pathologists is an aberrant focus of cytologically altered/atypical cells in an otherwise ordinary nevus. Such a finding is of concern for early transformation to melanoma or even fully evolved melanoma (Table 8-5). The latter histologic alteration, as already mentioned, is present most commonly in the dermis. However, as discussed in Chapter 10, the development of melanoma in the dermal component of a nevus is highly unusual. Therefore, such a diagnosis must be weighed carefully and based on sufficient criteria of atypicality, mitotic activity, and nodular (confluent) proliferation.

Although combined nevi are heterogeneous, they tend to be present in fairly young individuals (<40 years of age), measure less than 5 or 6 mm, and exhibit an overall symmetry and regular appearance. As mentioned previously, the presence of a focal aggregate of pigment-laden epithelioid/spindle cells is usually the feature of concern. Although occasional aggregates of epithelioid cells are large, many are small and well circumscribed. Cytologic atypia is usually low grade or insignificant compared with melanoma. The surrounding nevus, which commonly is of ordinary type, is generally unremarkable with reference to atypicality. An occasional mitosis may be observed in such a focus without undue concern; however, the presence of two or more mitoses per high-power field should prompt careful inspection for melanoma.

TABLE 8-4
Précis: Melanocytic Nevus with Focal Atypical Epithelioid Cell Component

Clinical features
Age mean 31.3 years (1 month to 78 years)
Women = men
Site—head and neck, trunk
Size—6.2 mm mean with central 1–5 mm dark brown or black macule or papule of recent onset
Histopathology
Ordinary nevus
Central focus containing large epithelioid melanocytes
Heavily pigmented
Cytologically atypical
Occupying about 5–80% of nevus
Associated melanophages
Differential diagnosis
Melanoma

*See Table 8-1.

TABLE 8-5
Comparison of Combined Nevus and Melanoma*

	Combined Nevus	*Melanoma*
Symmetry	Frequent	Uncommon
Size	< 6 mm often	> 1 cm often
Lateral borders	Sharply defined	Poorly defined
Focus, foci of altered cells	Present, well demarcated	Variable
Cytologic atypia	Usually absent or low grade	High grade
Mitotic activity	Absent or minimal	Frequent
Mononuclear cell infiltrates	Uncommon	Frequent

*Focus of epithelioid/spindle cells in ordinary nevus (as also observed in inverted type A nevi and melanocytic nevi with focal atypical epithelioid cell components).

DEEP PENETRATING NEVUS

The term *deep penetrating nevus* (DPN) was introduced in 1989 with the report of 70 unusual nevi with disturbing morphologic features.[13] The authors alleged that although deep penetrating nevus was related to blue nevus, cellular blue nevus, and Spitz nevus, it seemed to occupy a reasonably well defined niche among the latter entities. One particular point emphasized by the authors in reporting DPN was its frequent confusion with melanoma.[13] DPN also shows features in common with plexiform spindle cell nevus[14,15] (see below).

Clinical Features

In the single report of DPN, most patients ranged in age from 10 to 30 years[13] (Table 8-6). The most common sites of DPN included the face, upper trunk, and proximal extremities. Most lesions measured less than 1 cm in greatest diameter and were diagnosed clinically as blue nevus or cellular blue nevus. On follow-up ranging from 1 to 23 years (mean 7 years), none of the lesions had recurred or metastasized.[13]

Histopathology

Scanning magnification discloses in most instances a symmetric, well-circumscribed lesion with involvement of the deep reticular dermis and possibly subcutis[13] (see Table 8-6). The overall architecture is usually that of an inverted wedge extending into the deep dermis (Fig. 8-5). The superficial dermal portion is characterized by a diffuse proliferation of pigmented spindle cells that show progressive organization as discreet fascicles or nests with descent into the deep dermis. Junctional nests are noted in some lesions. The fascicles of spindle cells tend to be associated with neurovascular and adnexal structures of the lower reticular dermis. These cellular aggregates often exhibit bulbous contours and may bulge into the subcutis, as do cellular blue nevi (see Fig. 8-5A). Melanophages are usually intimately associated with the spindle cells. Some nevi may show cytologic atypia.

TABLE 8-6
*Précis: Deep Penetrating Nevus**

- Clinical features
  - Age range 10–30 years
  - Site—face, upper trunk, proximal extremities
  - Size < 1 cm
  - Raised lesions with bluish color
- Histopathology
  - Symmetric
  - Well circumscribed
  - Inverted-wedge configuration
  - Extension of cellular fascicles into deep dermis or subcutis
  - Pigmented spindle cells in fascicles associated with neurovascular bundles
  - Occasional junctional nests
  - Diffuse involvement of superficial dermis
  - Occasional cytologic atypia
- Differential diagnosis
  - Spindle and epithelioid cell nevus
  - Cellular blue nevus
  - Melanoma

*Plexiform spindle cell nevus is similar to deep penetrating nevus but shows a striking plexiform configuration not always present in deep penetrating nevus. Neither does the plexiform nevus always extend as deeply as deep penetrating nevus.

PLEXIFORM SPINDLE CELL NEVUS

Plexiform spindle cell nevi are notable for a plexiform arrangement of pigmented spindle cells often involving the deep reticular dermis.[14–16] The recognition of this unusual nevus is important so that it is distinguished from melanoma. A close relationship with superficial pigmented spindle cell nevus, Spitz nevus, blue nevus, and DPN has been emphasized.[15]

Clinical Features

The lesions thus far reported occurred in young adults (mean age 22.5 years) and involved the shoulders and back primarily.[15] Clinically, the lesions were described as raised, bluish or black, suggesting blue nevus, an atypical nevus, or melanoma.

Histopathology

Most lesions are slightly raised, symmetric, and exhibit a wedge-shaped configuration in the reticular dermis.[14–16]

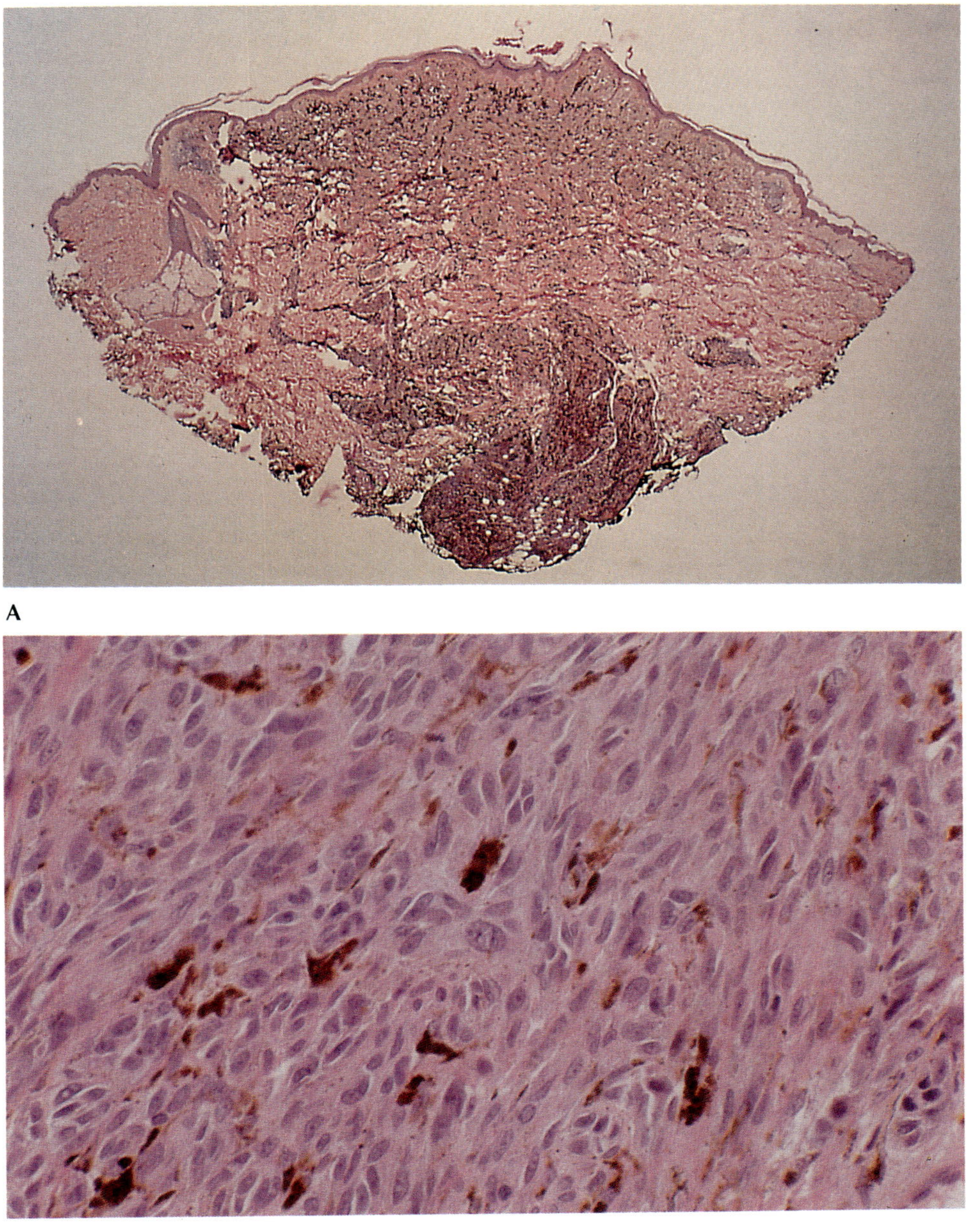

A

B

FIGURE 8-5

Deep penetrating nevus. (A) Note inverted-wedge configuration and deep extension of rounded bundles of pigmented spindle cells (H&E, × 20). (B) Tightly packed fascicles of fusiform cells and scattered melanophages. The nuclei within the fusiform cells have dispersed chromatin patterns (H&E, × 400).

The most striking feature is the plexiform arrangement of fascicles of pigmented spindle cells that track along adnexal structures and neurovascular bundles (Fig. 8-6). Other common features include junctional nests, diffuse involvement of the superficial dermis, and infiltration of cutaneous nerves and arrector pili muscles. The spindle cells contain abundant granular melanin and oval or elongate nuclei with delicate chromatin patterns and inconspicuous nuclei (see Fig. 8-6D). Occasional low-grade cytologic and rare mitotic figures are observed. Melanophages are often present in association with the spindle cell elements.

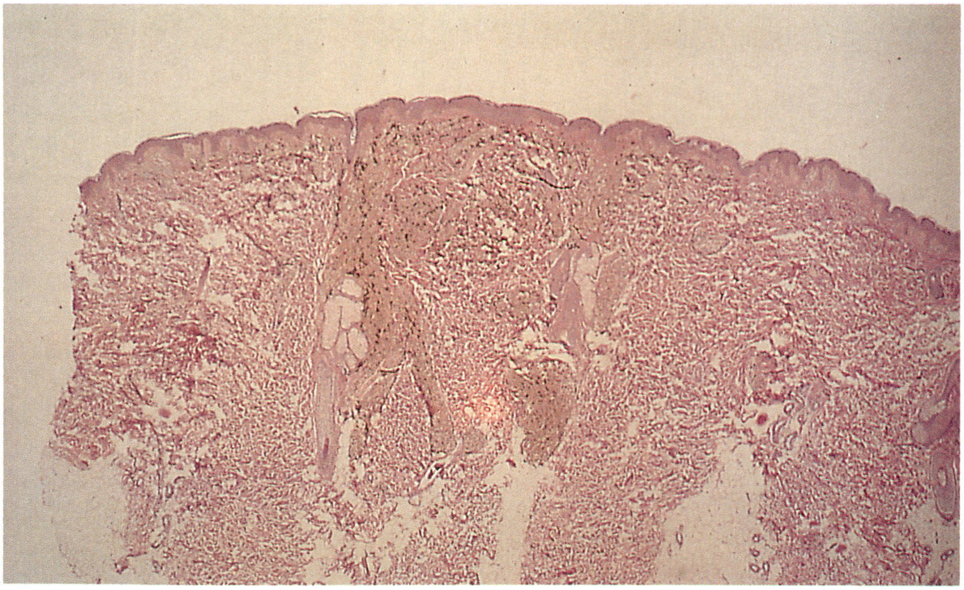

A

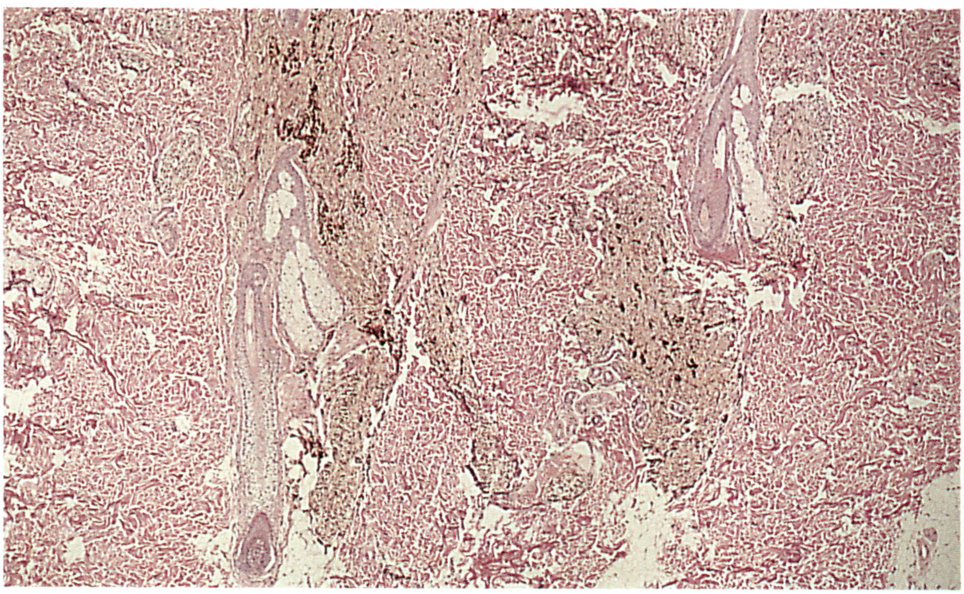

B

FIGURE 8-6

Plexiform pigmented spindle cell nevus. (A) Characteristic appearance at scanning magnification is notable for fascicles of pigmented spindle cells in plexiform arrangement (H&E, × 20). (B) The fascicles are associated with appendages, blood vessels, and nerves. There is normal collagen separating these cellular aggregates (H&E, × 40). (C) Compact bundles of spindle cells near a hair follicle infiltrate collagen in an orderly nondisruptive pattern (H&E, × 100). (D) This field shows a bundle of uniform-appearing fusiform cells. The cells contain fine granular melanin and monotonous nuclei with dispersed chromatin. There is a striking resemblance to the spindle cells of superficial pigmented spindle cell nevus (H&E, × 400).

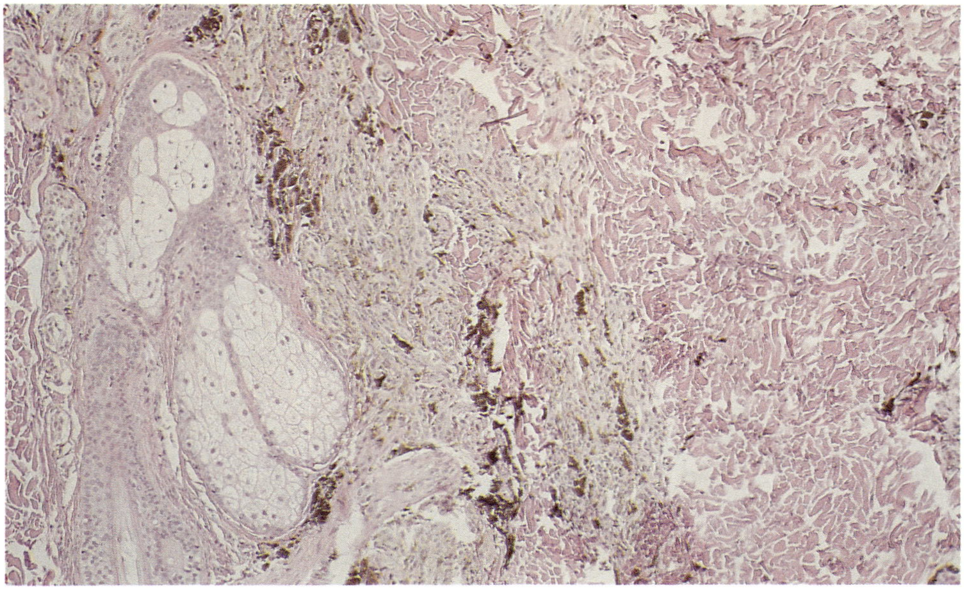

C

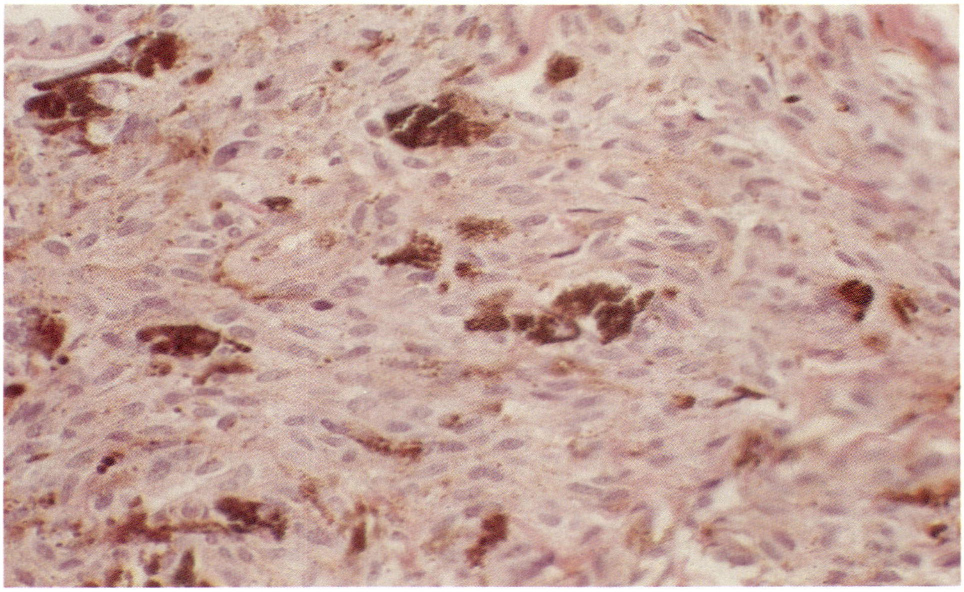

D

FIGURE 8-6 *(Continued)*

Differential Diagnosis

Because of the presence of pigmented spindle cells and frequent deep involvement, plexiform spindle cell nevi are closely related to DPN. However, they are discriminated from DPN by their striking plexiform configuration (often lacking in DPN) and frequent absence of bulbous cellular aggregates and deep involvement.

Because of the unusual nature of nevi described as deep penetrating or plexiform, the immediate concern is to discriminate such lesions from melanoma, whether primary or metastatic (Table 8-7). The most worrisome features include the depth of involvement, the presence of fascicles of pigmented spindle cells, perineurial infiltration, the plexiform or lobular configuration of such lesions, and especially cytologic atypia and mitoses, if present. Particular features aiding in this differential diagnosis include the usual size less than 6 or 7 mm (almost always < 1 cm), overall symmetry, nondisruptive growth

TABLE 8-7
Comparison of Deep Penetrating Nevus, Plexiform Spindle Cell Nevus, and Melanoma

	Deep Penetrating Nevus	*Plexiform Spindle Cell Nevus*	*Melanoma*
Symmetry	Frequent	Frequent	Uncommon
Size	< 1 cm often	< 1 cm often	> 1 cm often
Lateral borders	Sharply defined	Sharply defined	Often ill-defined
Dermal configuration	Inverted-wedge, lobular	Inverted wedge, plexiform	Variable, irregular
Deep extension	Present, often into subcutis	Variable, occasionally into subcutis	Variable
Rounded lobular aggregates in dermis	Frequent	Variable	Uncommon
Cytologic atypia	Absent to low grade	Absent to low grade	High grade
Mitotic activity	Absent or minimal	Absent or minimal	Frequent

patterns, lack of high-grade atypia, and lack of significant mitotic activity in such nevi. Nonetheless, some of these nevi are quite challenging because of their large size, confluent masses of cells without evidence of maturation, and cytologic atypia. As a result, the biologic potential of a small minority of such lesions may be difficult to predict. Rare instances of lymph node metastases have been observed.[10] The most appropriate management of these lesions is to communicate to the clinician the uncertain but possibly aggressive potential of such tumors and to ensure that they are excised with uninvolved surgical margins. The patient also should have careful periodic examinations for possible recurrence or metastasis. If sufficient criteria for unequivocal melanoma are lacking, our policy is to avoid labeling a patient with that diagnosis.

As discussed below, these nevi show overlap with cellular blue nevus and atypical variants of spindle and epithelioid cell nevus.

PHENOTYPIC HETEROGENEITY AND NOMENCLATURE

The nevi described above are related because of depth, architecture, and the presence of pigmented cells that may be oval, elongate, spindled, or perhaps dendritic. Discriminating features that might be of help are listed in Table 8.1 and include, for example, superficial or deep disposition, configuration (i.e., plexiform, bulbous), cell type (i.e., pigmented spindle cell, epithelioid cell, dendritic cell), and two or more populations of cells.

Also as noted in Table 8-1, deep penetrating nevus and plexiform spindle cell nevus (and combined nevus showing components of the latter two nevi) are related to both spindle and epithelioid cell nevi and blue nevi. For example, occasional Spitz nevi may extend deeply into the reticular dermis in an inverted-wedge pattern, and some may even involve subcutaneous fat (see Chap. 6). Such nevi also may be characterized by bulbous lobular aggregates of cells that protrude into the deep dermis or the subcutis. In some instances, one may have difficulty deciding whether such a nevus is a variant of Spitz nevus, pigmented spindle cell nevus, deep penetrating nevus, plexiform nevus, or blue nevus. Thus a distinction among these various nevi might simply be based on depth of involvement by the nevus and perhaps nuances of cell type and architecture.

Generally speaking, the designation of a lesion as blue nevus has been based on a constellation of clinical and histologic features. A major criterion is the presence of a bluish color, accompanied by localization to certain anatomic sites, such as the dorsal aspects of the hands and feet, buttocks and sacrococcygeal area, and a certain spectrum of histologic features. If one applies the clinical criterion of blue color for the diagnosis of blue nevi, the resulting spectrum of lesions would be rather large and would include ordinary and cellular blue nevi and "bluish" nevi with varying proportions of pigmented spindle cells, epithelioid cells, and intermediate cells. The latter nevi probably include plexiform spindle cell nevus, deep penetrating nevus, and various types of combined nevus.

With regard to histologic features, the limits of blue nevus have not been clearly delineated. The most prototypic blue nevi contain aggregates of heavily melanized dendritic melanocytes, circumscribed fibrosis, and melanophages. Cellular blue nevi encompass dermal lesions containing not only dendritic melanocytes but also less heavily melaninized spindle cells. Blue nevi rigorously characterized by bundles of dendritic melanocytes containing heavy melanin granules may exhibit an inverted wedge configuration, plexiform architecture, and deep extension into the reticular dermis. Thus even unequivocal blue nevi may show overlap with deep penetrating nevus and plexiform nevus. One may encounter melanocytic nevi with varying admixtures of pigmented spindle

TABLE 8-8
Proposed Classification of Melanocytic Proliferations

Intraepidermal melanocytic proliferation,
Lentiginous type (elongated rete)
Basilar type
Pagetoid type
Nested type
Intraepidermal and dermal melanocytic proliferation, superficial type (no deeper than upper half of reticular dermis)
Intraepidermal and dermal melanocytic proliferation, superficial and deep type
Dermal melanocytic proliferation, superficial type
Dermal melanocytic proliferation, superficial and deep type
Architectural characteristics of dermal component
Wedge-shaped pattern
Plexiform pattern
Expansile nodular pattern
Desmoplasia
Cytologic characteristics
Round or oval cell
Dendritic cell
Epithelioid cell
Spindle/fusiform cell
Small, intermediate, large with or without pigment
Degree of cytologic atypia, if any

cells, epithelioid cells, and dendritic melanocytes. Such nevi might be considered blue nevi or combined nevi, depending on the stringency of one's criteria. For similar nevi without dendritic melanocytes, one confronts particular problems of nosology. It is possible that one might define such lesions as either blue nevi using rather broad criteria (i.e., blue color and the presence of heavily melanized spindle cells and/or epithelioid cells and any of the following features: inverted-wedge configuration, plexiform morphology, and deep extension), spindle and epithelioid cell nevi (because of the presence of both spindled and epithelioid cells), deep penetrating nevi, or plexiform pigmented spindle cell nevi. Thus categorization of such lesions may be quite arbitrary.

CLASSIFICATION OF MELANOCYTIC LESIONS WITH PHENOTYPIC OVERLAP

Because of overlapping morphologic features, reproducible diagnosis of some of the lesions described in this chapter may not be possible. A reasonable approach is a descriptive diagnosis of such lesions according to the guidelines in Table 8-8. For example, a lesion involving the deep reticular dermis might be characterized as a superficial and deep pigmented spindle cell nevus (or, alternatively, melanocytic proliferation) or superficial and deep plexiform nevus (melanocytic proliferation) composed of pigmented dendritic cells and spindle cells. With this approach, one would be able to avoid forcing a lesion not easily classified into one particular category or another. Certain lesions fulfilling sufficient criteria for diagnosis may be classified under standardized terminology, e.g., Spitz nevus, blue nevus, etc. Use of the term *combined nevus* is also acceptable for nevi with two or more distinct cell types. However, we advise that the particular cell types should be specified in the diagnosis or an appended note.

REFERENCES

1. Tèiche M: Über benigne melanome ("chromatophorome") der hart-blaue naevi. *Virchows Arch [A]* 186:212–229, 1906.
2. Dubreuilh W, Petges G: Le naevus bléu. *Ann Dermatol* 2:552, 1912.
3. Allen AC, Spitz S: Malignant melanoma: A clinicopathologic analysis of the criteria for diagnosis and prognosis. *Cancer* 6:1–45, 1953.
4. Evans RW: Histologic appearance of tumors. *Med J Edinb Lond* 1:230, 1956.
5. Leopold JG, Richards DB: The interrelationship of blue and common naevi. *J Pathol Bacteriol* 95:37–46, 1968.
6. Gartmann H, Müller H: Über das gemeinsame vorkommen von blauem naevus und naevuszell-naevus in ein und derselben geschwulst ("combined nevus"). *Z Hautkr* 52:389–398, 1977.
7. Weedon D, Little JA: Spindle and epithelioid cell nevi in children and adults. *Cancer* 40:217–225, 1977.
8. Fletcher V, Sagebiel RW: The combined nevus: Mixed patterns of benign melanocytic lesions must be differentiated from malignant melanomas. In Ackerman AB (ed): *Pathology of Malignant Melanoma.* New York, Masson, 1981, pp 273–283.
9. Rogers GS, Advani H, Ackerman AB: A combined variant of Spitz's nevi. *Am J Dermatopathol* 7:61–78, 1985.
10. Pulitzer DR, Martin PC, Cohen AP, Reed, RJ: Histologic classification of the combined nevus: Analysis of the variable expression of melanocytic nevi. *Am J Surg Pathol* 15:1111–1122, 1991.
11. Mihm MC Jr, Googe PB: *Problematic Pigmented Lesions.* Philadelphia, Lea & Febiger, 1990, pp 76–77.
12. Ball NJ, Golitz LE: Melanocytic nevi (with focal atypical epithelioid cell components): A review of 73 cases. *J Am Acad Dermatol* 30:724–729, 1994.
13. Seab JA Jr, Graham JH, Helwig EB: Deep penetrating nevus. *Am J Surg Pathol* 13:39–44, 1989.
14. Barnhill RL, Barnhill MA, Berwick M, Mihm MC Jr: The histologic spectrum of pigmented spindle cell nevus: A review of 120 cases with emphasis on atypical variants. *Hum Pathol* 22:52–58, 1991.

15. Barnhill RL, Mihm MC Jr, Magro CM: Plexiform spindle cell naevus: A distinctive variant of plexiform melanocytic naevus. *Histopathology* 18:243–247, 1991.
16. Cooper PH: Deep penetrating (plexiform spindle cell) nevus: A frequent participant in combined nevus. *J Cutan Pathol* 19:172–180, 1992.
17. Smith KJ, Barrett TL, Skelton HG III, et al: Spindle cell and epithelioid cell nevi with atypia and metastasis (malignant Spitz nevus). *Am J Surg Pathol* 13:931–939, 1989.
18. McGovern VJ: Spitz nevus. In Blaustein A (ed): *Melanoma: Histological Diagnosis and Prognosis.* New York: Raven Press, 1982, pp 37–44.
19. Rodriguez HA, Ackerman LV: Cellular blue nevus. Clinicopathologic study of forty-five cases. *Cancer* 21:393–405, 1968.

9

Melanocytic Proliferations with Architectural Disorder and Cytologic Atypia (Melanocytic Dysplasia and Dysplastic Nevi)

Synonyms: atypical nevus, B-K mole, Clark's nevus, nevus with architectural disorder, cytologic atypia

Melanocytic proliferations with disordered arrangements and cytologic atypia of melanocytes are an important but highly controversial subject.[1-102] Broadly defined, this category of lesions is in essence a continuum of morphologic abnormality extending from "typical," e.g., basilar melanocytes or ordinary nevi, to melanoma[74,90] (Table 9-1). The immediate significance of such lesions is related to whether they are markers of increased melanoma risk, whether they are precursors of melanoma, and in practical terms, their histologic distinction from outright melanoma (Table 9-2).

The search for precursors to melanoma has intrigued both clinicians and pathologists for many years, since a sizable proportion of cutaneous melanomas (perhaps 18 to 85 percent) are associated with a preexisting nevus by clinical history and approximately a third of melanomas show the presence of a nevus remnant histologically.[11,61,99] In addition, many melanoma patients have been noted to have an increased number of normal and/or unusual moles.[1,2,5-8]

THE DYSPLASTIC NEVUS

The formal description[6-8] of the dysplastic melanocytic nevus (DMN) has stimulated rather intense interest in this curious association between nevi and melanoma by providing new information about and insights into the tumor progression of at least a subset of cutaneous melanomas. However, the advent of the DMN also has unleashed a maelstrom of unparalleled controversy and debate and has resulted in many unanswered questions about the relationship of nevi, both typical and atypical, and melanoma.[17,34,48,55,56,60,61]

The DMN is not a new entity; the presence of multiple nevi was noted on individuals in hereditary melanoma kindreds as early as 1820[1,2] (Table 9-3). In addition, nevi with atypical histologic features consonant with DMN had been described previously as "active," "activated," or "atypical" junctional nevus.[3-5] In fact, Lund and Kraus[4] outlined a sequence of progression of the atypical junctional nevus (or premalignant lentigo) to melanoma very similar to what has been proposed for the DMN.[17] Despite the latter observations, the significance of the DMN did not begin to become evident until the descriptions of individuals bearing these peculiar nevi in hereditary melanoma kindreds by Frichot et al.,[6] Lynch et al.,[7] and Clark et al.[8] (Table 9-4).

The legitimacy of the DMN as an intermediate lesion between common acquired nevi and melanoma has been confirmed over the past 15 years by a body of clinical, histopathologic, and experimental information[1-102] (Table 9-6). However, because there is in effect a continuum from ordinary nevi to melanoma (Fig. 9-1), it has been difficult to define the upper and lower limits that distinguish the DMN from ordinary nevi on the one hand and melanoma on the other.[74] This has resulted in considerable controversy as to the criteria for and prevalence of DMN. At present, there is no consensus as to the minimal essential histologic or clinical criteria for DMN, and consequently, there is considerable latitude in the diagnostic criteria for these lesions.

TABLE 9-1
Melanocytic Proliferations with Architectural Disorder and Cytologic Atypia (Melanocytic Dysplasia)

- Intraepidermal
  - Without dermal nevus remnant
    - Intraepidermal melanocytic proliferation with architectural disorder and cytologic atypia (junctional dysplastic nevus)
    - Lentiginous melanocytic proliferation with architectural disorder and cytologic atypia (melanocytic dysplasia) of acral skin
    - Lentiginous melanocytic proliferation with architectural disorder and cytologic atypia (melanocytic dysplasia) of sun-damaged skin
    - Lentigo maligna
    - Other intraepidermal melanocytic proliferations with architectural disorder and cytologic atypia not otherwise specified
  - With dermal nevus remnant
    - Intraepidermal melanocytic proliferation with architectural disorder and cytologic atypia (compound dysplastic nevus)
    - Other intraepidermal melanocytic proliferations with architectural and cytologic atypia
      - Spindle and epithelioid cell nevi
      - Pigmented spindle cell nevi
      - Congenital nevi
      - Genital nevi
      - Acral nevi
- Dermal
  - Dermal melanocytic proliferations with architectural disorder and cytologic atypia

TABLE 9-2
Summary of Prevalence, Melanoma Risk, and Genetics Associated with Dysplastic Nevi

1. Prevalence of dysplastic nevi		
Hereditary melanoma	54%	
Sporadic melanoma	33%	
General population	7%	
2. Melanoma risk		*Relative risk*
Hereditary melanoma kindreds		
Patient with previous melanoma and dysplastic nevi		500
Patient with dysplastic nevi		150
Individual with no dysplastic nevi		2–12
No family history		
Patient with previous melanoma and no dysplastic nevi		9
Individual with sporadic dysplastic nevi		7–20
3. Genetics		
Autosomal dominant mode with incomplete penetrance proposed versus two or more genes or polygenic inheritance		
Linkage analysis shows relationship to chromosome 1p		

TABLE 9-3
Chronology of Dysplastic Nevi

1820	Norris	First description of hereditary melanoma and observation that family members have numerous moles
1977	Frichot et al.	Cutaneous phenotype of atypical moles in family members of hereditary melanoma kindreds reported
1978	Clark et al.	B-K mole syndrome—individuals in familial melanoma kindreds have atypical moles (termed *B-K moles*) introduced
1978	Lynch et al.	Familial atypical multiple mole—melanoma syndrome (FAMMM) introduced
1980	Greene et al.	Dysplastic nevus syndrome introduced
1980	Elder et al.	Sporadic dysplastic nevus syndrome introduced
1992	NIH Consensus conference	Nevus with architectural disorder and/or cytologic atypia introduced to replace dysplastic nevus

Another source of controversy has arisen from the term *dysplastic* or *dysplasia*.[21,44] To some authors, the term is ambiguous and refers to a developmental anomaly as well as architectural and cytologic atypicality of tissue. Because of the latter controversy, an NIH Consensus Conference has recently recommended that the term *dysplastic nevus* be abandoned in favor of *nevus with architectural disorder and/or cytologic atypia*.[89] Without becoming too involved with issues of terminology, it should be pointed out that the term *dysplasia* as applied to melanocytic proliferations has probably encompassed both usages mentioned above.[74] First of all, the term has been used to indicate abnormal development of nevi, persistent lentiginous melanocytic proliferation with less tendency to undergo the typical maturational sequence or regression of nevi.[17] However, the predominant use of the term has been to signify a stage of tumor progression from common acquired nevi to melanoma.[17] Based on histopathologic features and biologic behavior, DMN do fulfill the general criteria for dysplasia.[74] DMN have cellular organizational (architectural) abnormalities, cytologic atypia, evidence of increased proliferation, and evidence of occasional progression to melanoma.[74]

Because of the attention promulgated by DMN, there has been a groundswell of interest in all aspects of melanocytic nevi and melanoma risk. As a result, it has become evident that total number of melanocytic nevi has

Low	*Melanoma Risk*	*High*
No nevi →	Increasing number of nevi →	Numerous nevi
No atypical nevi →	Increasing number of atypical nevi →	Atypical nevi
No family history of melanoma or dysplastic nevi →	Increasing genetic component →	Hereditary melanoma

FIGURE 9-1

Continuum of melanoma risk associated with particular clinical phenotypes.

TABLE 9-4

Categories of Individuals with Dysplastic Nevi Devised for Potential Risk Stratification

1. Hereditary melanoma
   a. Individuals with DMN phenotype* and at least one blood relative with melanoma ("D_1")
   b. Individuals with DMN phenotype and at least two blood relatives with melanoma ("D_2")†
2. Familial DMN: Individual with DMN phenotype and at least two blood relatives having DMN phenotype but not melanoma
3. Personal history of melanoma: Individual with both DMN phenotype and personal history of melanoma
4. Sporadic DMN: Individual with DMN phenotype but no personal or family history of melanoma or a family history of DMN‡

*The minimum criteria for this phenotype have not been quantified. The classic presentation is one of increased numbers of both typical and clinically atypical nevi.

†Highest-risk category.

‡Lowest-risk category.

TABLE 9-5

Observations Supporting the Concept that Dysplastic Nevi Are Intermediate to Common Acquired Nevi and Melanoma

Clinical behavior	Occasional progression to melanoma
Clinical features	Intermediate in size, asymmetry, complexity of coloration
Histologic features	Intermediate in architectural disorder and cytologic atypia
Histomorphology	Intermediate in intraepidermal melanocyte area, nuclear area, and variation in nuclear shape
Melanocyte-associated antigens	Intermediate in expression of antigens such as HLA-DR, EGF receptor, NGF receptor, gangliosides
DNA content	Intermediate
Cytogenetics	Intermediate in number of nonrandom chromosome abnormalities
Melanosomal alterations	Intermediate in frequency of abnormal melanosomes

TABLE 9-6

Risk Factors for Cutaneous Melanoma

Factor	*Estimated Relative Risk**
Changing pigmented lesion	Very high
Xeroderma pigmentosum	500
FAMMM† kindred: prior melanoma	500
FAMMM kindred: atypical nevi but no prior melanoma	150
Numerous common nevi	5–65
Atypical nevi	7–20
Giant congenital nevus	5–15
Previous melanoma	9
Lentigo maligna	5–10
Immunosuppression	4–7
Red or blond hair	2–7
Tendency to freckle	2–4
Sun sensitivity	2–3
Excessive sun exposures	2–4
Melanoma in first-degree relative	2–12
Few or no common nevi	0.3
Asian, Hispanic, or African-American pigmentation	0.08–0.15
Age <15 years	0.01

*Average risk = 1. Estimates derived from references.

†FAMMM, Familial atypical multiple mole–melanoma

Source: Adapted from Williams ML, Sagebiel RW: Melanoma risk factors and atypical moles. *West J Med,* 160:343–350, 1994.

been established as one of the most significant risk factors for melanoma[19,23,36,39,55,84,88,99] (Tables 9-6 and 9-7). The relative risks have varied from 1.6 to 64 in several case-control studies and show a dose-response effect (see Table 9-7). It is estimated that number of nevi may be a risk factor for as many as 29 to 79% of all melanomas.[55] It also has been shown that clinically atypical nevi, i.e., nevi with features such as size greater than 5 to 7 mm, irregular borders, and variegated color, irrespective of histologic findings, are associated with increased melanoma

TABLE 9-7
Relative Risk of Melanoma in Relation to Numbers of Benign Nevi

Study	*Country*	*Nevus Definition*	*Number of Nevi*	*Relative Risk*
Holly, 1987	USA	≥ 2 mm, whole body "nondysplastic"	11–25	1.6
			26–50	4.4
			51–100	5.4
			> 100	9.8
Weiss, 1991	Germany	"Benign" nevi	10–50	4.3
			> 50	15
Krüger, 1992	Germany	≥ 2 mm, trunk (males)	5–10	2.9
			11–20	5.5
			> 20	33
			> 40	133
Swerdlow and Green, 1987	Scotland	≥ 2 mm, whole body	10–24	4.4
			25–49	8.7
			≥ 50	64
Green, 1985	Australia	≥ 2 mm, left arm	2–4	16
			5–10	15
			> 10	20

Source: Adapted from Williams ML, Sagebiel RW: Melanoma risk factors and atypical moles. *West J Med.* 160:343–350, 1994.

TABLE 9-8
Melanoma Risk Associated with Clinically Atypical (Dysplastic) Nevi: Comparison of Occurrence in Melanoma Patients versus Controls

			One or More Dysplastic Nevi (%)		
Study	*Country*	*Definition*	*Melanoma Patients*	*Controls*	*Relative Risk*
Roush, 1986 and Nordlund, 1985	Australia	5 mm, irregular border, and haphazard pigmentation	34%	7%	7.7
MacKie, 1985	Scotland	> 5 mm and either irregular borders, irregular pigmentation, or inflammation	38%	20%	2.1–4.5*
Holly, 1987	USA	At least 3 of 6 criteria: ill-defined border, irregular border, irregular pigmentation, > 5 mm, erythema, accentuated skin markings	55%	17%	3.8–6.3†
Halpern, 1991	USA	> 4 mm, macular component, variegation of color, and irregular or indistinct border	39%	7%	8.8
Garbe, 1989	Germany	At least 3 of 5 criteria: > 5-mm irregular margins, ill-defined border, color variation, macular and papular components	45%	5%	7

*Relative risks for 1 or 2 atypical nevi, 2.1; for 3 or more atypical nevi, 4.5.
†Relative risks for 1 to 5 atypical nevi, 3.8; for 6 or more atypical nevi, 6.3.
Source: Adapted from Williams ML, Sagebiel RW: Melanoma risk factors and atypical moles. *West J Med* 160:343–350, 1994.

risk[26,36,39,55,56,59,62,79,99] (Table 9-8). In general, a dose-response relationship with melanoma risk also has been shown for these lesions. Furthermore, each of these abnormal "nevus parameters," i.e., large size, irregular borders, and haphazard color, also correlates with elevated melanoma risk.[36,42] The increased melanoma risk associated with clinically atypical nevi tends to parallel that associated with total numbers of normal nevi but in most studies has been reported as an independent risk factor for melanoma.[39,55,56] The term *clinically atypical nevus* is used to signify a nevus with the gross morphologic abnormalities mentioned above, regardless of whether the histologic features are dysplastic or not. The poor correspondence between clinical and histologic diagnosis of dysplastic nevus has been reported.[74,85] Based on these various investigations, it is apparent that there is a complex relationship between melanocytic nevi and melanoma[74,98,99] (see Fig. 9-1) Both quantitative and qualitative attributes of nevi correlate with increased melanoma risk.[42,55,74,99]

THE SIGNIFICANCE OF THE DMN

Markers of Increased Melanoma Risk

Based on studies of hereditary melanoma kindreds already referred to,[6–8,16,25,95,96] it has been noted that the presence of DMN on individuals in these kindreds confers a significantly increased risk for the development of melanoma (see Tables 9-2, 9-6, and 9-8). In fact, the presence of DMN in this setting confers a 48.9 percent cumulative risk for melanoma by age 50 years.[96] In prospective follow-up, only family members with DMN developed melanoma, whereas those without DMN did not develop melanoma. It also has been observed that individuals in the general population have dysplastic nevi[10] that also serve as markers for increased melanoma risk, although not nearly so great as in familial melanoma.[16,27,33,36,39,54–56,62] Estimates of the relative risk for melanoma in persons with sporadic DMN may be in the range of 7 to 20. The prevalence in individuals with sporadic DMN has been difficult to gauge accurately but may be in the range of 7 to 20 percent[18,27,36,59,79] (see Tables 9-2 and 9-8). As already mentioned, one particular reason for the difficulty in estimating prevalence of DMN has been the lack of standardized clinical and histopathologic criteria for DMN and also what constitutes the minimum essential criteria for the DMN phenotype, e.g., 50 or 100 or more clinically atypical nevi[74,99] (Table 9-9). Classifications have been devised for individuals with DMN and the extent to which they have a personal or family history of melanoma and DMN[16,54] (see Table 9-4). Although much more information is needed on this subject, risk-stratification protocols have been formulated to facilitate assessment of melanoma risk and the management of patients[16,54,62] (see Tables 9-2 and 9-6). As outlined in Figure 9-1, melanoma risk is probably a continuum, with risk directly related to family history of melanoma (especially for individuals with at least two first-degree blood relatives with melanoma), total number of nevi on the skin surface, total number of clinically atypical nevi, and personal history of melanoma.

Dysplastic Nevi as Precursors to Melanoma

In addition to the global melanoma risk conferred on the patient by the presence of clinically atypical nevi, DMN occasionally progress to melanoma and thus serves as a precursor to melanoma[17] (Fig. 9-2). This progression has been observed through the use of serial photographs and the documentation histologically of focal melanoma developing in an otherwise stable DMN[17,24] (seeTable 9-2). Various authors also have reported remnants of DMN associated with melanoma with an average frequency of about 33 percent.[11,17,48,50,61,99] A confounding problem in this situation is the inability in all instances to clearly distinguish in situ or microinvasive melanoma from DMN. Although DMN do undoubtedly progress to melanoma, the frequency of this progression has probably been overestimated.

TABLE 9-9
Nevus Phenotypes

	Normal Nevus Pattern	*Abnormal Nevus Phenotype*
Number	None to few (<25) nevi	Many (>50) nevi
Size	<5 mm	Variable: small to large, often several >5 mm
Color/ borders	Uniform or homogeneous color, well circumscribed	Some to many nevi with irregular or haphazard color, erythema, irregular or ill-defined borders

Source: Adapted from Williams ML, Sagebiel RW: Melanoma risk factors and atypical moles. *West J Med* 160:343–350, 1994.

GENERAL CLINICAL FEATURES

The numbers of clinically atypical nevi on the individual patient may vary from only one or two to several hundred or more.[6–8,24,25,32,48] As has already been mentioned, the minimum number of nevi and degree of clinical atypicality that constitute the abnormal mole phenotype have not been formulated (see Table 9-8). In all likelihood, the trait may be a continuous variable. Some authors nonetheless have suggested an arbitrary number such as 50 or 100 nevi as the minimum number for the "atypical nevus phenotype."[99] The distribution of nevi is also an important feature. Although the majority of DMN occur on the trunk, these nevi show a peculiar propensity for the scalp, female breasts, buttocks, and dorsal surfaces of the feet (Table 9-10). Another attribute of these nevi is their

TABLE 9-10
Clinical Features of Dysplastic Nevi

General
- Increased numbers of typical and atypical nevi
- Variation in gross morphologic features among nevi
- Increased numbers of nevi on scalp, female breasts, buttocks

Nevus characteristics:
- Increased size (4–12 mm, but not always)
- Asymmetry
- Macular component
- Irregular border
- Ill-defined border
- Altered topography, pebbled or cobblestone surface
- Haphazard, variegated, or greater complexity of coloration

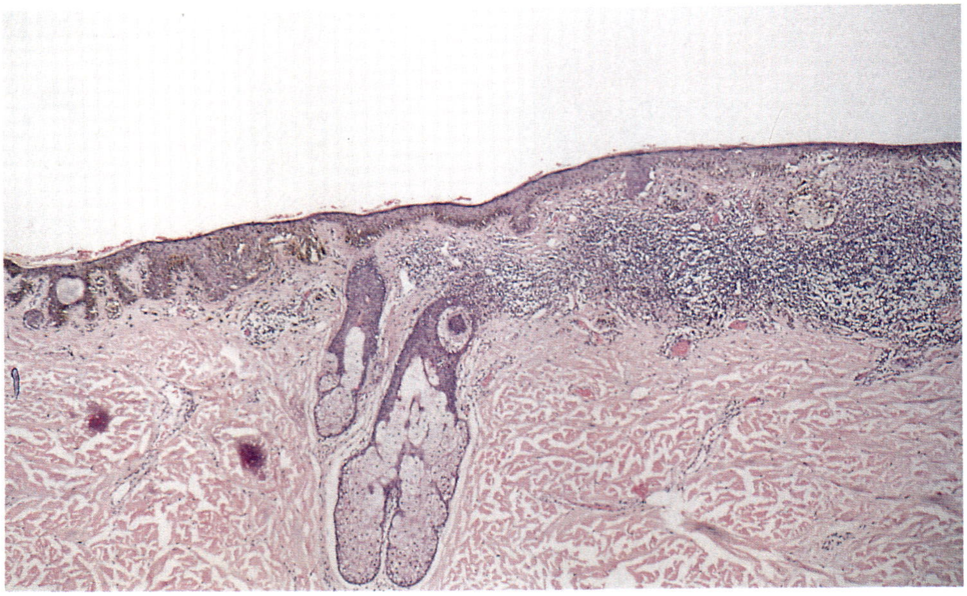

A

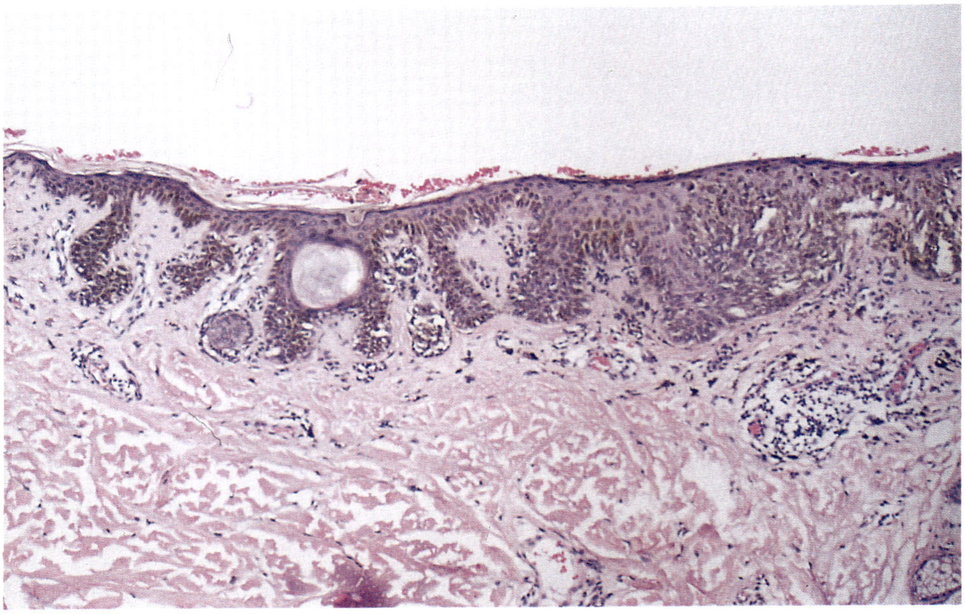

B

FIGURE 9-2

Malignant melanoma arising in association with dysplastic nevus. (A) Scanning magnification discloses a dysplastic nevus on the left side of the field (to the left of the hair follicle) and a superficially invasive melanoma on the right (H&E, × 40). (B) Higher magnification showing the dysplastic nevus occupying most of the field and the transition to melanoma in the right part of the field (H&E, × 100).

tendency to show considerable variation in size, shape, and coloration from nevus to nevus.

CLINICAL FEATURES OF THE INDIVIDUAL NEVUS

As mentioned previously, DMN exhibit clinical features intermediate to common nevi and melanoma[6–8,24,48,74,75] (see Table 9-10). In general, they tend to be larger than common nevi and smaller than melanoma (but not necessarily so) and generally range from 4 to 12 mm in greatest diameter. They are usually characterized by some degree of asymmetry, often irregular and ill-defined borders, and a relatively flat surface topography (at least part of the lesion is entirely flat). The surface also may be "pebbled" or have a cobblestone appearance. DMN in general have a more complex color than do ordinary nevi. There are often more than two colors present (i.e., tan, brown, dark brown) and the colors have an irregular or haphazard pattern.

HISTOPATHOLOGY

The histologic criteria for DMN have included parameters of architectural disorder, cytologic atypia, and host response[8–11,17,20,22,24,28,29,34,47–50,57,61,63,64,67–70,74,77] (Figs. 9-3 to 9-10 and Table 9-11). There has been considerable controversy as to which of these various parameters are the most important for the recognition of DMN and which are simply secondary (correlative) features.[69] A fundamental issue in the discussion of the histology of DMN has been the debate over cytologic atypia in DMN. From this author's perspective, cytologic atypia, or more specifically, nuclear atypia, is a fundamental part of the phenomenon of histologic dysplasia as has been described in other organ systems. In its well-developed stage, such nuclear atypia can be recognized by most well-trained observers. However, the existence of nuclear atypia in DMN has been questioned, and architectural disorder has been emphasized to the exclusion of nuclear atypia in some formulations of histologic criteria for DMN.[20,21,44,63] Undoubtedly, the central issues in this controversy relate to the fact that there is a continuum of nuclear atypia (ranging from minimal to severe) in DMN, objective criteria for recognizing nuclear atypia have not been standardized, and defining the threshold at which point nuclear atypia first appears is difficult and possibly not easily reproducible.[74] The recent documentation of a spectrum of abnormal DNA content (aneuploidy) and nuclear area by image analysis that parallels grade of nuclear atypia in DMN provides objective evidence for nuclear atypia in DMN.[91,101] It seems reasonable to conclude at this time that nuclear atypia does exist in DMN.

In order to address the issue of the importance of various histologic features in DMN, various architectural and host-response parameters have been correlated with unequivocal nuclear atypia of intraepidermal melanocytes in a series of clear-cut DMN versus nondysplastic nevi.[69] On multivariate analysis, (1) lentiginous melanocytic proliferation and (2) variation in size, shape, and placement of junctional nests showed a statistically significant correlation with nuclear atypia after adjustment for 14 other histologic features. Certain features typically ascribed to DMN such as lateral extension of the intraepidermal component (the "shoulder phenomenon"), lymphocytic infiltrates, and papillary dermal fibroplasia failed to show a significant correlation with nuclear atypia. Two other studies examining histologic criteria for DMN, although different in experimental design, reached fairly similar conclusions.[47,57] Based on these observations, one may conclude that the most important histologic features of DMN are in essence (1) disordered intraepidermal melanocytic proliferation and (2) nuclear atypia of intraepidermal melanocytes[74] (see Table 9-11). Other features, although undoubtedly strongly correlated with the latter two features and helpful in the recognition

TABLE 9-11
Histologic Features of Dysplastic Nevi

Architectural features
Lentiginous melanocytic proliferation*
Variation in size, shape, location of junctional nests with bridging or confluence*
Lack of cellular cohesion of junctional nests
Lateral extension (the "shoulder phenomenon") of junctional component
Asymmetry often
Intraepidermal component often poorly circumscribed
Cytologic features
Spindled cell (with prominent retraction artifact of cytoplasm) pattern
Epithelioid cell pattern
Discontinuous nuclear atypia (not all nuclei atypical)*
Nuclear enlargement
Nuclear pleomorphism
Nuclear hyperchromatism
Prominent nucleoli
Prominent pale or "dusty" cytoplasm
Large melanin granules
Host response
Lymphocytic infiltrates
Fibroplasia
Concentric eosinophilic pattern
Lamellar pattern
Prominent vascularity

*Essential features needed for diagnosis. Either lentiginous melanocytic proliferation or variation in junctional nesting is acceptable.

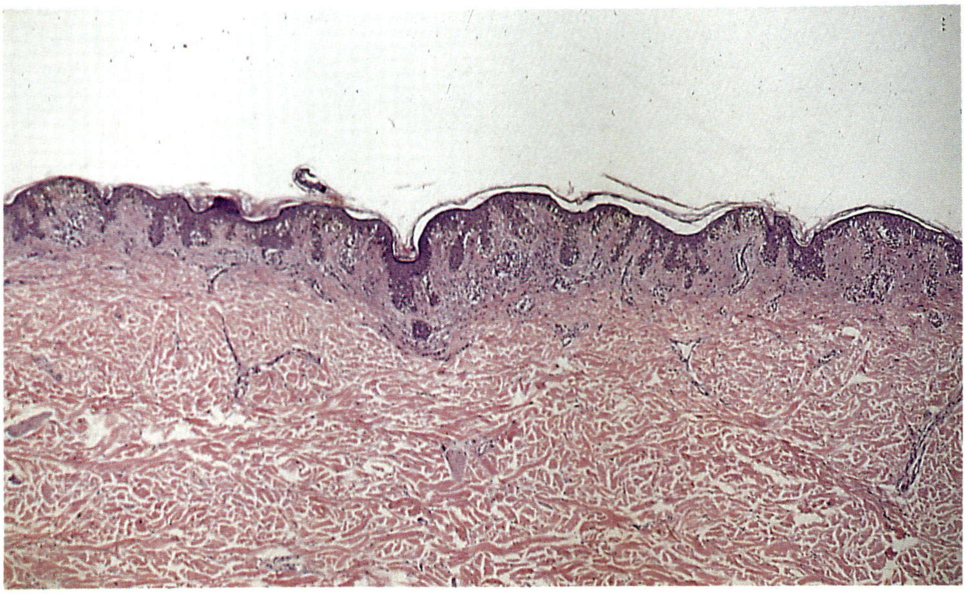

A

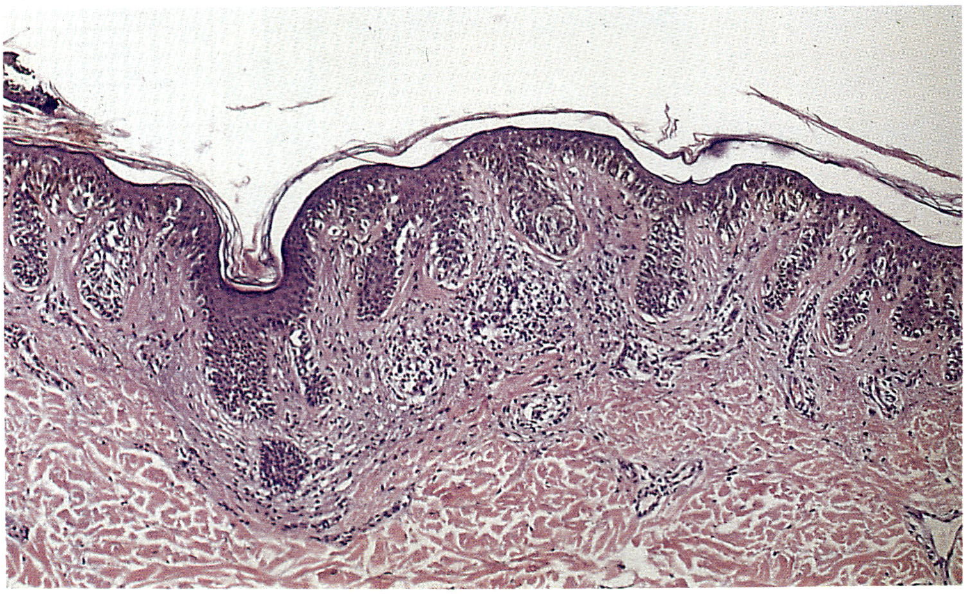

B

FIGURE 9-3

Compound dysplastic nevus. (A) Scanning magnification shows the typical flat topography of a dysplastic nevus. As with many dysplastic nevi, the lesion is poorly circumscribed and there is a dearth of dermal nevus elements in the papillary dermis (H&E, × 40). (B) This field demonstrates the lentiginous architecture of a dysplastic nevus. The rete ridges are elongated. Lymphocytic infiltrates are present in the papillary dermis (H&E, × 100). (C) Higher magnification discloses prominent lentiginous melanocytic proliferation and some variation in the nesting pattern. Concentric fibroplasia about rete ridges and lymphocytic infiltrates are evident (H&E, × 200).

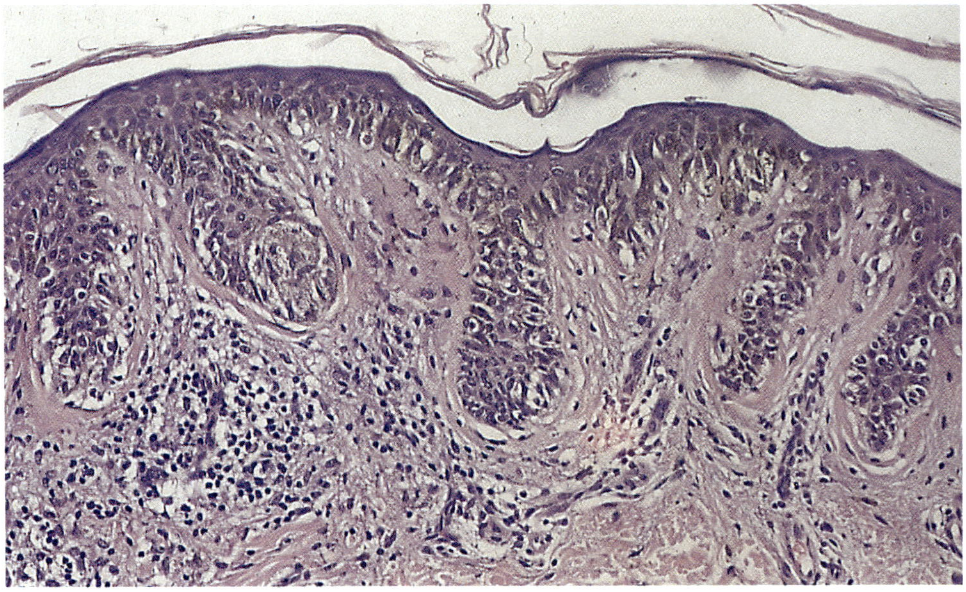

C

FIGURE 9-3 *(Continued)*

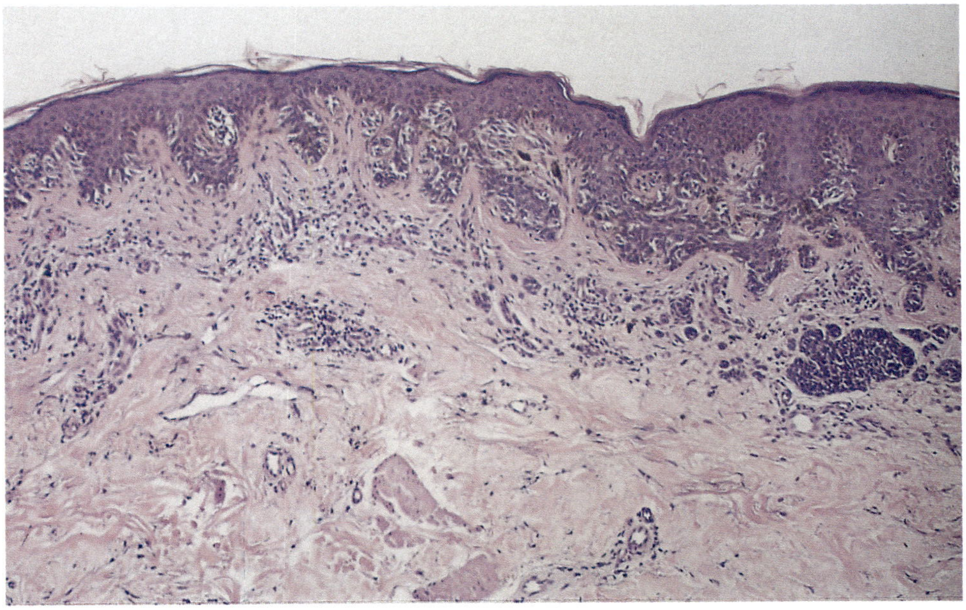

FIGURE 9-4
Compound dysplastic nevus. This field demonstrates the lateral extension of the intraepidermal component (to the left) beyond the dermal nevus component (right side of the field) (H&E, × 100).

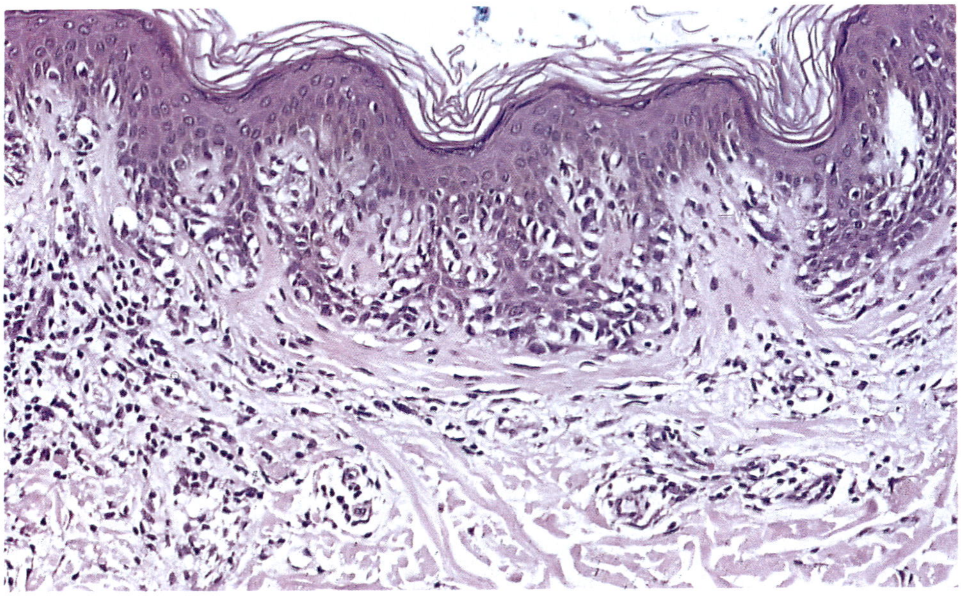

A

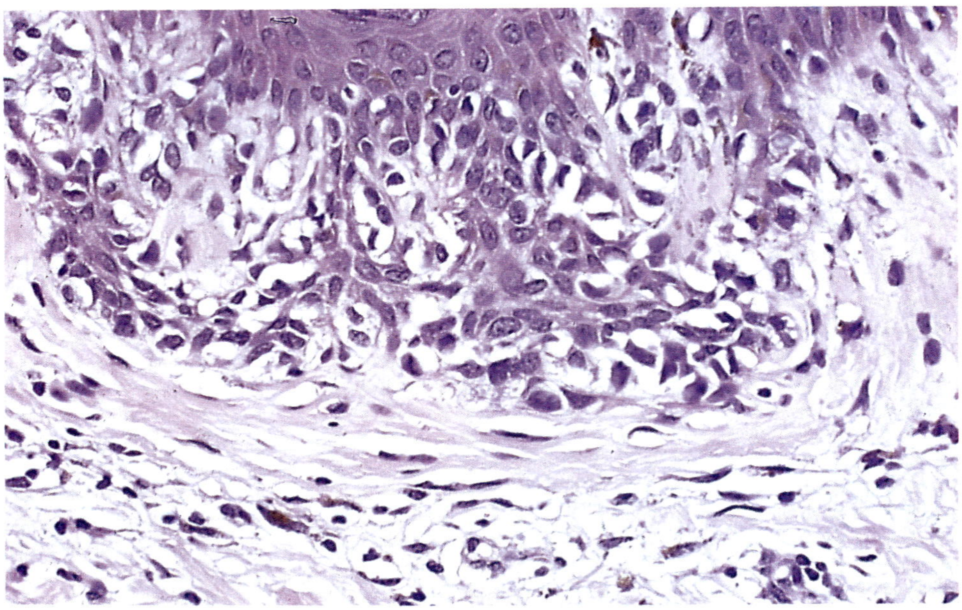

B

FIGURE 9-5

Junctional dysplastic nevus. (A) Predominant lentiginous pattern of dysplastic nevus. The basilar melanocytes reach confluence along the rete ridges. This lesion also demonstrates concentric eosinophilic fibrosis (H&E, × 200). (B) Higher magnification discloses variation in size, shape, and staining of nuclei of basilar melanocytes. Some melanocytes have nuclei larger than those in spinous layer keratinocytes. Note again concentric eosinophilic fibrosis (H&E, × 400).

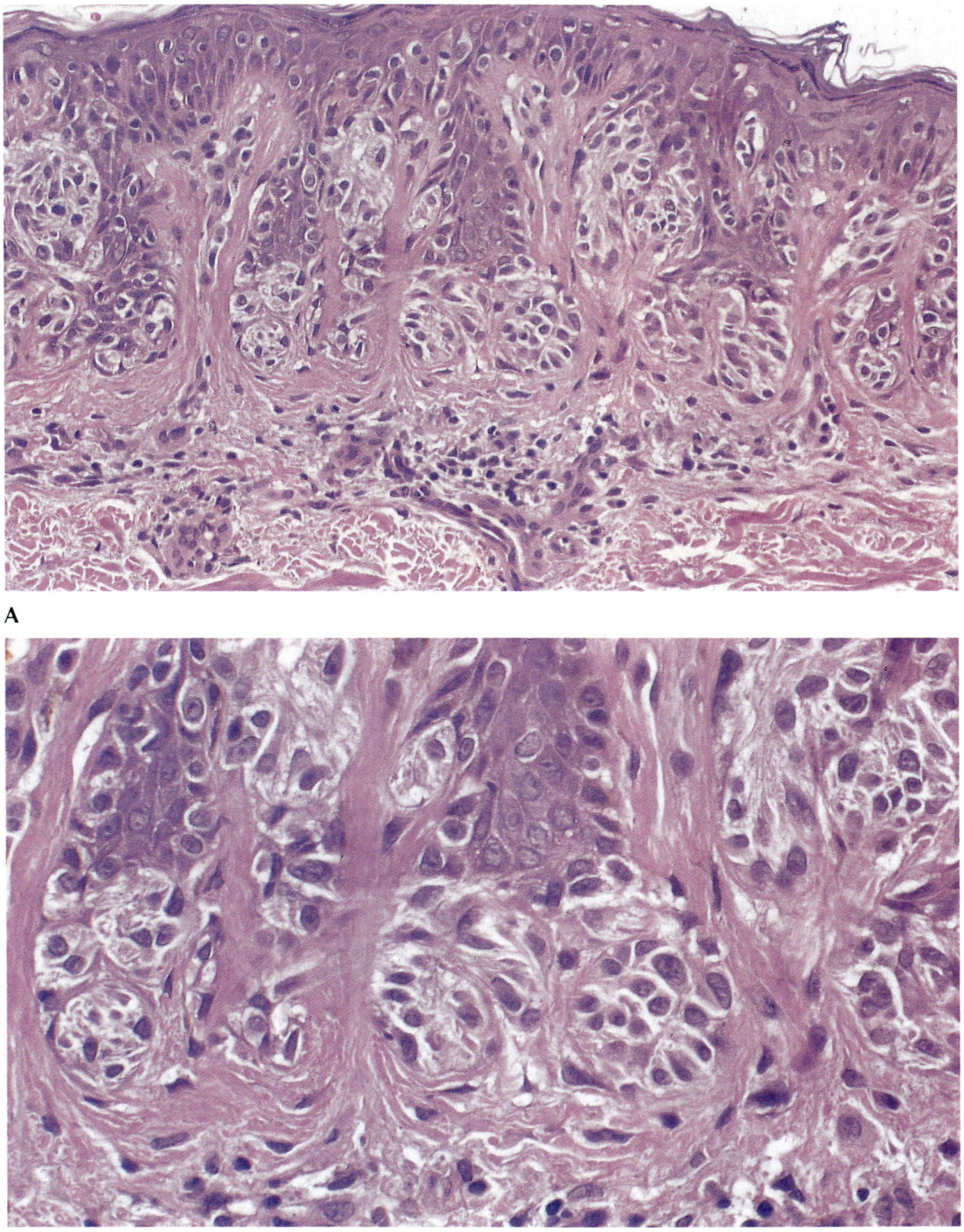

A

B

FIGURE 9-6

Compound dysplastic nevus. (A) Mainly junctional nested pattern. There is some variation in the size, shape, and placement of junctional nests (H&E, × 200). (B) High magnification shows variation in nesting and nuclear characteristics of melanocytes (H&E, × 400).

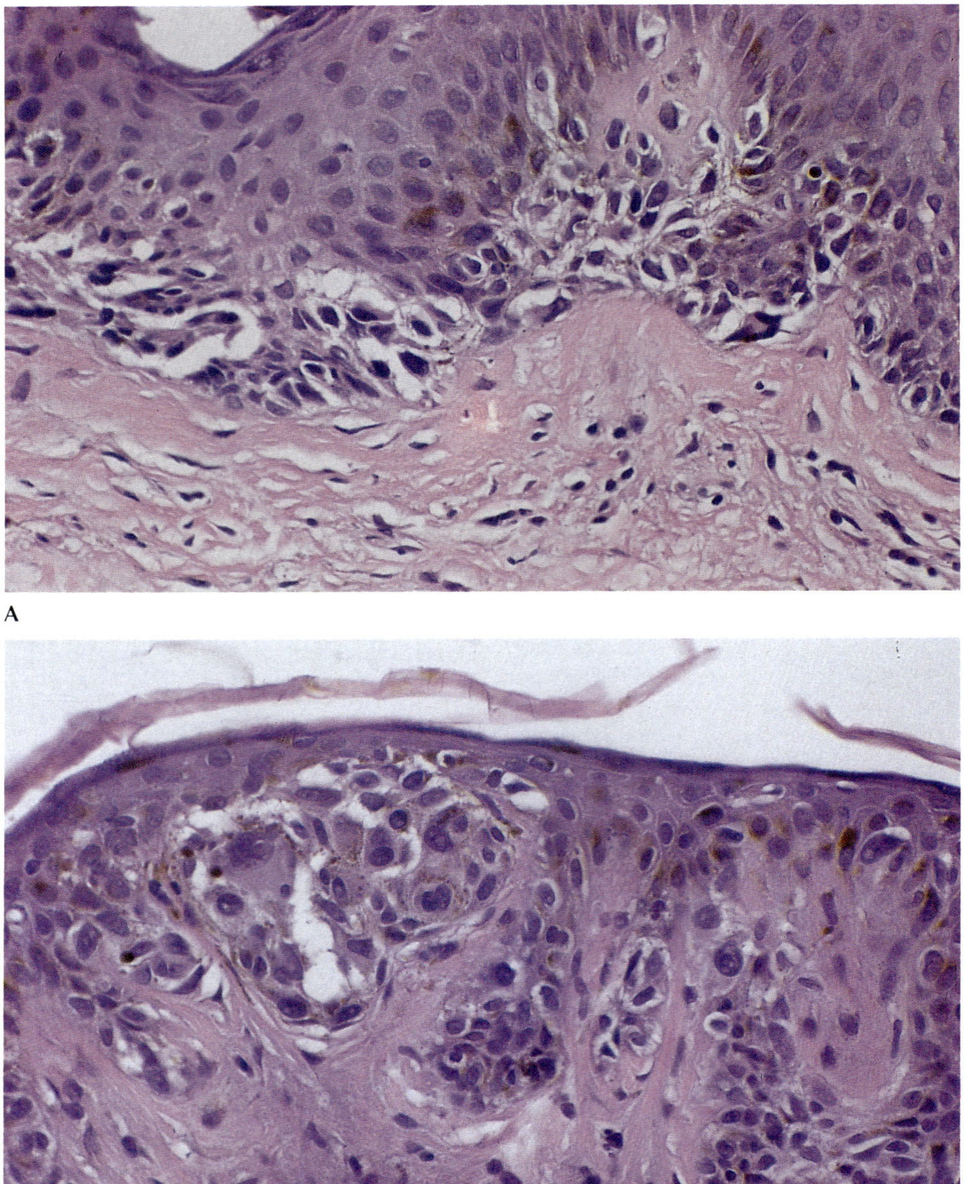

A

B

FIGURE 9-7

Architectural variation in nesting patterns of a dysplastic nevi. (A) There is confluence of irregular nests along the dermoepidermal junction of this compound dysplastic nevus. Note variation in nuclear size, shape, and staining of basilar melanocytes (H&E , × 400). (B) Note large nest of melanocytes between rete ridges in this dysplastic nevus. Some melanocytes exhibit severe cytologic atypia (H&E, × 400). (C) This dysplastic nevus shows marked confluence and bridging of junctional nests. There is cytologic atypia of melanocytes within the nest. The subjacent dermis also demonstrates lamellar fibroplasia (H&E, × 400).

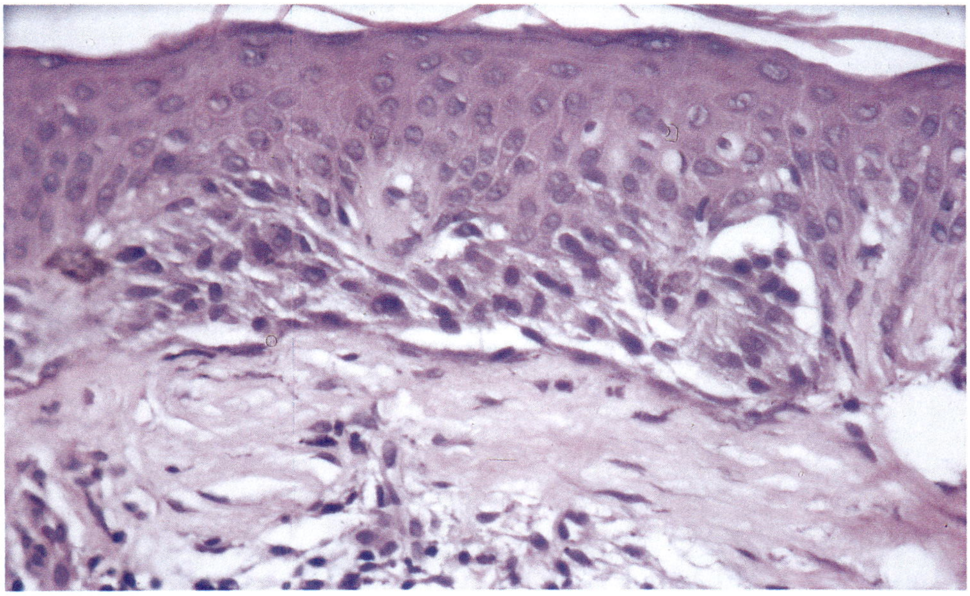

C

FIGURE 9-7 *(Continued)*

of DMN (or melanocytic dysplasia), are secondary or dependent variables. The latter two features are in fact the essential criteria of histologic dysplasia as proposed for other tissue domains: disordered proliferation or arrangements of cells and cellular atypia.

A General Description of the Histologic Features of DMN

Architecture. The majority of DMN, perhaps 80 percent, are compound and the remainder junctional.[68] Most are best described as relatively flat with only slight expansion of the papillary dermis by limited dermal components (see Fig. 9-3A). Many (but not all) DMN are lentiginous (i.e., the epidermal rete ridges are elongated and often club-shaped), accompanied by melanocytic proliferation and increased melanin content of the epidermis[69,74] (see Fig. 9-3B and C). Many heavily pigmented DMN also contain melanin macroglobules in the basilar epidermis, an entirely nonspecific finding.[69] Many (perhaps the vast majority of) compound DMN have lateral extension and poor circumscription of the intraepidermal components (see Fig. 9-4). The latter features refer to the intraepidermal melanocytic component, i.e., lentiginous melanocytic proliferation and/or junctional nesting, extending laterally or peripherally beyond the papillary dermal nevus elements (the "shoulder phenomenon") by at least three rete ridges and gradually diminishing in cellularity without clear-cut demarcation. Although not a fundamental component of dysplasia as outlined above, lateral extension is a useful feature in recognizing most compound DMN, particularly at scanning magnification, and does correlate with the peripheral macular annulus observed clinically in many DMN. Junctional DMN, by definition, do not display lateral extension; however, in common with compound DMN, they tend to be poorly circumscribed at their peripheries.

As discussed earlier, the predominant architectural feature of DMN is disordered intraepidermal melanocytic proliferation.[69,74] As already mentioned, the two patterns of disordered proliferation include: (1) lentiginous melanocytic proliferation and (2) disordered or irregular junctional nesting. Both patterns are often present to varying degrees in many DMN, but either pattern may be present in isolation. As discussed in Chapter 3, lentiginous melanocytic proliferation is essentially the pattern of a lentigo, an increased frequency of solitary basilar melanocytes most concentrated along the lower-most poles of elongated epidermal rete (see Fig. 9-5). The numbers of melanocytes tend to be least frequent above the dermal papillae. The frequency of melanocytes in DMN is as a rule greater than in a lentigo, often reaching confluence and replacing basilar keratinocytes. In its most extreme version, the proliferation of melanocytes may result in multilayered confluence of cells along the dermoepidermal junction, often "bridging" between rete ridges. Such lentiginous patterns also may result in the so-called moth-eaten appearance of the epidermal rete[9] ridges (Figs. 9-3C and 9-5B). Although cytologic features are discussed below, the melanocytes present

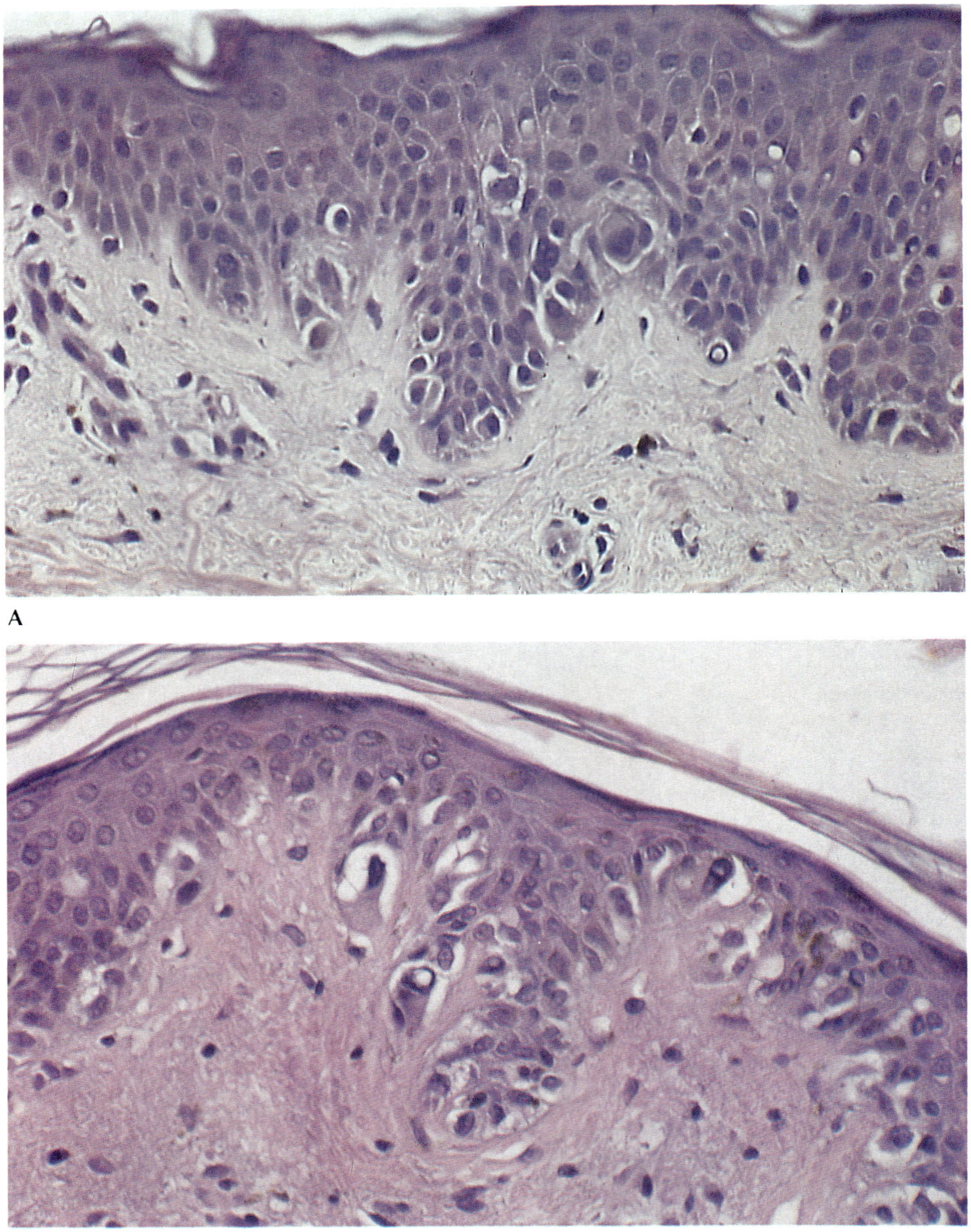

FIGURE 9-8

Cytologic atypia in dysplastic nevi. (A) There is significant nuclear enlargement and pleomorphism of basilar melanocytes (H&E, × 400). (B) Severe cytologic atypia in a compound dysplastic nevus. Note strikingly enlarged and hyperchromatic nuclei of basilar melanocytes. This dysplastic nevus shows discontinuous variable nuclear atypia, whereas melanoma demonstrates a monotonous or continuous atypia. Nonetheless, a lesion such as this should be evaluated carefully for melanoma (H&E, × 400). (C) Melanoma in situ developing in a severely atypical dysplastic nevus. Note large cells with abundant cytoplasm that contain large nuclei. Occasional prominent nucleoli can be observed (H&E, × 400).

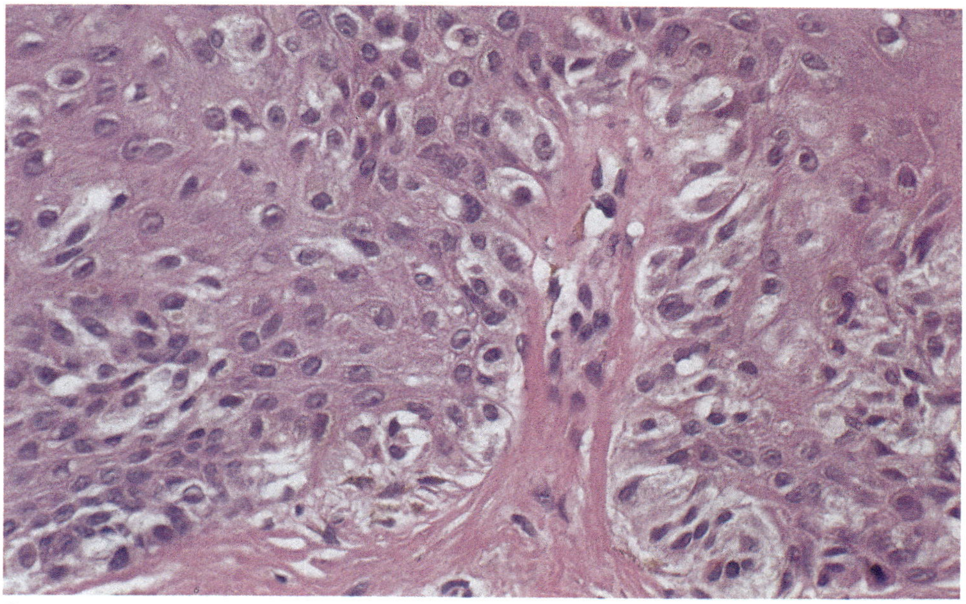

C

FIGURE 9-8 *(Continued)*

in this pattern commonly exhibit retraction of cytoplasm resulting in a vacuolated appearance of the basal layer, almost suggesting basal layer vacuolopathy. The nuclei within these vacuolated cells are commonly pleomorphic with angulated contours[69,74] (see Fig. 9-5B).

The second architectural pattern is characterized by variation in intraepidermal nesting of melanocytes (see Figs. 9-6 and 9-7). Compared with the description of junctional nests in typical nevi in Chapter 4, the patterns of nesting in DMN are more asymmetric and chaotic. Individual nests tend to vary significantly in size, shape (ovoid, elongate, or confluent along the dermal-epidermal junction), and spacing (nests are not present at equidistant intervals). Junctional nests, instead of being located at the tips of rete ridges in ordinary nevi, are irregularly distributed on the sides and between rete ridges, often with no regular pattern ("irregularly irregular").

Bridging of nests between rete ridges is another feature of the abnormal nesting pattern, as with lentiginous melanocytic proliferation. In some instances, there may be bridging or confluence of nests along the bases of three or four consecutive epidermal rete ridges (see Fig. 9-7B).

Often paralleling the variation in nesting is the loss of cellular cohesion in junctional nests of DMN. The individual nevus cells literally appear to fall apart, with clear spaces forming between individual cells and aggregates of cells (see Fig. 9-7A).

Although upward migration of melanocytes throughout the epidermis is not a common feature of DMN, it is seen on occasion but is often limited, focal, or orderly in appearance.

In summary, when assessing the architectural disorder of a melanocytic nevus/proliferation, one must judge the degree to which the nevus deviates from the well-ordered morphology of an ordinary melanocytic nevus (Table 9-12). Thus, one must be cognizant of (1) a continuum of basilar melanocytic proliferation varying from sparse numbers of solitary basilar melanocytes to multilayered cellular confluence and (2) a continuum ranging from cohesive, round, regular, uniform junctional nests located at the tips of rete ridges and regularly spaced, to marked variation in the nesting pattern. At the extreme end of the latter spectrum, junctional nests tend to become enlarged, pleomorphic (i.e., marked variation in size and shape of nests, elongated nests, serpentine nests) irregularly distributed, and discohesive. Other global attributes at scanning magnification that are useful in assessing the degree of disorder include the degree of asymmetry, if any, and the degree of circumscription of the lesion (i.e., well-demarcated versus poorly demarcated). With experience, the overall gestalt of the lesion will enable one to immediately categorize the lesion as slightly or minimally disordered versus more highly disordered. After this assessment of architectural disorder, one must proceed to higher magnification to assess cytologic characteristics of the intraepidermal melanocytes.

Cytologic Features. One of the fundamental criteria for DMN is the presence of variable (or discontinuous) cytologic atypia of intraepidermal melanocytes.[22,68,69,74] The latter refers to intraepidermal melanocytes that are not uniformly atypical but tend to vary from cell to cell as to

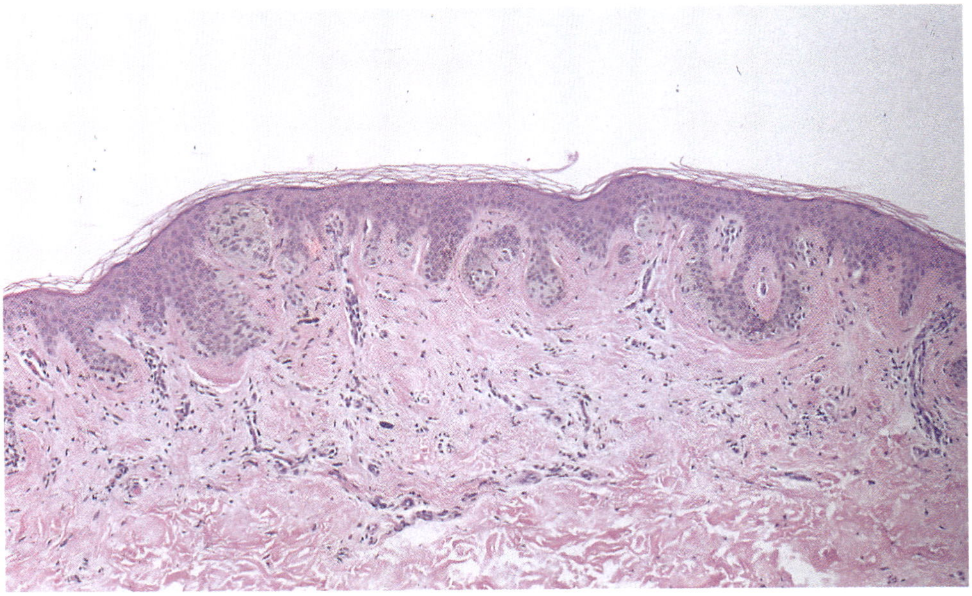

A

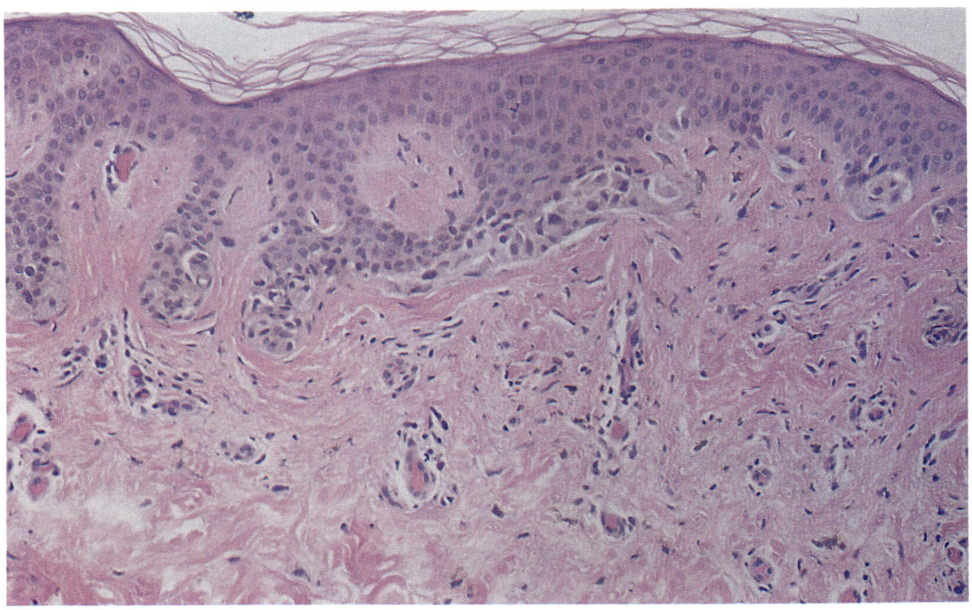

B

FIGURE 9-9

Compound dysplastic nevus, epithelioid cell variant. (A) Junctional nests contain epithelioid melanocytes. There is variation in the junctional nesting pattern (H&E, × 100). (B) Note abundant "dusty" cytoplasm of the epithelioid cells. There is striking confluence of junctional nests in this field. The papillary dermis also shows prominent fibrosis (H&E, × 200). (C) High magnification of part B. In addition to abundant cytoplasm, the melanocytes display variation in nuclear size, shape, and staining properties of nuclei (H&E, × 400).

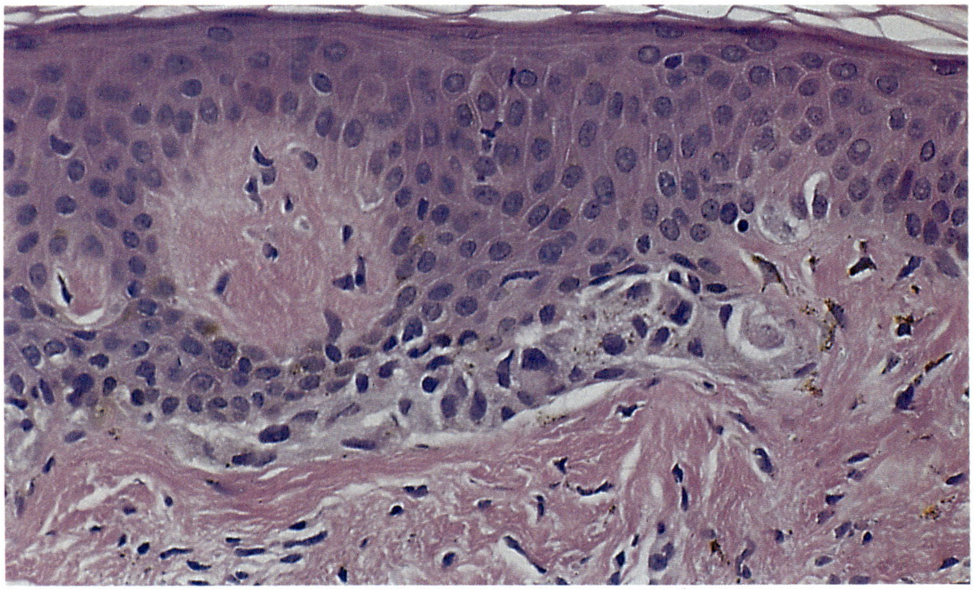

C

FIGURE 9-9 *(Continued)*

the degree of nuclear atypia. In general, this nuclear atypia is a continuum characterized by gradual nuclear enlargement, pleomorphism, variation in nuclear chromatin pattern, and the eventual development of prominent nucleoli. As has been mentioned, the beginnings of nuclear atypia may be almost imperceptible and may not be reproducibly recognized. Commonly with slight or low-grade cytologic atypia, the cells show retraction of cytoplasm and thus have a vacuolated or clear cell appearance. The nuclei often are oval, rhomboidal, triangular, spindled, or angulated in shape (see Fig. 9-5B). The chromatin tends to be evenly dispersed, and nucleoli are inconspicuous or small. The size of the melanocytic nuclei is increased and approximates that of or is slightly larger than the nuclei of spinous layer keratinocytes[64] (see Figs. 9-5b and 9-6B). With greater (moderate) atypia, the cells may continue to have scant cytoplasm or may begin to show abundant cytoplasm (see Figs. 9-7C and 9-9C). The nuclei continue to display prominent pleomorphism, and it should be emphasized that this is one of the most important characteristics of the nuclear atypia in DMN. The nuclei of some cells are somewhat larger than the nuclei of spinous layer keratinocytes, and nucleoli are more commonly visible. With severe cytologic atypia, the melanocytes may contain abundant cytoplasm which often has a granular eosinophilic appearance or may contain finely divided ("dusty") melanin[64] (see Fig. 9-8). However, the amount of cytoplasm may be minimal. The nuclei are pleomorphic and may be enlarged to twice the size of keratinocyte nuclei in the spinous layer, or larger (see Fig. 9-8B). Nucleoli are often enlarged and may be eosinophilic (see Fig. 9-8C). The ultimate endpoint is a uniformly atypical population of cells which marks the development of melanoma. In this formulation, moderate and severe atypia are considered high-grade atypia.

The cell types that comprise DMN include variations of basilar melanocytes with retracted cytoplasm, small rounded nevus cells, spindle cells, sometimes pigmented to some degree, and epithelioid cells[17,22,69,74] (see Fig. 9-9). The basilar melanocytes with retraction of cytoplasm are often observed in predominantly lentiginous forms of DMN, while the epithelioid cell type is often present in a much less prevalent, predominantly nested form of DMN (so-called epithelioid cell dysplasia).

Host Response. Of the three variables that generally constitute the host response in DMN, mononuclear cell infiltrates, fibroplasia, and prominent vascularity, the first two have received considerable attention as criteria for DMN.[17,22,24,28,29,69,74] Lymphocytic infiltrates are present in the overriding majority of DMN but probably not in all. These infiltrates vary from sparse perivascular lymphoid infiltrates (see Fig. 9-6A) to dense bandlike infiltrates filling the papillary dermis, as in halo-like DMN (see Fig. 9-10). In most instances, easily observed perivascular infiltrates are present. It should be pointed out that monocytes/macrophages constitute a portion of these infiltrates and that melanin-laden macrophages (melanophages) are present in many melaninized DMN.

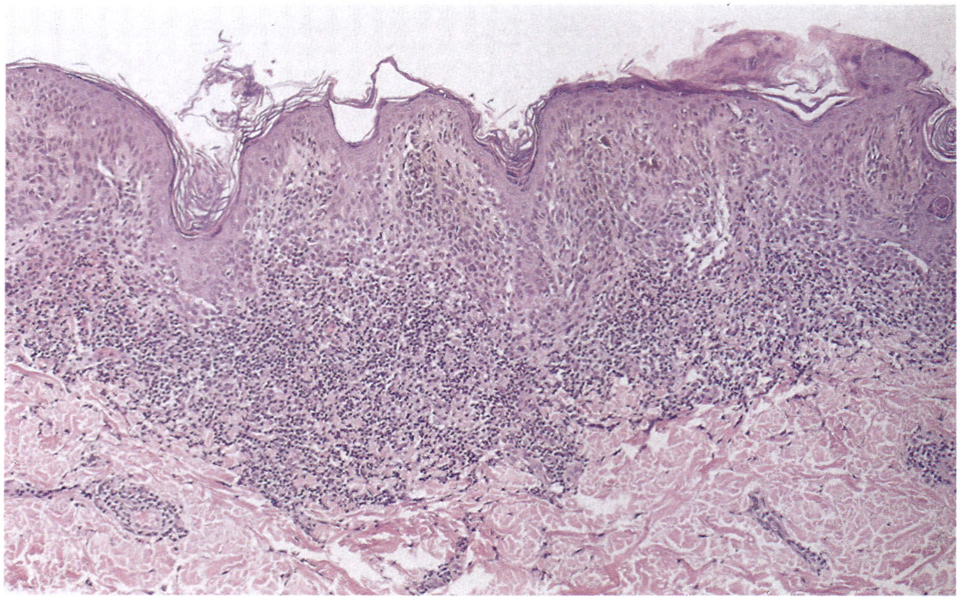

A

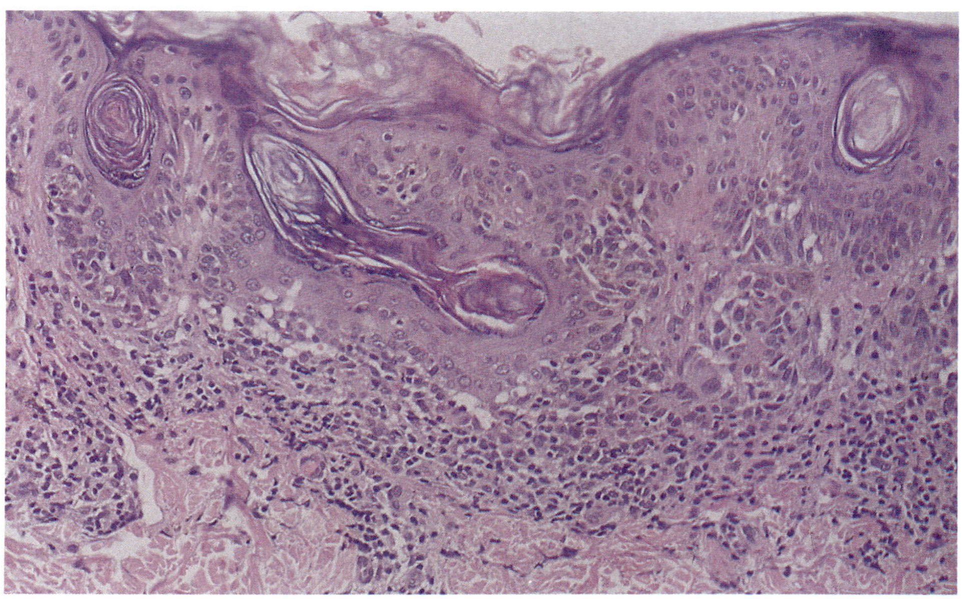

B

FIGURE 9-10

Compound dysplastic nevus, halo variant. (A) There is a dense lymphocytic infiltrate filling the papillary dermis in this dysplastic nevus (H&E, × 100). (B) There is confluence of variably atypical basilar melanocytes in addition to the prominent mononuclear cell infiltrate in the papillary dermis (H&E, × 200). (C) Higher magnification of part B showing variation in nuclear characteristics of melanocytes. The lesion fulfills the architectural and cytologic criteria for dysplastic nevus, as well as demonstrating a band-like infiltrate characteristic of halo nevus (H&E, × 400).

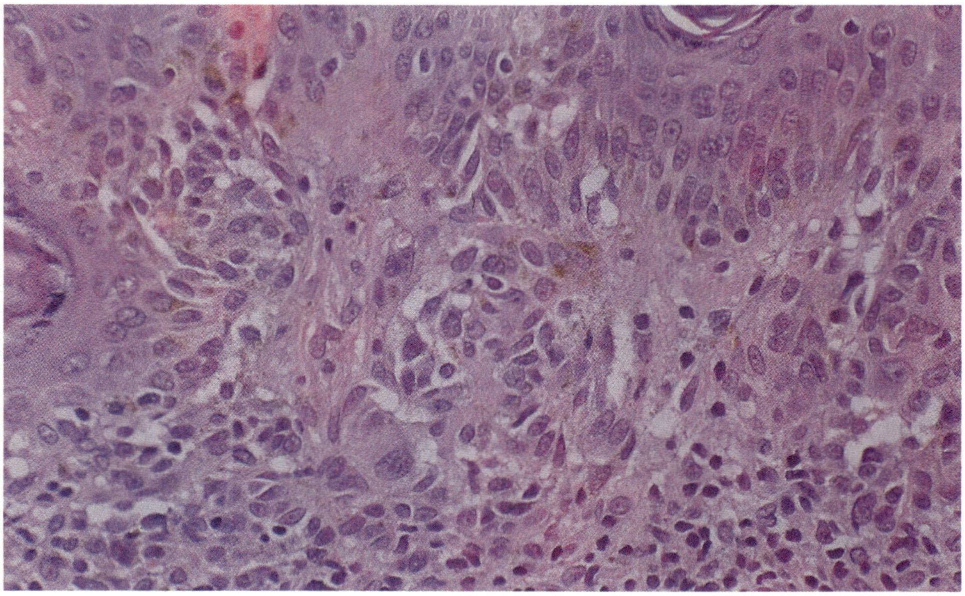

C

FIGURE 9-10 *(Continued)*

The papillary dermal fibroplasia observed in DMN is of two types. The more common form has been termed *concentric eosinophilic fibrosis* and is characterized by hyalinized collagen that is compactly disposed about the epidermal rete ridges (see Fig. 9-5). On the other hand, *lamellar fibroplasia* is less prevalent and notable for delicate stacking of horizontally disposed collagen subjacent to the epidermal rete ridges (see Fig. 9-7C). Mesenchymal spindle cells typically line these filamentous strands of collagen. Both patterns of fibroplasia may be present in the same lesion, or they may occur separately.

For many years, the prominence of the papillary dermal vascular plexus has been commented on in DMN. Recent quantification of papillary dermal microvessels using *Ulex europaeus* agglutinin I in a series of melanocytic nevi including DMN has shown that, except for severely atypical DMN, DMN do not differ from ordinary nevi in terms of numbers of microvessels in the papillary dermis.[103] Severely atypical DMN do in fact have significantly less vascularity than melanoma. Thus the appearance of prominent vascularity in most DMN is most likely secondary to vascular dilation and hypertrophy rather than true angiogenesis.

Histologic Variants of Dysplastic Nevus

Epithelioid Cell Variant. This variant is relatively uncommon but has distinctive cytologic features[17,22] (see Fig. 9-9). The "epithelioid" cells in these nevi resemble the cell type in superficial spreading (or pagetoid) melanoma except that they tend to be less cytologically atypical. The cells are round or polygonal and contain abundant pink or "dusty" (finely divided melanin) cytoplasm. Relatively small round nuclei are usually present in the center of the cell. The cells tend to have an almost exclusively nested distribution, often without an associated lentiginous element.

Halo Nevus Variant. In contrast to the typical halo nevus (see Chapter 4), there are variants of DMN that display dense mononuclear cell infiltrates filling the papillary dermis and obscuring any nests of nevus cells present there (see Fig. 9-10). These nevi are distinguished from benign halo nevi by the aberrant architectural features and cytologic atypia of DMN.

Specificity of Histologic Features of Dysplastic Nevus

The observations that nevi with histologic features of DMN are present in 53 percent of Caucasians in a study from Utah and in clinically normal appearing nevi have suggested that DMN are prevalent lesions and thus lack significance as markers of increased melanoma risk.[63,73] To address this issue, one must again remember that there is a continuum from common nevi to melanoma and that prevalence of nevi declines as nevi become increasingly atypical.[74] Therefore, if one uses histologic criteria based simply on architectural abnormalities without definite cytologic atypia, one will include many more nevi in the category of DMN and diminish its power as a marker of melanoma risk. It is likely that a certain threshhold of

TABLE 9-12
Guidelines for Grading Architectural Disorder and Cytologic Atypia in Melanocytic Proliferations

	*Spectrum of Changes**		
	Low-grade	⟶	*High-grade*
Architectural features		Asymmetry† Lateral extension	
	Lentiginous melanocytic proliferation†		Confluence of cells along basal layer
	Little or no upward migration†	Intraepidermal upward migration of cells	Fully developed pagetoid spread
	Little variation in nesting†	Variation in junctional nesting, bridging	Confluence of nests; marked variation in size, shape, location, spacing of nests
	Cohesion of cells in nests		Diminished cohesion of cells
	Elongated rete		Effacement (loss) of rete pattern
	Little disturbance in dermal maturation†	Failure of maturation of dermal cellular component	Rounded expansile nests of dermal cells
Cytologic features	Discontinuous atypia† (few cells atypical)		Continuous atypia (most cells atypical)
		Cellular enlargement† Nuclear enlargement† Nuclear pleomorphism† Prominent nucleoli† Hyperchromatism†	
	Uniform, nongranular cytoplasm	Abundant cytoplasm	Abundant granular eosinophilic or dusty cytoplasm

*Each variable or parameter below is a continuous variable from low-grade to high-grade, e.g., the variable "asymmetry" would represent a spectrum from little or no asymmetry (low-grade) to prominent or marked asymmetry (high-grade). Thus either the extremes for each parameter are specifically indicated or the parameter is simply stated without qualification of the extremes.
†A principal feature for grading architectural and cytologic atypia.

architectural and cytologic atypia (dysplasia) must be achieved to have significance in terms of melanoma risk. If nevi do not have unequivocal architectural abnormality and cytologic atypia, they should not be diagnosed as DMN. Such nevi might be designated as junctional or compound nevi with architectural disorder.

It is evident from examining a variety of melanocytic proliferations that disordered arrangements of cells and cytologic atypia are encountered in a number of lesions thought to be distinct from conventional DMN.[90] The latter findings are often similar to those observed in DMN and provide evidence that almost any melanocytic proliferation may progress to an "intermediate" or dysplastic stage and possibly have some potential for giving rise to melanoma. Because these other "dysplastic" melanocytic lesions, such as congenital nevi, Spitz nevi, and vulvar nevi have received considerably less attention than conventional DMN, essentially no information is available concerning their melanoma risk.[90] As outlined in Table 9-12, it is proposed that these various lesions may be subjected to the same guidelines as DMN (see below).

The same exposition holds for intraepidermal melanocytic proliferations developing de novo, i.e., without an associated nevus.[90] For example, lentiginous melanocytic proliferations of acral skin, sun-exposed skin, and mucosa may exhibit a comparable spectrum of atypicality. It is apparent that criteria for and grading of these various lesions have not been standardized as they have not been for conventional DMN.

The evaluation of atypical melanocytic lesions in the dermis or connective-tissue stroma has received little attention, except perhaps in the context of congenital nevi or "minimal-deviation" melanoma. Features of architectural disorder might include an expansile or cohesive nodule, whether the nodule is sharply demarcated or blends with surrounding melanocytes, degree of cellularity (cells crowded together), and degree of maturation.[90] Cytologic features would include cytologic atypia, necrosis, and mitotic figures, typical or atypical.

DIFFERENTIAL DIAGNOSIS

The DMN must be distinguished from fully developed in situ or invasive melanoma, lentigo maligna, lentiginous nevi, pigmented spindle cell nevus, Spitz nevus, halo nevus, congenital nevus, and recurrent nevus. One of the

TABLE 9-13
Comparison of Severely Atypical Dysplastic Nevus and Melanoma

*Severely Atypical Dysplastic Nevus**	*In Situ or Microinvasive Melanoma**
Some asymmetry	Prominent asymmetry
Poorly circumscribed	Poorly circumscribed
Rete ridges preserved	Tendency to loss or effacement of rete ridges
Some maintenance of nevus nesting pattern and order	Loss of orderly nesting pattern
Some diminished cohesion of nests	Diminished cohesion of tests may be prominent
Lentiginous melanocytic proliferation concentrated on rete ridges	Loss of rete-oriented melanocytic proliferation
Pagetoid spread absent, miminal, or not prominent	Pagetoid spread prominent
Discontinous cytologic atypia	Fairly uniform (continuous) cytologic atypia
Often some maturation of dermal component	Often no maturation of dermal component
Usually no mitoses in dermal component	Uncommon mitoses in dermal compoment (microinvasive melanoma)
Usually perivascular but occasionally band-like lymphocytic infiltrates	Tendency to band-like lymphocytic infiltrates

*The histologic guidelines listed in this table represent the most common presentation. However, there is considerable variation among these features.

most difficult problems is the discrimination of severely atypical DMN from in situ or microinvasive melanoma. This differential diagnosis is discussed at length in Chapter 10, and the most salient points are summarized in Table 9-13. In one sense, this distinction is somewhat arbitrary and subjective, since no consensus has been reached regarding criteria for separating the two entities. However, in another sense, the central issue is whether a particular lesion retains some degree of growth control, an orderly nevic appearance, and variable or discontinuous nuclear atypia versus loss of growth control, loss of an orderly nevic appearance, and continuous nuclear atypia.

DMN and lentigo maligna (LM) show histologic similarities on occasion and may be difficult to separate. This is understandable, since both are melanocytic dysplasias (see Table 9-1). As discussed in Chapter 10, many consider LM to be melanoma in situ. However, LM exhibits a spectrum of atypicality, some of which does not warrant diagnosis as melanoma in situ.

LM is distinguished from DMN in most instances because LM is a dysplasia secondary to cumulative sun exposure and consequently develops on markedly sun-exposed skin of the elderly (average age 60 years) (Table 9-14). The most common locations are the cheek and nose, which are unusual sites for conventional DMN. LM is usually a de novo melanocytic dysplasia, since dermal nevus components are uncommon, whereas approximately 80 percent of DMN contain dermal nevus cells.[61]

LM developing on the central face most commonly shows a basilar proliferation of variably atypical melanocytes that often involve the appendageal epithelium (see Table 9-14). The epidermis is usually effaced, i.e., has no rete ridge pattern, and there is prominent solar elastosis in the dermis. In contrast, the DMN generally has elongated rete ridges with concentration of basilar melanocytes and many junctional nests along the rete ridges, and solar elastosis is usually minimal. LM also may have junctional nests, but they are often discohesive elongate nests composed of pigmented spindled cells. The latter nests

TABLE 9-14
Comparison of Dysplastic Nevus and Lentigo Maligna

Dysplastic nevus	*Lentigo maligna*
Age 10 years and up	Mean age: 60 years
Site: intermittently sun-exposed or covered skin–trunk > buttock, scalp, extremities > face (unusual)	Site: markedly sun-exposed skin—face (cheek, nose) most common
Histopathology	
Poorly circumscribed	Poorly circumscribed
Elongated rete ridges	Effaced epidermis (loss of rete ridges)
Usually lentiginous and junctional nesting	Mainly lentiginous pattern but occasional nesting
Involvement of adnexal structures not prominent	Striking involvement of adnexal structures by melanocytic proliferation
Spindle cells on occasion	Pigmented spindle cells common
Papillary dermal fibroplasia common	Papillary dermal fibroplasia not prominent
Solar elastosis usually inconspicuous	Solar elastosis prominent

on occasion show striking involvement of hair follicles and eccrine ducts, a finding not typically observed in DMN.

LM arising on other sun-exposed sites may show a rete ridge pattern and thus present an even greater problem in differential diagnosis. Discriminating features favoring LM include a mainly lentiginous pattern of melanocytic proliferation, prominent involvement of appendages, presence of pigmented spindle cells, and solar elastosis. Overlap with DMN on occasion may be so great that separation may be difficult and often arbitrary. The various clinical and histologic features present must be assessed (see Table 9-13). If discrimination is not possible, a reasonable approach is a descriptive diagnosis, e.g., intraepidermal melanocytic proliferation with features of both lentigo maligna and dysplastic nevus and degree of cytologic atypia.

Another conundrum is the distinction of DMN from lentiginous nevi, particularly those from acral skin. Here, the main problem is one of threshold; i.e., is there sufficient disordered architecture and cytologic atypia for the diagnosis of DMN? Such lesions should be evaluated for poor circumscription, asymmetry, substantially increased frequency of basilar melanocytes, irregularity of junctional nesting with elongated, confluent nests, bridging of nests between rete ridges, and finally, cytologic atypia of intraepidermal melanocytes. Lesions having equivocal changes should not be diagnosed as DMN. It is reasonable to designate the latter lesions as showing some architectural disorder or, alternatively, as not having clear-cut or unequivocal melanocytic dysplasia.

As discussed below, a number of types of melanocytic nevi such as pigmented spindle cell nevus, Spitz nevus, and congenital nevus may on occasion demonstrate disordered architectural patterns and cytologic atypia, i.e., show evidence of melanocytic dysplasia. Yet, at the same time, these various nevi retain many of the histologic features that make them distinctive, e.g., fascicles of slender pigmented spindle cells in pigmented spindle cell nevus, large epithelioid cells in Spitz nevus, and extensive involvement of the reticular dermis in congenital nevus. Some might argue that these various abnormal histologic changes are not distinctive or dysplastic and have no association with increased melanoma risk. The fact of the matter is that these various features have not been the subject of sufficient investigation, and thus their significance has not been determined. From the perspective of this author, these histologic features must be acknowledged, if present beyond a certain threshold, and communicated in the pathology report. In some instances, there may be such striking overlap with conventional DMN that classification of a lesion may be difficult and arbitrary. This problem has been discussed at length in a study of atypical variants of pigmented spindle cell nevus[104] (see Chap. 6). A subset of such lesions is characterized by peripheral extension of the intraepidermal component, poor circumscription, prominent lentiginous melanocytic proliferation, irregular junctional nesting, horizontal confluence and bridging of intraepidermal nests, and cytologic atypia. Thus whether such lesions are termed *dysplastic nevi, atypical spindle cell nevi,* or *spindle cell nevi with architectural disorder and cytologic atypia* is perhaps subjective. As mentioned, the melanoma risk associated with such nevi is unknown. It is logical to assume that such nevi with high-grade or severe atypia have increased risk for progression to melanoma and should be treated accordingly. The same discussion applies to other nevi, such as Spitz, congenital, and genital nevi, and, in reality, all nevi.

Recurrent melanocytic nevi may on occasion enter into the differential diagnosis of DMN and may in fact be recurrent DMN (see Chap. 4). Such nevi are characterized by a typical history of recurrence approximately 6 weeks to 6 months after a shave biopsy of a banal nevus. Histologically, such nevi may show a variable intraepidermal component localized to the area of the scar and not beyond. There is usually effacement of the epidermis, and often a dermal nevus remnant lies beneath the scar. There may be irregular nesting, single-cell hyperplasia, and occasional pagetoid spread of the intraepidermal component. Cytologically, the melanocytes often take on an epithelioid appearance, but cytologic atypia is usually minimal or absent. As discussed in Chapter 4, it is incumbent on the pathologist to review the previous biopsy and to ensure the absence of significant atypicality. DMN occasionally recur and must be evaluated carefully for possible progression to melanoma. Extension of the intraepidermal component beyond the scar is a worrisome feature and should prompt particular scrutiny to rule out melanoma.

CORRELATION OF HISTOLOGIC MELANOCYTIC DYSPLASIA WITH INCREASED MELANOMA RISK

Although the DMN as a clinicopathologic entity has been shown to correlate with increased melanoma risk, histologic melanocytic dysplasia in isolation has not been sufficiently studied at this time to conclude that it is a definite risk factor for melanoma. However, one would expect that a certain threshold of atypia must be reached in order to have a significantly increased risk for progression to melanoma.[74] In fact, two recent studies have shown that DMN in patients with melanoma demonstrate greater atypia than do DMN in patients without melanoma.[49,70] Although the grading of atypia differed in the latter two studies, these findings provide corroborative but preliminary evidence that histologic dysplasia of a sufficient grade may be a risk factor for melanoma. Some studies have not shown this relationship, but such an outcome might be attributed to variation in histologic criteria for DMN.[67,100]

GRADING OF DYSPLASTIC NEVI

The aim of grading dysplastic lesions in any cellular system should have relevance to the management of patients. Specifically, this means that lesions that are risk markers or with significant risk for progression to malignancy are identified and distinguished from lesions with lesser degrees of risk. Such a grading scheme also should guide clinicians in the practical management of individual lesions, e.g., which lesions should be excised with particular margins or simply left alone. For a grading scheme to be useful, it also must be reproducible among pathologists. The grading system outlined below has been subjected to interobserver agreement studies. The latter investigations were conducted without prior discussion of criteria for grading.[92] The kappa values recorded for three paired readings, i.e., grading of DMN by experienced dermatopathologists working at the same institution, indicated fair to good agreement. The latter results suggest that grading of DMN is feasible and reproducible and is likely to improve significantly with standardized criteria and training. Additional studies are underway to verify the utility of grading DMN.

TABLE 9-15
Histopathologic Reporting of Dysplastic Nevi

Grade of Lesion	*Reexcision if Margins Involved*
Low-grade lesions	
Junctional or compound nevus with architectural disorder (no cytologic atypia)	No
Junctional or compound dysplastic nevus with slight atypia* (or nevus with architectural disorder and slight cytologic atypia)	No, if bulk of lesion removed
High-Grade Lesions	
Junctional or compound dysplastic nevus with moderate atypia (or nevus with architectural disorder and moderate cytologic atypia)	Yes
Junctional or compound dysplastic nevus with severe cytologic atypia (or nevus with architectural disorder and severe cytologic atypia)	Yes, with at least 5 mm margins

*See text for criteria for grades of cytologic atypia.

In lieu of standardized grading, the following guidelines are suggested: (1) It is important that severely atypical or high-grade DMN are recognized because of their overlap with melanoma in situ. This recognition is of paramount significance because melanoma in situ may potentially undergo rapid progression to invasive melanoma. Severely atypical DMN are characterized by markedly disordered growth and cytologic atypia (see earlier discussion). Such lesions should be excised completely with margins of at least 5 mm. (2) DMN with moderate atypia (see earlier discussion) should be removed completely with clear margins. Because DNA aneuploidy has been documented in such lesions, there may possibly be a greater potential for progression to melanoma than less atypical lesions.[101] (3) DMN with slight or minimal atypia need not have reexcision if the bulk of the lesion has been removed, even if the margins are involved. Such lesions are common, and reproducible distinction from lentiginous nevi with architectural disorder and no cytologic atypia may not be possible. In general, slightly atypical DMN seem not to exhibit DNA aneuploidy.[101] In the author's experience, recurrence as melanoma has not been observed with such lesions.

HISTOPATHOLOGIC REPORTING OF DYSPLASTIC NEVI

The most important point in reporting melanocytic lesions is that the pathologist communicates clearly to the clinician the nature of the lesion and its significance, regardless of terminology used. In one sense, the significance of the individual lesion is related to the degree of atypicality in that lesion. The immediate concern of the pathologist is to ensure proper management of the individual lesion, i.e., the degree of atypicality is properly assessed and recorded and the need for additional therapy, if any, is communicated to the clinician (Table 9-15). In another sense, the significance of a DMN must be viewed from the perspective of global melanoma risk in the patient. Thus the significance of the individual DMN can be viewed in quantitative terms and is directly related to family history of melanoma (number of blood relatives with melanoma), family history of DMN, personal history of melanoma, the patient's nevus phenotype (total number of typical and atypical nevi on the skin surface), degree of atypia of previously removed nevi, and other risk factors for melanoma such as immunosuppression or history of sunburn. Based on the histologic findings of the individual DMN placed in the context of the preceding parameters, management of the individual patient can be formulated by the pathologist and clinician functioning as a team. Such cooperation works in the best interests of patients and ensures the best possible risk stratification.

REFERENCES

1. Norris W: A case of fungoid disease. *Edinb Med Surg J* 16:562–565, 1820.
2. Cawley EP: Genetic aspects of malignant melanoma. *AMA Arch Dermatol* 65:440–450, 1952.
3. Allen AC, Spitz S: Malignant melanoma: A clinicopathological analysis of the criteria for diagnosis and prognosis. *Cancer* 6:1–45, 1953.
4. Lund HZ, Kraus JM: Melanotic tumors of the skin. In *Atlas of Tumor Pathology*, sec 1, fasc 3. Washington, Armed Forces Institue of Pathology, 1962, pp 86–89.
5. Munro DD: Multiple active junctional naevi with family history of malignant melanoma. *Proc R Soc Med* 67:594–595, 1974.
6. Frichot BV, Lynch HT, Guirgis HA, et al: A new cutaneous phenotype in familial malignant melanoma. *Lancet* 1:864–865, 1977.
7. Lynch HT, Frichot BC III, Lynch JF: Familial atypical multiple mole–melanoma syndrome. *J Med Genet* 15:352–356, 1978.
8. Clark WH Jr, Reimer RR, Greene M, et al: Origin of familial malignant melanomas from heritable melanocytic lesions: The B-K mole syndrome. *Arch Dermatol* 114:732–738, 1978.
9. Sagebiel RW: Histopathology of borderline and early malignant melanomas. *Am J Surg Pathol* 3:543–552, 1979.
10. Elder DE, Goldman LI, Goldman SC, et al: Dysplastic nevus syndrome: A phenotypic association of sporadic cutaneous melanoma. *Cancer* 46:1787–1794, 1980.
11. Elder DE, Greene MH, Bondi EE, Clark WH Jr: Acquired melanocytic nevi and melanoma: The dysplastic nevus syndrome. In Ackerman AB (ed): *Pathology of Malignant Melanoma.* New York, Masson, 1981, pp 185–215.
12. Greene MH, Young J, Clark WH Jr: Malignant melanoma in renal-transplant recipients. *Lancet* 1:1196–1199, 1981.
13. Reynolds P, Austin D, Thomas J: Familial and occupational risks associated with malignant melanoma of the skin. *Am J Epidemiol* 116:570, 1982.
14. Beral V, Evans S, Shaw H: Cutaneous factors related to the risk of melanoma. *Br J Dermatol* 109:165–172, 1983.
15. Greene MH, Goldin LR, Clark WH Jr, et al: Familial cutaneous malignant melanoma: Autosomal dominant trait possibly linked to the Rh locus. *Proc Natl Acad Sci USA* 80:6071–6075, 1983.
16. Kraemer KH, Greene MH, Tarone R, et al: Dysplastic naevi and cutaneous melanoma risk (letter). *Lancet* 2:1076–1077, 1983.
17. Clark WH Jr, Elder DE, Guerry D IV, et al: A study of tumor progression: The precursor lesions of superficial spreading and nodular melanoma. *Hum Pathol* 15:1147–1165, 1984.
18. Crutcher WA, Sagebiel RW: Prevalence of dysplastic nevi in a community practice (letter). *Lancet* 1:729, 1984.
19. Holman CDJ, Armstrong BK: Pigmentary traits, ethnic origin, benign nevi, and family history as risk factors for cutaneous malignant melanoma. *J Nath Cancer Inst* 72:257–266, 1984.
20. NIH Consensus Conference: Precursors to malignant melanoma. *JAMA* 251:1864–1866, 1984.
21. Ackerman AB, Mihara I: Dysplasia, dysplastic melanocytes, the dysplastic nevus syndrome, and the relation between dysplastic nevi and malignant melanoma. *Hum Pathol* 16:87–91, 1985.
22. Elder DE. The dysplastic nevus. *Pathology* 17:291–297, 1985.
23. Green A, MacLennan R, and Siskind V: Common acquired naevi and the risk of malignant melanoma. *Int J Cancer* 35:297–300, 1985.
24. Greene MH, Clark WH Jr, Tucker MA, et al: Acquired precursors of cutaneous malignant melanoma: The familial dysplastic nevus syndrome. *N Engl J Med* 312:91–97, 1985.
25. Greene MH, Clark WH Jr, Tucker MA, et al: High risk of malignant melanoma in melanoma-prone families with dysplastic nevi. *Ann Intern Med* 102:458–465, 1985.
26. MacKie RM, English J, Aitchison TC, et al: The number and distribution of benign pigmented moles (melanocytic naevi) in a healthy British population. *Br J Dermatol* 113:167–174, 1985.
27. Nordlund JJ, Kirkwood J, Forget BM, et al: Demographic study of clinically atypical (dysplastic) nevi in patients with melanoma and comparison subjects. *Cancer Res* 45:1855–1861, 1985.
28. Sagebiel RW: Histopathology of precursor melanocytic lesions. *Am J Surg Pathol* 9:41–52, 1985.
29. Sagebiel RW: Diagnosis and management of premalignant melanocytic proliferations. *Pathology* 17:285–290, 1985.
30. Bale SJ, Chakravarti A, Greene MH: Cutaneous malignant melanoma and familial dysplastic nevi: Evidence for autosomal dominance and pleiotropy. *Am J Hum Genet* 38:188–196, 1986.
31. Elwood JM, Williamson C, Stapleton PJ: Malignant melanoma in relation to moles, pigmentation, and exposure to fluorescent and other lighting sources. *Br J Cancer* 53:65–74, 1986.
32. Kelly JW, Crutcher WA, Sagebiel RW: Clinical diagnosis of dysplastic melanocytic nevi: A clinicopathological correlation. *J Am Acad Dermatol* 14:1044–1052, 1986.
33. Kraemer KH, Tucker MA, Tarone R, et al: Risk of cutaneous melanoma in dysplastic nevus syndrome types A and B. *N Engl J Med* 315:1615–1616, 1986.
34. Roush GC, Barnhill RL, Duray PH, et al: Diagnosis of the dysplastic nevus in different population. *J Am Acad Dermatol* 14:419–425, 1986.
35. Seywright MM, Doherty VR, MacKie RM: Proposed alternative terminology and subclassification of so-called "dysplastic naevi." *J Clin Pathol* 39:189–194, 1986.
36. Swerdlow AJ, English J, MacKie RM, et al: Benign melanocytic naevi as a risk factor for malignant melanoma. *Br Med J (Clin Res Ed)* 292:1555–1559, 1986.
37. Caporaso N, Greene MH, Tsai S, et al: Cytogenetics in hereditary malignant melanoma and dysplastic nevus syndrome: Is dysplastic nevus syndrome a chromosomal instability disorder? *Cancer Genet Cytogenet* 24:299–314, 1987.
38. Herlyn M, Clark WH, Rodeck U, et al: Biology of tumor progression in human melanocytes. *Lab Invest* 56:461–474, 1987.
39. Holly EA, Kelly JW, Shpall SN, Chiu SH: Number of melanocytic nevi as a major risk factor for malignant melanoma. *J Am Acad Dermatol* 17:459–468, 1987.

40. Holzmann B, Bröcker EB, Lehmann JM, et al: Tumor progression in human malignant melanoma: Five stages defined by their antigenic phenotypes. *Int J Cancer* 39:466–471, 1987.
41. Rhodes AR, Weinstock MA, Fitzpatrick TB, et al: Risk factors for cutaneous melanoma: A practical method of recognizing predisposed individuals. *JAMA* 258:3146–3154, 1987.
42. Swerdlow AJ, Green A: Melanocytic naevi and melanoma: An epidemiological perspective. *Br J Dermatol* 117:137–146, 1987.
43. Weinstock MA, Sober AJ: Risk of progression of lentigo maligna to lentigo maligna melanoma. *Br J Dermatol* 16:303–310, 1987.
44. Ackerman AB: What naevus is dysplastic, a syndrome and the commonest precursor of malignant melanoma? A riddle and an answer. *Histopathology* 13:241–256, 1988.
45. Aronson PJ, Ito K, Fukaya T, et al: Monoclonal antibody (AFH1) immunoreactive on morphologically abnormal basal melanocytes within dysplstic nevi, nevocellular nevus nests, and melanoma. *J Invest Dermatol* 90:452–458, 1988.
46. Bain C, Colditz GA, Willett WC, et al: Self-reports of mole counts and cutaneous malignant melanoma in women: Methodological issues and risk of disease. *Am J Epidemiol* 127:703–712, 1988.
47. Balkau D, Gartmann H, Wischer W, et al: Architectural features in melanocytic lesions with cellular atypia. *Dermatologica* 177:129–137, 1988.
48. Barnhill RL, Hurwitz S, Duray PH, Arons MS: The dysplastic nevus: Recognition and management. *Plast Reconstr Surg* 81:280–289, 1988.
49. Bergman W, Ruiter DJ, Scheffer E, van Vloten WA: Melanocytic atypia in dysplastic nevi: Immunohistochemical and cytophotometrical analysis. *Cancer* 61:1660–1666, 1988.
50. Black WC: Residual dysplastic and other nevi in superficial spreading melanoma: Clinical correlations and association with sun damage. *Cancer* 62:163–173, 1988.
51. Evans RD, Kopf AW, Lew RA, et al: Risk factors for the development of malignant melanoma: I. Review of case-control studies. *J Dermatol Surg Oncol* 14:393–407, 1988.
52. Osterlind A, Tucker MA, Hou-Jensen K, et al: The Danish case-control study of cutaneous malignant melanoma: I. Importance of host factors. *Int J Cancer* 42:200–206, 1988.
53. Rhodes AR, Seki Y, Fitzpatrick TB, Stern RS: Melanosomal alterations in dysplastic melanocytic nevi: A quantitative, ultrastructural investigation. *Cancer* 61:358–369, 1988.
54. Rigel DS, Rivers JK, Friedman RJ, Kopf AW: Risk gradient for malignant melanoma in individuals with dysplastic nevi. *Lancet* 1:352–353, 1988.
55. Roush GC: Abnormal nevi, excess total nevi, and melanoma: An epidemiologic perspective. *Cancer Treat Rev* 43:85–100, 1988.
56. Roush GC, Nordlund JJ, Forget B, et al: Independence of dysplastic nevi from total nevi in determining risk for nonfamilial melanoma. *Prev Med* 17:273–279, 1988.
57. Steijlen PM, Bergman W, Hermans J, et al: The efficacy of histopathological criteria required for diagnosing dysplastic naevi. *Histopathology* 12:289–300, 1988.
58. Bale SJ, Dracopoli NC, Tucker MA, et al: Mapping the gene for hereditary cutaneous malignant melanoma: Dysplastic nevus syndrome to chromosome 1p36. *N Engl J Med* 320:1367–1372, 1989.
59. Garbe C, Krüger S, Stadler R, et al: Markers and relative risk in a German population for developing malignant melanoma. *Int J Dermatol* 28:517–523, 1989.
60. Green A, Swerdlow AJ: Epidemiology of melanocytic nevi. *Epidemiol Rev* 11:204–221, 1989.
61. Gruber SB, Barnhill RL, Stenn KS, Roush GC: Nevomelanocytic proliferations in association with cutaneous malignant melanoma: A multivariate analysis. *J Am Acad Dermatol* 21:773–780, 1989.
62. MacKie RM, Freudenberger T, Aitchison TCd: Personal risk-factor chart for cutaneous melanoma. *Lancet* 2:487–490, 1989.
63. Piepkorn M, Meyer LJ, Goldgar D: The dysplastic melanocytic nevus—A prevalent lesion that correlates poorly with clinical phenotype. *J Am Acad Dermatol* 20:407–415, 1989.
64. Rhodes AR, Mihm MC Jr, Weinstock MA: Dysplastic melanocytic nevi: A reproducible histologic definition emphasizing cellular morphology. *Mod Pathol* 2:306–319, 1989.
65. Rigel DS, Rivers JK, Kopf AW, et al: Dysplastic nevi markers for increased risk of melanoma. *Cancer* 63:386–389, 1989.
66. van Haeringen A, Bergman W, Nelen MR, et al: Exclusion of the dysplastic nevus snydrome (DNS) locus from the short arm of chromosome 1 by linkage studies in Dutch families. *Genomics* 5:61–64, 1989.
67. Ahmed I, Piepkorn MW, Rabkin MS, et al: Histopathologic characteristics of dysplastic nevi: Limited association of conventional histologic criteria with melanoma risk group. *J Am Acad Dermatol* 22:727–733, 1990.
68. Barnhill RL, Roush GC: Histopathologic spectrum of clinically atypical melanocytic nevi: Studies of nonfamilial melanoma, part II. *Arch Dermatol* 126:1315–1318, 1990.
69. Barnhill RL, Roush GC, Duray PH: Correlation of histologic and cytoplasmic features with nuclear atypia in atypical (dysplastic) nevomelanocytic nevi. *Hum Pathol* 21:51–58, 1990.
70. Black WC, Hunt WC: Histologic correlations with the clinical diagnosis of dysplastic nevus. *Am J Surg Pathol* 14:44–52, 1990.
71. Cannon-Albright LA, Goldgar DE, Wright EC, et al: Evidence against the reported linkage of the cutaneous melanoma: Dysplastic nevus syndrome locus to chromosome 1p36. *Am J Hum Genet* 46:912–918, 1990.
72. Grob JJ, Gouvernet J, Aymar D, et al: Count of benign melanocytic nevi as a major indicator of risk for nonfamilial nodular and superficial spreading melanoma. *Cancer* 66:387–395, 1990.
73. Klein LJ, Barr RJ: Histologic atypia in clinically benign nevi: A prospective study. *J Am Acad Dermatol* 22:275–282, 1990.
74. Barnhill RL: Current status of the dysplastic melanocytic nevus. *J Cutan Pathol* 18:147–159, 1991.
75. Barnhill RL, Roush GC: Correlation of clinical and histopathological features in clinically atypical melanocytic nevi. *Cancer* 67:3157–3164, 1991.
76. Clark WH Jr: Tumour progression and the nature of cancer. *Br J Cancer* 64:631–644, 1991.

77. Clemente C, Cochran AJ, Elder DE, et al: Histopathologic diagnosis of dysplastic nevi: Concordance among pathologists convened by the World Health Organization Melanoma Programme. *Hum Pathol* 22:313–319, 1991.
78. Goldgar DE, Cannon-Albright LA, et al: Inheritance of nevus number and size in melanoma and dysplastic nevus syndrome kindreds. *J Natl Cancer Inst* 83:1726–1733, 1991.
79. Halpern AC, Guerry D, Elder DE, et al: Dysplastic nevi as risk markers of sporadic (nonfamilial) melanoma. *Arch Dermatol* 127:995–999, 1991.
80. Roush GC, Barnhill RL: Correlation of clinical pigmentary characteristics with histopathologically-confirmed dysplastic nevi in nonfamilial melanoma patients: Studies of melanocytic nevi, part IX. *Br J Cancer* 64:943–947, 1991.
81. Roush GC, Barnhill RL, Ernstoff MS, Kirkwood, JM: Interclinician agreement on the recognition of clinical pigmentary characteristics of patients with cutaneous malignant melanoma: Studies of melanocytic nevi, part VI. *Br J Cancer* 64:373–376, 1991.
82. Titus-Ernstoff L, Ernstoff MS, Duray PH, et al: A relation between childhood sun exposure and dysplastic nevus syndrome among patients with nonfamilial melanoma. *Epidemiology* 2:210–214, 1991.
83. Traupe H: Polygenic vs. monogenic inheritance of dysplastic nevi and malignant melanoma. In Lynch HT, Tantu P (eds): *Recent Progress in the Genetic Epidemiology of Cancer.* New York, Springer-Verlag, 1991, pp 102–113.
84. Weiss J, Bertz J, Jung EG: Malignant melanoma in southern Germany—Different predictive value of risk factors for melanoma subtypes. *Dermatologica* 183:109–113, 1991.
85. Barnhill RL, Roush GC, Ernstoff MS, Kirkwood JM: Interclinician agreement on the recognition of selected gross morphologic features of pigmented lesions: Studies of melanocytic nevi, part V. *J Am Acad Dermatol* 26:185–190, 1992.
86. Barnhill RL, Roush GC, Titus-Ernstoff L, et al: Comparison of nonfamilial and familial melanoma. *Dermatology* 184:2–7, 1992.
87. Duray PH, DerSimonian R, Barnhill RL, et al: An analysis of interobserver recognition of the histopathologic features of dysplastic nevi from a mixed group of nevomelanocytic lesions. *J Am Acad Dermatol* 27:741–749, 1992.
88. Krüger S, Garbe C, Büttner P, et al: Epidemiologic evidence for the role of melanocytic nevi as risk markers and direct precursors of cutaneous malignant melanoma. *J Am Acad Dermatol* 26:920–926, 1992.
89. NIH Consensus Development Panel on Early Melanoma: Diagnosis and treatment of early melanoma. *JAMA* 268:1314–1319, 1992.
90. Barnhill RL: Melanocytic nevi and tumor progression: Perspectives concerning histomorphology, melanoma risk, and molecular genetics. *Dermatology* 187:86–90, 1993.
91. Bruijn JA, Berwick M, Mihm MC Jr, Barnhill RL: Common acquired melanocytic nevi, dysplastic melanocytic nevi and malignant melanomas: An image analysis cytometric study. *J Cutan Pathol* 20:121–125, 1993.
92. Duncan LM, Berwick MA, Bruijn JA, et al: Histopathologic recognition and grading of dysplastic melanocytic nevi: An interobserver agreement study. *J Invest Dermatol* 100:318S–321S, 1993.
93. Roush GC, Dubin N, Barnhill RL: Prediction of histologic melanocytic dysplasia from clinical observation. *J Am Acad Dermatol* 29: 555–562, 1993.
94. Titus-Ernstoff L, Barnhill RL, Duray PH, et al: Dysplastic nevi in relation to superficial spreading melanoma. *Cancer Epidemiol Biomarkers Prev* 2:99–101, 1993.
95. MacKie RM, McHenry P, Hole D: Accelerated detection with prospective surveillance for cutaneous malignant melanoma in high-risk groups. *Lancet* 341:1618–1620, 1993.
96. Tucker MA, Fraser MC, Goldstein AM, et al: Risk of melanoma and other cancers in melanoma-prone families. *J Invest Dermatol* 100:350S–355S, 1993.
97. Halpern AC, Guerry DP IV, Elder DE, et al: A cohort study of melanoma in patients with dysplastic nevi. *J Invest Dermatol* 100: 346S–349S, 1993.
98. Barnhill RL: Moles and melanoma—New method in the madness. *West J Med* 160:381–383, 1994.
99. Williams ML, Sagebiel RW: Melanoma risk factors and atypical moles. *West J Med* 160:343–350, 1994.
100. Piepkorn MW, Barnhill RL, Rabkin MS, et al: A multiobserver, population-based analysis of histological dysplasia in melanocytic nevi, phenotype, and prevalence in population controls. *J Am Acad Dermatol*. 30:707–714, 1994.
101. Schmidt B, Hollister K, Weinberg D, Barnhill RL: Analysis of melanocytic lesions by DNA image cytometry. *Cancer* 73:2971–2977, 1994.
102. Kang S, Barnhill RL, Mihm MC Jr, et al: Melanoma risk in individuals with clinically atypical nevi. *Arch Dermatol* 130:999–1001, 1994.
103. Barnhill RL, Fandrey K, Levy MA, et al: Angiogenesis and tumor progression of melanoma: Quantification of vascularity in melanocytic nevi and cutaneous malignant melanoma. *Lab Invest* 67:331–337, 1992.
104. Barnhill RL, Barnhill MA, Berwick MA, Mihm MC Jr: The histologic spectrum of pigmented spindle cell nevus: A review of 120 cases with emphasis on atypical variants. *Hum Pathol* 22:52–58, 1991.
105. Greene MH, Clark WH Jr, Tucker MA, et al: Precursor naevi in cutaneous malignant melanoma: A proposed nomenclature (letter). *Lancet* 2:1024, 1980.

10

Malignant Melanoma

In recent years, malignant melanoma of the skin has become a major public health issue for many Western countries (Table 10-1). The reasons for this heightened concern are that incidence rates of cutaneous melanoma are currently rising rapidly (perhaps more so than for any other form of cancer among Caucasians), death rates from melanoma are also rising, though not as rapidly, and there are currently no effective treatments for metastatic melanoma.[1-3] Despite this seemingly dismal outlook, melanoma generally can be recognized at an early stage of development and the patient cured by complete excision of the lesion. Major campaigns have thus been initiated for the early detection of melanoma.

The purpose of this chapter is to describe the histopathology of primary melanoma of the skin. Emphasis is placed not only on the major forms of melanoma and their differential diagnosis but also on unusual variants that are difficult to recognize histologically. Congenital and childhood melanoma and melanoma developing in congenital nevi are covered in Chapter 5. Metastatic melanoma is discussed in Chapter 11.

TUMOR PROGRESSION OF MELANOMA

Human cancers are thought to progress through a series of discrete stages in which each successive step confers a growth advantage.[4-6] The endpoint of this cascade is a tumor endowed with properties requisite for metastasis (the metastatic phenotype). Because cutaneous melanocytic lesions are readily visible and accessible, it has been relatively easy to study their biology (see Table 10-1).

Melanoma is thought to arise through two principal pathways of tumorigenesis[7,8] (Table 10-2). The most common (~67 percent cutaneous malignant melanoma) involves the de novo proliferation of basilar epidermal melanocytes, and the other major paradigm of tumor progression occurs via melanocytic nevi.[9] Both sequences involve intermediate stages of atypicality that have been termed *dysplastic*; the latter term refers to histologic patterns of architectural and cytologic atypia intermediate between basilar melanocytes or common nevi and melanoma[10,11] (see Chap. 9).

CLASSIFICATION OF MELANOMA BASED ON STAGE OF TUMOR PROGRESSION

The currently accepted classification of cutaneous malignant melanoma (CMM) is based on the recognition of two distinct phases of tumorigenesis: the radial or horizontal growth phase and the vertical or tumefactive growth phase[5,6,12-16] (Tables 10-3 and 10-4).

The Radial or Horizontal Growth Phase (RGP)

Intraepidermal Proliferation (Melanoma in Situ). There is mounting evidence that almost all melanomas begin with a proliferation of melanocytes initially confined to the epidermis.[17] The duration of this intraepidermal phase ranges from months to many years, during which these proliferative lesions show progressive degrees of architectural and cytologic atypicality. The architectural abnormalities include basilar proliferation of melanocytes reaching confluence and upward migration (pagetoid

TABLE 10-1
Summary of Malignant Melanoma of the Skin

1. Melanoma represents 3% of all cancers by incidence (excluding nonmelanoma skin cancers).*
2. Incidence is latitude-dependent; crude incidence rates (whites), 1990, per 100,000 population per year:

Northern United States (Connecticut)	12.4*
Southern United States (Arizona)	26

3. Total new cancer cases estimated* in the United States for 1994:

Malignant melanoma	32,000
Primary brain tumor	17,500
Thyroid	13,000
Multiple myeloma	12,700
Pharynx	9,200
Hodgkin's disease	7,900

4. Incidence of melanoma: Connecticut Registry,* per 100,000 population per year:

1935–1940	1.1
1946–1949	2.4
1956–1960	3.3
1966–1970	5.2
1976–1980	8.5
1986–1990	12.4

5. Overall deaths (United States) 6451; melanoma accounts for 1 percent of all cancer deaths.*
6. Overall 10-year survival[34] (clinical Stage I): 71%
7. Ten-year survival based on Clark's anatomic levels of invasion, percent (clinical Stage I) (34):

II (into papillary dermis)	95%
III (filling papillary dermis)	75%
IV (into reticular dermis)	70%
V (into subcutaneous fat)	45%

8. Ten-year survival[34] of clinical stage I tumors based on primary tumor thickness in mm:

<0.76	95%
0.76–1.49	84%
1.50–2.49	69%
2.50–3.99	58%
4–7.99	47%
>8.0	30%

9. Most frequent sites[15] in whites:
   Males: back, anterior torso, upper extremity, head and neck
   Females: back, lower leg, upper extremity, head and neck
10. Most frequent sites in blacks and Asians: soles, mucous membranes, palms, nail beds
11. Frequency of melanoma by type of tumor,[15] %:

Superficial spreading melanoma	67
Nodular melanoma	10
Lentigo maligna melanoma	9
Acral melanoma	4
Unclassified	5
Rare and unknown forms of melanoma	5

12. Important features[35] in recognition:
   Variegation in color and pigmentation pattern (mixtures of colors in addition to brown and tan)
   Irregularity of border, presence of notching

*Weinstock MA, personal communication, 1994.

TABLE 10-2
Two Principal Pathways of Tumor Progression of Melanoma

1. Basilar melanocytes	1. Basilar melanocytes
2. Intraepidermal melanocytic proliferation	2. Acquired melanocytic nevus
3. Intraepidermal melanocyte proliferation with atypia (dysplasia)	3. Dysplastic nevus

4. Melanoma, radial growth phase
   a. Melanoma in situ (intraepidermal)
   b. Microinvasive melanoma
5. Melanoma, vertical growth phase
6. Metastatic melanoma

spread) of melanocytes (Fig. 10-1*A*). In general, such proliferations display a predominance of single cells, initially basilar, but with time scattered randomly throughout the epidermis and frequently extending into the granular layer and stratum corneum (see Fig. 10-1*A*). Commonly, there is extension of these proliferations along the basilar zones of appendageal structures, a feature most developed in lentigo maligna.[18]

Increasing cytologic atypia of melanocytes accompanies the aberrant architectural appearance. The melanocytes vary in degree of atypia and the proportion of cells with nuclear atypia. For the most part, criteria for nuclear atypia are subjective and lack reproducibility. However, atypical melanocytes usually have nuclei as large as or larger than nearby keratinocytes, exhibit variation in nuclear shapes and chromatin patterns, and may have large nucleoli. Thickening of nuclear membranes and irregular nuclear contours are also characteristic of atypical melanocytes. The cytoplasm of such melanocytes may be abundant, pink, may contain granular or finely divided ("dusty") melanin, or show retraction, resulting in a clear space around the nuclei (see Fig. 10-1*B*). Melanocytes with scant cytoplasm typically have high nuclear-to-cytoplasmic ratios. Such proliferations have been variously labeled *atypical melanocytic hyperplasia, premalignant melanosis, melanocytic dysplasia*, and recently *pagetoid melanocytic proliferation*, as well as *melanoma in situ*.[13,19–21] The use of an assortment of terms reflects the spectrum of these lesions, the lack of reliable criteria for their diagnosis, uncertainty as to the biologic potential of these lesions, and reluctance to render a diagnosis of malignancy in face of the latter uncertainty.

Microinvasive Melanoma. After the period of intraepidermal proliferation, many of these in situ melanomas invade the papillary dermis,[5,13,15,18] primarily as single cells and small aggregates of cells with histologic characteristics similar to the intraepidermal cells (Table 10-3 and Fig. 10-2*A*). There is evidence at this stage that the invad-

TABLE 10-3
A Comparison of Histomorphologic Characteristics of Melanomas in the Radial (or Horizontal) Growth Phase versus Those in the Vertical Growth Phase

Radial Growth Phase, Microinvasive	*Vertical Growth Phase*
Invasion of papillary dermis as single cells and small aggregates of melanoma cells of similar size (usually under 5–10 cells in greatest diameter)	Formation of single cohesive cellular nodule or plaque or multiple nests of cells in papillary dermis (usually over 15–25 cells in diameter)
Dermal nests no larger than intraepidermal nests	Individual cellular nests larger than those nests observed in radial growth phase
The constituent cells in dermis cytomorphologically similar to the intraepidermal melanoma cells	The melanoma cells in general cytomorphologically different from the cells in the radial growth phase
Mitotic figures absent or rare	Mitotic figures common
Usually no induction of stroma	Induction of stroma common
Usually prominent mononuclear cell infiltrates	Mononuclear cell infiltrates less prominent
Focal or partial regression common	Regression less common

TABLE 10-4
Classification of Malignant Melanoma

- Characteristics of intraepidermal component
  - Presence of radial (or horizontal) growth phase
    - Superficial spreading (pagetoid) melanoma
    - Lentiginous melanomas
      - Lentigo maligna
      - Acral lentiginous
      - Mucosal lentiginous
    - Unclassified
  - Absence of radial growth phase
    - Nodular melanoma
- Characteristics of invasive dermal component
  - Most common cytologic variants
    - Epithelioid cell
    - Spindle cell
    - Small cell or nevus-like cell
- Unusual histologic and cytologic variants
  - Desmoplastic
  - Neurotropic
  - Minimal deviation
  - Nevoid
  - Verrucous
    - Verrucous and pseudonevoid
    - Verrucous-keratotic
    - Verrucous nevoid and keratotic
  - Malignant blue nevus
  - Clear cell sarcoma
    - Malignant melanoma of soft parts
  - Melanoma arising in dermal nevi
  - Balloon cell
  - Spitzoid
  - Myxoid
  - Melanomas resembling experimentally induced and spontaneous melanomas in animals

ing melanocytic cells lack significant proliferative attributes and the capacity for cohesive nodular growth (and probably for metastasis).[16] Microinvasive melanoma is also remarkable for a striking host response in the papillary dermis, typically a dense cellular infiltrate of lymphocytes and monocytes/macrophages in a perivascular or bandlike pattern (Fig. 10-2*A* and *B*). Melanin-containing macrophages and vascular proliferation typically accompany the mononuclear cell infiltrates. Presumably, in consequence of this host reaction, regression, often focal, is common in up to 50 percent of microinvasive melanomas[22] (see below).

Intraepidermal proliferation of melanoma and subsequent microinvasion have been termed the *radial or horizontal growth phase* of tumor progression. *Radial* indicates a peripherally extending (presumably clonal) growth of intraepidermal melanocytes or, as described by Clark, Elder, and colleagues,[5,13,15] "extending along the radii of an imperfect circle." This proliferation may be characterized by upward migration of cells throughout the epidermis (*pagetoid* spread) or mainly basilar (*lentiginous*) proliferation of melanocytes (in lentigo maligna, acral, and mucosal lentiginous melanomas) and eventual downward growth (microinvasion) into the dermis.

The Vertical Growth Phase (VGP)

This phase of tumor progression is characterized by the focal proliferation of melanoma cells as a cohesive aggregate in the dermis (Fig. 10-3) and supervenes on an RGP in about 90 percent of melanomas[5,13,15,16] (see Table 10.3). It is theorized that the VGP develops de novo, or from rapid progression of the intraepidermal component, in approximately 10 to 15 percent of tumors (see Nodular Melanoma, below). Hypothetically, the genesis of the VGP as described above does not rule out an origin from the dermis or the adnexa (eccrine sweat ducts or hair follicles).

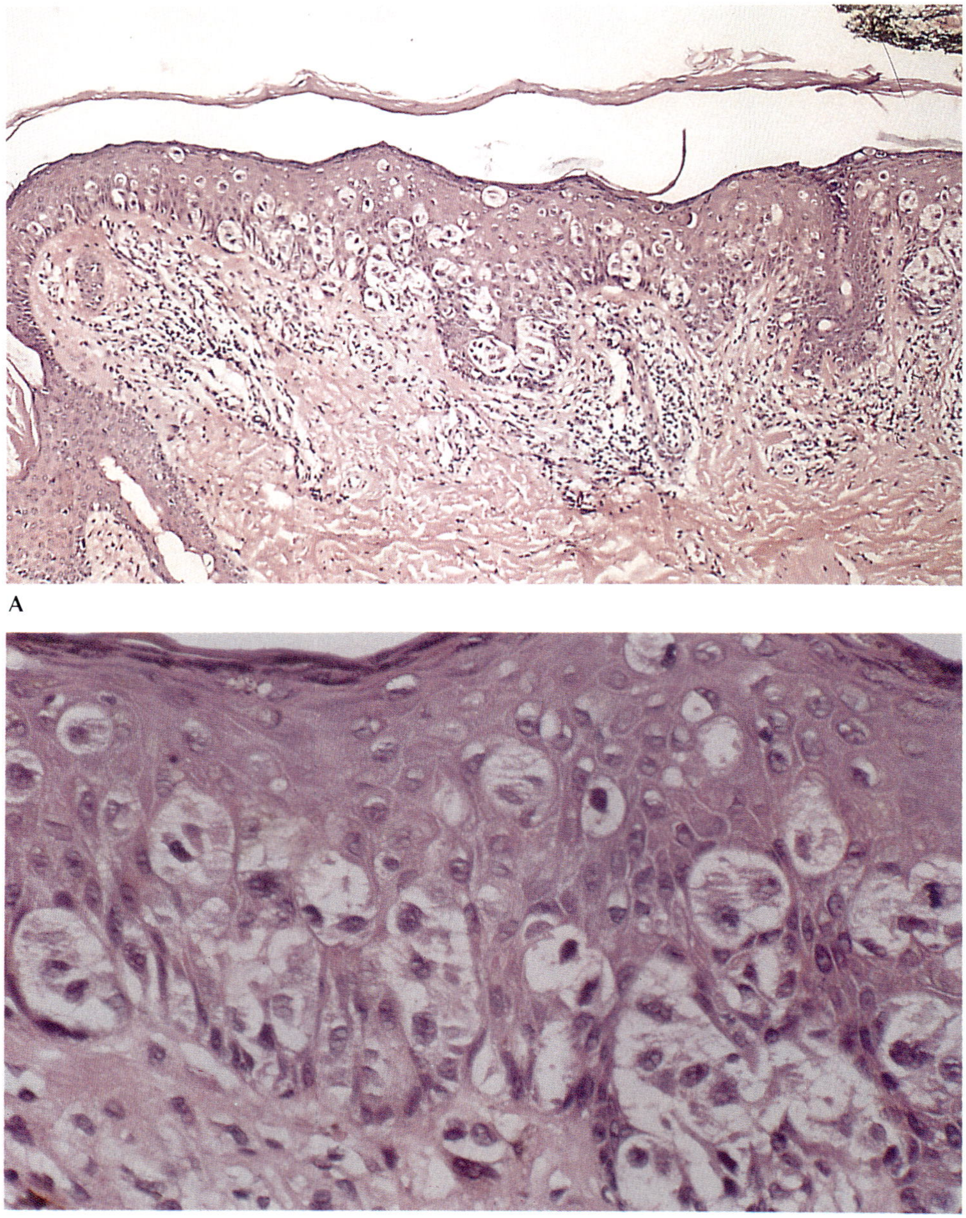

A

B

FIGURE 10-1
Melanoma in situ, superficial spreading (pagetoid) type. (A) Pagetoid spread of epithelioid cells throughout epidermis (H&E, × 100). (B) Higher magnification of part A (H&E, × 400).

The VGP apparently signals a qualitative change in the histomorphology and biology of a tumor.[5,13,15,16,20] There is evidence that the VGP may signify the onset of the metastatic phenotype, since it is indistinguishable from the histomorphology of metastatic melanoma. Such tumoral foci are characterized by a single-cell nodule or plaque or a nodule or plaque composed of smaller cohesive nests[16] (see Table 10-3). The constituent cells within the latter configurations are tightly packed, are frequently monomorphous with marked cytologic atypia, and commonly display mitotic activity and individual-cell necrosis (Fig. 10-4). In general, mononuclear cell infiltrates

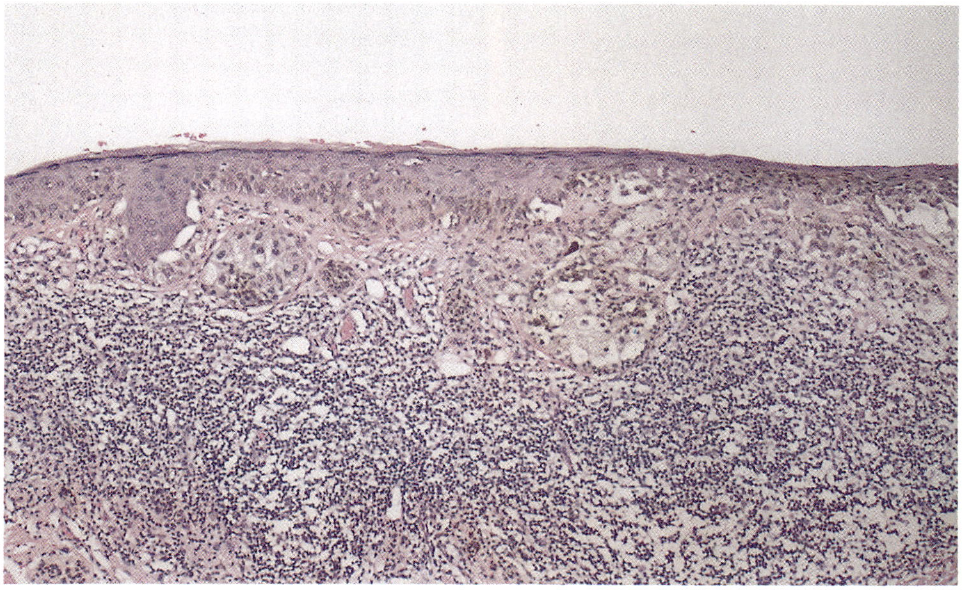

A

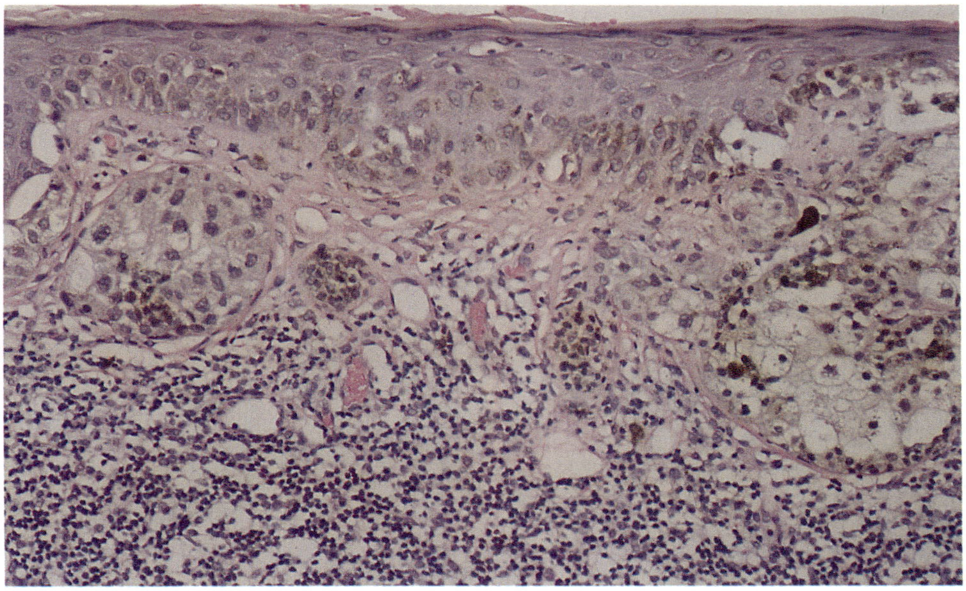

B

FIGURE 10-2

Superficial spreading melanoma, superficially invasive. (A) The lesion shows nests of melanoma cells in the papillary dermis with effacement (loss) of the elongated epidermal rete pattern. A dense mononuclear cell infiltrate expands the papillary dermis (H&E, × 100). (B) Higher magnification showing expansile nests of melanoma cells possibly representing the early vertical growth phase (H&E, × 200).

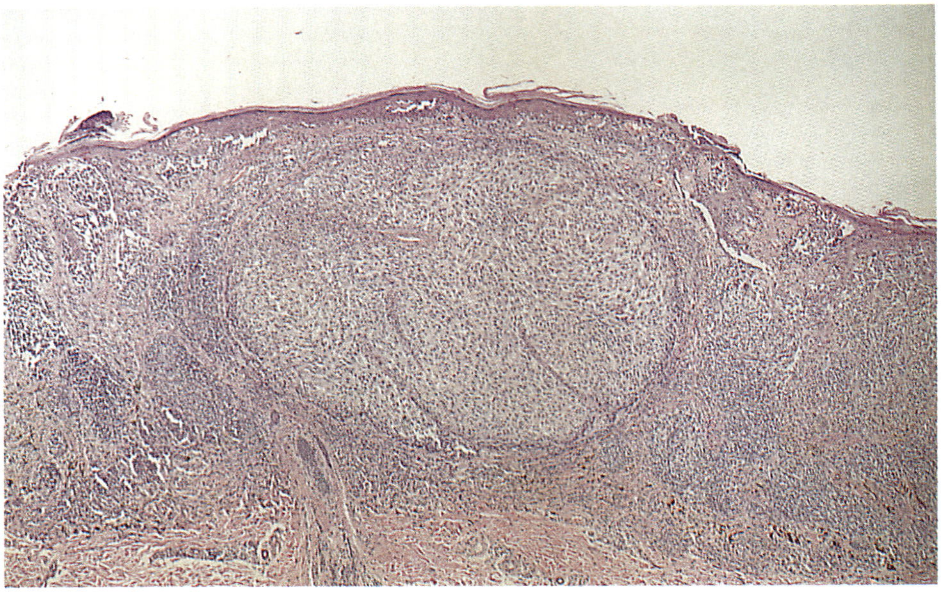

FIGURE 10-3
Malignant melanoma, vertical growth phase. Cohesive aggregate of epithelioid melanoma cells is present in the papillary dermis (H&E, × 400).

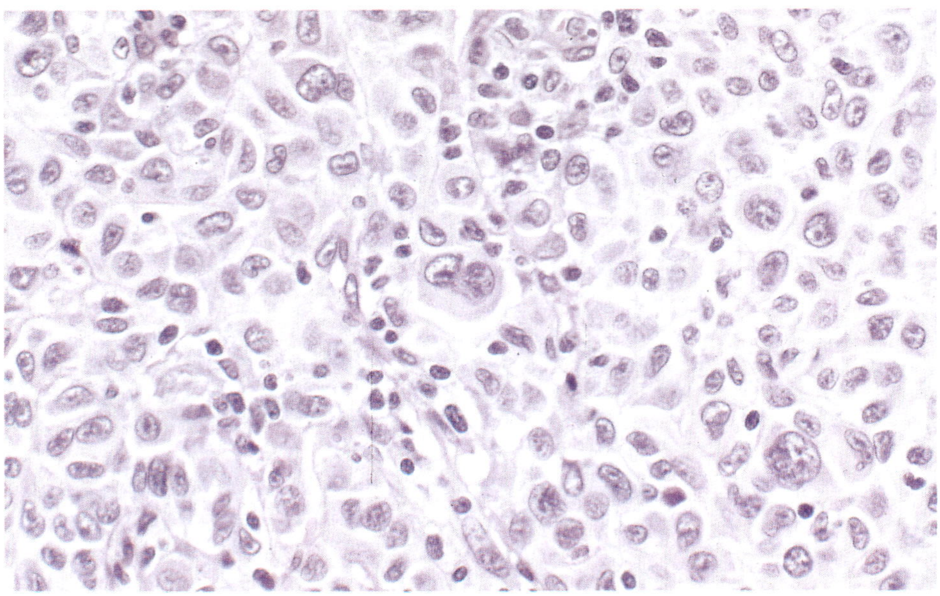

FIGURE 10-4
Vertical growth phase melanoma. This field shows a sheet of epithelioid cells in the dermis. Such a field might be observed in any subtype of melanoma but more commonly in superficial spreading or nodular melanoma. The cells have a monotypic appearance and are characterized by plentiful cytoplasm (H&E, × 400).

and regression are less conspicuous in the VGP than in the RGP (see below). However, junction of the radial and vertical components often discloses a zone of histologic regression.

Experimental work has verified differential properties between the latter two phases of tumor progression. Cell surface antigen phenotype, cytogenetics, and growth of isolated cells in soft agar and in cell culture are some of the experimental characteristics that have confirmed differences between the RGP and VGP, as well as melanocytic nevi.[23] These experimental studies, added to clinicopathologic features, support the putative multistep cascade of melanocytic tumor progression.

CURRENT CLASSIFICATION OF CUTANEOUS MELANOMA

The current system of classifying most melanomas is based on the presence or absence of a recognizable RGP and, if present, the pattern of the RGP[12–15] (Table 10-4). In general, there has probably been too much emphasis placed on the classification of intraepidermal histomorphologic patterns of melanoma and insufficient attention paid to the characteristics of the invasive dermal component which largely determines prognosis. Intraepidermal patterns generally include two major subtypes: (1) the pagetoid pattern (see above), as in superficial spreading melanoma, and (2) the lentiginous pattern, as described in lentigo maligna, acral lentiginous, and mucosal lentiginous melanoma. The latter two patterns are not mutually exclusive since overlapping patterns may occur. In addition, some intraepidermal patterns are difficult to categorize, hence the *unclassified* designation. Despite problems in classification, recognition of a particular intraepidermal pattern may relate more to the pathogenesis of particular forms of melanoma rather than necessarily to issues such as prognosis. For the latter reason, there still may be some justification for classifying intraepidermal (radial growth phase) patterns.

The characteristics of the invasive or dermal component of melanoma have begun to receive more attention in recent years. The importance of studying the dermal component has been recognized since prognosis is directly a function of tumor thickness and undoubtedly other attributes that have not received sufficient investigation. As outlined in Table 10-4, the current classification of the invasive or dermal component of melanoma has not been standardized; and is based largely on descriptions of cell type and distinctive or unusual histologic features. For example, melanomas developing in the dermis may be categorized as to predominant cell type(s) whether an epithelioid cell, spindle cell, small cell, or other cell type. Some melanomas have been classified according to their cytologic resemblance to melanocytic nevi, *vis-a-vis* minimal deviation melanoma, nevoid melanoma, spitzoid melanoma. Particular melanomas have also been distinguished arbitrarily on their origin from the dermal portion of both acquired and congenital nevi and blue nevi, e.g., melanomas arising in dermal nevi and malignant blue nevi.

Other melanomas have been recognized because of peculiar and unique histologic characteristics of their epidermal, invasive, or dermal components, e.g., the presence of a verrucous or papillomatous epidermal surface (verrucous melanoma), a fibrotic or desmoplastic stroma (desmoplastic melanoma), a myxoid stroma (myxoid melanoma), neural appearance (neurotropic and neural-transforming melanoma), and perineurial and endoneurial invasion (neurotropic melanoma).

It is apparent that a number of these unusual patterns of melanoma show considerable overlap. The case can be made that the current classification of melanoma needs reevaluation and perhaps revision and simplification.

Four clinicopathologic subtypes of melanoma are generally accepted (Tables 10-5 and 10-6) based on clinical, pathologic, and epidemiologic evidence.[12–15,18,20,24–29] There is compelling epidemiologic evidence that lentigo maligna melanoma (LMM) is distinct from the superficial spreading and acral lentiginous melanoma (ALM) because of its strong correlation with cumulative sunlight exposure, onset in older persons, and uncommon association with melanocytic nevi.[9,26–29] Superficial spreading melanoma (SSM) is notable for its correlation with intermittent sunlight exposure, occurrence in fairly young adults (fourth and fifth decades), and frequent association with melanocytic nevi (usually dysplastic) and familial melanoma.[9,26–29] ALM develops in relatively sun-protected sites and, similar to LMM, is seldom associated with melanocytic nevi.[15,24–26] Nodular melanoma (NM) is remarkable for the absence of a RGP and is thought by some to be a final common pathway of rapid tumor progression of potentially any subtype of melanoma.[20,26,27,30] Nonetheless, NM shares several properties with SSM: frequent occurrence at the same sites as SSM, greater continuity with nevi than LMM or ALM, and predominance of epithelioid cells in the VGP.[15,26–28] Both LMM and ALM differ from SSM (and most NM) because of the lentiginous characteristics of the RGP, predominance of spindle cells in the VGP, and higher prevalence of desmoplasia and neurotropism.[15,20] However, the mechanisms of the unique growth properties of NM deserve further attention.[15,26]

As already mentioned, there has probably been too much emphasis on the classification of RGP to the detriment of other histopathologic aspects of CMM, such as the histologic and cytologic characteristics of the invasive

TABLE 10-5
Clinical Features of Major Types of Malignant Melanoma of the Skin

Type	*Median Age (years)*	*Location*	*Size*	*Duration of Radial Growth Phase*	*Topography*	*Color*
Superficial spreading	44	All sites, often on trunk of men, legs of women	2.5 cm	1–7 years	Palpable	Various shades of brown, black, gray, red
Nodular	53	All sites as for superficial spreading	1–2 cm	Months to 2 years*	Palpable	Bluish, black, pink (amelanotic)
Lentigo maligna	65	Sun-exposed sites, usually head and neck	3–6 cm	5–15 years	Flat	Various shades of tan, brown, black with frequent hypopigmentation
Acral lentiginous	65	Palms, soles, nail beds	3 cm	1–3 years	Flat or palpable	Various shades of tan, brown, black

*Period of evolution (theoretically no radial growth phase).

TABLE 10-6
Salient Histologic Features in Four Major Subtypes of Melanoma

	SSM	*NM*	*LMM*	*ALM*
Pattern of radial growth phase (RGP)	Pagetoid	—	Lentiginous	Lentiginous
Epidermis of RGP	Hyperplastic	—	Atrophic	Marked hyperplasia
Usual cell type of RGP	Epithelioid	—	Spindle, epithelioid	Spindle, epithelioid
Papillary dermis of RGP	Inflamed, thickened	—	Variably inflamed	Inflamed, thickened
Frequency of regression	Common (38%)	Uncommon	Common	Common
Solar elastosis of dermis	Slight	Slight	Marked	None
Usual cell type of vertical growth phase	Epithelioid	Epithelioid	Spindle	Spindle, highly pleomorphic cell
Desmoplasia	Uncommon	Uncommon	Common	Common
Neurotropism	Uncommon	Uncommon	Common	Common
Precursor nevus	Common (20–33%)	Less common (8%)	Uncommon (3%)	Uncommon

component. Some RGPs are difficult to categorize, and their classification is arbitrary.[17,31,32] It also should be pointed out that any RGP pattern may occur in any anatomic location. It is possible that the particular anatomic site may have more to do with the actual pathogenesis of a melanoma than the histologic pattern of the RGP.

Although there has been accumulating evidence that melanoma thickness has much greater prognostic significance than the RGP pattern,[33] the histogenetic type of melanoma may still have some effect on biologic behavior.[34] In particular, lentigo maligna may be less aggressive on the one hand and ALM more aggressive than SSM of equivalent thicknesses.[34] However, it must be pointed out again that anatomic site may possibly influence biologic behavior more than actual histopathologic pattern of the RGP.

If a proliferation does not fulfill the necessary criteria for one or another particular type of RGP, it is best left unclassified. A tumor that has a limited intraepidermal component may be a nodular melanoma, but it also may be a subtype of an RGP neoplasm.[15] In all likelihood, the rapidity of progression to VGP from an intraepidermal component varies among tumor types.[9] Detection of this intraepidermal component depends on its extent, the adequacy of sampling, and at what point in its evolution the lesion is excised.

MAJOR SUBTYPES OF MELANOMA BASED ON CLASSIFICATION OF THE INTRAEPIDERMAL COMPONENT

Superficial Spreading Melanoma

Synonym: pagetoid melanoma

Superficial spreading melanoma (SSM) is the most common (~70%) form of melanoma in Caucasians[12–15,20]

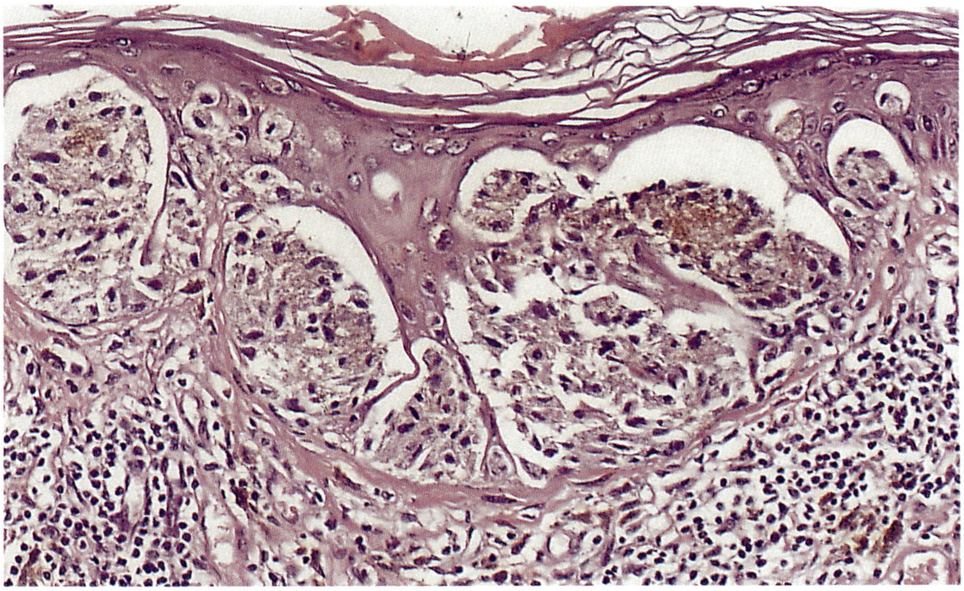

FIGURE 10-5
Superficial spreading melanoma, radial growth phase. There are large nests of epithelioid cells within the thickened epidermis (H&E, × 200).

(see Table 10-5). The tumor is associated with a history of intermittent sun exposure, is most common on the backs of males and lower extremities of females,[15,29] and is commonly associated with dysplastic nevi, familial melanoma, and multiple primary melanomas.[15]

Clinical Features. SSM in the radial or horizontal growth phase is characterized by a slightly elevated plaque, usually over 1 cm in diameter, with irregular borders and variegation of pigmentation.[12,13,15] The VGP is heralded by the development of a focal papule or nodule, often dusky blue, blue-black, or pink in color.[13,15,25]

Histologic Features. Examination at scanning magnification usually will disclose a broad lesion (often > 1 cm in diameter) displaying asymmetry and possible ulceration, particularly in thick melanomas.[36]

The RGP is remarkable for the presence of pagetoid spread (transepidermal migration of cells in a manner analogous to Paget's disease of the breast).[5,12–15] Single cells and small groups of cells are randomly scattered throughout the epidermis, reaching the granular layer and stratum corneum. Typical melanoma cells in SSM have an epithelioid cell appearance; i.e., they resemble epithelial cells because of abundant cytoplasm that is usually granular and eosinophilic or contains finely divided ("dusty") melanin (see Table 10-6). The cells are usually larger than (sometimes two to three times) the surrounding keratinocytes. The epidermis is commonly hyperplastic in SSM, the epidermal rete pattern is often lost (effaced), and the surface of the epidermis abutting the intraepidermal tumor may exhibit a characteristically scalloped contour (see Fig. 10-2*A*). Melanoma cells often proliferate as variably sized nests and horizontally disposed aggregates immediately underneath this scalloped epidermis. These aggregates are frequently large in size and have diminished cohesion of cells (Fig. 10-5). In some instances, the latter proliferative pattern may predominate with little or no pagetoid spread. Melanoma confined to the epidermis has been classified conventionally as in situ or level I melanoma[12] (Table 10-7).

TABLE 10-7
Anatomic Levels of Invasion and Relationship to Growth Phase

Radial or horizontal growth phase	
Level I:	entirely intraepidermal, melanoma in situ
Level II:	microinvasive into papillary dermis
Vertical growth phase	
Level III:	expansion of papillary dermis by cohesive cellular nodule or plaque (but confined to papillary dermis)
Level IV:	invasion of reticular dermis
Level V:	invasion of subcutaneous fat

Invasion of the papillary dermis begins as single cells and small nests of melanoma cells[5,12–15] (see Fig. 10-2*A* and *B* and Tables 10-3 and 10-7). Melanoma in this early stage of development typically is associated with variable perivascular or dense mononuclear cell infiltrates filling the papillary dermis and producing a bandlike pattern and variable numbers of melanin-containing macrophages. Focal regression is a prevalent finding at this step of development (see below). The papillary dermis is commonly thickened by the tumor cell invasion, mononuclear cell infiltrates, and stromal alterations, including fibroplasia, vascular ectasia, and angiogenesis.

The formation of cohesive nests or plaques of melanoma cells or aggregates of individual nests of cells characterizes the VGP[15,16] (see Tables 10-3 and 10-7). The nests of cells in the papillary dermis are generally larger than the intraepidermal nests, and the cells of the VGP are usually larger and more atypical than those of the RGP (see Fig. 10-3). The nuclei are enlarged, pleomorphic, hyperchromatic, and have irregular nuclear membranes and often prominent nucleoli. Necrotic cells and mitotic figures are also commonly found in the dermal component of melanomas. If the tumor is confined to the papillary dermis, the tumor is classified as level III (see Table 10-6). More advanced melanomas invade the reticular dermis and exhibit discrete foci of tumor in the reticular dermis and/or subcutaneous fat ("microscopic" satellites),[37] and they may occasionally infiltrate blood and lymphatic vessels and nerves (neurotropism).

The most common cell in the VGP is epithelioid or polygonal[15] (see Fig. 10-4). Less frequently, spindle cells, small cells resembling nevus cells, or large, bizarre mononuclear or multinucleate cells may predominate or are admixed with the other cell types. Many melanomas of all subtypes during vertical growth are characterized by heterogeneity of cell type, such that the cells vary in nuclear size and shape and amount of cytoplasm from one focus to another.

Approximately one-third of SSMs are associated with a contiguous melanocytic nevus,[9] a junctional or compound nevus (occasionally atypical or dysplastic), or most commonly, a dermal nevus remnant. There has been controversy as to whether atypical intraepidermal components identified as dysplastic nevi are truly precursor lesions or simply the peripheral, less atypical portion of the melanoma.[9] Such distinctions are difficult, arbitrary, and subjective.

Differential Diagnosis The differential diagnosis of SSM includes various melanocytic proliferations (Table 10-8): LMM, markedly atypical dysplastic nevi, halo nevi, spindle and epithelioid cell (Spitz) nevi, pigmented spindle cell nevi, recurrent melanocytic nevi, and congenital nevi, particularly in the first year of life. Nevi associated with prominent pagetoid spread are commonly confused with SSM.

SSM must frequently be discriminated from LMM, since LMM may display junctional nesting, variable pagetoid spread, and the presence of epithelioid cells in either the intraepidermal or dermal components or both, all of which are features suggesting SSM.[20,27,28] The presence of SSM-like findings may signify tumor progression of LMM to a higher-grade tumor equivalent to SSM.[20] The application of strict criteria should allow distinction of SSM from LMM in most instances. Thus, in the case of LMM, one usually observes epidermal atrophy and effacement, marked solar elastosis, prominent involvement of adnexal units by the melanocytic proliferation, and strikingly pleomorphic melanoma cells with scant cytoplasm in at least some portion of the lesion.[18] However, some authors designate melanomas with features of both SSM and LMM as unclassifiable.[28]

Dysplastic nevi with pronounced atypia may be misdiagnosed as SSM because of appearances suggestive of early pagetoid spread, confluence of cellular aggregates along the dermoepidermal junction, prominent variation in nesting pattern, significant cytologic atypia, entrapment of nests of dermal nevus cells in the papillary dermis, and dense mononuclear cell infiltrates. On occasion, the distinction of dysplastic nevi from SSM is exceedingly difficult. Nonetheless, discrimination of SSM from dysplastic nevi is usually possible because of the greater asymmetry and disorder encountered in melanoma. Usually dysplastic nevi will maintain an overall symmetry, a nevic appearance, as exemplified by fairly organized junctional nesting, a basilar proliferation of melanocytes that is still concentrated along the epidermal rete ridges and with greater density toward the lower poles of the rete ridges. Thus, the intervening epidermis between rete ridges will contain a lesser density of melanocytes compared with that on the epidermal rete ridges. If pagetoid spread is present, this architectural pattern usually shows a predilection for the epidermal rete ridges and is confined to the lower-most epidermis. Occasional dysplastic nevi exhibit effacement of the epidermal rete pattern andconfluence of melanocytic cells along the dermoepidermal junction in this zone. The latter changes are commonly associated with dense mononuclear cell infiltrates, may strongly suggest melanoma, and must be carefully interpreted in the overall context of the lesion. Dysplastic nevi are generally characterized by variable or discontinuous cytologic atypia; i.e., the degree of nuclear enlargement, pleomorphism, and hyperchromatism varies from cell to cell.[10] This cytologic feature is very helpful in discriminating dysplastic nevi from the more uniform or contiguous cytologic atypia of melanoma.

TABLE 10-8
Differential Diagnosis of Major Subtypes of Malignant Melanoma

Superficial spreading melanoma	Nodular melanoma	Lentigo maligna melanoma	Acral lentiginous melanoma
Melanocytic tumors	Melanocytic tumors	Melanocytic tumors	Melanocytic tumors
Lentigo maligna melanoma	Metastatic melanoma	Solar lentigo	Melanocytic nevi of acral skin
Dysplastic melanocytic nevus	Spindle and epithelioid cell nevus	Dysplastic nevus	Lentiginous melanocytic proliferations of acral skin
Halo nevus	Pigmented spindle cell nevus	Pigmented spindle cell nevus	Pigmented spindle cell nevus
Spindle and epithelioid cell nevus	Cellular blue nevus	Superficial spreading melanoma	Nonmelanocytic tumors
Pigmented spindle cell nevus	Nonmelanocytic tumors	Nonmelanocytic tumors	Squamous cell carcinoma, spindle cell type
Recurrent melanocytic nevus	Squamous cell carcinoma	Squamous cell carcinoma, spindle cell type	Atypical fibroxanthoma
Other melanocytic nevi with prominent pagetoid spread	Atypical fibroxanthoma	Atypical fibroxanthoma	Cellular neurothekeoma
Nonmelanocytic tumors	Malignant fibrous histiocytoma	Cellular neurothekeoma	Malignant peripheral nerve sheath tumor
Squamous cell carcinoma	Cellular neurothekeoma	Malignant peripheral nerve sheath tumor	Angiosarcoma
Paget's disease, mammary or extramammary	Malignant peripheral nerve sheath tumors		Kaposi's sarcoma
Sebaceous carcinoma	Angiosarcoma		Histiocytoid hemangioma
Cutaneous T-cell lymphoma	Kaposi's sarcoma		Leiomyosarcoma
Epidermotropic eccrine carcinoma	Histiocytoid hemangioma		
Metastatic carcinoma, other	Leiomyosarcoma		
Angiosarcoma			
Kaposi's sarcoma			
Leiomyosarcoma			
Atypical fibroxanthoma			
Malignant fibrous histiocytoma			

A finding that raises the possibility of melanoma is entrapment of atypical nevus cells in a fibrotic papillary dermis of a dysplastic nevus. Such findings may even suggest partial regression of melanoma. A distinction from melanoma should be based on an assessment of all the cytologic and architectural characteristics of the lesion. Importantly, the dermal nevus cells in question usually lack the marked and uniform cytologic atypia, especially manifested as hyperchromasia, of melanoma cells.

In general, halo nevi have dense mononuclear cell infiltrates, histologic regression in some instances, and varying degrees of architectural and cytologic atypia that may suggest SSM. The typical halo nevus of children and adolescents is characterized by overall symmetry, orderly appearance, and little or no cytologic atypia. The lymphoid cells that permeate the dermal nevus have a uniform density and regular horizontal contour. The nevus cells of halo nevi may demonstrate cellular enlargement with prominent eosinophilic cytoplasm, but their nuclear details are usually little altered. In contrast, there is a variant of halo nevus that has prominent pattern and cellular atypia and is perhaps best categorized as a dysplastic nevus. The discussion of dysplastic nevi is relevant to this form of (atypical) halo nevus (see Chap. 9).

The misdiagnosis of other melanocytic nevi, including spindle and epithelioid cell nevi, pigmented spindle cell nevi, congenital nevi, recurrent melanocytic nevi, and nevi in children, as melanoma is related primarily to misinterpretation of patterns of minor pagetoid spread. Overall symmetry and a well-organized appearance, as well as little or no cytologic atypia, favor a benign melanocytic proliferation. Pagetoid spread in benign melanocytic nevi is generally characterized by an orderly pattern, is generally limited to the lower epidermis, and aggregates of cells predominate over single cells.

Spindle and epithelioid cell nevi pose particular diagnostic problems because of the overall resemblance of their large epithelioid cells to melanoma cells, the presence

TABLE 10-9

Histochemical and Immunohistochemical Evaluation of Pagetoid Involvement of the Epidermis

	Superficial Spreading Melanoma	*Mammary Paget's Disease*	*Squamous Cell Carcinoma in Situ*	*Cutaneous T-Cell Lymphoma*	*Sebaceous Carcinoma*
PAS + D	−	±	−	−	−
Alcian blue	−	±	−	−	−
Fontana-Masson (melanin)	+	±	±	−	−
S-100 protein	+	−	−	−	−
HMB-45	+	−	−	−	−
CAM 5.2	−	+	−	−	−
Keratin	±	±	+	−	±
21N	−	+	−	−	−
EMA	±	+	+	−	+
CEA	±	±	−	−	−
GCDFP-15	−	+	−	−	−
LCA	−	−	−	+	−
CD_3 (panT)	−	−	−	+	−

**Note:* PAS + D, periodic acid–Schiff and diastase for neutral glycosaminoglycans; Alcian blue, for acidic glycosaminoglycans (nonsulfated); CAM 5.2, monoclonal antibody against cytokeratins 8,18,19,39,43,52 KD; 21N, polyclonal antibody against c-*erb* B_2 protein; EMA, epithelial membrane antigen; CEA, carcinoembryonic antigen; GCDFP-15, gross cystic disease fluid protein-15; LCA, leukocyte common antigen; CD_3 (pan T), surface markers common to all T lymphocytes.

of confluent nests of cells, and occasional striking cytologic atypia. However, spindle and epithelioid cell nevi generally differ from melanoma because of symmetry and an orderly architectural appearance, a monotonous character of the constituent cells, and the presence of benign nuclear characteristics in a majority of the nevus cells. The nuclear features in the epithelioid cells include an even dispersion of chromatin, delicate nuclear membranes, and nucleoli of uniform size from cell to cell. Spindle and epithelioid cell nevi also display in general a characteristic maturation of cells with infiltration into the dermis. The cells are remarkable for a diminution in cellular and nuclear sizes as well as a diminution in size of aggregates of cells descending into the dermis. The cells also typically infiltrate the stroma in an orderly and regular pattern.

Pigmented spindle cell nevi similarly are frequently confused with SSM, and criteria similar to those discussed above should be applied for their discrimination.

On occasion, nonmelanocytic lesions are considered in the differential diagnosis of SSM. The principal conditions include Paget's disease, either mammary or extramammary, squamous cell carcinoma in situ, sebaceous carcinoma, epidermotropic eccrine carcinoma, cutaneous T-cell lymphoma, and other epidermotropic carcinomas. In most instances, the dilemma can be resolved simply by careful attention to histologic details in routinely stained sections.[38] For example, the absence of melanin (with exceptions), the presence of mucin-containing cells in Paget's disease, and the presence of cells with intercellular bridges and dyskeratotic cells in squamous cell carcinoma in situ argue against melanoma. In some instances, adjunctive studies such as mucin and melanin stains or immunohistochemistry[38] (Table 10-9) may provide additional help in diagnosis. For example, the antibodies against S-100 protein[39,40] and the HMB-45 antigen[41] are fairly specific for melanoma, whereas the CAM 5.2 and 21N antibodies are specific for mammary Paget's disease. CAM 5.2 is a monoclonal antibody directed against cytokeratins with molecular weights 8,18,19,39,43, and 52 kDa, which are expressed in glandular epithelium.[42] The polyclonal antibody 21N reacts with the c-*erb* B_2 protein, which is found in many adenocarcinomas.[43] Guidelines for the further delineation of proliferations with a pagetoid pattern are outlined in Table 10-9 (see also Chap. 2).

Nodular Melanoma

Nodular melanoma (NM) accounts for 10 to 15 percent of melanomas in white individuals[12–15] (see Table 10-5). NM is distinctive if strictly defined as a tumor exclusively in vertical growth (i.e., lacking an associated RGP).[23–28] In all likelihood, moreover, NM includes an assortment of melanomas either originating from the rapid clonal progression of a short-lived RGP no longer recognizable or the de novo development of a VGP of intraepidermal, adnexal, or dermal origin.[20–30] One hypothesis holds that NM

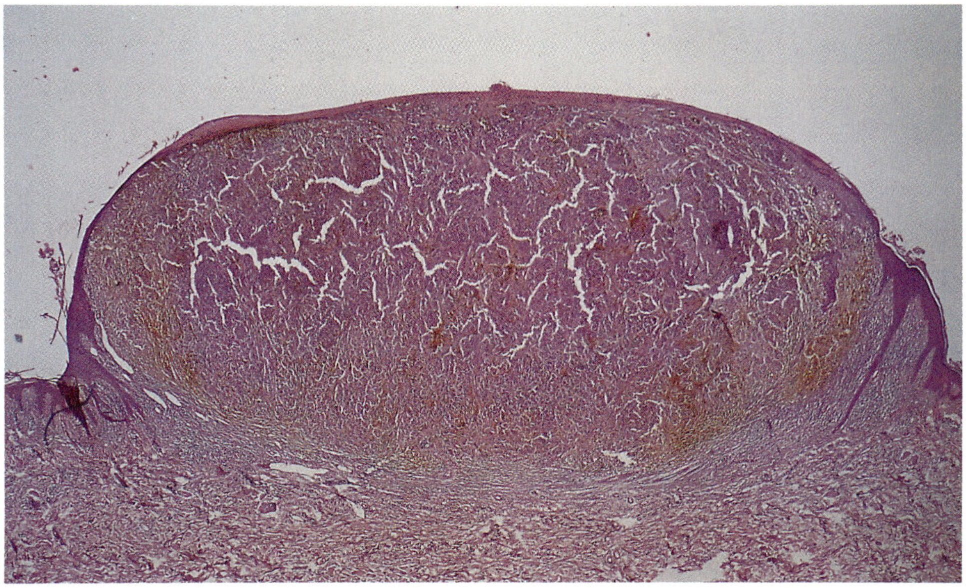

FIGURE 10-6
Nodular melanoma. The tumor has a polypoid configuration with virtually all the tumor above the horizontal plane of the epidermis (H&E, × 20).

represents a final common pathway of very rapid tumor progression from a brief intraepidermal proliferative phase of superficial spreading, lentigo maligna, or acral lentiginous type. This notion has considerable merit, since NM may develop on any anatomic site, the VGP of NM lacks specificity, and the RGP in any given melanoma may vary from a small remnant to an extensive area several centimeters in diameter. It appears that NM is a heterogeneous collection of melanomas of diverse origins that merit more study because of the unique property of rapid tumorigenesis.[15]

Nonetheless, NM shares epidemiologic characteristics with SSM, possibly because NM may often represent a rapidly evolving form of SSM.[27,28] Although NM may occur in any location, it is most common on the trunk.[15]

Clinical Features. The tumor usually presents as a protuberant or polypoid blue-black papule or nodule associated with obliteration of skin markings and frequent ulceration and crust.[12,13,15] A subset of NM lacks pigment and presents as a pink (amelanotic) tumor. A high index of suspicion is needed to diagnose amelanotic NM.

Histologic Features. Scanning magnification discloses a raised, dome-shaped, or polypoid tumor often but not always exhibiting some asymmetry[12–15] (Fig. 10-6 and Table 10-6). Melanoma cells usually occupy the papillary dermis, exhibiting VGP characteristics (Fig. 10-7). The epidermis over the tumor is usually thin, effaced, and may be ulcerated. Variable upward migration of melanoma cells in the epidermis may be present, but intraepidermal spread should not extend beyond the margins of the VGP. If a well-defined adjacent intraepidermal pagetoid component with or without microinvasion is present, the melanoma should be categorized according to the characteristics of the RGP; if not, the tumor should be classified as NM.

The dermal component is typified by a cohesive nodule or smaller nests of tumor cells that have a pushing or expansile pattern of growth[5,15,16] (Figs. 10-8 and 10-9). The tumor cells most frequently are epithelioid (see Fig. 10-7), but other cell types, including spindle cells (see Fig. 10-8), small epithelioid cells resembling nevus cells, and giant mononuclear or multinucleate ("monstrocellular") forms, may predominate or be admixed with other cell types.[15] The cell population usually appears monomorphous, but closer examination reveals frequent cellular enlargement, nuclear enlargement, variation in nuclear size and shape, hyperchromatism, and prominent nucleoli. High nuclear-to-cytoplasmic ratios are often noted. The cytoplasm of epithelioid cells has eosinophilic granular qualities or contains melanin granules that may vary in size. Epithelioid cells often contain finely divided "dusty" melanin granules; but melanin may be absent.

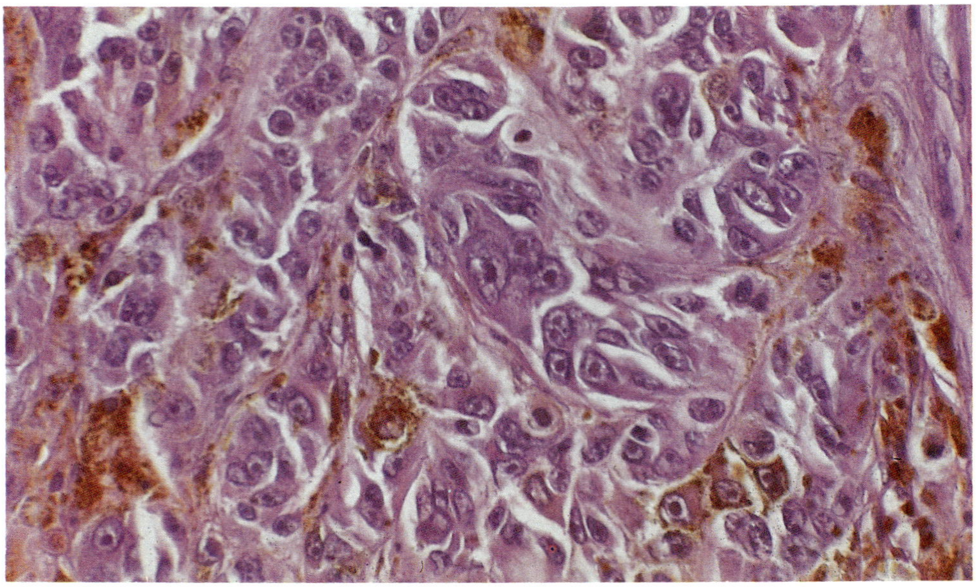

FIGURE 10-7
Nodular melanoma. Typical nest of epithelioid cells in dermis (H&E, × 500).

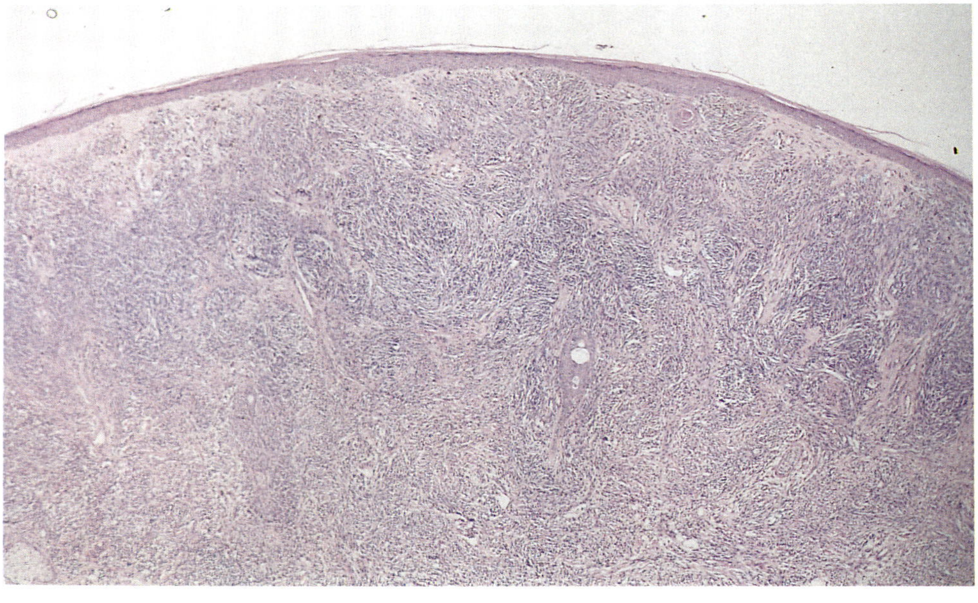

FIGURE 10-8
Nodular melanoma. Fascicles of spindle cells in dermis (H&E, × 40).

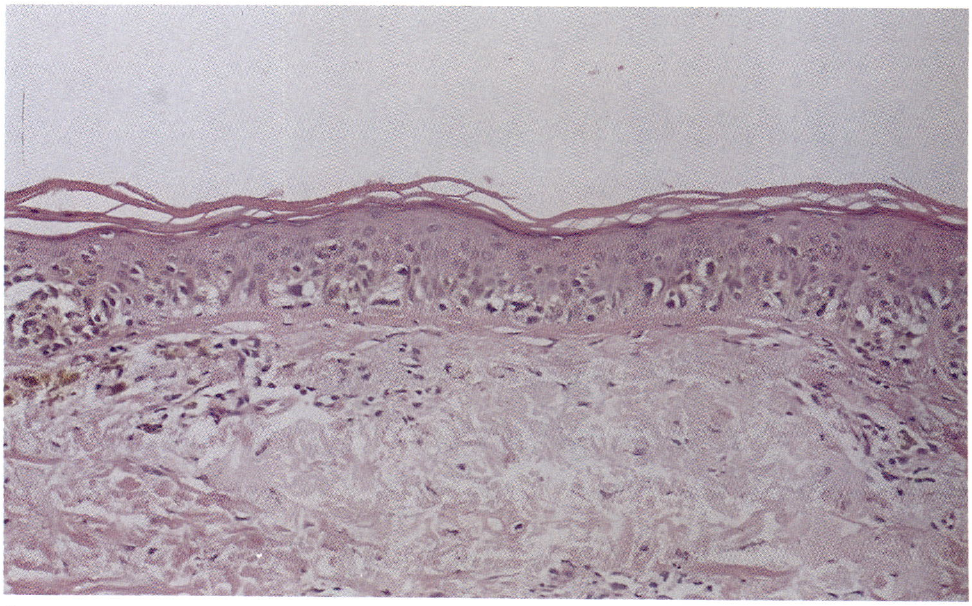

A

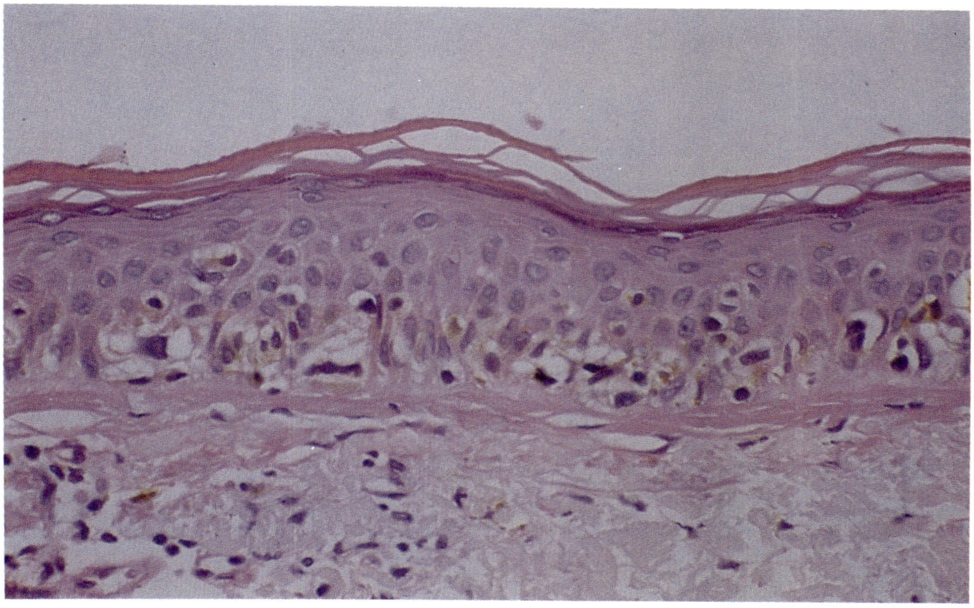

B

FIGURE 10-9

Lentigo maligna and lentigo maligna melanoma. (A) Lentigo maligna. The key features include effacement of epidermis, increased frequency of basilar melanocytes that are atypical, and prominent solar elastosis (H&E, × 200). (B) Higher magnification of part A showing variable atypia of basilar melanocytes. The changes are not sufficiently developed for melanoma in situ but instead are those of a melanocytic dysplasia (H&E, × 400). (C) Lentigo maligna melanoma. There is basilar proliferation of variably atypical melanocytes in both the epidermis and the follicular epithelium (H&E, × 200). (D) Higher magnification showing prominent involvement of a hair follicle by the atypical proliferation of melanocytes. Note highly pleomorphic and hyperchromatic character of nuclei (H&E, × 400). (E) Confluent nesting of melanoma cells along dermoepidermal junction (H&E, × 200). Invasive melanoma cells are also present throughout the papillary dermis. (F) Higher magnification showing prominent nuclear atypia of invasive melanoma cells (H&E, × 400). (G) The vertical growth phase of lentigo maligna melanoma commonly consists of bundles of monomorphous spindle cells as noted in this field (H&E, × 400).

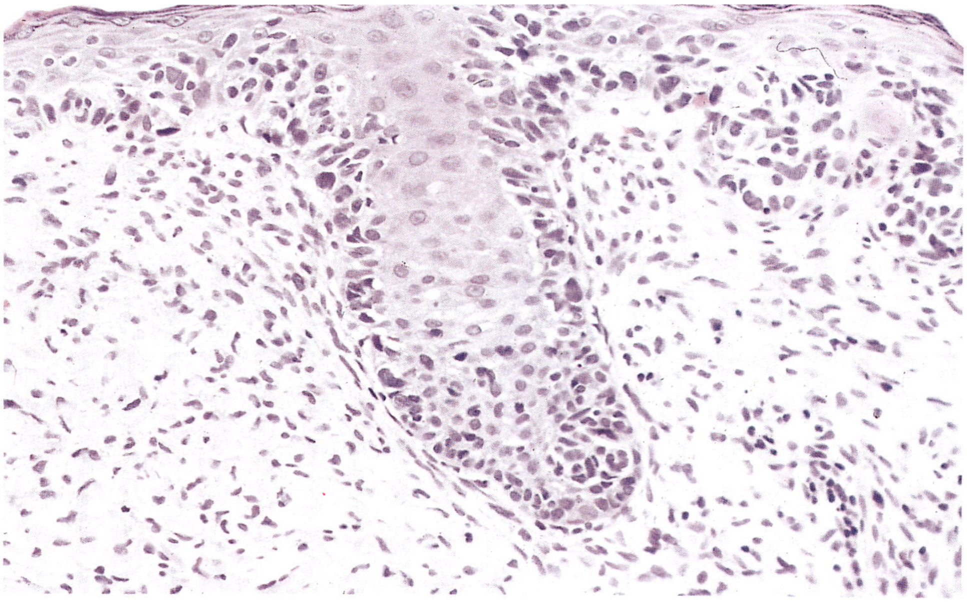

C

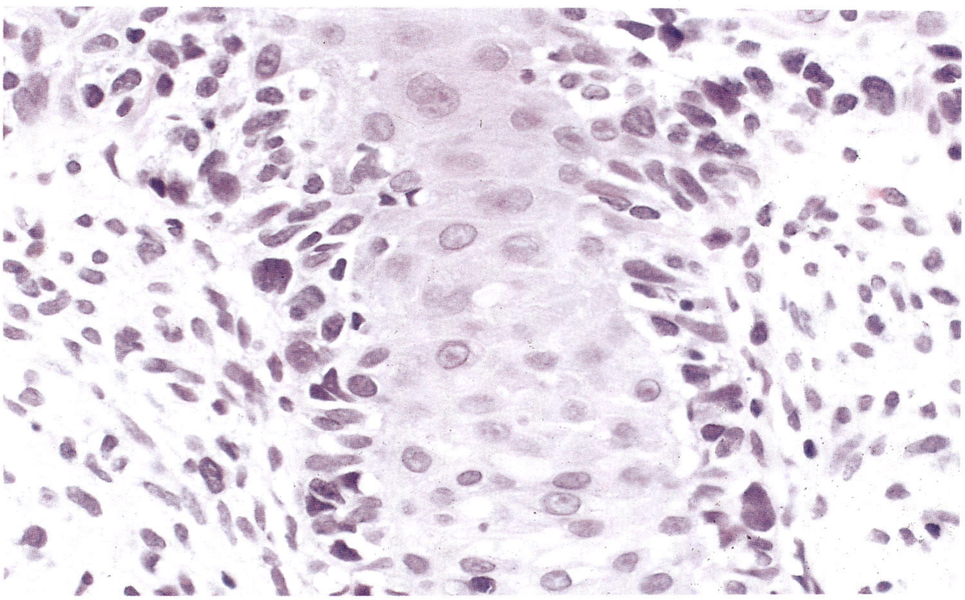

D

FIGURE 10-9 *(Continued)*

The surrounding stroma may demonstrate variable mononuclear cell infiltrates, fibroplasia, telangiectasia, and melanophages.

Differential Diagnosis NM may be confused with metastatic melanoma, spindle and epithelioid cell nevus, atypical cellular blue nevus, squamous cell carcinoma, atypical fibroxanthoma, fibrous histiocytoma, leiomyosarcoma, myoid fibroma, cellular capillary hemangioma, and Kaposi's sarcoma (see Table 10-8). Epidermotropic metastatic melanoma involving the papillary dermis may prove difficult to distinguish from NM (see Chap. 11).[44] Metastatic melanoma is often fairly monomorphous with little stromal response, while NMs are often polymorphous and exhibit greater stromal response. However, distinction may be impossible in certain cases, and

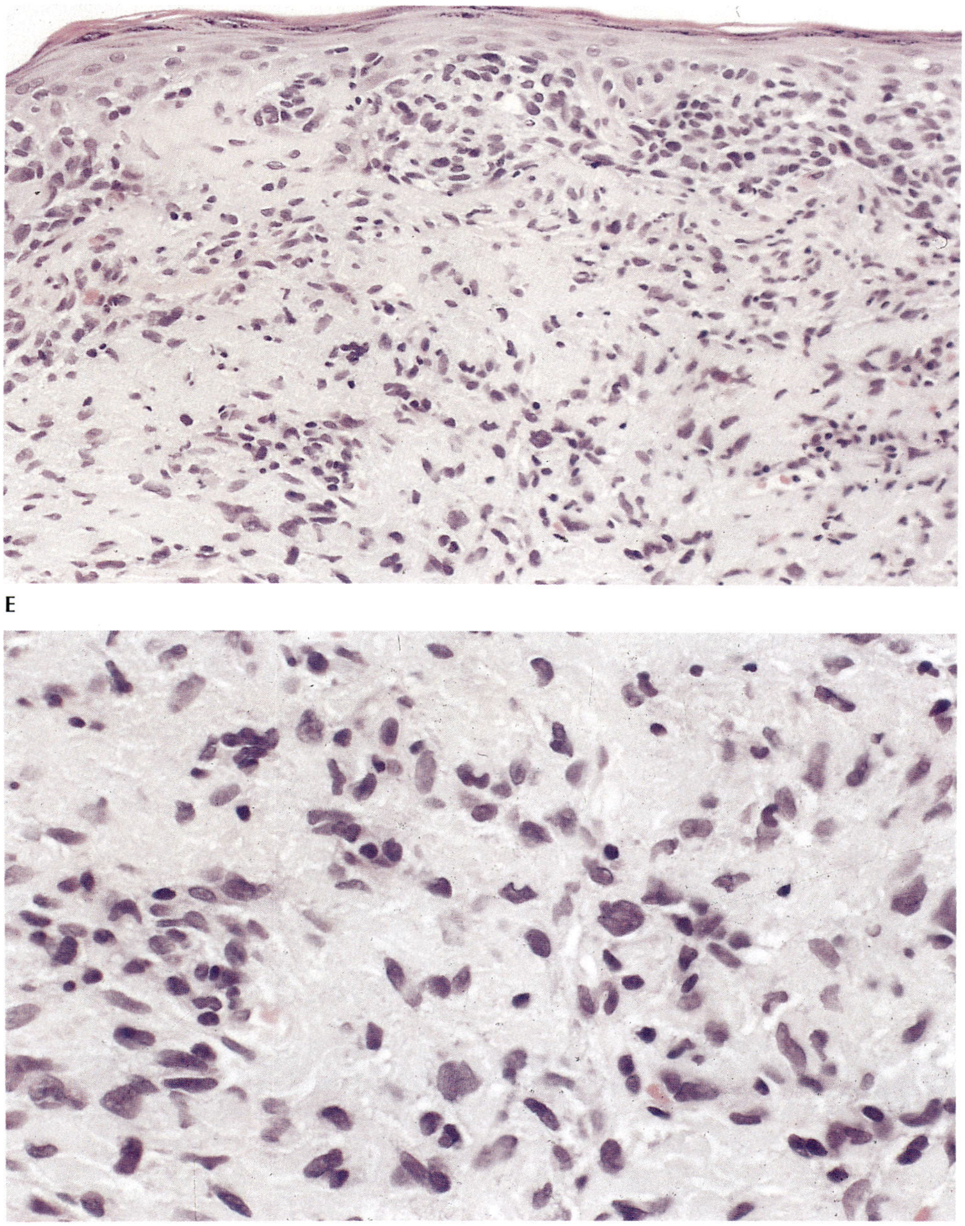

E

F

FIGURE 10-9 *(Continued)*

discrimination must rely on clinical information and clinical course.

Certain spindle and epithelioid (Spitz's) cell nevi, particularly those with atypia, enter into the differential diagnosis of NM, and this is discussed in Chapter 6. Clinical information is pertinent to the diagnosis, since melanoma is uncommon in the young, whereas atypical lesions are more suspicious for melanoma in adults.

Lentigo Maligna Melanoma

Synonyms: melanoma arising in Hutchinson's melanotic freckle; melanoma arising in precancerous melanosis of Dubreuilh

Lentigo maligna melanoma (LMM) is a distinctive form of melanoma arising on sun-exposed (mainly cheek)[15] skin of the elderly and is associated with cumulative sunlight exposure[12–15,18] (see Table 10-5). The most common

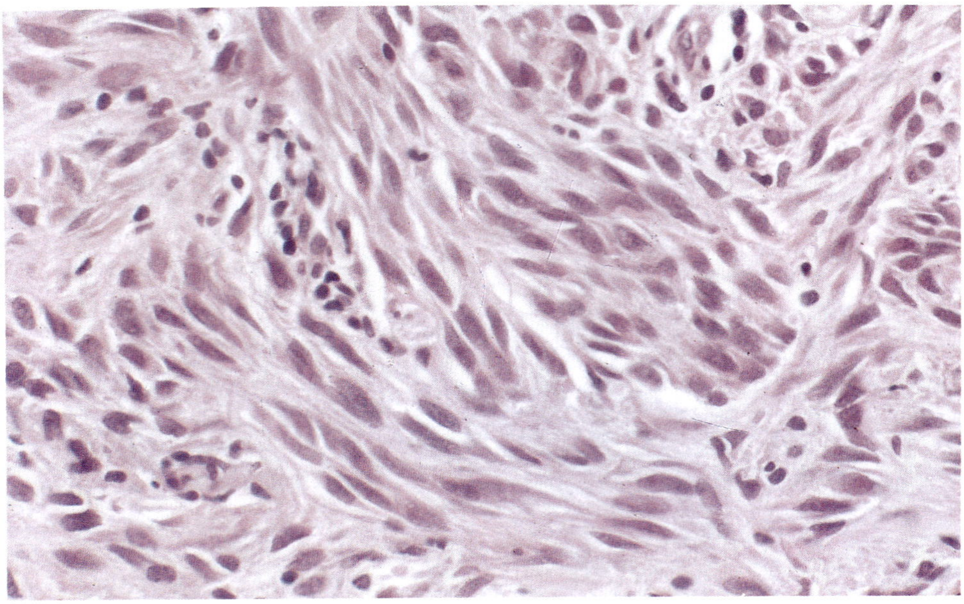

G

FIGURE 10-9 *(Continued)*

age of onset is in the seventh decade, although it may be seen in the thirties and fourties in high-sun areas. Approximately 5 to 10 percent of melanomas of Caucasians are of the lentigo maligna subtype.[15] LMM is the most common form of melanoma occurring in patients with xeroderma pigmentosum, a rare genetic disease associated with defective DNA repair.

Clinical Features. LMM often develops after an indolent period of growth (up to 20 to 30 years) as its precursor lesion LM (Hutchinson's melanotic freckle). The lesion often begins as a brown macule that enlarges with considerable irregularity and variegation of the pigment pattern. Shades of tan, brown, dark brown, and black are often present. The VGP of LMM occurs in 5 to 30 percent of LMs[45] and is often a black, raised focus, or pink (amelanotic) tumor.

Histologic Features. Lentigo maligna is characterized by a histologic spectrum from slightly increased numbers of basilar melanocytes with variable, low-grade cytologic atypia (see Figs. 10-9*A* and *B*) to a contiguous and often nested intraepidermal proliferation of highly pleomorphic melanocytic cells[18] (see Fig. 10-9*C* and Table 10-6). The latter histologic picture is that of melanoma in situ. Some pathologists consider all LMs as melanoma in situ; however, this author and other authorities do not. In addition to a mainly basilar proliferation of melanocytes (see Fig. 10-9*A* and *B*), LM is also characterized by atrophy and effacement of the epidermis (see Fig. 10-9*A*), involvement of appendageal structures (see Fig. 10-9*C* and *D*), and marked solar elastosis.[12–15,18] However, the presence of the latter changes may simply be related to anatomic site; i.e., the skin of the cheek in older individuals usually exhibits a flattened epidermis and prominent solar elastosis in the dermis. The evolution of LM is typified by progressively increased frequency of basilar melanocytes eventually reaching confluence and the development of nests of cells with diminished cohesion (see Fig. 10-9*E*). There may be prominent involvement of appendageal epithelium in some cases with large cellular nests. Recognition of prominent appendageal involvement by LM, or any melanoma, is of critical importance so that the lesion is not misdiagnosed as invasive melanoma rather than simply as an intraepithelial or in situ component. One of the most difficult problems associated with LM is undoubtedly the distinction of invasive tumor from both intraepidermal and appendageal intraepithelial nests of melanoma cells. Careful serial sections may be of help in resolving this dilemma. With progression of LM, there is a tendency for upward migration of cells and microinvasion of the papillary dermis. The cell type typical for LM is a cell with retracted cytoplasm, an often elongate, stellate, or spindled configuration,[18] and a high nuclear-to-cytoplasmic ratio. The nuclei are commonly pleomorphic and hyperchromatic (see Fig. 10-9*E* and *F*). Multinucleate giant cells with peripherally arranged nuclei in a wreath-like pattern are frequent but are not unique to LM. With progression, the cells become more epithelioid in appearance and exhibit nuclear enlargement and prominent nucleoli (see Fig. 10-1*B*). Epidermal hyperplasia also may be encountered in the latter context. A characteristic feature of LM in many instances is the presence of prominent spindle cell differentiation with formation of confluent fascicles of spindle cells along the dermoepidermal junction and also involving appendages[18] (Fig. 10-9*E*). The discohesive qualities of some aggregates of these cells have been likened to a "nest of swallows."

Extension of LMM into the dermis may be difficult to recognize because of prominent cellularity of the stroma and activation of mesenchymal cells (Fig. 10-9*E* and *F*). The invasive dermal component of LMM is frequently composed of spindle cells occurring either singly or in bundles[20] (Fig. 10-9*G*) with varying stromal desmoplasia and invasion of nerve twigs (see Desmoplastic Melanoma, below). It is important to emphasize that invasion of the dermis may originate from appendageal-associated melanoma cells or nests. In the latter instances, depth of invasion (Breslow thickness) should not be measured from the granular layer of the epidermis, since this value would overestimate tumor depth. The measurement of tumor thickness instead ideally should be taken from the granular layer of the hair follicle or sweat gland. The stromal response usually includes lymphocytic infiltrates, prominent vascularity, and melanin-containing macrophages.

The VGP of LMM is most often composed of cohesive nodules of spindle cells (Fig. 10-9*G*), but epithelioid cells and small nevus-like cells are also occasionally observed. The invasive component of LMM may be so well-differentiated that one may consider the lesion to be an unusual nevus, whether composed of spindle cells or small nevus-like cells. Usually the abnormal intraepidermal component, irregular patterns of growth in the dermis, mitotic figures, and necrotic cells should favor melanoma.

Differential Diagnosis. LM and LMM must be distinguished from solar lentigo, dysplastic nevus, pigmented spindle cell nevus, and superficial spreading melanoma (see Table 10-8). LM may in fact develop from some varieties of solar lentigo. Solar lentigo is usually characterized by elongated epidermal rete ridges, an increased frequency of basilar melanocytes but not as great as that seen in LM, and minimal or no cytologic atypia. Well-differentiated forms of LMM with spindle cells may cause confusion with pigmented spindle cell nevus (PSCN). Typical PSCN usually involves covered skin and commonly occurs in children and young adults,[46] whereas LMM invariably develops in sun-exposed skin and usually in older persons. An effaced epidermis, cellular nests with diminished cohesion, and a prominent basilar single-cell proliferation of markedly atypical spindle cells argue in favor of LMM. Pigmented spindle cell nevi are usually well circumscribed with well-formed, orderly, and regular fascicles of pigmented spindle cells. Epidermal hyperplasia usually encountered in PSCN contrasts with the atrophy of LMM. Cytologically, PSCN is usually composed of monotonous fusiform cells with nuclei containing delicate chromatin. Nonetheless, atypical varieties of PSCN may show considerable overlap with LMM.

Advanced LMM may exhibit epithelioid cells with some upward migration through the epidermis, suggesting SSM. Careful evaluation of such tumors usually will disclose a predominance of basilar melanocytic cells, effacement of the epidermis, marked solar elastosis, and prominent involvement of skin appendages. A small minority of cases display overlapping features and are best left unclassified (see under SSM).

Acral Lentiginous Melanoma

Synonym: plantar lentiginous melanoma

Acral lentiginous melanoma (ALM), although accounting for 5 percent or less of melanomas among Caucasians, is the most frequent form of melanoma among Asians, blacks, and other ethnic groups of color[15,20,24,25,47] (see Table 10-5). It should be emphasized, however, that approximately the same incidence of ALM occurs in all ethnic groups. The cause of ALM is the least understood among the various subtypes of melanoma, since sunlight would not seem to be a risk factor. Although poorly documented, trauma has been implicated, and viruses and chemical carcinogens also have been suggested as possible etiologic agents for ALM. This subtype of melanoma usually occurs in older individuals on the palms, soles, and subungual sites.[15] The tumor is usually diagnosed at an advanced stage because of neglect and failure to seek medical attention or misdiagnosis as traumatic injury or a banal process such as verrucae.

Clinical Features. ALM usually evolves through an intraepidermal macular phase, characterized by increasing size, irregularity of borders, and variegation of color.[15,20,24,25,47–49] However, the macular RGP often has a striking black color. The VGP is usually associated with a focal elevated portion that is often dusky blue, black, or amelanotic, and ulceration is common.

Histologic Features. These tumors are usually advanced, often ulcerated, and characterized by a tumor nodule frequently extending deeply into the stroma.[15,20,24,25,47] Scanning magnification usually will reveal an RGP with a hyperplastic epidermis and lentiginous proliferation of variably atypical melanocytic cells (Figs. 10-10 and 10-11 and Table 10-6). These cells are commonly contiguous with occasional clustering, appear to lie within lacunae, and display prominent dendrites that extend through the epidermis (see Fig. 10-11*A* and *B*). The nuclei are enlarged, hyperchromatic, and often

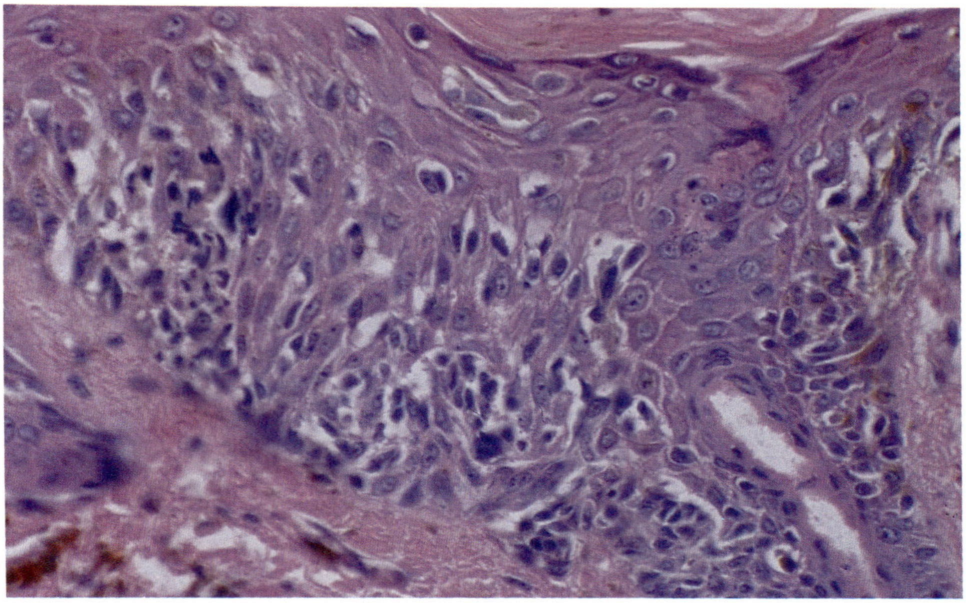

FIGURE 10-10
Acral lentiginous melanoma in situ. There is a disorderly proliferation of atypical basilar melanocytes with some pagetoid spread (H&E, × 400).

highly pleomorphic (see Fig. 10-11*B*). With tumor progression, there is a tendency for upward migration and dermal invasion (see Fig. 10-10). Variable degrees of melanization are present. From the center of the lesion toward the periphery, there is commonly a diminution in both the frequency and atypia of intraepidermal melanocytes such that the diagnosis of melanoma may legitimately be in doubt (this point holds for all melanomas in radial growth). The RGP is usually typified by relatively dense mononuclear cell infiltrates in a thickened, fibrotic papillary dermis and foci of regression.[25]

The dermal component is most often composed of spindle cells (see Fig. 10-14*A* and *B*), but epithelioid cells, small nevus-like cells, and highly pleomorphic cell types are occasionally noted.[25] A small proportion of ALMs exhibit desmoplasia and neurotropism (see below). The VGP consists of a cohesive proliferation of melanoma cells, most often spindle cell in character (Fig. 10-12).

Subungual Melanoma

Synonym: melanoma of the nail apparatus

Subungual melanoma (SM) is a distinctive variant of ALM that involves the nail apparatus.[48,50,51] References to this form of melanoma are present in the medical literature as early as 1854. However, Sir Jonathan Hutchinson first described the entity as "melanotic whitlow" and is credited with the observation that hyperpigmentation extending onto periungual skin, Hutchinson's sign, often indicates subungual melanoma.[48] The median age of patients with subungual melanoma is approximately 64 years.[48] These tumors most often involve the nail bed of the great toe or thumb, where they often present as an ulcerated tumor of the nail bed. However, the initial manifestations may include a longitudinal pigmented band of the nail plate (frequently $\geq$ 9 mm in width) or a mass under the nail plate.[52] The presence of hyperpigmentation extending onto periungual skin should strongly suggest subungual melanoma. Subungual melanomas are often treated initially as infections, granulation tissue, or verrucae.[48] Other clinical findings include shedding of the nail, pain, and bleeding.

Histologic Features. (As described for ALM.) Approximately 50 percent of these tumors exhibit an adjacent RGP[48,50,51] (Fig. 10-13). The VGP, as in other forms of ALM, is usually composed of spindle cells, but epithelioid cells are also occasionally noted. Some tumors may exhibit deep extension with invasion of bone, a number are desmoplastic-neurotropic, and some may exhibit a prominent fibrovascular stromal alteration.[48]

Differential Diagnosis. The differential diagnosis for ALM (including SM) includes primarily lentigines and lentiginous melanocytic nevi of acral skin (see Table 10-8).

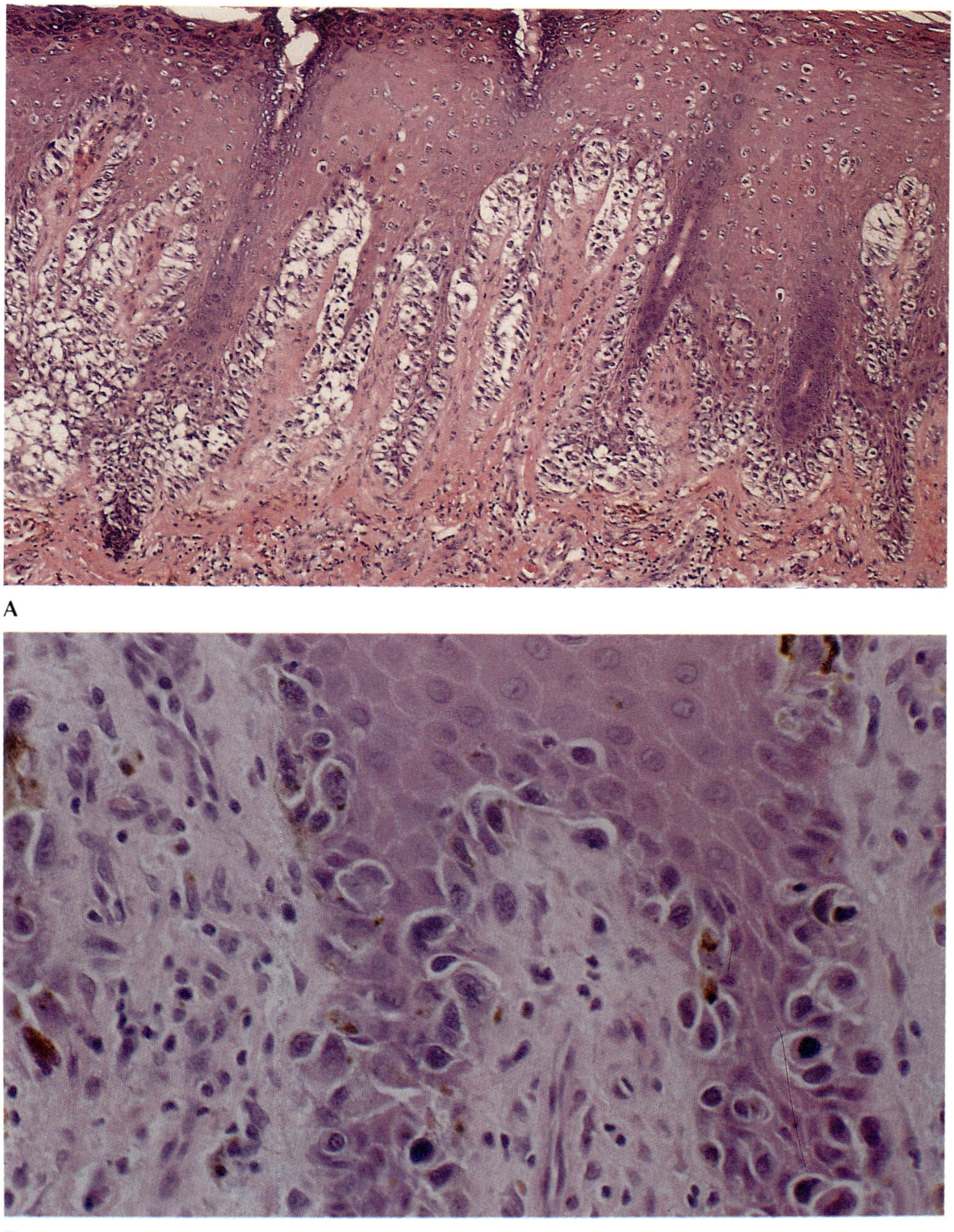

FIGURE 10-11
Acral lentiginous melanoma, radial growth phase. (A) The epidermis is hyperplastic and exhibits characteristic lentiginous proliferation of pleomorphic melanoma cells. There is minimal upward migration of cells throughout epidermis (H&E, × 100). (B) There is confluence of highly atypical melanocytes along the basal layer of the epidermis (H&E, × 400).

Lentigines of acral skin usually do not exhibit the frequency of melanocytic proliferation or cytologic atypia that is typical of ALM.[25,48] Occasional acral nevi may have alarming features such as upward migration of cells throughout the epidermis, prominent lentiginous melanocytic proliferation, and some degree of cytologic atypia. Although upward migration may be noted in acral nevi, particularly in children, the constituent cells seldom reveal more than low-grade cytologic atypia, and the pattern of pagetoid spread is usually orderly and confined to the lower-most epidermis. Other characteristics of acral nevi include regular size, spacing, and cohesive qualities

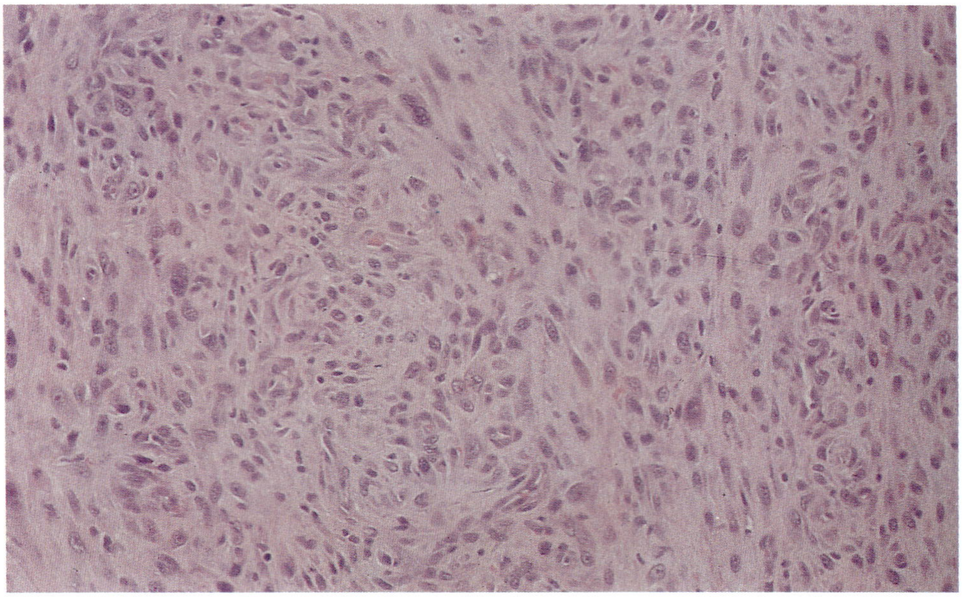

FIGURE 10-12
Acral lentiginous melanoma, vertical growth phase. Fascicles of plump spindle cells are distributed throughout the dermis (H&E, × 200).

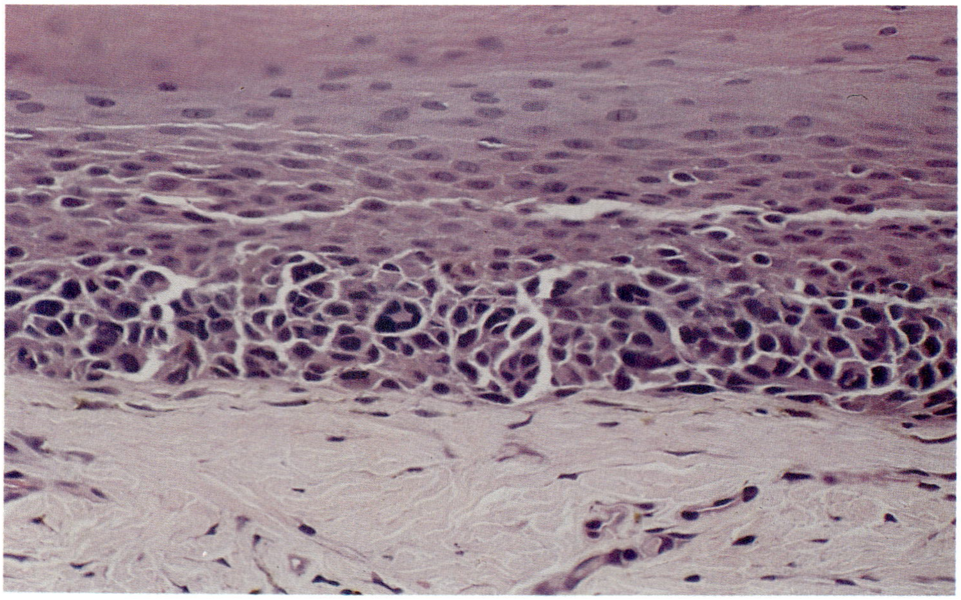

FIGURE 10-13
Subungual melanoma in situ. The basilar portion of the squamous epithelium is replaced by atypical melanocytes (H&E, × 200).

of the junctional nesting. One particular note of caution is that well-differentiated ALM may exhibit dermal components with little or no inflammatory response. In such cases, careful evaluation for cytologic atypia, necrotic cells, and mitotic activity is helpful in recognizing melanoma.

Mucosal Lentiginous Melanoma

Synonyms: mucosal melanoma; mucocutaneous melanoma.

Primary melanomas of mucosal sites such as the oral cavity, nasal cavity, vulva, vagina, and anorectum often share clinical and histologic features in common with acral lentiginous (and lentigo maligna) melanoma (see above).[53] In general, many of these mucosal lentiginous melanomas appear to develop from atypical lentiginous melanocytic proliferations of mucosal epithelium and often subsequently exhibit lentiginous RGPs. The most common cell type comprising these lesions is a pleomorphic spindled or dendritic melanocyte. Some mucosal melanomas also show intraepithelial pagetoid spread. Nodular melanomas may involve mucosal surfaces and, as with all nodular melanomas, must be distinguished from metastatic melanoma. The invasive component of mucosal lentiginous melanoma is often composed of pleomorphic or small round cells,[54] but spindle cells and epithelioid cells are also observed. As with other lentiginous melanomas, the invasive component is not uncommonly desmoplastic-neurotropic (see below). In general, mucosal melanomas are highly aggressive tumors and are associated with a dismal prognosis.

UNUSUAL HISTOLOGIC AND CYTOLOGIC VARIANTS OF THE INVASIVE DERMAL COMPONENT OF MELANOMA

Desmoplastic Melanoma

This rare variant of melanoma is defined primarily by a distinctive histomorphologic pattern of invasive melanoma typified by a fibrous nodule filling the dermis and commonly extending into subcutaneous fat, corresponding to a firm or indurated nodule clinically.[55-74] In reality, desmoplastic melanoma exhibits a continuum of histologic features corresponding to the neuroectodermal origin of the melanocyte. The phenotype of the tumor may thus include any combination of the following: desmoplasia—fibroblast-like spindle cells usually in fascicles (predominant pattern), neurotropism (perineurial invasion)—invasion of nerve structures by tumor cells (see Neurotropic Melanoma, below); neural differentiation (both schwannian and perineurial)—formation of nervelike structures recapitulating perineurium and endoneurium or delicate sheets of spindle cells reminiscent of neurofibroma (see Neurotropic Melanoma, below); and less commonly neuroendocrine differentiation—as in Merkel cell carcinoma. Desmoplastic melanoma (DM) most frequently arises in association with the lentiginous melanomas, notably LMM, but also the acral and mucosal lentiginous subtypes.[15,20,55-74] However, de novo variants of desmoplastic melanoma also occur. Some of the latter are recurrent tumors,[57-64,70] but some may result from the regression of an intraepidermal component or originate from appendageal melanocytes. Because of the frequent linkage to LMM, these tumors have a predilection for sun-exposed skin of the head and neck and usually affect individuals at least 60 years of age[55-74] (Tables 10-10 and 10-11). From the number

TABLE 10-10

*Précis: Desmoplastic Melanoma**

Clinical features	
	Age 60–65 years
	Men ≥ women
	Sun-exposed skin, head and neck, but also acral, mucosal sites
	Firm nodule
	Flesh-colored or with pigmented lesion (29–43%)
	1 to 3 cm
	Occasional dysesthesias, nerve palsies
Histopathology	
	Intraepidermal melanocytic proliferation in 75 to 85%
	Lentigo maligna, most common
	Fibrous nodule in dermis and possibly subcutis†
	Often absence of pigment
	Atypical spindle cells, usually in fascicles (atypia varies from slight to marked)†
	Schwannian, perineurial differentiation
	Neurotropism common (perineurial and endoneurial invasion)
	Patchy lymphoid infiltrates common
	Variable myxoid stroma
	Occasional mitoses in dermis
Differential diagnosis	
	Sclerosing blue nevi including variants with hypercellularity
	Desmoplastic (sclerosing) Spitz nevus
	Neurothekeoma, particularly cellular variants
	Malignant peripheral nerve-sheath tumors
	Myxoma
	Dermatofibroma
	Dermatofibrosarcoma protuberans
	Atypical fibroxanthoma
	Malignant fibrous histiocytoma
	Scar
	Fibromatosis
	Spindle cell squamous cell carcinoma
	Leiomyosarcoma

*Neurotropic melanoma shows considerable overlap with desmoplastic melanoma but uncommonly may occur as a separate entity.

†Essential feature needed for diagnosis of desmoplastic melanoma.

TABLE 10-11
Previously Reported Series of Desmoplastic Melanoma

Author	*No. of Cases*	*Mean Age (years)*	*Thickness, Level*	*Follow-up Period (years)*	*Local Recurrence*	*Distant Metastasis*	*Survival*
Reed and Leonard*[73]	22	59.1	NA	2–9 (mean 3.4)	77%	32%	44%
Reiman[56]	9	64.7	NA	1.3–10	22%	56%	34%
Egbert[57]	25	61.2	Level IV or V	0.1–9 (mean 2.7)	52%	22%	87%
Walsh[58]	14	55.4	Level III—7% Level IV—64% Level V—21%	0.4–23 (median 4.6)	43%	14%	86%
Beenken[59]	16	62.7	5.75 mm	2–12 (mean 1.5)	46.2%	38%	69.2%
Jain[60]	45	71	NA	0.3–15 (mean 4.6)	55%	40%	64%
Smithers[61]	45	61	4.5 mm Level II—2% Level IV—42% Level V—49%	0.1–9	27%	11%	89%

*Mainly neurotropic melanoma.
NA, not available.

of cases seen in our own referral center and the frequency of reports of such cases (<400 cases), desmoplastic melanomas and their variants are rare.

Although the natural history of DM has not been fully characterized, DM may differ from conventional melanoma by showing a greater propensity for local recurrences, a lower rate of lymph node metastasis, and possibly a more favorable prognosis; however, this has not been rigorously validated.[59-61,70,72]

Clinical Features. The usual presentation is as a raised, firm nodule that is flesh-colored or associated with variable pigmentation[55-74] (Table 10-10). The irregular and variegated features of an associated RGP or intraepithelial component such as LM may be the most visible component of desmoplastic melanoma. Difficulty in recognizing desmoplastic melanoma, clinically and histologically, usually causes a delay in diagnosis and appropriate surgery.

Histologic Features. Scanning magnification usually discloses a fibrous nodule displacing the normal dermal collagen or lamina propria and often extending into subcutaneous fat[70-72] (Table 10-10 and Fig. 10-14*A*). An intraepidermal melanocytic proliferation is usually observed in approximately 75 to 85 percent of DMs reported in the literature.[72] In a recent series of 28 cases, 48 percent of DMs had an intraepidermal component of LM as compared with 15 percent in the literature.[72] An additional 33 percent of the latter cases and 56 percent from the literature showed a component best described as a lentiginous proliferation of atypical melanocytes rather than LM.[72] Four percent of the cases exhibited an intraepidermal pattern consistent with superficial spreading melanoma. Fifteen percent of the DMs did not show any evidence of an intraepidermal melanocytic component, and this has been similarly observed in 13 percent of cases reported from the literature. With increasing depth of DM, there is a tendency for the intraepidermal component to become disassociated from the dermal component or completely lost.[72] In sum, intraepidermal melanocytic proliferation, whether sufficiently developed for LM or not, is often present, usually in sun-exposed skin (see Fig. 10-10*A*). Marked solar degeneration of collagen is an almost invariable finding in these sun-exposed sites.[72]

As mentioned earlier, the most common histologic pattern of DM is a predominantly desmoplastic presentation.[70-72] Interspersed among dense collagenous fibers are individual spindle cells and variably sized fascicles of cells (see Fig. 10-14*B*). The nuclei may show slight to pronounced pleomorphism and wavy or serpiginous morphology (Fig. 10-15*A* and *B*), though most nuclei are enlarged and exhibit tapering contours. However, some nuclei are plump, and occasional bizarre multinucleate giant cell forms are noted. Most desmoplastic melanomas lack pigment, but occasional cells may contain fine melanin granules within cellular processes. The tumor stroma is usually fibrous, but myxoid alteration is occasionally encountered and uncommonly may be prominent.[70]

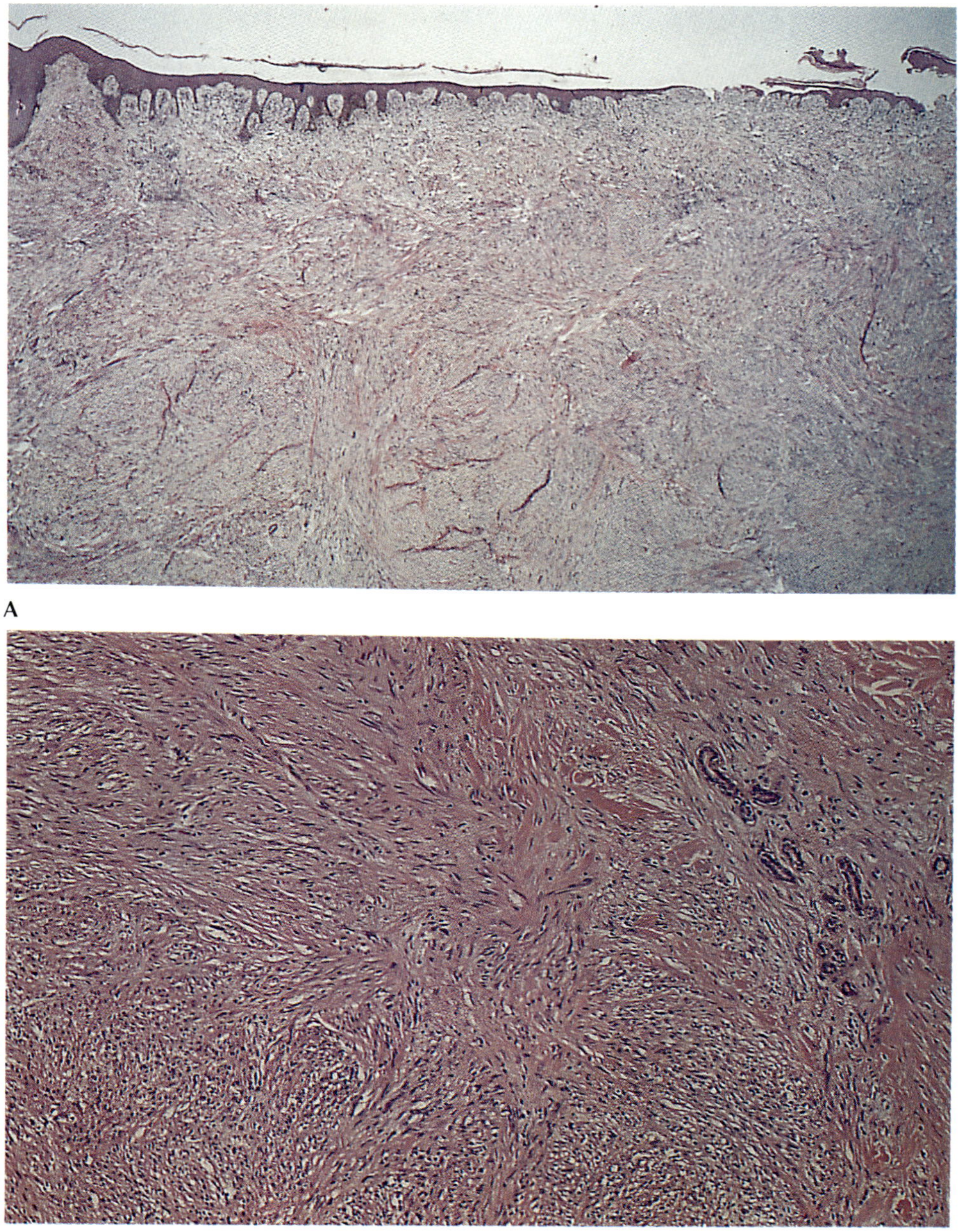

FIGURE 10-14

Desmoplastic melanoma. (A) Fibrotic nodule occupies dermis (H&E, × 20). (B) Intersecting fascicles of spindle cells with dense fibrous stroma (H&E, × 100).

The fascicles of spindle cells may blend with the perineurium of cutaneous nerves such that tumor cells comprise the perineurium. Tumor cells also may infiltrate the endoneurium (neurotropism).[57,60,61,70,72,73] Care must be exercised in assessing neurotropism because the tumor cells may be arranged in wavy fascicles and resemble neural tissue[57–61,72,73] (see Fig. 10-15C). Concentric, whorled arrangements of cells may resemble a neuroma.[70] The tumor cells in desmoplastic melanoma are also notable for infiltrating walls of blood vessels. Mitotic figures usually can be found even in the most paucicellular forms of this tumor.[70–72]

A finding typical of desmoplastic melanoma and useful in its recognition is the presence of variably dense

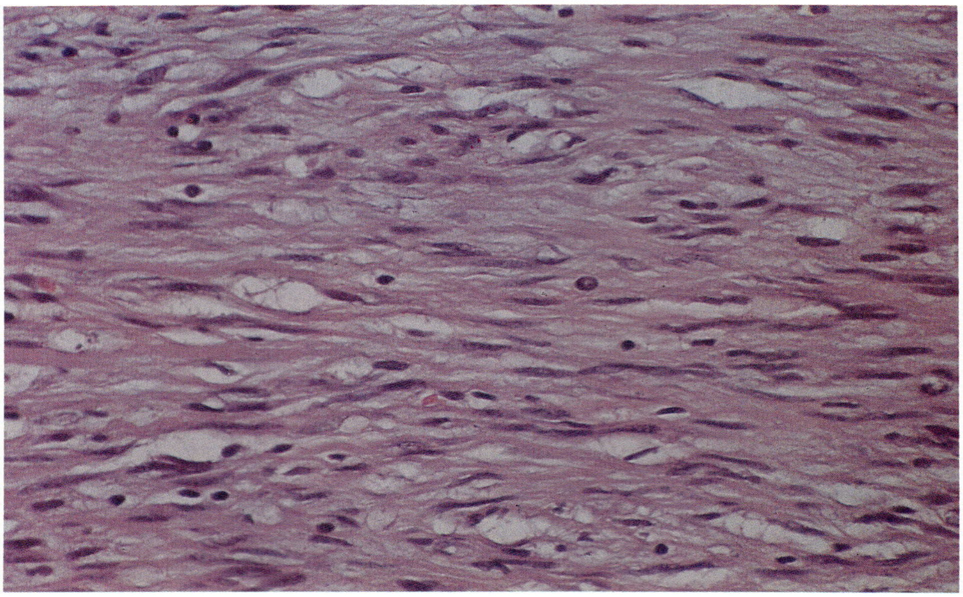

A

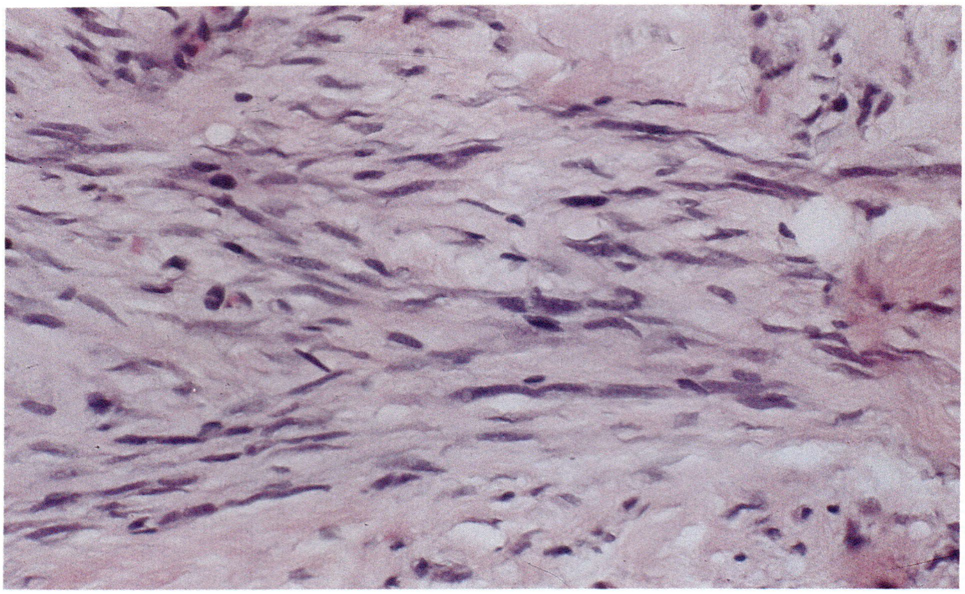

B

FIGURE 10-15

Desmoplastic-neurotropic melanoma. (A) Linear array of spindle cells disposed in dense fibrotic matrix (H&E, × 400). (B) Fascicles of spindle cells contain elongated, wavy, hyperchromatic nuclei (H&E, × 400). (C) This field shows nuclei dispersed in delicate matrix resembling a neurofibroma (schwannian differentiation) (H&E, × 200).

perivascular lymphocytic infiltrates usually scattered throughout the tumor.[70]

Desmoplastic melanoma is usually diagnosed at an advanced stage, since they are usually at least 4 or 5 mm in thickness and level IV or V[55–74] (Tables 10-10 and 10-11). Because of misdiagnosis, they are commonly first recognized as recurrent or metastatic tumors. Desmoplastic melanomas frequently recur (range 25 to 82 percent).[55–61,70] Based on a series of 45 cases, local recurrence was associated with the following factors: failure to diagnose the tumor correctly, inadequate surgery (resection margins less than 1 cm), location on the head and neck,

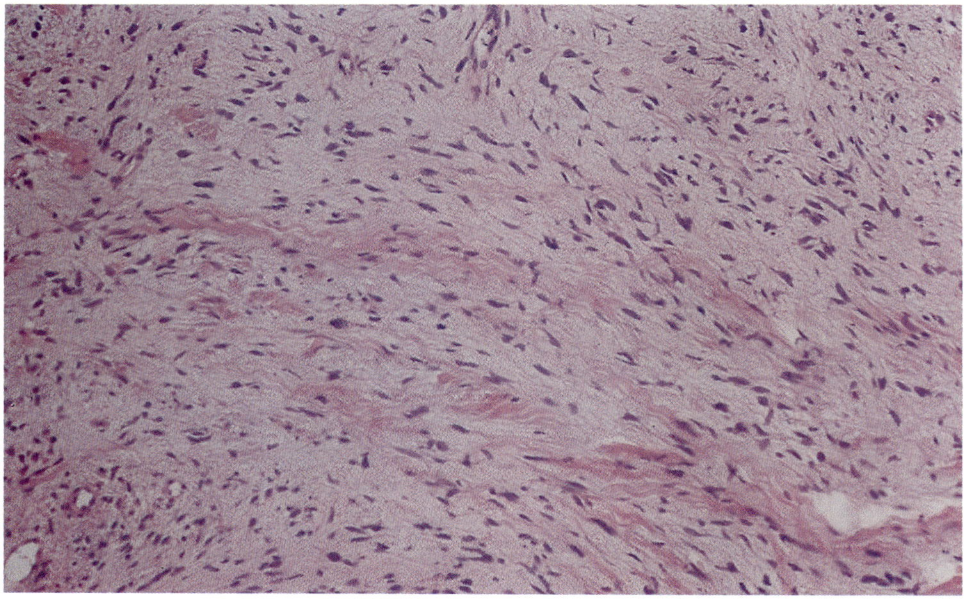

C

FIGURE 10-15 *(Continued)*

anatomic level V, and thickness greater than 4 mm.[61] Failure to completely extirpate desmoplastic melanoma is related to the difficulty of assessing margins, infiltration of nerves, and the fact that they are usually amelanotic.

Histogenesis. The pathogenesis of desmoplasia and the true nature of the spindle cells in desmoplastic melanoma remain a subject of controversy and debate.[55,65,66,68,69] Some authors maintain that the fibroplasia results from the induction of collagen synthesis by benign fibroblasts, while others believe that melanoma cells function as adaptive fibroblasts to promote collagenization in these tumors.[66]

Recent experimental work utilizing human melanoma cell lines injected into nude mice provides new information possibly relevant to the natural history and pathogenesis of DM.[75] One particular cell line, UCT-Mel7, when injected into nude mice, results in a tumor with many characteristics of DM: desmoplastic stroma and indolent growth in contrast to the inexorable proliferation and dissemination associated with other melanoma cell lines. It is of interest that the desmoplasia elicited by UCT-Mel7 correlated with slow growth; i.e., the collagen content of the tumor was inversely related to cell growth. In additional studies, coculture of UCT-Mel7 cells with fibroblasts resulted in a twofold increase in collagen synthesis solely by the fibroblast population.[76] Increased mRNA expression for collagen was observed in the cultured fibroblasts. These data support the origin of collagen production in DM from fibroblasts rather than melanoma cells.

Nevertheless, many authorities counter that the spindle cells in DM are true melanoma cells that have undergone metaplasia to adaptive fibroblasts and thus are themselves capable of collagen synthesis.[65] The latter conclusion results from immunohistochemical and ultrastructural studies[56,66,68–70] (Tables 10-12 and 10-13), and the fact that because of their neural crest origin, melanocytes are capable of collagen production as well as melanin synthesis and schwannian differentiation.[71,72]

By electron microscopy, the spindle cells of DM contain premelanosomes and/or melanosomes, according to some studies (Table 10-13).[64,65] However, other investigators have not detected evidence of melanin synthesis in the tumor cells of DM.[59,67,69,70,72] From and coworkers[65] studied DM by electron microscopy and noted a progressive transition from large, pleomorphic melanocytes near the dermoepidermal junction to fusiform cells in middermis and to predominantly spindle-shaped cells in a desmoplastic stroma in the deep dermis. All these cell types contained non-membrane-bound melanosomes and were positive for S-100 protein. Some of the spindle-shaped cells displayed myofibroblastic differentiation.[66] Valensi, in ultra structural studies of DM,[68,69] reported macular desmosomes between the tumor cells and cited this as evidence that the tumor cells were dedifferentiated melanocytic cells with fibroblastic characteristics rather than true fibroblasts.

TABLE 10-12
Results of Immunohistochemistry Reported for Desmoplastic Melanoma

	Carlson et al[72]	*Literature*
S100	100%	94% (165/175)
Vimentin	100%	92% (23/25)
HMB-45	21%	5% (5/92)
NSE	42%	96% (22/23)
EMA	43%	0 (0/1)
FXIIIa	39%	100% (15/15)
Actin, smooth muscle	52%	—
Leu-7	0	—
Keratins AE1.3	0	0 (0/14)
Cam 5.2	0	—

TABLE 10-13
Results of Electron Microscopy Reported for Desmoplastic Melanoma

	Carlson et al.[72]	*Literature*
Intertwining cell processes	100%	45%
Cell junctions	100%	55%
Basal lamina	57%	39%
Lysosomal-like dense bodies	43%	16%
Premelanosomes	0	19%
Melanosomes	0	26%
Long spacing collagen	28%	0
Myodense bodies	0	26%

Neurotropic Melanoma

Any form of melanoma may show some degree of desmoplasia, neurotropism, or both (Table 10-10).[57-61] To be categorized as DM, the *predominant pattern* of the invasive dermal component should be desmoplastic. The same criterion applies to melanomas designated as *neurotropic.* Most desmoplastic melanomas have some degree of neurotropism or neuroid differentiation. When prominent desmoplasia *and* neurotropism are present, the tumor is designated as *desmoplastic-neurotropic.*

Although the term *neurotropic melanoma*[73] was introduced to describe a specific variant of desmoplastic melanoma that showed infiltration of cutaneous nerves, neural differentiation, or neuroma-like patterns, new terms, recently introduced, emphasize different features in the spectrum of neurotropic melanoma. Jain and Allen[60] described a "nerve-centered" form of desmoplastic melanoma to depict a principally perineural localization of tumor.[60] Smithers et al.[61] have designated melanomas with neural differentiation as "neural transforming." Such tumors have spindle cells with serpiginous morphology dispersed singly or in paucicellular bundles in a delicate, frequently myxoid stroma.

Clinical Features. The clinical presentation of neurotropic melanoma closely parallels that of desmoplastic melanoma because of their frequent association.[70-74] However, melanomas with significant neurotropism often show cranial nerve involvement with consequent palsies and paresthesias.[59] Recurrence and extension of tumor into the brain are more frequent in neurotropic melanoma than in conventional desmoplastic melanoma.[59]

Histologic Features. Neurotropic melanoma is often associated with lentiginous proliferation of atypical melanocytes or lentiginous forms of melanoma within the epidermis and skin appendages.[55-61,72] However, some neurotropic melanomas may arise de novo without an intraepidermal component.[57,72] The skin appendages may be the source of some of these tumors.

The term *neurotropism* refers to the involvement of perineurium and endoneurium of cutaneous nerves by melanoma (spindle) cells[73] (Fig. 10-16*A*, *B*, and *C*). There may be considerable thickening of the perineurium and expansion of the endoneurial space by the tumor involvement.[60,61,70-72] Extension of tumor along the cutaneous nerves, however, may be extensive and subtle. Histologic clues to nerve involvement include the presence of hyperchromatic spindle cells in the perineurium or endoneurium and mucinous alteration of the nerve. Careful examination of cutaneous nerves at the surgical margins is mandatory to assess adequate excision. Melanoma spindle cells involving cutaneous nerves usually show nuclear enlargement, hyperchromatism, and pleomorphism.

The term *neurotropism* also describes neural or schwannian differentiation in a pattern resembling peripheral nerve sheath tumors such as neurofibromas or neuromas and the recapitulation of perineurium and endoneurium[70-74] (see Fig. 10-16*A*, *B*, and *C*). The tumor cells in such areas are characterized by serpiginous or wavy nuclear configurations and filamentous cytoplasmic processes. The cells are embedded in a variably mucinous and fibrous stroma (see Fig. 10-15*C*). In some instances, the stroma may be so sufficiently myxoid to suggest a myxoma. However, the tumor cells demonstrate loose fascicular arrangements, cytologic atypia, and occasional mitotic figures.

Differential Diagnosis. The spectrum of tumors potentially confused with desmoplastic and neurotropic melanoma is varied and includes spindle cell proliferations and tumors with a fibrous appearance[55-74,77] (see Table 10-10). The principal lesions to be considered include sclerosing blue nevus,[70] desmoplastic Spitz nevus,[78]

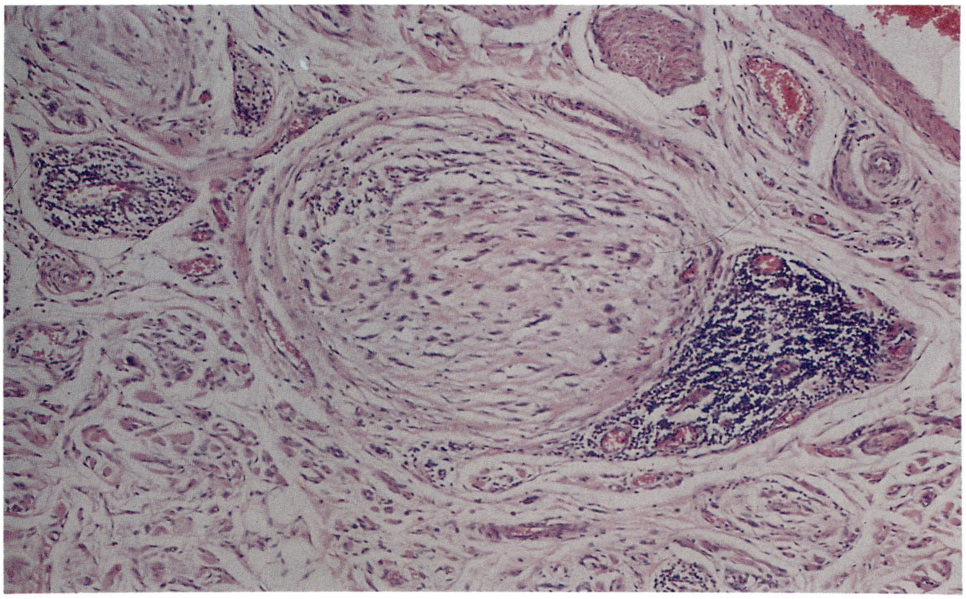

A

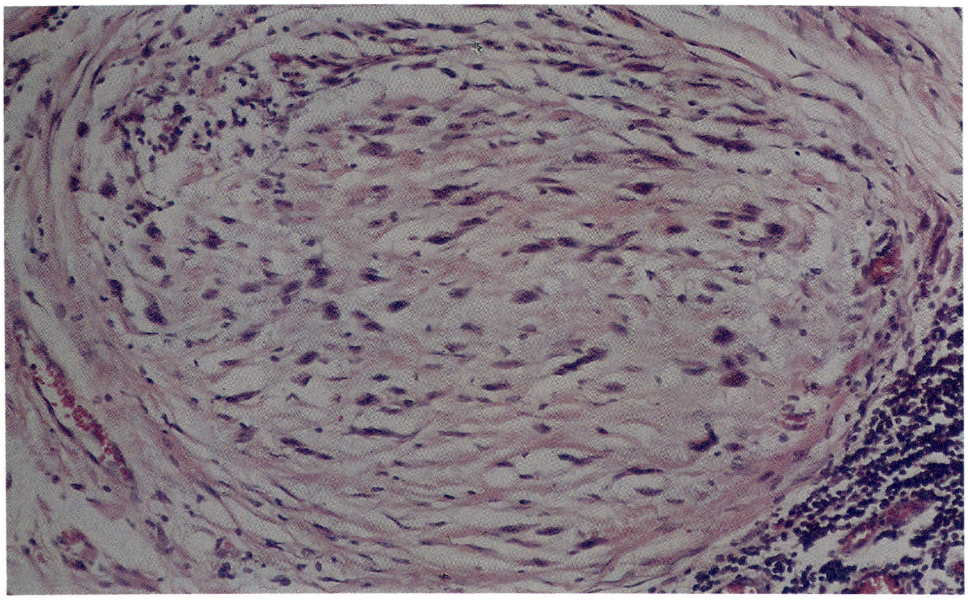

B

FIGURE 10-16

Desmoplastic-neurotropic melanoma. (A) A cutaneous nerve shows prominent perineurial and endoneurial infiltration by melanoma cells (neurotropism) (H&E, × 200). (B) Higher magnification reveals neurotropism by spindle cells with hyperchromatic nuclei (H&E, × 400).

neurothekeoma,[79] malignant peripheral nerve sheath tumor, dermatofibroma, atypical fibroxanthoma, malignant fibrous histiocytoma, scar, fibromatosis, myxoma, spindle cell squamous cell carcinoma, and leiomyosarcoma.[70–74,77] The lentiginous melanocytic proliferation commonly found in desmoplastic melanoma is usually absent in the other conditions.

Sclerosing blue nevus and desmoplastic Spitz nevus[70,78] both are characterized by an orderly infiltration of the fibrotic stroma and an overall benign cytologic appearance. Mitotic figures, usually encountered in desmoplastic melanoma, are exceedingly rare or absent in sclerosing blue nevus, but early forms of desmoplastic melanoma may be exceedingly difficult to distinguish from sclerosing blue nevus,[70,71] and it is vital to weigh all clinical and histologic features. For example, the occurrence of desmoplastic melanoma in a young individual on an anatomic site other than the head and neck or acral areas would be highly unusual, and such circumstances would argue against a diagnosis of desmoplastic melanoma.

The desmoplastic Spitz nevus is characterized by symmetry, an inverted wedge-shaped configuration, and infiltration of the dermis by relatively monotonous epithelioid or spindle cells,[78] allowing its distinction from desmoplastic melanoma in most instances. Desmoplastic melanoma also may show a fascicular arrangement of cells that is generally lacking in desmoplastic Spitz nevus.

Relatively cellular variants of neurothekeoma (nerve sheath myxoma) may suggest desmoplastic melanoma.[79] Neurothekeoma commonly arises in the head and neck region, as does desmoplastic melanoma. Neurothekeoma generally occurs in young individuals (average age 20 years), does not demonstrate an intraepidermal melanocytic proliferation, and is typified by a lobular architecture in the dermis.[79] Concentric and fascicular arrangements of cells are often noted in neurothekeoma, the constituent cells may be epithelioid or bipolar, and stellate and multinucleate forms are seen. Low-grade nuclear pleomorphism and occasional mitotic figures are encountered. Distinction from desmoplastic melanoma is based on a regular, organized appearance, orderly infiltration of the dermis, and a lesser degree of cytologic atypia.[79]

Because of prominent schwannian differentiation, discrimination of desmoplastic-neurotropic melanoma from peripheral nerve sheath tumors may be difficult or impossible. Except for the presence of intraepidermal proliferation of atypical melanocytes, tumors designated as malignant epithelioid schwannoma of superficial soft tissue may be indistinguishable from desmoplastic-necrotropic melanoma. All clinical and histologic characteristics must be considered. Tumors developing in association with intraepidermal proliferation of atypical melanocytes or lentiginous melanomas are usually not a diagnostic problem and should be considered to be melanoma. Tumors without an intraepidermal component will cause difficulty and immunohistochemistry may be of particular value in them (see below).[62,63,80,81]

Lesions demonstrating fibrous or fibrohistiocytic differentiation figure prominently in the differential diagnosis of desmoplastic melanoma and include dermatofibroma (fibrous histiocytoma), juvenile xanthogranuloma, dermatofibrosarcoma protuberans, atypical fibroxanthoma, superficial forms of malignant fibrous histiocytoma, scar, and fibromatosis. These lesions generally lack intraepidermal melanocytic proliferation, melanin pigment, and neurotropism. Atypical fibroxanthoma and malignant fibrous histiocytoma enter the differential diagnosis and often require immunohistochemical evaluation, though they may contain xanthoma cells, which are not usually seen in desmoplastic melanoma. Fibrohistiocytic tumors as a general rule do not display neurotropism.

Desmoplastic melanomas with extensive mucin may raise problems of differential diagnosis, suggesting, for example, a myxoma. However, myxomas generally lack the cytologic atypia and neurotropism of desmoplastic-neurotropic melanoma, and the mxyomatous variants of desmoplastic melanoma usually have zones of prominent cellularity.

Spindle cell squamous carcinoma and cutaneous leiomyosarcoma may be confused with desmoplastic melanoma, but neither of the former two lesions show intraepidermal melanocytic proliferation or melanin synthesis. Squamous cell carcinoma may show keratinization, dyskeratosis, and intercellular bridges. Leiomyosarcoma may exhibit the cytologic characteristics of smooth-muscle cells, but immunohistochemistry may be essential to finalize the diagnosis.

Because of the serious consequences of this tumor, immunohistochemistry is needed in most desmoplastic melanomas to confirm the diagnosis (see Table 10-12). Almost 100 percent of desmoplastic-neurotropic melanomas demonstrate immunoreactivity with antibodies against vimentin and S-100 protein,[57–63,65] but uniquely, almost all are negative for HMB-45.[72,81] In recent studies, we have found that if there is positive immunostaining for HMB-45 in DM, it involves nondesmoplastic foci only, i.e., an intraepidermal component or superficial dermal focus of conventional melanoma cells.[72] A battery of markers must be utilized to evaluate such tumors. Other antibodies with variable reactivity with desmoplastic melanoma are neuron-specific enolase and NK1/C3. Antibodies against keratin, desmin, actin, and Leu-7 (specific for peripheral nerve-sheath differentiation but negative in melanocytic tumors), in general, are negative in desmoplastic melanoma.[62,63,72]

Minimal-Deviation Melanoma

This section will discuss the conceptual basis of minimal-deviation melanoma (MDM) without attempting to resolve the controversies of nomenclature, biologic course, or very legitimacy of the entity. From precedents in other neoplastic systems, the idea that the biologic behavior of melanomas may correlate with cytomorphology and degree of differentiation seems plausible.

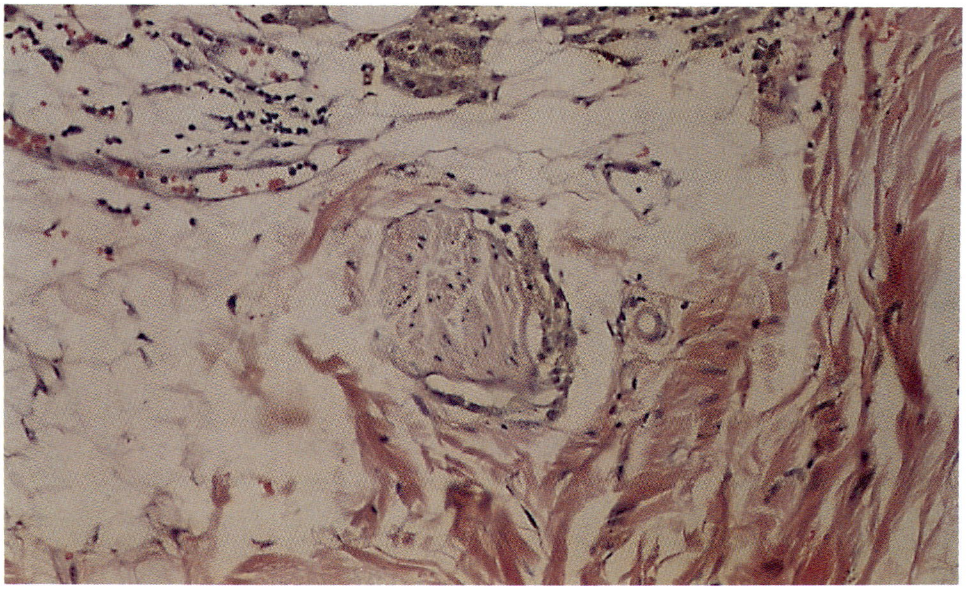

FIGURE 10-17
Neurotropism in conventional melanoma. There is perineurial infiltration of a small nerve in the subcutaneous fat (H&E, × 200).

The term MDM was introduced to embrace the concept that a subset of melanomas in the VGP is characterized by lesser cytologic atypia and a better prognosis than conventional melanomas of the same thickness.[82–88] Thus central to the concept of MDM is the presence of a cohesive nodule of dermal tumor cells. The growth pattern of such a nodule potentially indicates aggressive properties, such as recurrence or metastasis. Also implicit is the presence of a cell type lacking the characteristics of "fully evolved" melanoma cells of the VGP of SSM or NM.[85–87] Such cells express nuclear and cytoplasmic abnormalities intermediate between a typical basilar melanocyte or nevus cell and a melanoma cell. The cell types presumed to occur in MDM resemble ordinary nevus cells, spindled melanocytes, and epithelioid cells as from Spitz nevi.[85–88]

The central problem of MDM is the reliability and significance of recognizing different grades of cytologic atypia and different cell types. At present, there are no specific criteria that clearly distinguish MDM from conventional melanomas or atypical nevi. Neither has the biologic potential of these melanocytic proliferations been sufficiently and objectively correlated with cytologic characteristics, i.e., cellular and nuclear morphology (e.g., spindle cell versus epithelioid cell), nuclear area or volume, and nuclear pleomorphism. However, a few studies suggest that prognosis may relate to cell type; e.g., spindle cell melanomas may be associated with a better outcome than those composed of epithelioid cells.[89–91] Measurement of nuclear volume may have prognostic significance in melanoma.[92]

Because of the lack of specific histologic criteria and objective markers, data are not available that confirm or refute MDM as an entity. The diagnosis of MDM has probably been applied to a heterogeneous collection of tumors of widely varying biologic potential from atypical nevi to conventional melanomas. Until sufficient numbers of MDMs have been identified using standardized histologic criteria and patients followed for adequate periods, the legitimacy of MDM remains in question.

Nevoid Melanoma

The term *nevoid melanoma* was first used by Schmoeckel et al.[93] to describe a group of melanomas with histologic features suggesting a melanocytic nevus. It is quite likely that some of these lesions also might be considered to be minimal-deviation melanoma by some observers. However, in their description of 33 patients with nevoid melanoma, Schmoeckel and colleagues noted that 15 patients developed metastases. They did not consider nevoid melanoma to have any better prognosis than conventional melanomas.[93]

Clinical Features. In the latter series of 33 patients, the mean age at diagnosis was 47 years, and 76 percent of the patients were women (Table 10-14)[93]. Seventy percent of

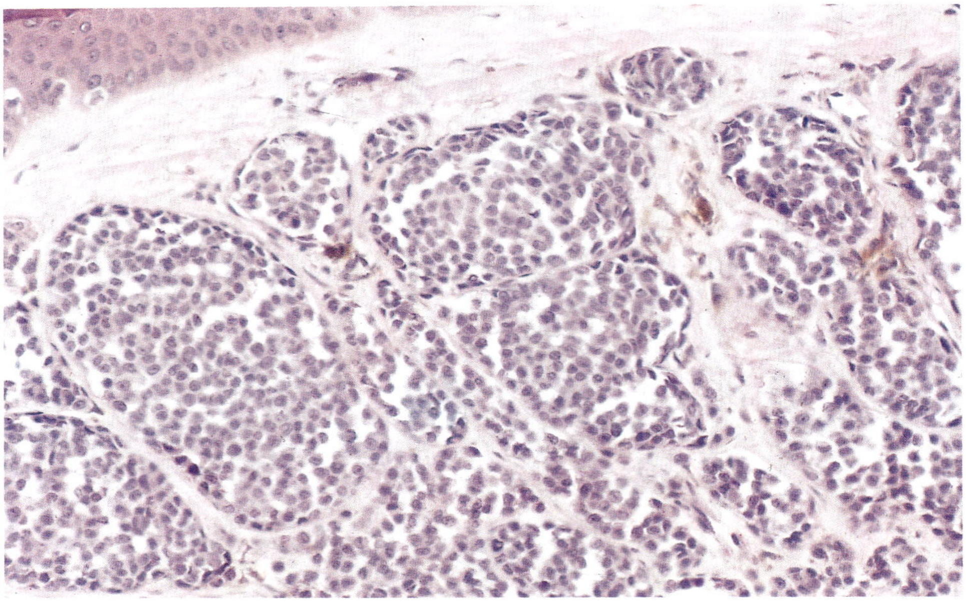

FIGURE 10-18
Nevoid melanoma. The dermis contains nests of relatively small nevus-like cells that are monotypic, show discohesion of nests, and lack maturation, all features suggestive of melanoma (H&E, × 200).

the tumors occurred on the lower extremities. There were no distinctive clinical features compared with conventional melanomas.

Histopathology. At scanning magnification, the most striking feature is a close resemblance to a nevus[93] (Fig. 10-18). Most of these lesions exhibit an overall symmetry, minimal or no intraepidermal pagetoid spread, and a monomorphous population of nevus-like cells in the dermis (Table 10-14) (see Fig. 10-18). Although the base of the melanoma is often poorly defined, the lateral margins may be well demarcated. In most instances, there is no host inflammatory response or surface ulceration. Histologic features favoring melanoma generally include the lack of maturation of dermal tumor cells, prominent cytologic atypia, mitoses in the dermal component, and infiltrative growth of cells into the deep dermis[93] (Fig. 10-19).

TABLE 10-14
Précis: Nevoid Melanoma

Clinical features
Affects women > men
Mean age 47 years
Occurs anywhere, but lower extremities most common
No distinctive features
1–2 cm
Histopathology
Symmetry common
Well-circumscribed lateral margins
Pagetoid spread not common
Nevus-like cells, monomorphous appearance
Lack of maturation
Cytologic atypia
Mitoses in dermal component
Infiltration of adnexal structures
Infiltration of deep dermis
Little or no inflammation
Differential diagnosis
Melanocytic nevus, especially papillomatous dermal nevus

Differential Diagnosis. The principal dilemma is discrimination of such melanomas from melanocytic nevi, especially papillomatous dermal nevi.[93] As outlined in Table 10-15, a constellation of factors must be considered in arriving at a final diagnosis. In some cases, it may be difficult to reach a final diagnosis. It is reasonable in such situations to communicate this uncertainty to the clinician and advise that the patient have appropriate treatment and periodic follow-up examinations as for melanoma.

Verrucous Melanoma

Although verrucous melanoma was described initially in his classification of melanoma in 1967 (Table 10-16),[12] Clark subsequently discarded the term because he believed that its features could be present in any of the major subtypes of melanoma.[13] In his depiction of verrucous melanoma, Clark called attention to its striking

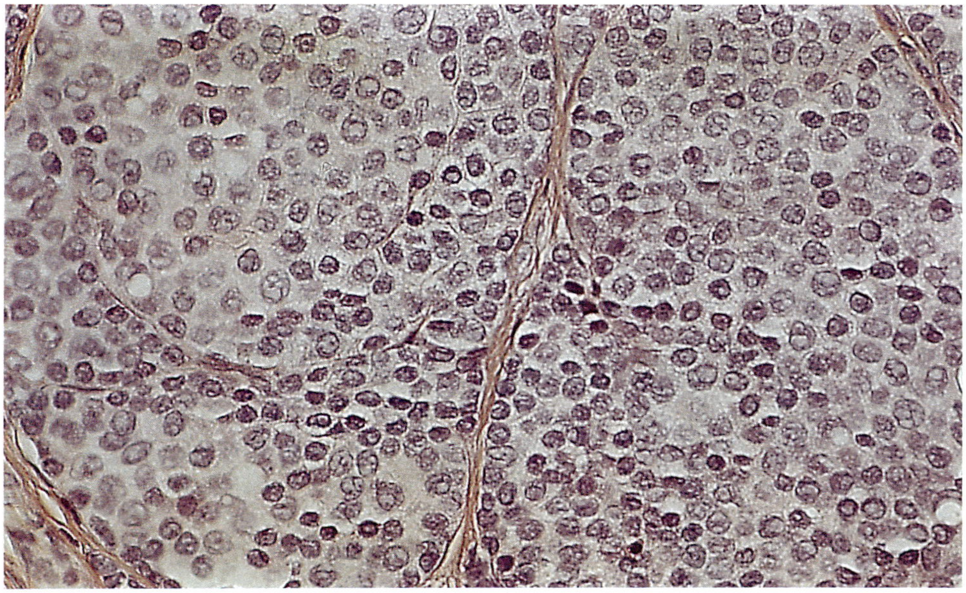

FIGURE 10-19
Nevoid melanoma. The vertical growth phase of this melanoma contains cohesive nests of nevus-like cells. Some nuclei are hyperchromatic, while others contain nucleoli (H&E, × 250).

keratotic surface and prominent epidermal hyperplasia on histologic examination.[12] Over the past decade or so, additional cases of verrucous melanoma have been reported,[94] some under a number of closely related terms such as *verrucous* and *pseudonevoid melanoma*,[95,96] *verrucous-keratotic melanoma*,[97] and *verrucous nevoid* and *keratotic melanoma*.[98] All the latter reports have emphasized the prominent clinical and histologic verrucous features of such melanomas as well as the difficulty in classifying many of these lesions. Some authors also have called attention to the striking resemblance to papillomatous dermal nevi. The latter features thus suggest that some of these melanomas also might be classified as nevoid melanoma.

According to Kuehl-Petzoldt and colleagues,[97] verrucous melanomas have the same biologic behavior and prognosis as conventional melanomas when matched pairs are analyzed. It should be noted, however, that tumor depth may be inappropriately thick in many cases because of epidermal hyperplasia or a papillomatous configuration. Anatomic level thus may provide a more accurate assessment of the biologic potential of the tumor.

Clinical Features. Some studies have reported a greater frequency of these lesions on the lower extremities of women[94,97] (Table 10-16). However, this has not been corroborated in all studies, since the backs of men also may be affected commonly.[98] The majority of patients have been in their sixth decade at the time of diagnosis.[94,97,98] Most lesions are described as well circumscribed, 1 to 2 cm

TABLE 10-15
Comparison of Nevoid Melanoma and Melanocytic Nevus

Nevoid Melanoma	*Melanocytic Nevus*
Clinical Features	
Older age	Younger age
Larger size, i.e., 1–2 cm	Smaller size, i.e., < 6 mm
Some variation in color	More homogeneous color
Greater asymmetry	Less asymmetry
Histopathology	
Greater asymmetry	Symmetry
Less well circumscribed	Well circumscribed
Greater likelihood of pagetoid spread	Little or no pagetoid spread
Intraepidermal basilar melanocytic proliferation common	Basilar proliferation less common
Infiltration of adnexae	No infiltration of adnexae
Little or no maturation	Maturation
Mitoses in dermis	Usually no dermal mitoses
Atypical mitoses	No atypical mitoses
Deep infiltration of dermis	No deep infiltration

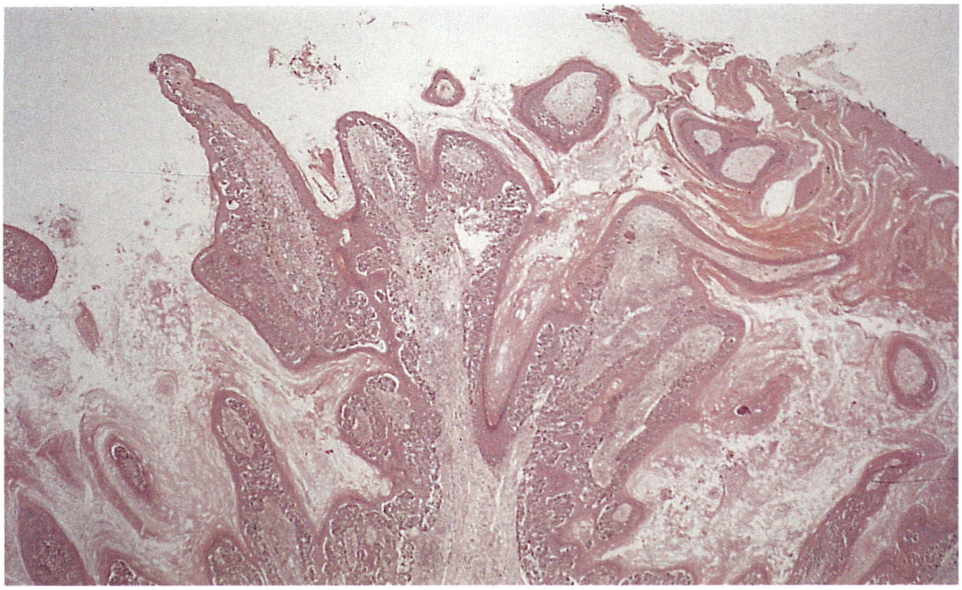

A

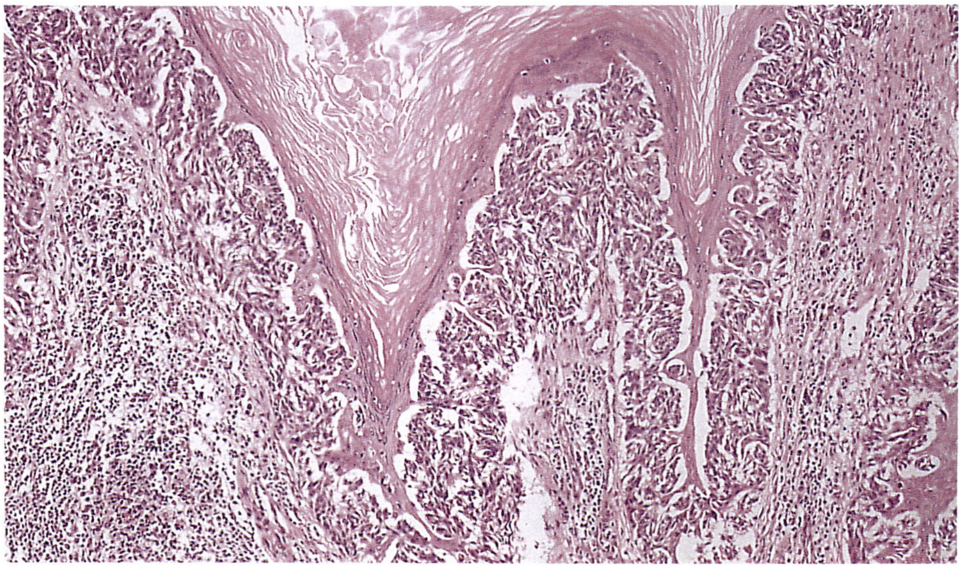

B

FIGURE 10-20

Verrucous melanoma. (A) Note prominent papillomatous configuration of lesion suggesting a papillomatous dermal nevus (H&E, × 20). (B) Confluent intraepidermal proliferation of melanoma cells is a striking feature of verrucous melanoma (H&E, × 100). (C) Higher magnification of part B showing irregular confluent intraepidermal nesting of pleomorphic melanoma cells (H&E, × 400). (Courtesy of Karen Blessing, M.D., University of Aberdeen, U.K.)

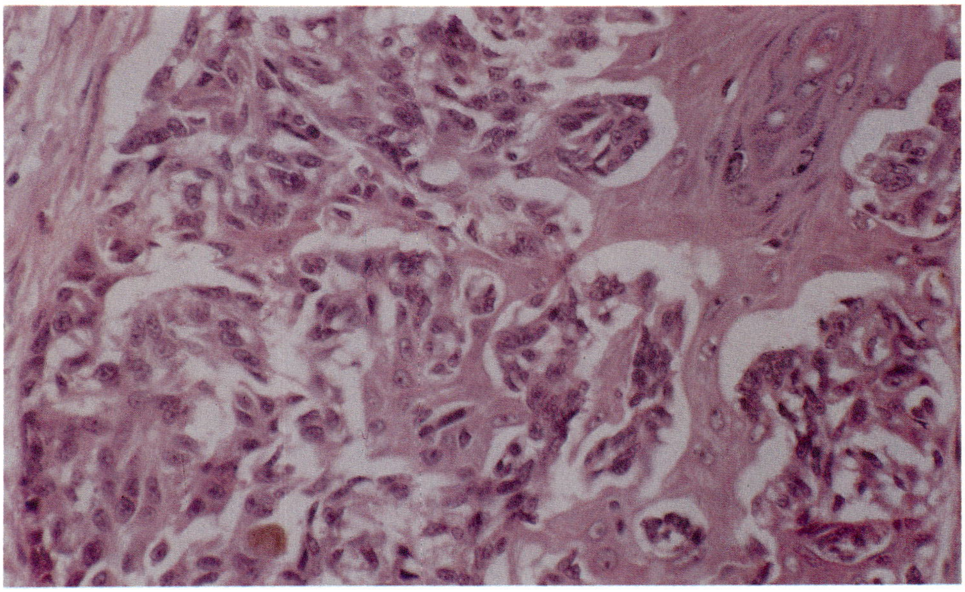

C

FIGURE 10-20 *(Continued)*

TABLE 10-16
Précis: Verrucous Melanoma

Clinical features	
	Age 50–60 years
	Affects women > men
	Location anywhere but lower extremities favored
	Well circumscribed
	1–2 cm
	Dark brown, black, grayish
	Verrucous hyperkeratotic surface
	Ulceration uncommon
Histopathology	
	Hyperkeratosis
	Papillomatous epidermal hyperplasia
	Occasional pseudoepitheliomatous hyperplasia
	Symmetry on occasion
	Epidermal involvement
	None
	Pagetoid spread
	Contiguous basilar melanocytic proliferation
	Involvement of adnexal structures
	Dermal component
	Occasional striking nevus-like appearance
	Little or no maturation
	Confluent sheets or nests of cells
	Mitoses in dermis
	Necrotic cells
	Little or no inflammation common
	May resemble any other histogenetic type of melanoma
Differential diagnosis	
	Papillomatous dermal nevus
Prognosis	
	Same as for other types of melanoma

in diameter, and characterized by a dark-brown, black, or grayish appearance and hyperkeratotic verrucous surface. Whitish or bluish color suggesting regression is distinctly uncommon.[94,97] Many such lesions are diagnosed clinically as seborrheic keratoses or papillomatous nevi.[94,98]

Histopathology. The most striking feature at scanning magnification is the prominent papillomatous or verrucoid epidermal hyperplasia suggesting a seborrheic keratosis, epidermal nevus, verruca, or papillomatous melanocytic nevus[94–98] (Table 10-16 and Fig. 10-20*A*). Many such lesions also exhibit some degree of symmetry, although this feature should not be so common as in a benign process. Hyperkeratosis and parakeratosis also may be prominent.[94] The degree of epidermal hyperplasia may be marked and have a pseudoepitheliomatous pattern in some instances.[98] The intraepidermal melanocytic component may vary from minimal or none to pagetoid spread indistinguishable from superficial spreading melanoma (see Fig. 10-20*B* and *C*). Also in common with superficial spreading melanoma is the frequent presence of a laterally extending intraepidermal component (radial growth phase).[98] As noted by Levene,[95] some of these tumors may show a contiguous basilar and suprabasilar proliferation of atypical melanocytes, often involving adnexal epithelium (see Fig. 10-20*B*). In common with nevoid melanoma, the dermal component in some melanomas may show a startling resemblance to a dermal nevus.[96] The cell type in the latter tumors resembles a small nevus cell, but careful inspection should disclose prominent cellular pleomorphism, little or no maturation, and cells dispersed in confluent nests and sheets without orderly infiltration of stroma. The presence of mitotic figures (e.g., more than two or three per section) and necrotic cells in the dermal component also argues against a benign process.

Differential Diagnosis. On cursory examination, verrucous melanoma may suggest nonmelanocytic tumors such as seborrheic keratosis, verruca, and epidermal nevus. However, the melanocytic nature of the lesion should become clear with careful inspection. Of particular concern is the potential misdiagnosis of verrucous melanoma as a benign nevus, especially a papillomatous dermal nevus.[96] Many of the same characteristics as outlined in Table 10-15 must be weighed in assessing problematic lesions. A host of factors are potentially relevant: age of the patient (older age more common in melanoma), size of the lesion (size > 6 mm and especially > 10 mm), clinical asymmetry, variegation of color, histologic asymmetry, pagetoid or contiguous basilar melanocytic proliferation, confluent sheets of cells in dermis, lack of maturation, and dermal mitoses.

TABLE 10-17
Précis: Melanoma Arising in Association with Dermal Nevus

Clinical features
Age 40–60 years
Head and neck most common site
Often 1–2 cm
Resembles dermal nevus
Often uniform pink, tan, or brown
Often history of recent enlargement
Histopathology
Focal cohesive nodules of atypical melanocytes
Background of ordinary dermal nevus
Monomorphous cells in nodules
Cellular and nuclear enlargement
Nuclear pleomorphism
Melanin content variable
Mitotic figures usually present
Differential diagnosis
Dermal nevus
"Combined," "inverted type A," nevus with focal dermal component of atypical epithelioid cells

Melanoma Arising in Association with Dermal Nevi

The development of melanoma in the dermal component of an acquired nevus is an uncommon or rare event judging from the number of cases reported to date.[99–101] This phenomenon may overlap to some degree with nevoid melanoma and verrucous melanoma. It is also possible that some of these melanomas may originate from adnexal-associated nevus elements.

Clinical Features. Most patients reported thus far have been approximately 40 to 60 years of age, and the most common site of involvement has been the head and neck area (Table 10-17)[99–101]. The general clinical appearance is usually rather innocuous and in fact rather similar to that of a dermal nevus, i.e., uniform pink or tan color. However, the lesions are often larger than ordinary dermal nevi, e.g., 1 to 2 cm, and there is usually a history of recent change or enlargement.

Histopathology. Usually within an otherwise ordinary dermal nevus one encounters a distinct nodule of cytologically atypical melanocytes[99–101] (Table 10-17) (Fig. 10-21*A*). There is usually a transition from the ordinary dermal nevus component to the nodular aggregate of atypical cells (see Fig. 10-21*B*). The latter cells are most commonly enlarged with abundant cytoplasm and pleomorphic nuclei. Mitotic figures are usually easily found within the cellular nodule.

Differential Diagnosis. The most obvious dilemma is the differentiation of a focus of melanoma from dermal nevus, especially a nevus with cytologically bizarre nevus cells, as in ancient schwannoma or a distinct focus of epithelioid or fusiform cells, i.e., so-called combined nevus, inverted type A nevus, or nevus with a focal atypical epithelioid cell component in the dermis.[82,102] First of all, the nodular area in question should demonstrate a cohesive or expansile aggregate of cells with unequivocal cytologic atypia. Although these melanocytic cells will usually have a monomorphous or clonal appearance, inspection of individual cells should disclose substantial nuclear pleomorphism and often prominent nucleoli and hyperchromatism. Mitotic figures also should be present in this focus. A dermal nevus with bizarre or ancient cytologic features usually will not show mitoses. One also should consider clinical factors such as age of the patient (melanoma usually in persons greater than 40 years of age), size (such lesions often > 1 cm in diameter), and history of recent change or enlargement. On the other hand, so-called combined nevi are often present in younger individuals, are characterized by a small dark nodule or papule in a relatively small symmetric nevus, and usually show low-grade or no cytologic atypia of the epithelioid/fusiform cells. Often the latter cells display prominent melaninization of melanocytes and are accompanied by melanophages.

Malignant Blue Nevus

Malignant blue nevus (MBN) is an extremely rare form of melanoma originating from or associated with a preexisting blue nevus and characterized by a dense proliferation of variably pigmented spindle cells without involvement

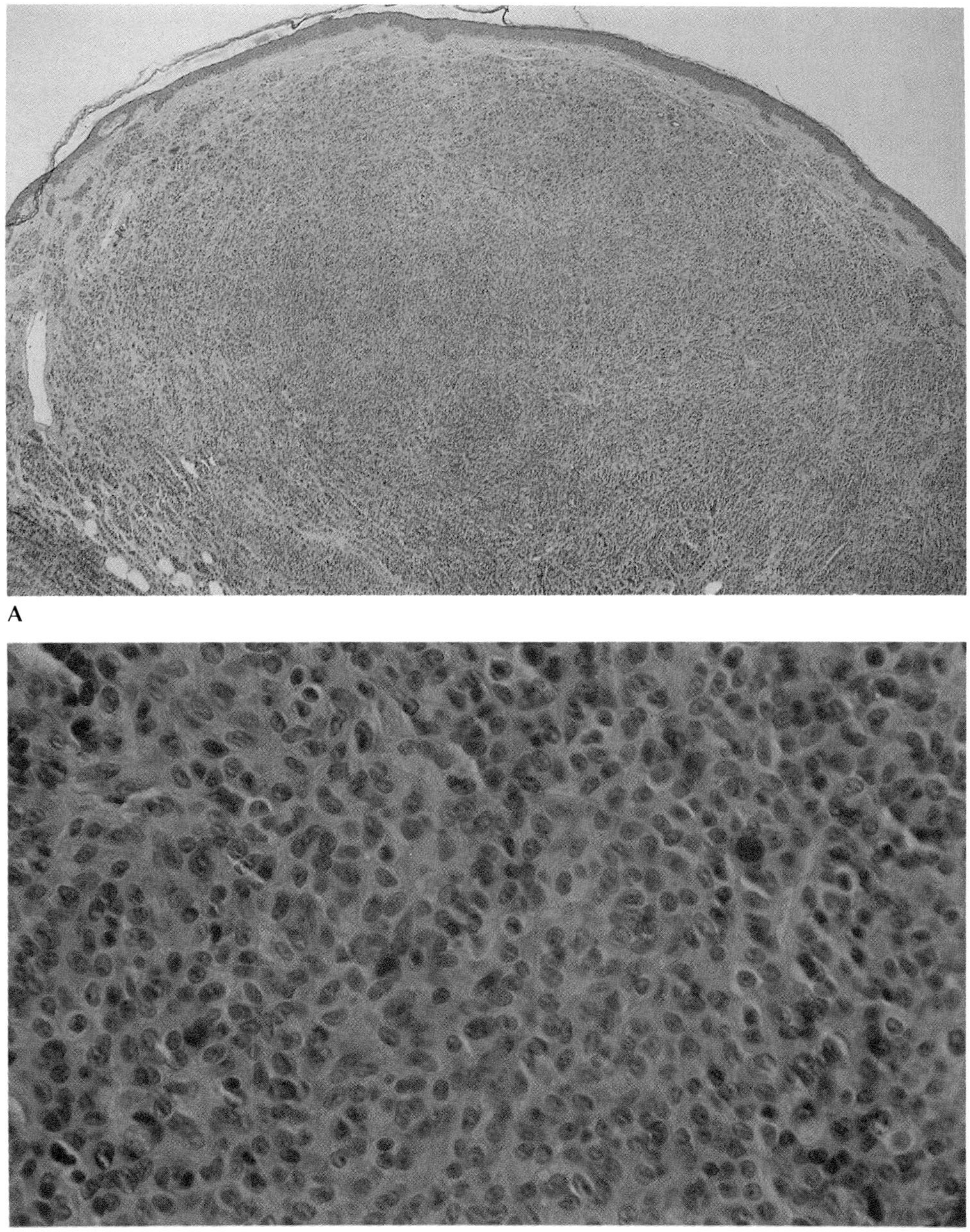

FIGURE 10-21

Melanoma arising in the dermal component of a nevus. (A) Dome-shaped expansile nodule in dermis with surrounding dermal nevus (H&E, × 40). (B) Central expansile nodule notable for high cellularity, nuclear pleomorphism, and mitotic activity (H&E, × 400).

of the epidermis.[103–112] Because of its rarity and potential confusion with atypical cellular blue nevus (Table 10-18), NM, and metastatic melanoma, many have doubted the existence of MBN. If strict criteria are applied, as outlined above, only 33 cases of MBN have been reported.[109,110] The largest series was published recently by Connelly and Smith[110] and included 12 patients. The average age at diagnosis is 45 years, two-thirds of the patients are men, and the most common site of origin is the scalp.

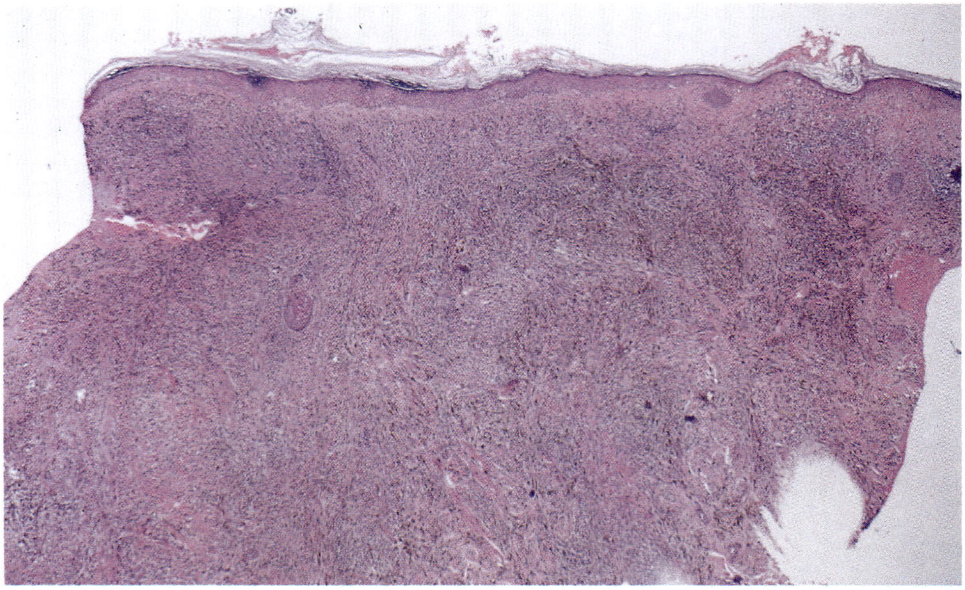

A

FIGURE 10-22

Malignant blue nevus (malignant melanoma arising in association with blue nevus). (A) Malignant melanoma occupies the dermis without connection to the overyling epidermis. This melanoma can only be distinguished from conventional melanoma by the association with or history of a previous blue nevus at this site. (H&E, × 40). (B) Fascicular arrangements of spindle cells, many of which contain melanin, can be observed in this field (H&E, × 200). (C) High magnification showing compact aggregates of plump fusiform and epithbelioid melanoma cells. Marked cytologic atypia is present (H&E, × 400).

Clinical Features. Malignant blue nevi most frequently present as blue or blue-black plaques or nodules ranging from 1 to 4 cm (most > 3 cm),[110] that are often multinodular. There is usually a history of recent enlargement or change in a previously stable blue nevus.

Histologic Features. Malignant blue nevi are characterized by nodular or multinodular aggregations of spindle cells in tightly packed fascicles in the dermis and often the subcutis[103-110] (Table 10-18) (Fig. 10-22*A–C*). By definition, there is sparing of the epidermis (see Fig. 10-22*A*). Occasional epithelioid cells and multinucleate giant cells are encountered. Melanin pigment (see Fig. 10-22*B*) and cytoplasmic vacuolization are noted in approximately two-thirds of cases. However, in the M.D. Anderson series, only about a third were heavily melaninized.[110] Necrosis, a feature previously thought characteristic of MBN, was observed in only 4 of 12 cases reported by Connelly and Smith.[110] In general, there is striking cytologic atypia (see Fig. 10-22*C*), prominent nuclear pleomorphism, infrequent mitotic figures (approximately 1

TABLE 10-18
Précis: Malignant Blue Nevus

Clinical features
- Age 45 years
- Affects men > women
- Scalp most common site
- 1–4 cm (usually > 3 cm)
- Blue or blue-black plaque or nodules
- Multinodular
- Often recent change in stable blue nevus

Histopathology
- Nodular or multinodular aggregates of spindle cells
- Sparing of epidermis
- Highly variable cytologic atypia
- Pigmentation in one-third of cases
- Necrosis in one-third of cases
- Mitotic figures infrequent
- Component of cellular blue nevus and less often ordinary blue nevus

Differential diagnosis
- Cellular blue nevus and atypical variants
- Nodular melanoma
- Metastatic melanoma

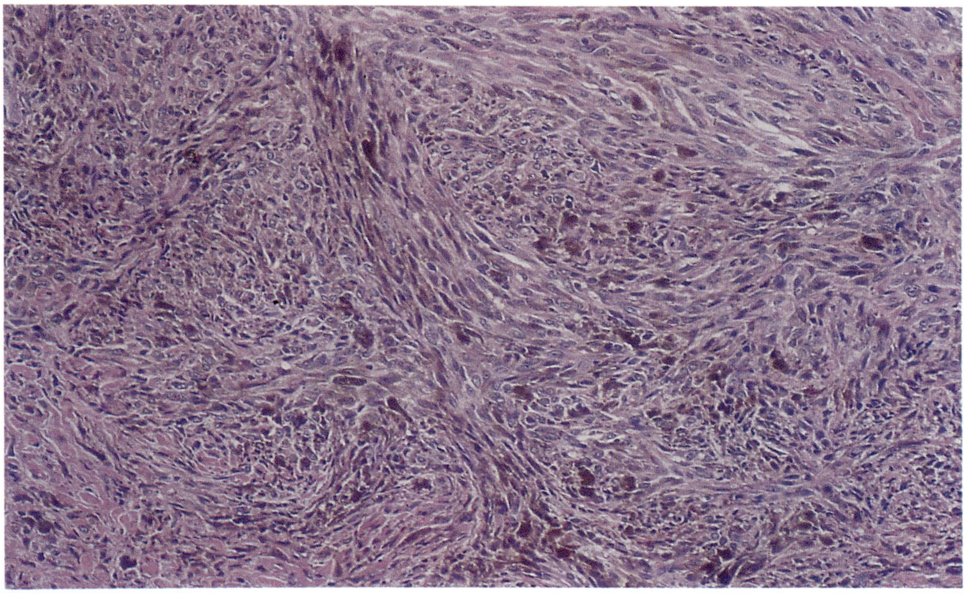

B

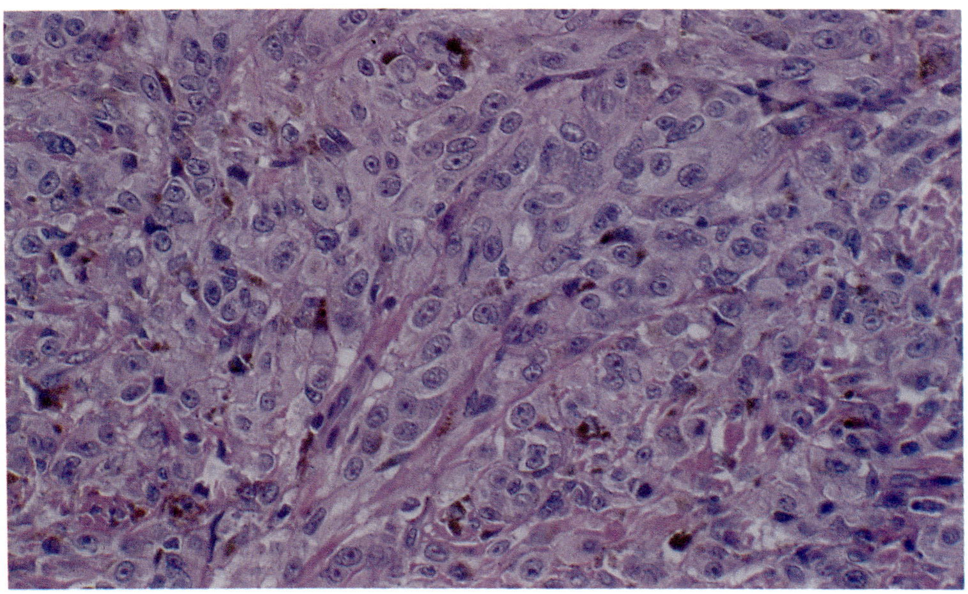

C

FIGURE 10-22 *(Continued)*

mitosis per 10 high-power fields, but some have more), and uncommonly atypical mitoses. Most MBN have a component of cellular blue nevus (CBN), but elements of common blue nevus (pigmented dendritic melanocytes, fibrosis, and melanophages) and rarely nevus of Ota may be observed.[109,110]

Differential Diagnosis. Malignant blue nevus must be distinguished from CBN[111] or atypical CBN,[112] NM,[110] and metastatic melanoma.[109,110] The discrimination of MBN from CBN is based on clinical and histologic characteristics. MBN are usually greater than 3 cm in longest diameter, whereas CBN are usually less than 2 cm.[109,110]

TABLE 10-19
Précis: Clear Cell Sarcoma

Clinical features
- Ages 20–40 years
- Affects women ≥ men
- Distal extremities, the foot most commonly involved
- Deep location—tendons and aponeuroses
- Slowly enlarging mass
- Tenderness, pain

Histopathology
- Multilobulated tumor
- Oval or fusiform cells in nests and fascicles
- Fibrous trabeculae separate cellular aggregates
- Clear or eosinophilic cytoplasm
- Multinucleate giant cells
- Melanin in over half of cases

Immunohistochemistry
- S-100protein +
- HMB-45 +

Electron microscopy
- Premelanosomes
- Melanosomes

Differential diagnosis
- Metastatic melanoma
- Cellular blue nevus
- Malignant blue nevus
- Malignant peripheral nerve sheath tumor
- Epithelioid sarcoma
- Synovial sarcoma
- Fibrosarcoma

MBN are often typified by a markedly irregular, asymmetric, and frequently multinodular appearance in contrast to the more symmetric and regular CBN.[111] Histologically, MBN usually display greater asymmetry, hypercellularity, frankly malignant cytologic characteristics, and more mitoses and necrosis than are found in CBN. Atypical mitoses are characteristic of MBN. Less commonly MBN may demonstrate rather banal cytologic features, and occasional atypical CBN show necrosis.[109] Distinction of MBN from atypical CBN is occasionally exceedingly difficult. Lesions designated as atypical CBN should therefore have adequate surgical margins and long-term follow-up.[110]

Because there are no histologic features specific for MBN, a contiguous remnant of blue nevus should be identified or a history of an antecedent blue nevus documented to distinguish MBN from either NM or metastatic melanoma.[110]

MBN are aggressive, with metastasis to lymph nodes and a variety of visceral sites in 82 percent of the 33 cases mentioned above.[110] MBN are remarkable for metastases developing after intervals as long as 10 years.

Clear Cell Sarcoma

Synonym: malignant melanoma of soft parts

Clear cell sarcoma (CCS) has been a perplexing tumor because of its origin in soft tissue, classification in the past as synovial sarcoma or fibrosarcoma,[113-116] and a pattern of biologic behavior that is consistent with a sarcoma.[116] However, at present, CCS is best considered an unusual variant of malignant melanoma. It develops in young adults between the ages of 20 and 40 and most commonly involves the distal extremities (the foot being the most common site) (Table 10-19). The tumor typically presents as a slowly enlarging, deep-seated mass because of its association with tendons and aponeuroses, and there may be occasional tenderness or pain. CCS is slightly more prevalent in women.

Histologic Features. The tumor is characterized by a well-circumscribed, multilobulated appearance (Table 10-19).[113-116] Oval or fusiform cells with clear or eosinophilic granular cytoplasm are arranged in well-defined nests and fascicles (Fig. 10-23*A* and *B*). Tumor aggregates are generally compartmentalized by fibrous tissue of variable thickness that merges with aponeurotic or tendinous structures (see Fig. 10.23*A*). There is variation in nuclear size and shape, and the nuclei are notable for vesicular qualities and prominent nucleoli. Distinctive multinucleate giant cells occur in about two thirds of cases.[113,114] Melanin may be detected in approximately half these tumors. Special stains will yield more tumors containing melanin. Most tumors react with antibodies to vimentin, S-100 protein, HMB-45, and neuron-specific enolase.[115] There is no staining with antibodies against cytokeratin, epithelial membrane antigen, or leukocyte common antigen.[115] Melanosomes and premelanosomes are noted on electron microscopy.[115]

Local recurrences are frequent with 70 percent of patients in one series experiencing at least one recurrence during a mean period of 4.2 years.[114] The recurrences are often multiple and followed by less frequent regional node and lung metastases. In the preceding series, 43 percent of the individuals died of metastases.[114]

Differential Diagnosis. CCS may be confused with CBN, MBN, metastatic melanoma, malignant peripheral nerve-sheath tumor, epithelioid sarcoma, synovial sarcoma, and fibrosarcoma.[113-116] The tumor probably most closely resembles CBN with atypia and MBN, but the latter do not usually occur in soft tissue. CCS is distinguished by the typical clinical presentation in young adults, involvement of distal extremities, typical histology, and immunohistochemistry. On occasion, CCS must be discriminated from metastatic melanoma involving soft tissue sites of the extremities. The latter distinction is predicated upon the absence of primary and/or metastatic melanoma at another location (or other locations) and, if

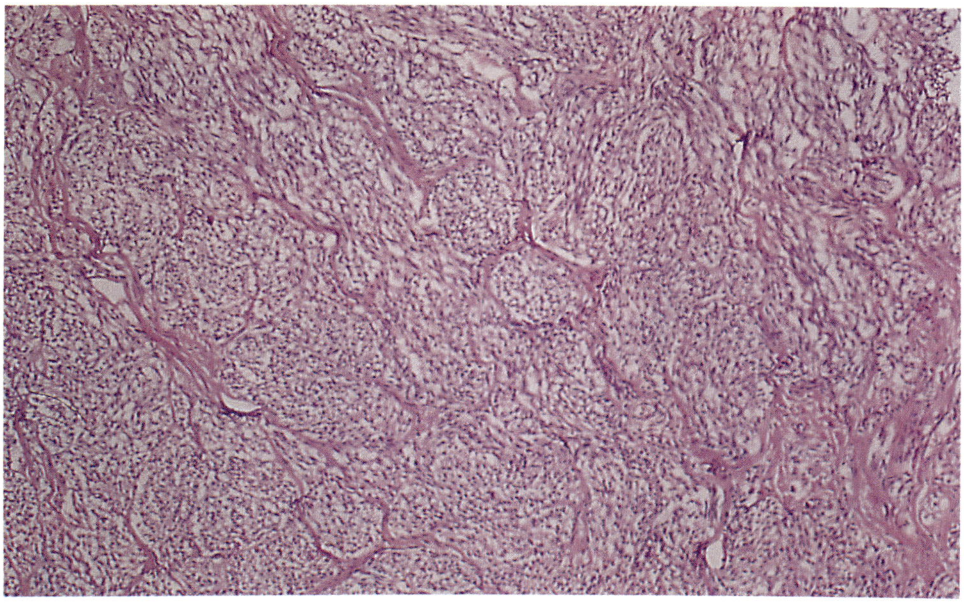

A

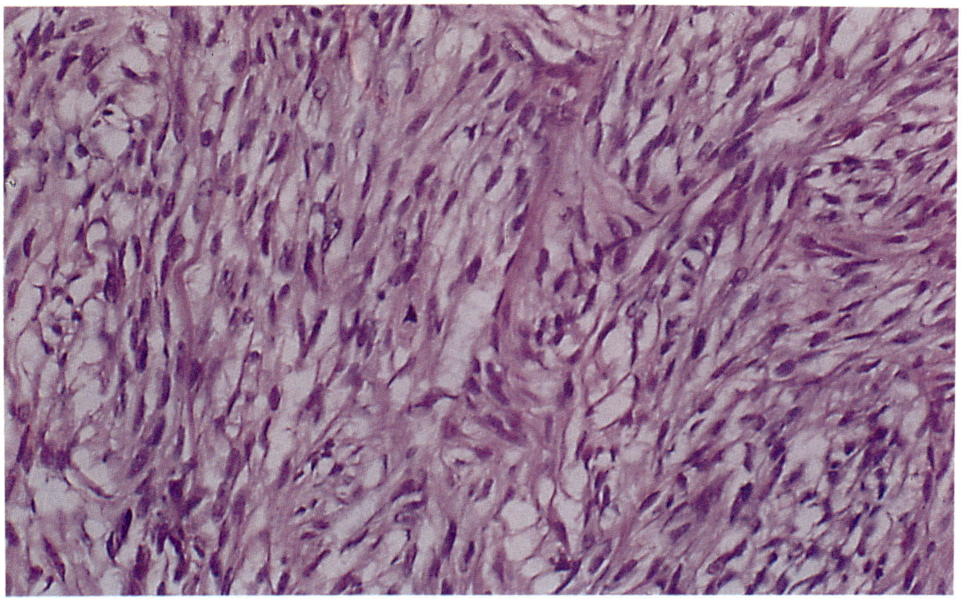

B

FIGURE 10-23

Clear cell sarcoma. (A) The tumor is remarkable for intersecting fascicles of spindle cells, compartmentalized by fibrous tissue focally (H&E, × 125). (B) The spindle cells are characterized by clear cytoplasm. The nuclei are pleomorphic with hyperchromatism (H&E, × 313).

necessary, cytogenetic studies. CCS exhibits a characteristic chromosomal translocation t(12;22)(q^{13};q^{12}) whereas cutaneous melanoma does not.[117] Epithelioid sarcoma and synovial sarcoma immunostain with cytokeratin and epithelial membrane antigen but not with S-100 protein and HMB-45.

UNUSUAL OR RARE VARIATIONS OF MELANOMA AND PARTICULAR HISTOLOGIC ALTERATIONS

Polypoid Configuration of Melanoma

Melanomas in the VGP, whether accompanied by an RGP component or not, occasionally are polypoid (see Fig. 10-6). In a large series of melanomas from Australia, 21.5 percent were polypoid,[118] either pedunculated or sessile. Virtually all the tumor is located above the epidermal surface in pedunculated melanomas, whereas sessile tumors have more than half the tumor above the epidermal surface (see Fig. 10-6). Polypoid tumors usually have an ulcerated, friable surface and epidermal collarettes at the tumor base. Approximately two-thirds are of nodular type.[118] Originally, an adverse prognosis was assigned to polypoidal melanoma, but subsequent studies have failed to confirm this.

Amelanotic Melanoma

Uncommonly, primary melanomas develop without associated pigmentation (1.8 percent in a series of 2881 melanomas).[119] Most such tumors are NM; however, an amelanotic VGP may supervene on a pigmented RGP. Rarely, the RGP also may be devoid of pigment. Such tumors are difficult to diagnose clinically because they lack important clues such as variegated pigmentation.

In fact, melanin pigment is almost always present in some portion of a primary melanoma, and careful scrutiny of tumors apparently lacking pigment will often demonstrate finely granular melanin in some tumor cells. Special silver stains such as the Fontana-Masson stain frequently will yield a positive result with even small amounts of melanin. Finally, immunohistochemistry will verify the melanocytic nature of a tumor (see Chap. 2). Metastatic melanoma is amelanotic much more frequently than primary melanoma and thus often enters into the differential diagnosis of metastatic cancer.

Balloon Cell Melanoma

Analagous to balloon cell nevus (see Chap. 4), balloon cell melanoma (BCM) is defined by a distinctive cellular alteration, i.e., ballooning, in at least 50 percent of the melanoma cells.[120,121] The individual "balloon cells" have abundant vacuolated cytoplasms that impart a clear cell appearance. Although BCM is extremely rare, knowledge of BCM is important for its distinction from the much more common balloon cell nevus and from other clear cell tumors of the skin. The prognosis in BCM appears to be directly related to tumor thickness and to be no different from that of conventional melanoma. In a recent series of 34 cases of BCM, the 5-year survival was 37.5 percent (close to half the tumors were >2.0 mm in thickness).[121] BCM is reported to have a particular propensity for multiple skin and subcutaneous metastases.[120]

Clinical Features. In the recently reported series of 34 cases of BCM, the median age of patients was 54 years (range 19 to 91) (Table 10-20).[120] BCM was located most commonly on the head, neck, and upper trunk. Compared with conventional melanoma, there were no distinctive

TABLE 10-20
Précis: Balloon Cell Melanoma

Clinical features
- Exceedingly rare
- Median age 54 years
- Head, neck, and upper trunk most common sites
- No distinctive clinical features
- Size 3–35 mm

Histopathology
- Enlarged polygonal cells containing vacuolated (clear) cytoplasm in ≥ 50% of melanoma cases
- Occasional pagetoid spread of balloon cells
- Large nodular aggregates of balloon cells in dermis
- Irregular placement of nuclei
- In general, slight to moderate variation in nuclear characteristics and mitotic activity
- Multinucleate balloon giant cells

Immunohistochemistry
- S-100 protein +
- HMB-45 +
- Neuron-specific enolase + (weak)
- Carcinoembryonic antigen + (2/7 tumors)

Differential diagnosis
- Balloon cell nevus
- Clear cell sarcoma (malignant melanoma of soft parts)
- Xanthoma
- Hibernoma
- Metastatic clear cell carcinomas
  - Renal cell carcinoma
  - Clear cell carcinoma of lung, ovary, and endometrium
- Granular cell tumor
- Malignant eccrine acrospiroma
- Clear cell syringoma
- Sebaceous carcinoma
- Clear cell squamous cell carcinoma
- Atypical fibroxanthoma
- Lepromatous leprosy

Prognosis
- No different from conventional melanomas, directly related to tumor thickness
- Degree of balloon cell change does not alter prognosis
- Five-year survival 37.5% (melanomas of all thicknesses)

clinical features of BCM. These lesions ranged in size from 3 to 35 mm.

Histopathology. The characteristic balloon cells are large, round, or polygonal cells with clear or eosinophilic, slightly granular cytoplasm[120,121] (Table 10-20). The nuclei are irregularly placed and exhibit only slight to moderate atypia. Mitotic activity is also generally low. The balloon cells occasionally are associated with pagetoid spread in the epidermis (Fig. 10.24*A* and *B*) and often form large nodular aggregates and nests in the dermis. Melanin has been noted in about a quarter of cases.[121] Metastases from BCM often show balloon cell change but may be difficult to diagnose because of they are amelanotic and fail to exhibit nesting. Virtually all BCMs studied thus far show positive immunostaining with S-100 protein and HMB-45.[121] A small number may be positive for carcinoembryonic antigen (as may all melanomas).

Etiology. The balloon cell change has been attributed to (1) degeneration and coalescence of melanosomes, (2) defective melanosome formation and subsequent generation of large membrane-bound vesicles, (3) blocked melanin synthesis and subsequent accumulation of protyrosinase vesicles, and (4) lipoidal degeneration of melanocytes.[121] Recent ultrastructural studies have provided evidence supporting the first three explanations. In addition, the presence of abundant RNA in the balloon cells and immunostaining with HMB-45 suggest that the cells are metabolically active rather than degenerative.[121]

Differential Diagnosis. Because of the striking clear cell appearance and mild cellular atypia, BCM may be confused with balloon cell nevus, xanthoma, hibernoma, granular cell tumor, metastatic clear cell carcinomas such as renal cell or adenocarcinoma, liposarcoma, and clear cell appendage tumors[120,121] (Table 10-20). Clinical correlation is critical, since most balloon cell melanomas have the gross morphology of melanoma. Perhaps the greatest problem is distinction of BCM from a balloon cell nevus. Careful attention to the overall characteristics of the tumor should allow distinction of BCM from a balloon cell nevus. In general, balloon cell nevi occur in young individuals (under age 30 years), show "maturation" of nevus cells (decreased size of cells and nuclei with depth), and the presence of multinucleate giant cells (see Chap. 4), in contrast to BCM, which tends to develop in older patients, to lack "maturation" of melanoma cells, and to have cellular atypia and mitotic activity.[121]

Other rare and unusual variants of melanoma[122–126] are listed in Table 10-21 and shown in Figs. 10-24, 10-25, and 10-26.

Regression

Melanoma is notable for its frequency of spontaneous regression.[22] The prevalence of histologic regression varies according to the definition of regression used and the thickness range of the melanomas reported.[22,127,128] In a study of 563 cases of primary melanoma, histologic regression was noted in 46 percent of thin (<1.5 mm), 32 percent of intermediate (1.5–3.0 mm), and 9 percent of thick (>3.0 mm) melanomas.[128] McGovern[127,129] also has recorded regression in 58 percent of melanomas 0.70 mm or less in thickness. Complete regression of melanoma is uncommon and has been reported to occur with a frequency of 2.4 to 8.7 percent.[130,131] Many cases of metastatic melanoma with unknown primary are thought to be explained by regression of the primary melanoma.

Regression is thought to be immunologically mediated because of mononuclear cell infiltrates containing T lymphocytes and monocytes/macrophages at the site of regression.[132] Regression is seen most often in the RGP of melanoma and is present as focal, partial, and rarely complete regression of the tumor.[22,133] The changes of regression form a continuum but may be arbitrarily categorized into three stages[133] (Table 10-22). Early regression shows a rich, mononuclear infiltrate closely associated with the invasive dermal melanoma (Fig. 10-27*A*). It is necessary that actual tumor cell destruction be demonstrated, and careful inspection usually will disclose lymphoid cells closely opposed to tumor cells (satellitosis) in a pattern reminiscent of graft-

TABLE 10-21
Unusual or Rare Presentations of Primary Melanoma

Spitzoid melanoma[122]	Cellular composition resembles enlarged epithelioid/fusiform cells of Spitz nevus
Myxoid melanoma[123–125]	Prominent myxoid stroma suggesting mucinous carcinoma or peripheral nerve-sheath tumors (see Fig. 10-24)
Melanoma resembling experimentally induced and spontaneous melanomas in animals[126]	Raised dermal tumor composed of heavily melaninized epithelioid cells, fusiform cells often with dendrites, and histiocytes. The striking melanin content tends to obscure cytologic detail, and bleaching is often needed.
Small cell melanoma[123–126]	Melanoma composed of uniform small cells, sometimes in organoid arrangements (see Fig. 10-25), developing in congenital nevi and frequently mucosal sites such as vulva, vagina.

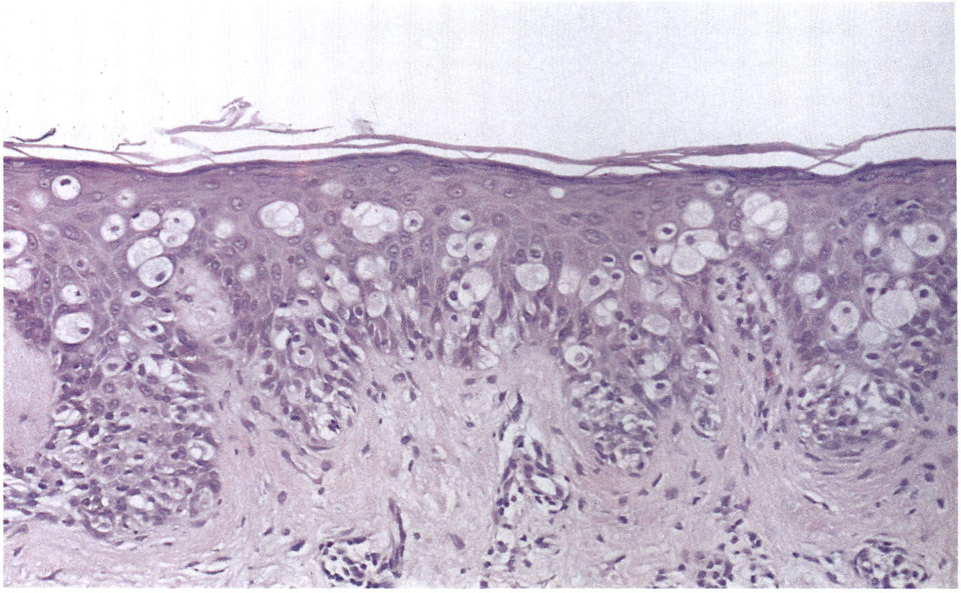

A

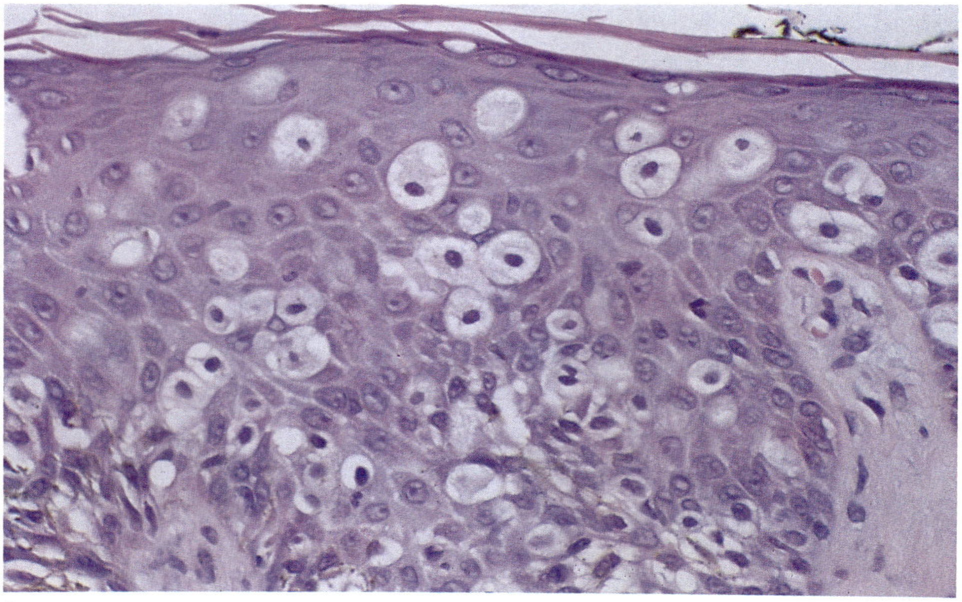

B

FIGURE 10-24

Balloon cell melanoma. (A) Pagetoid spread of balloon cells in this melanoma in situ (H&E, × 200). (B) Balloon melanoma cells are enlarged with abundant clear cytoplasm and pleomorphic nuclei (H&E, × 400). (Courtesy of T.-Y. Wong, M.D.)

versus-host disease. There also may be epidermal infiltration by the mononuclear cells.

Intermediate regression is characterized by loss or dropout of tumor in the papillary dermis, epidermis, or both and continued host response[133] (see Fig. 10-27*B* and Table 10-22). The loss of tumor is associated with variable thickening and fibroplasia of the papillary dermis, mononuclear cell infiltrates, prominent vascularity, and melanin-containing macrophages. In general, there is some diminution in the intensity of the infiltrate at this stage, and there may be effacement of the epidermal rete pattern.

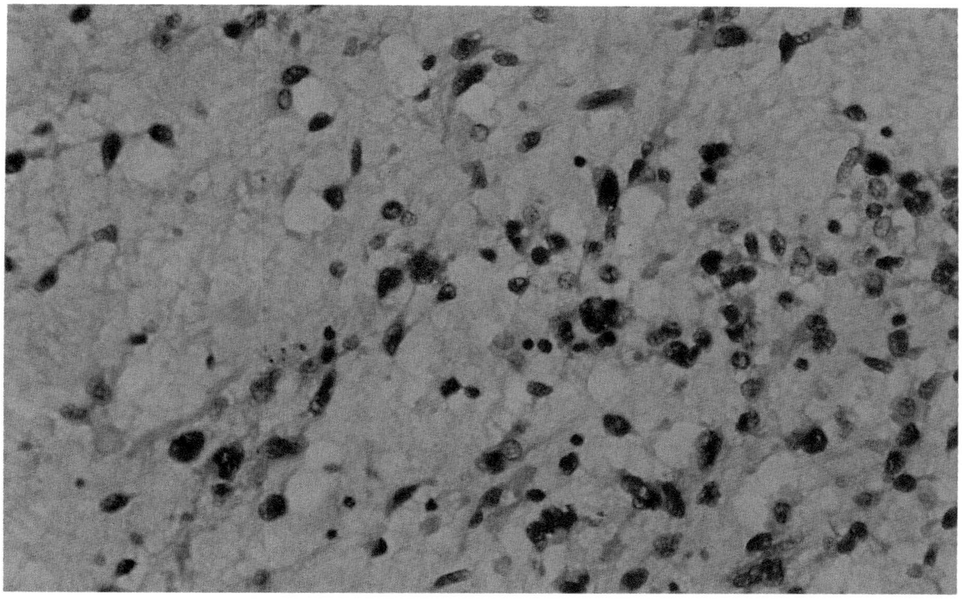

FIGURE 10-25
Myxoid melanoma. Melanoma cells dispersed in abundant mucinous stroma (H&E, × 400). (Courtesy of Mark Wick, M.D.)

Late-stage regression (see Fig. 10-27C) shows prominence of papillary dermal fibrosis[133] (see Table 10-22), characterized by dense layering of coarse fibrous tissue similar to scarring. There is absence of tumor in both epidermis and dermis and often complete effacement of the epidermal rete pattern. Residual single melanoma cells or small nests of cells may remain at the dermoepidermal junction or entrapped in the fibrosis. Mononuclear cell infiltrates are minimal or absent at this stage. There may be remarkable angiogenesis and ectasia of vessels in these zones of regression,[134] and melanophages may be present to a variable extent.

The changes of regression vary considerably from tumor to tumor and within a single tumor.[133] The proportion of the melanoma involved may range from a small focus (most common) to complete regression. All phases of regression may be found within the same tumor, resulting in several distinctive presentations of melanoma that are important to recognize.[22] Melanoma with prominent mononuclear cell infiltrates (early regression) may simulate a halo nevus clinically and histologically. However, in general regression in melanoma is distinct from inflammatory regression of melanocytic nevi. In halo nevi, the histologic changes are characterized by variable loss of nevus cells and delicate fibroplasia, which differs from the dense,

TABLE 10-22
Stages of Histologic Regression of Malignant Melanoma

Early (or active): Zone of papillary dermis and epidermis within a recognizable melanoma, characterized by dense infiltrates of lymphocytes disrupting/replacing nests of melanoma cells within the papillary dermis and possibly the epidermis as compared with adjoining zones of tumor; degenerating melanoma cells should be recognizable. There is no obvious fibrosis.

Intermediate: Zone of papillary dermis and epidermis within a recognizable melanoma, characterized by reduction (loss) in the amount of tumor (a disruption in the continuity of the tumor) or absence of tumor in papillary dermis and possibly within the epidermis compared with adjacent zones of tumor and replaced by varying admixtures of lymphoid cells and increased fibrous tissue (as compared with normal papillary dermis) in this zone. Variable telangiectasia (and new blood vessel formation) and melanophages may also be present.

Late: Zone of papillary dermis and epidermis characterized by marked reduction in the amount of tumor compared with adjacent areas of tumor or absence of tumor in this zone and replacement and expansion of the papillary dermis in this zone by extensive fibrosis (usually dense fibrous tissue, horizontally disposed) and variable telangiectasia (and new blood vessel formation), melanophages, sparse or no lymphoid infiltrates, and effacement of the epidermis (other than fibrosis, the latter features are frequently present but not essential for recognizing regression).

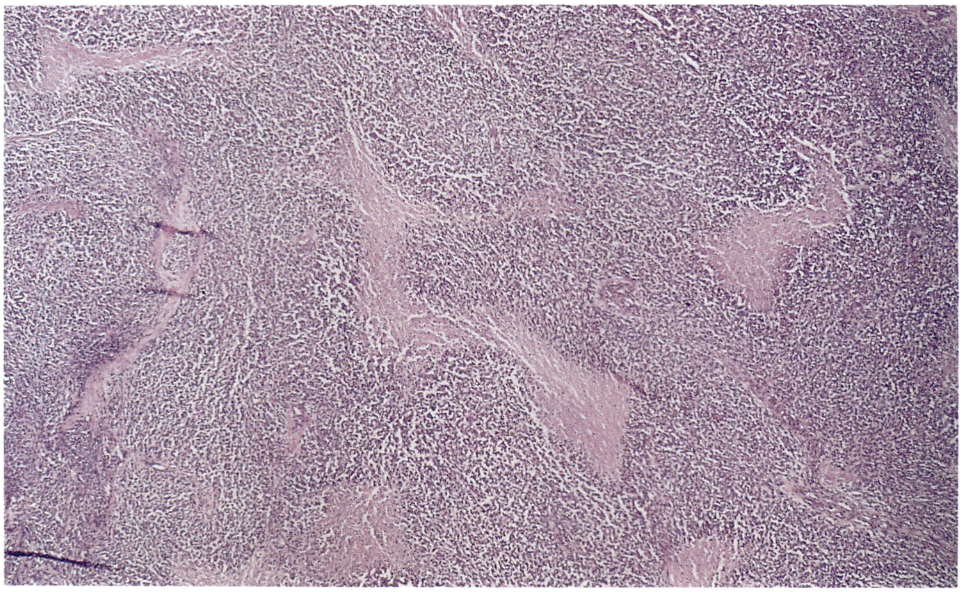

A

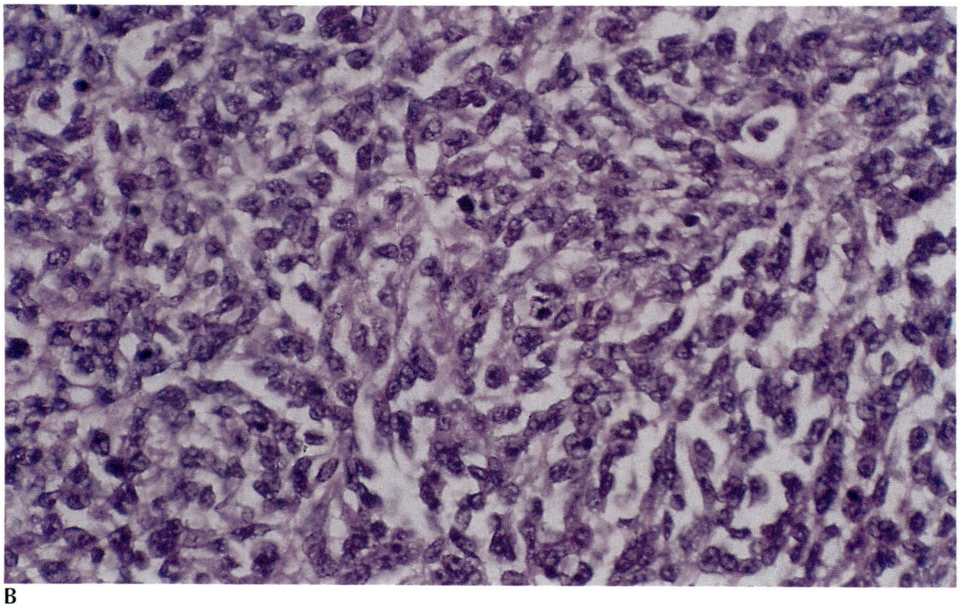

B

FIGURE 10-26

Small cell melanoma. (A) Arcuate zones of necrosis in melanoma composed of small "blue" cells (H&E, × 40). (B) Sheet of small monomorphous cells resembling lymphoma (H&E, × 400). (Courtesy of Mark Wick, M.D.)

coarse fibrosis of melanoma.[135] Nevic cells often display cytoplasmic eosinophilia and frequent binucleation. Other findings of regression of nevi include mononuclear cell infiltrates, telangiectasia, mucinous alteration of the stroma, and diminished or absent melanin in the epidermis.

Regression of the intraepidermal component of melanoma leaving residual melanoma in the dermis may strongly suggest metastatic melanoma or local satellites, solitary or multifocal.[22] Complete obliteration of the dermal component of melanoma occasionally leaves persistent junctional nests and dermal fibrosis,

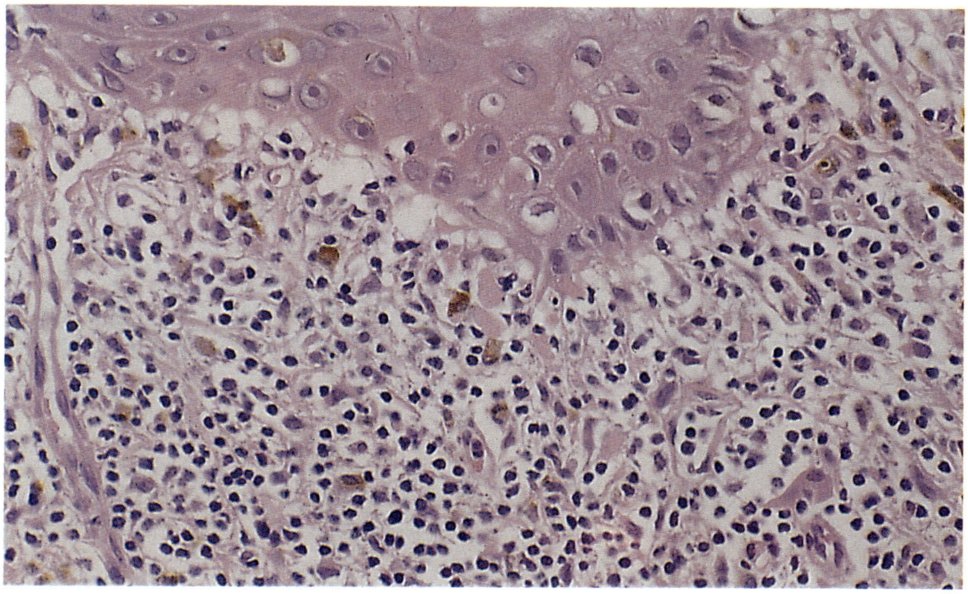

A

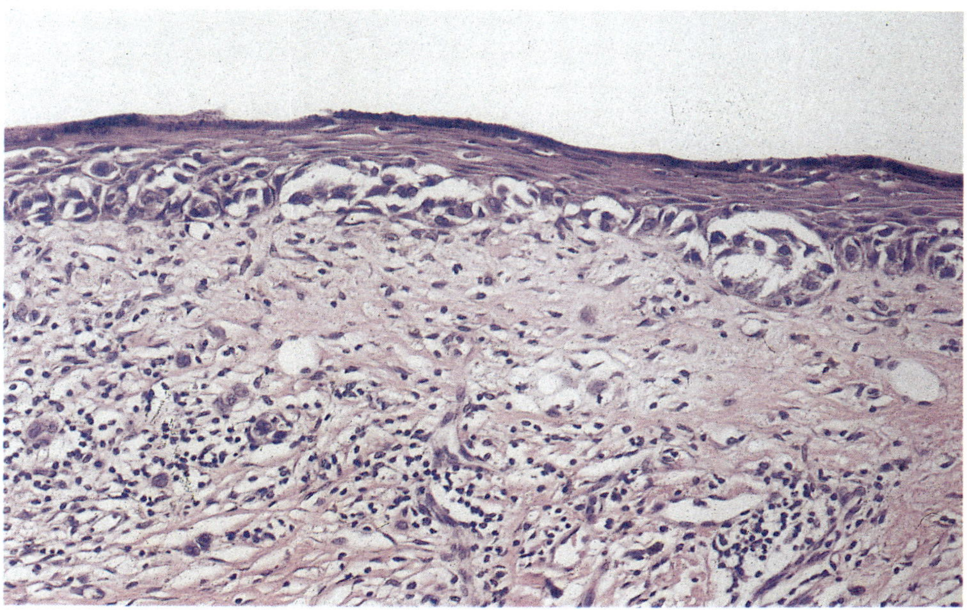

B

FIGURE 10-27

Three stages of regression in melanoma. (A) Early regression demonstrates dense mononuclear cell infiltrates in papillary dermis and apoptotic cells near dermo-epidermal junction (H&E, × 400). (B) Intermediate regression. There is effacement of epidermis but residual melanoma within both epidermis and dermis. Fibrosis of papillary dermis and patchy mononuclear infiltrates also can be observed (H&E, × 200). (C) Late-stage regression. This field shows almost complete absence of melanoma, effacement of the epidermal rete ridges, and thickening and fibrosis of the dermis (H&E, × 400).

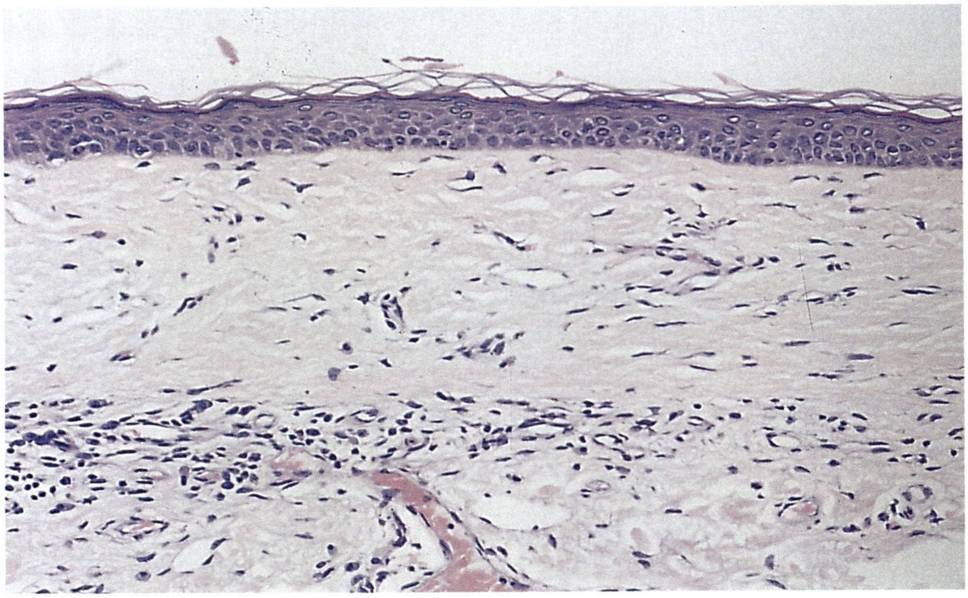

C

FIGURE 10-27 *(Continued)*

simulating in situ or microinvasive melanoma and falsely suggesting an excellent prognosis, when in reality the patient has a greater risk for metastasis.

THE HISTOLOGIC DIAGNOSIS OF MALIGNANT MELANOMA

The histologic diagnosis of malignant melanoma remains rather imprecise and depends on the recognition of a constellation of histologic features, no single feature in and of itself being diagnostic of melanoma. On the other hand, a large percentage of malignant melanomas are diagnosed correctly by a majority of knowledgeable histopathologists. It is also true that a small percentage of melanocytic tumors are histologically challenging and will produce no consensus even among expert histopathologists.

A number of architectural and cytologic characteristics are assessed in evaluating melanomas in the RGP and VGP (Table 10-23). Many histologic parameters hold for both growth phases. In general, melanomas are characterized by overall asymmetry, whereas benign melanocytic lesions tend to have symmetry and orderliness. Although there is no absolute size criterion, the larger the lesion in breadth (generally > 6 mm and especially > 10 mm), the greater is the likelihood that the lesion is melanoma. Melanomas are also characterized by poor circumscription of the peripherally extending intraepidermal component. Other architectural attributes suggesting melanoma include considerable variation in the sizes and shapes of intraepidermal cellular nests and diminished cohesiveness of the nests of cells. The elongated epidermal rete pattern that typifies melanocytic nevi is frequently lost in melanoma, and there may be an accompanying confluence of melanoma cells along the dermoepidermal junction.

One of the features most characteristic of malignant melanoma, yet one that is not specific to melanoma, is upward migration or pagetoid spread of melanocytes in a random pattern. A predominance of single cells over small aggregates or nests typifies this pattern in melanoma. Melanoma cells are usually present at all levels of the epidermis, including the granular and cornified layers.

Cytologic atypia is mandatory for a diagnosis of melanoma (Table 10-23). There is a uniformity or monomorphous quality of the atypia in melanoma rather than the discontinuous pattern of atypia found in dysplastic nevi and lentigo maligna. Melanoma is also notable for hypercellularity and high nuclear-to-cytoplasmic ratios of melanoma cells.

The VGP is a nodular cellular aggregate with pushing or expanding configuration without regard for stroma. In general, there is less host response associated with the VGP but greater mitotic activity and necrosis of cells compared with the RGP.

TABLE 10-23
Criteria for the Histologic Diagnosis of Melanoma

Radial (or horizontal) growth phase (melanoma in situ, melanoma with microinvasion)

Architecture
- Asymmetry
- Large size (>6 mm) but many exceptions
- Poor circumscription of proliferation
- Variation in size, shape, placement of nests
- Diminished cohesiveness of cells in nests
- Confluence of nests
- Loss of epidermal rete pattern (effacement)
- Upward migration of melanocytes (pagetoid spread) in random pattern, single cells predominate over nests, cells reach granular and cornified layers
- Rich mononuclear cell infiltrates, usually bandlike
- Fibroplasia of papillary dermis
- Regression frequently present

Cytology:
- Nuclear changes
  - Majority of melanocytes uniformly atypical
  - Nuclear enlargement
  - Nuclear pleomorphism (variation in sizes and shapes)
  - Nuclear hyperchromasia with coarse chromatin
  - One or more prominent nucleoli
- Cytoplasmic changes
  - Abundant granular eosinophilic cytoplasm in epithelioid cells
  - Finely divided ("dusty") melanin
  - Variation in size of melanin granules
  - High nuclear-to-cytoplasmic ratios in spindle cells
  - Retraction of cytoplasm
  - Mitoses (unusual in dermal component)
  - Atypical mitoses
  - Necrotic cells

Vertical growth phase

- Architecture
  - Tumefactive cellular aggregates
  - Pushing, expanding pattern without regard for stroma
  - Hypercellularity
  - Less host response in general
- Cytology
  - As for radial growth phase
  - Increased nuclear-to-cytoplasmic ratios
  - Mitoses in dermal component
  - Atypical mitoses
  - Necrotic cells

THE DIFFERENTIAL DIAGNOSIS OF MALIGNANT MELANOMA

The list of conditions potentially confused with melanoma has been discussed in the context of specific entities in this chapter. However, in this section, five histologic patterns of melanoma that cause particular difficulty in differential diagnosis will be examined.

1. *Upward migration or pagetoid spread of cells.* This histologic pattern probably causes the greatest difficulty in distinguishing benign simulants from melanoma (Fig. 10-28*A* and *B*). One also must rely on other histologic features such as the presence or absence of asymmetry, large size, poor circumscription, and maturation, among other features as outlined in Table 10-23. The principal melanocytic lesions entering into the differential diagnosis include melanocytic nevi in children, congenital nevi (particularly in the first year of life), spindle and epithelioid cell (Spitz) nevi, pigmented spindle cell nevi (see Fig. 10-28*A*), nevi from acral surfaces, and recurrent melanocytic nevi.

As recorded by Cullity,[136] 7 percent of melanocytic nevi in children under the age of 14 years had prominent pagetoid spread of cells. He found that the upward migration of melanocytes was independent of age, sex, or type of nevus. The pagetoid spread in such nevi is notable for limitation usually to the lower-most epidermis, aggregates of cells predominating over single cells, and low-grade or absent cytologic atypia. Other architectural characteristics will generally be present and include overall symmetry, small size, well-circumscribed margins, and maturation. A particular problem is the evaluation of small or partial biopsies in which other architectural parameters cannot be adequately assessed. In this circumstance, the histologic diagnosis should be deferred until the entire lesion can be evaluated fully. The clinical setting is also of paramount importance, since melanoma in childhood is rare.

The same comments are generally applicable to the presence of pagetoid spread in congenital nevi, spindle and epithelioid cell nevi, pigmented spindle cell nevi, and

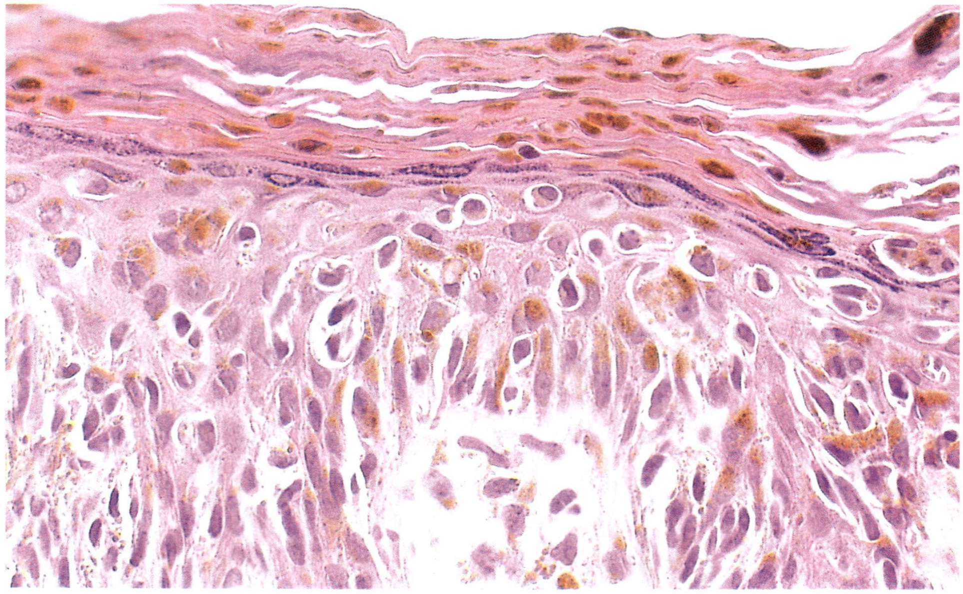

A

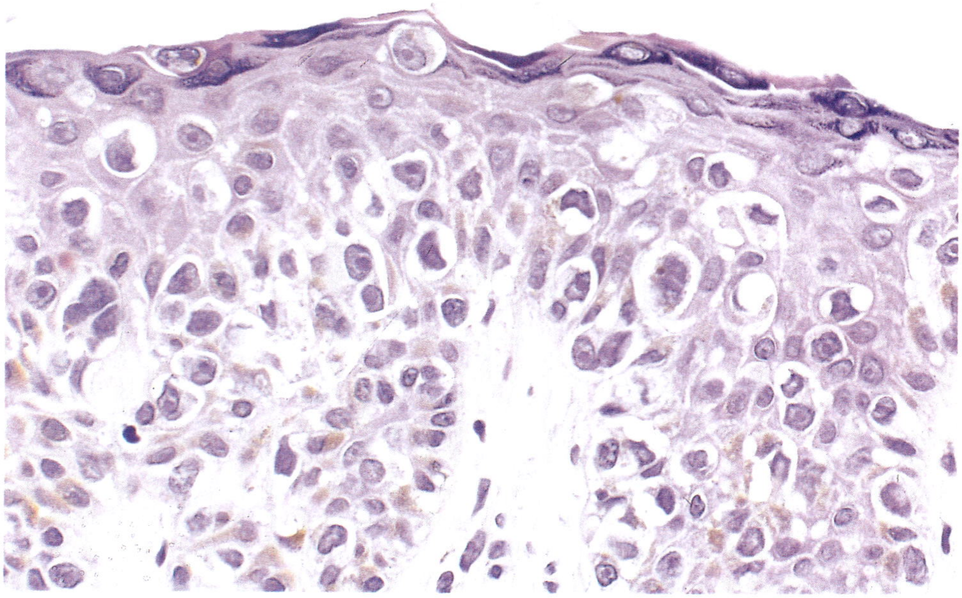

B

FIGURE 10-28

Pagetoid spread. (A) Individual melanocytes are scattered throughout the epidermis in this pigmented spindle cell nevus in a child. The lesion was small, symmetric, well circumscribed, and had an orderly arrangement of intraepidermal nests. The pagetoid cells lack the atypia of melanoma in situ as noted in part B (H&E, × 400). (B) Melanoma in situ. Note pagetoid spread of markedly atypical melanocytes compared with part A. The nuclei show prominent pleomorphism and enlargement (H&E, × 400).

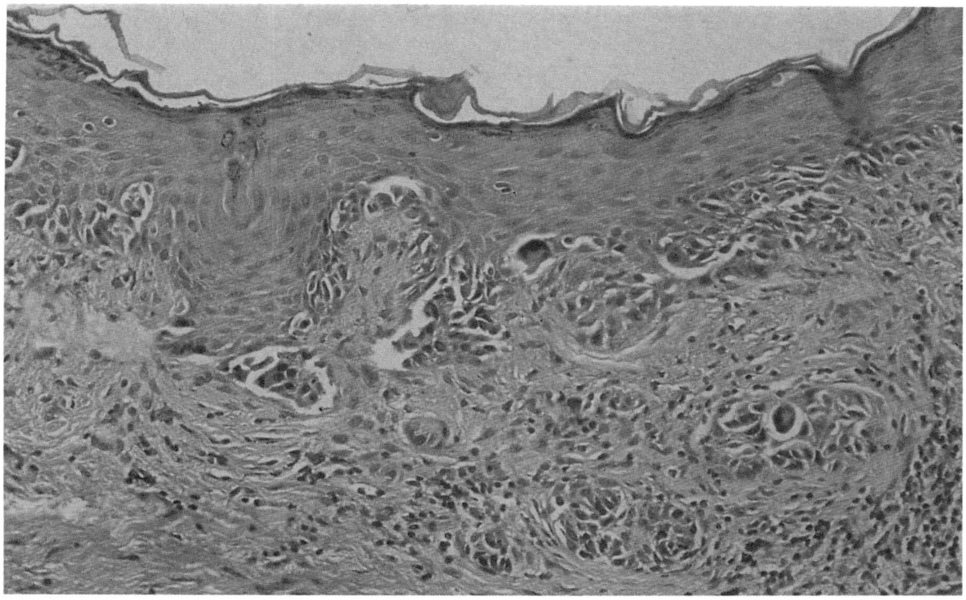

FIGURE 10-29
Horizontal confluence of junctional nests in dysplastic nevus. The rete ridge pattern has not been lost in this dysplastic nevus. There is variable cytologic atypia (H&E, × 200).

acral nevi. Congenital nevi usually will show an overall symmetry and orderly transmigration of cells. There is also maturation of nevus cells in the dermal component, if present. Spindle and epithelioid cell nevi and pigmented spindle cell nevi are also characterized by a usually orderly upward migration of cells, the predominance of nests over cells, regular and symmetric pattern within the epidermis, and the lack of marked cytologic atypia (see Fig. 10-28).

Recurrent melanocytic nevi on occasion have a disorderly pattern of junctional nesting with some upward migration of cells. However, these nevi are distinguished from melanoma because of the confinement of the intraepidermal proliferative elements to the epidermis above the scar and the presence of little or no cytologic atypia. The typical arrangement of intraepidermal nests above a fibrotic dermis and the original dermal nevus remnant provides the characteristic features of recurrent nevus.

Nonmelanocytic tumors that enter into the differential diagnosis of this pattern include squamous cell carcinoma in situ, mammary or extramammary Paget's disease, sebaceous carcinoma, epidermotropic eccrine carcinoma, neuroendocrine carcinoma, and cutaneous T-cell lymphoma.

2. *Large, confluent nests of atypical melanocytic cells disposed along the dermoepidermal junction.* Dysplastic nevus, spindle and epithelioid cell nevus, and pigmented spindle cell nevus are most likely to be confused with this pattern of melanoma. Melanoma is characterized by effacement of the epidermal rete pattern, whereas the typical configuration of the epidermis is maintained in the other three entities. Dysplastic nevus generally has elongated rete ridges, an organized nesting pattern, and discontinuous cytologic atypia (Fig. 10-29). Spindle and epithelioid cell nevus and pigmented spindle cell nevus may on occasion have prominent horizontally disposed fascicles of cells. However, there is an overall orderly and regular placement of nesting within the epidermis consistent with a benign process. The majority of cells in the latter lesions are fairly uniform with delicate chromatin patterns.

3. *Lentiginous pattern of melanocytic proliferation.* This pattern, describing single cell proliferation along the dermoepidermal junction, is the predominant type of proliferation observed in lentigo maligna and acral lentiginous melanoma (see Figs. 10-9 and 10-11). Occasional lentigines and dysplastic nevi may have this change and suggest melanoma. The criteria favoring melanoma include the various architectural features described in Table 10-23. The patterns noted in melanoma will include contiguous proliferation of melanocytes along the dermoepidermal junction reaching confluence and a uniformity of marked cytologic atypia. This frequency of melanocytic

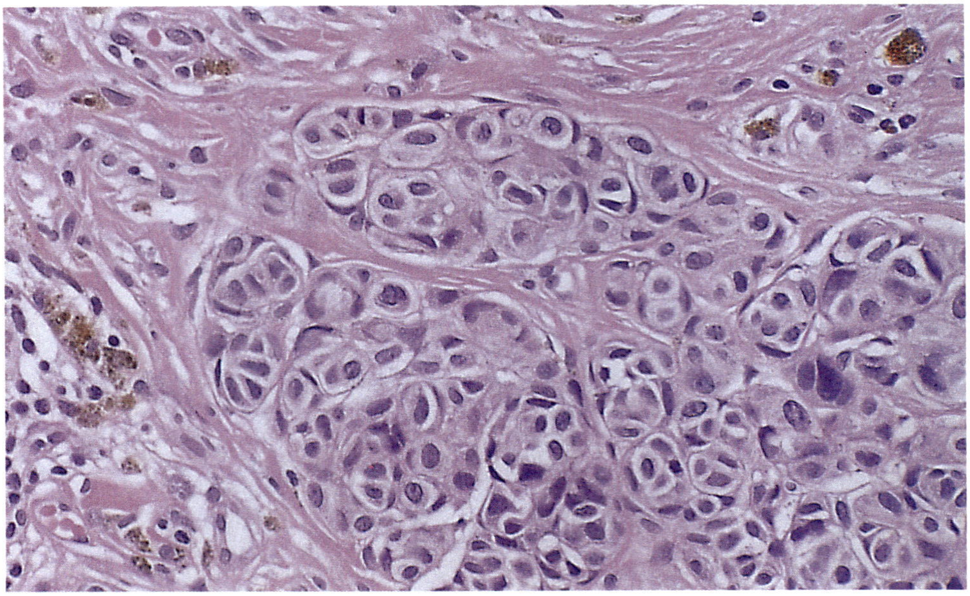

A

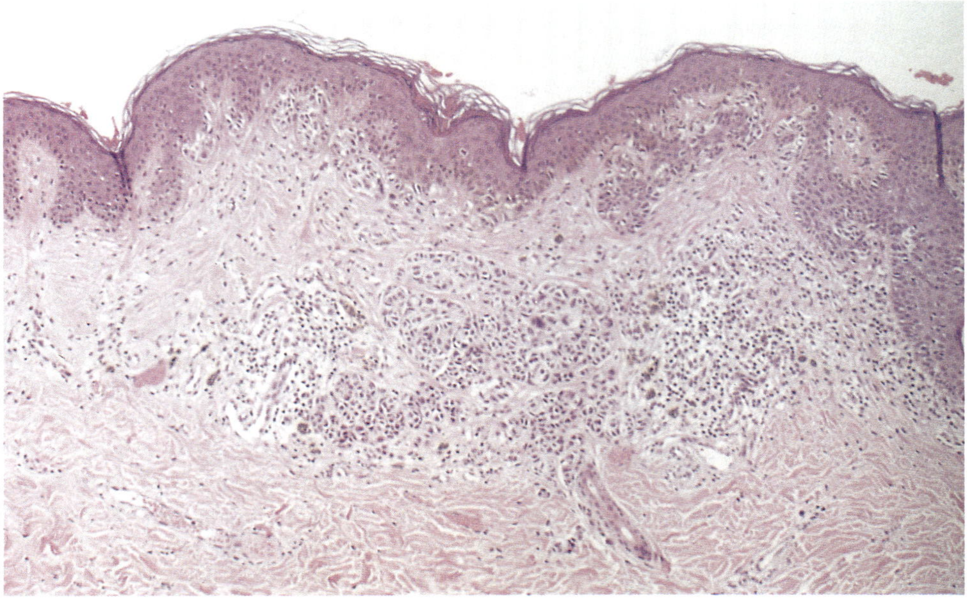

B

FIGURE 10-30

Cohesive cellular nodule in papillary dermis of compound dysplastic nevus. (A) The expansile nature of the nests in the papillary dermis suggests melanoma (H&E, × 400). (B) Overall, the lesion retains the appearance of a nevus with symmetry, junctional nesting, and absence of pagetoid spread (H&E, × 100). (C) Although the cells within the dermal nodule exhibit atypia, there is some degree of maturation, and mitotic figures are absent (H&E, × 200).

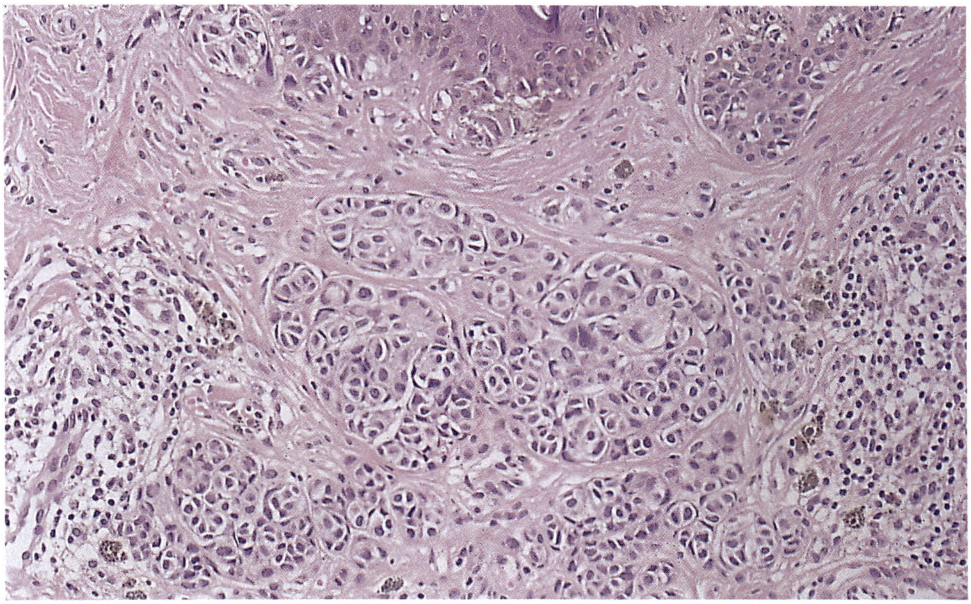

C

FIGURE 10-30 *(Continued)*

proliferation is not present in lentigines and usually not in dysplastic nevi. Lentigo maligna, furthermore, is notable for nesting of atypical cells with diminished cohesion and the basilar proliferation of melanocytes in appendageal epithelium. Acral lentiginous melanoma has epidermal hyperplasia and the presence of strikingly enlarged melanoma cells possessing prominent dendrites.

4. *Cohesive cellular nodules.* This histomorphologic feature typifies the VGP of melanoma, and certain melanocytic proliferations closely simulate this pattern. Cohesive cellular aggregates are occasionally noted in spindle and epithelioid cell nevi, pigmented spindle cell nevi, the dermal component of both acquired (often dysplastic) and congenital nevi, and cellular blue nevi and are considered architecturally atypical (Fig. 10-30). As has already been emphasized, all the architectural and cytologic characteristics of a particular proliferation must be assessed in the determination of whether a given lesion is benign, malignant, or indeterminant (see Table 10-23). Although the overall histologic picture may suggest a benign process, a focal nodular proliferation may indicate possible transformation to melanoma. Features strongly suggesting melanoma include hypercellularity and crowding of nuclei within the nodule, an abrupt transition from the nodule to the surrounding cellular elements rather than a gradual transition, an expanding or pushing quality with disregard of surrounding stroma, a uniformity of cytologic atypia, marked cytologic atypia, high nuclear-to-cytoplasmic ratios, easily found mitotic figures including atypical mitoses, and necrotic cells.

In general, primary melanoma may be distinguished from metastatic melanoma by the presence of larger size, host response and regression, the extension of an intraepidermal component lateral to a dermal component, and a polyclonal appearance (see Chap. 11). Metastatic melanoma, on the other hand, may exhibit epidermotropism, but this is generally confined to the epidermis immediately above the metastatic tumor.

5. *Distinction of melanoma in dermis from dermal nevus cells.* One of the most perplexing diagnostic problems encountered by the histopathologist is the discrimination of melanoma from nests of dermal nevus cells. Specific situations where this dilemma is encountered include nests of nevus-appearing cells either in continuity or discontiguous with invasive melanoma, entrapped in a fibrotic dermis of a markedly atypical dysplastic nevus (Fig. 10-31*A* and *B*), and in areas of regression.

Probably the easiest of these three problems is the discrimination of dermal melanoma cells from a discontiguous nevus-appearing focus. The presence of two distinct, spatially separate components, one clearly melanoma and the other suggesting nevus, is probably the best evidence favoring an associated remnant of dermal nevus. However, other characteristics of dermal nevus cells include envelopment of individual nevus cells and cellular

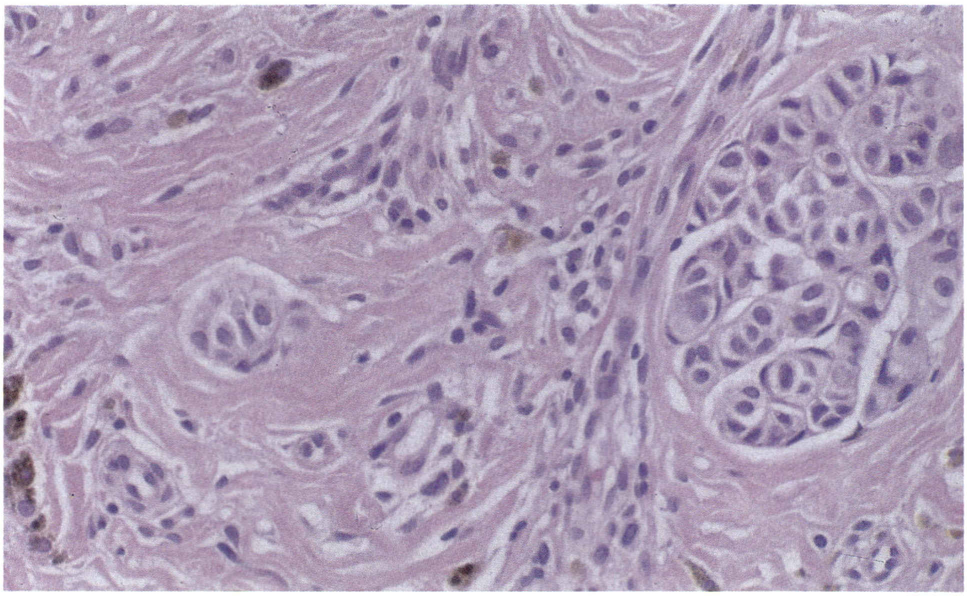

A

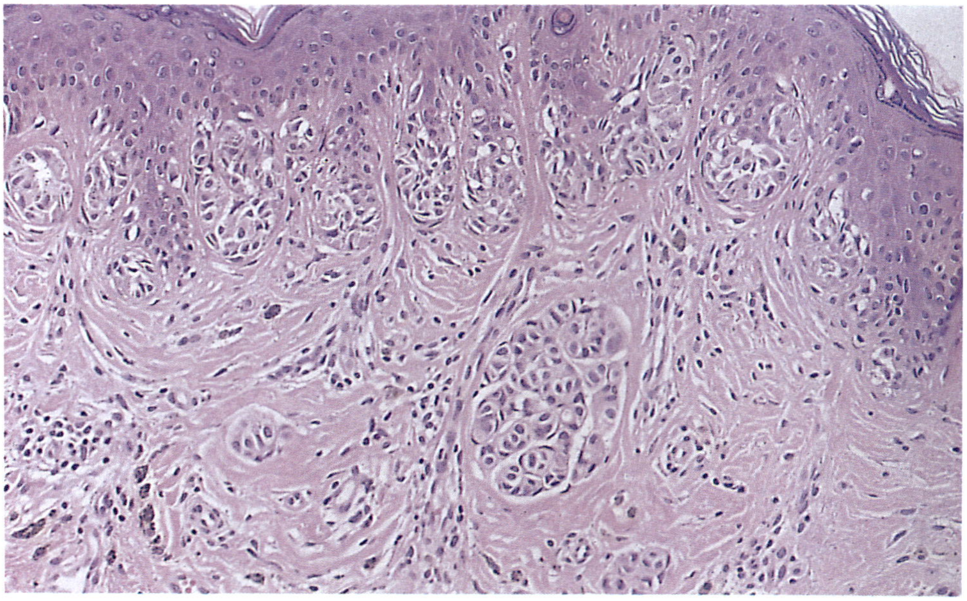

B

FIGURE 10-31

Atypical dermal nevus cells entrapped in fibrotic papillary dermis of dysplastic nevus. (A) The dermal component suggests melanoma (H&E, × 400). (B) However, the intraepidermal component lacks sufficient changes for melanoma. The lesion has an overall orderly pattern with well-formed junctional nests, no pagetoid spread, and moderate atypia (H&E, × 200). (C) Melanoma with tumor cells entrapped in fibrotic papillary dermis. Extensive regression has resulted in a horizontal disposition of melanoma cells. There is continuity of these cells with intraepidermal and superficial papillary melanoma cells (H&E, × 200).

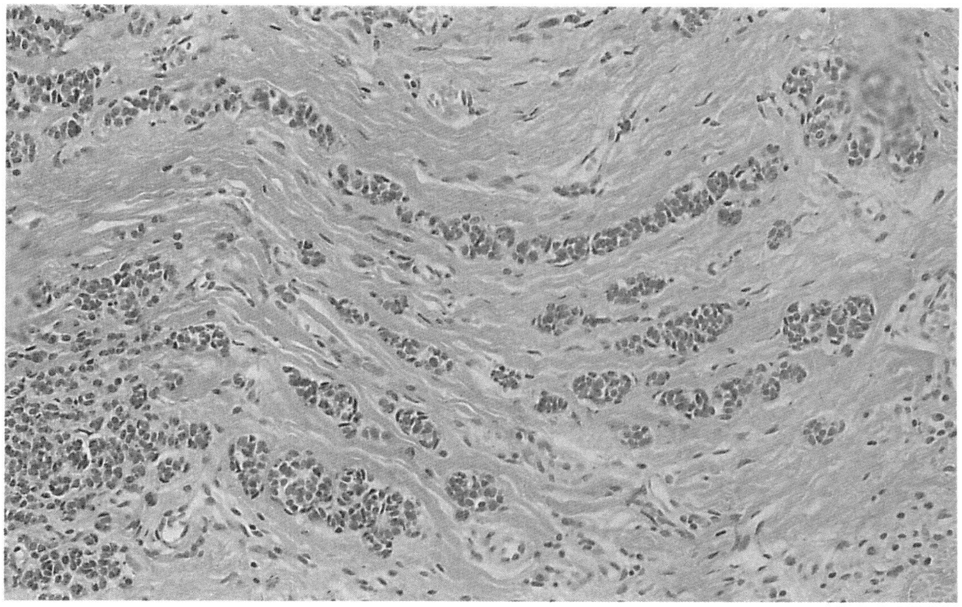

C

FIGURE 10-31 *(Continued)*

TABLE 10-24
Histopathologic Reporting of Melanoma

Essential information	
	Diagnosis: Malignant melanoma, in situ or invasive
	Measured depth (mm)
	Presence of desmoplasia, neurotropism, or both
	Presence of marked or virtually complete regression
	Presence of vascular/lymphatic invasion
	Adequacy of surgical margins
Other prognostic information	
	Histologic subtype, e.g., lentigo maligna
	Histologic ulceration
	Mitotic rate (per mm^2)
	Anatomic level, i.e., I, II, III, IV, V
	Radial or vertical growth phase
	Tumor-infiltrating lymphocytes
	Microscopic satellites

aggregates by collagenous fibers (as well as other basement membrane elements), lack of expansile qualities of the nests, lack of striking nuclear hyperchromasia, relatively low nuclear-to-cytoplasmic ratios of nevus cells, fairly uniform nuclei with inconspicuous or absence of nucleoli, and the usual absence of mitoses and necrotic cells. It must be emphasized that melanoma cells may on occasion display such pronounced nevus differentiation that careful consideration of all the preceding criteria is needed for separation of nevus from melanoma.

Certain melanomas demonstrate "maturation" or a gradient of increasing nevus differentiation of melanoma cells with depth in the dermis. The latter phenomenon refers to contiguous cells that appear most nevus-like in the lower-most portions of the dermal component (see Fig. 10-31*C*). Because the entire cellular mass is continuous, it is assumed (and seems logical to conclude) that all elements are melanoma (see Fig. 10-31*C*). This gradient in differentiation may in fact represent stages of tumor progression or possibly the inductive effects of stroma on the tumor cells. However, if the deepest portion of the nevomelanocytic proliferation qualifies as fully benign, then the atypical cells above this area should be interpreted as malignant only cautiously.

Nests of atypical melanocytic cells entrapped in a fibrotic matrix must be assessed in the overall context of the lesion. In the case of dysplastic nevus, the intraepidermal findings will usually support a benign diagnosis: maintenance of rete ridge patterns, cohesive junctional nesting of variably atypical melanocytic cells, overall orderly pattern with usually little or no pagetoid spread (see Fig. 10-31*A* and *B*). The presence of residual nests of cells in the setting of regression may prove to be exceedingly difficult if the cells are not obviously melanoma or nevus cells. One must weigh all the characteristics referred to above for discrimination of melanoma from nevus cells in the dermis.

HISTOPATHOLOGIC REPORTING OF MELANOMA

The pathology report should include the following minimum information: diagnosis, i.e., malignant melanoma, in situ or invasive; depth of tumor invasion in millimeters, measured vertically from the granular layer of the epidermis or from the surface of an ulcer with an ocular micrometer; and the adequacy of surgical margins (Table 10-24). The following histologic changes also should be mentioned if present: desmoplasia or neurotropism, marked or virtually complete regression; and true vascular/lymphatic invasion.

Other prognostic factors such as histologic type of melanoma, ulceration, mitotic rate per square millimeter, anatomic level, radial or vertical growth phase, tumor-infiltrating lymphocytes, and microscopic satellites might be reported as well. However, many of the latter factors are highly correlated with tumor thickness and thus may not add significant information beyond thickness alone (see Chap. 12 for additional discussion).

REFERENCES

1. Roush GC, Schymura MJ, Holford TR: Risk for cutaneous melanoma in recent Connecticut birth cohorts. *Am J Public Health* 75:679–682, 1985.
2. Roush GC, Holford TR, Schymura MJ, et al: *Cancer Risk and Incidence Trends: Connecticut Perspective.* Washington, Hemisphere Publishing, 1987, pp. 203–219.
3. Sondik EJ, Kessler LG, Ries LAG: *Cancer Statistics Review, 1973–1987* (Publication No. NIH 90-2789). Washington, U.S. Government Printing Office, 1990, pp. I.10–V.18.
4. Foulds L: *Neoplastic Development*, vol 1. New York, Academic Press, 1969, pp. 41–96.
5. Clark WH Jr, Elder DE, Guerry D IV, et al: A study of tumor progression: The precursor lesions of superficial spreading and nodular melanoma. *Hum Pathol* 15:1147–1165, 1984.
6. Clark WH: Tumor progression and the nature of cancer. *Br J Cancer* 64:631–644, 1991.
7. Mishima Y: Melanocytic and nevocytic malignant melanoma. Cellular and subcellular differentiation. *Cancer* 20:632–649, 1967.
8. Holman CDJ, Armstrong B, Heenan P: A theory of the etiology and pathogenesis of human cutaneous malignant melanoma. *J Natl Cancer Inst* 71:651–656, 1983.
9. Gruber SB, Barnhill RL, Stenn KS, Roush GC: Nevomelanocytic proliferations in association with cutaneous malignant melanoma: A multivariate analysis. *J Am Acad Dermatol* 21:773–780, 1989.
10. Barnhill RL, Roush GC, Duray PH: Correlation of histologic architectural and cytoplastic features with nuclear atypia in atypical (dysplastic) nevomelanocytic nevi. *Hum Pathol* 21:51–58, 1990.
11. Barnhill RL: Current status of the dysplastic melanocytic nevus. *J Cutan Pathol* 18:147–159, 1991.
12. Clark WH Jr: A classification of malignant melanoma in man correlated with histogenesis and biologic behavior. In Montagna W, Hu F (eds): *Advances in the Biology of the Skin*, vol VIII. New York, Pergamon Press, 1967, pp. 621–647.
13. Clark WH Jr, From L, Bernardino EA, Mihm MC: The histogenesis and biologic behavior of primary human malignant melanomas of the skin. *Cancer Res* 29:705–727, 1969.
14. McGovern VJ, Mihm MC Jr, Bailly C, et al: The classification of malignant melanoma and its histologic reporting. *Cancer* 32:1446–1457, 1973.
15. Clark WH Jr, Elder DE, Van Horn M: The biologic forms of malignant melanoma. *Hum Pathol* 17:443–450, 1984.
16. Clark WH Jr, Elder DE, Guerry D IV, et al: Model predicting survival in stage I melanoma based on tumor progression. *J Natl Cancer Inst* 81:1893–1904, 1989.
17. Ackerman AB: Malignant melanoma: A unifying concept. *Hum Pathol* 11:591–595, 1980.
18. Clark WH Jr, Mihm MC Jr: Lentigo maligna and lentigo maligna melanoma. *Am J Pathol* 55:39–67, 1969.
19. Ten Seldam R, Helwig E, Sobin L, et al: Histological typing of skin tumours. In *Histological Typing of Skin Tumours: International Histological Classification of Tumors, No. 12.* Geneva, WHO, 1974.
20. Reed RJ: The pathology of human cutaneous melanoma. In Costanzi JJ, (ed): *Malignant Melanoma I.* The Hague: Martinus Nijhoff, 1983, pp. 85–116.
21. Clark WH Jr, Evans HL, Everett MA, et al: Early melanoma: Histologic terms. *Am J Dermatopathol* 13:579–582, 1991.
22. McGovern VJ: Spontaneous regression of melanoma. *Pathology* 7:91–99, 1975.
23. Herlyn M, Clark WH, Rodeck U, et al: Biology of tumor progression in human melanocytes. *Lab Invest* 56:461–474, 1987.
24. Reed RJ: Acral lentiginous melanoma. In *New Concepts in Surgical Pathology of Skin.* New York, Wiley, 1976, pp. 89–90.
25. Arrington JH III, Reed RJ, Ichinose H, Krementz ET: Plantar lentiginous melanoma: A distinctive variant of human cutaneous malignant melanoma. *Am J Surg Pathol* 1:131–143, 1977.
26. Elder DE, Jucovy PM, Tuthill RJ, Clark WH Jr: The classification of malignant melanoma. *Am J Dermatopathol* 2:315–320, 1980.
27. English DR, Heenan PJ, Holman CD, et al: Melanoma in Western Australia in 1980–81: Incidence and characteristics of histological types. *Pathology* 19:383–392, 1987.
28. Heenan PJ, Armstrong BK, English DE, et al: Pathological and epidemiological variants of cutaneous malignant melanoma. In Elder DE (ed): *Pathobiology of Malignant Melanoma.* Basel, Karger, 1987, pp. 107–146.
29. Holman CDJ, Armstrong BK: Cutaneous malignant melanoma and indicators of total accumulated exposure to the sun: An analysis separating histogenetic types. *J Natl Cancer Inst* 73:75–82, 1984.
30. Heenan PJ, Holman CDJ: Nodular malignant melanoma: A distinct entity or a common end stage? *Am J Dermatopathol* 4:477–478, 1982.

31. Mishima Y, Matsunaka J: Pagetoid premalignant melanosis and melanoma: Differentiation from Hutchinson's freckle. *J Invest Dermatol* 65:434–440, 1975.
32. Heenan PJ, Matz LR, Blackwell JB, et al: Inter-observer variation between pathologists in the classification of cutaneous malignant melanoma in Western Australia. *Histopathology* 8:717–729, 1984.
33. Vollmer R: Pathology of melanoma. In Seigler H (ed): *Clinical Management of Melanoma.* The Hague: Martinus Nijhoff, 1982, pp. 9–40.
34. Balch CM, Soong S-J, Shaw HM, et al: An analysis of prognostic factors in 8,500 patients with cutaneous melanoma. In Balch CM (ed): *Cutaneous Melanoma* (ed 2). Philadelphia, Lippincott, 1992, pp. 165–187.
35. Mihm MC Jr, Fitzpatrick TB, Brown MM, et al: Early detection of primary cutaneous malignant melanoma. A color atlas. *N Engl J Med* 289:989–996, 1973.
36. Price NM, Rywlin AM, Ackerman AB: Histologic criteria for the diagnosis of superficial spreading malignant melanoma: Formulated on the basis of proven metastatic lesions. *Cancer* 38:2434–2441, 1976.
37. Day CL Jr, Harrist TJ, Gorstein F, et al: Malignant melanoma. Prognostic significance of "microscopic satellites" in the reticular dermis and subcutaneous fat. *Ann Surg* 194:108–112, 1981.
38. Fitzpatrick JE: The histologic diagnosis of intraepithelial pagetoid neoplasms. *Clin Dermatol* 9:255–259, 1991.
39. Cochran AJ, Wen D-R: S-100 protein as a marker for melanocytic and other tumors. *Pathology* 17:340–345, 1985.
40. Schmitt FC, Bacchi CE: S-100 protein: Is it useful as a marker in diagnostic immunocytochemistry. *Histopathology* 15:281–288, 1989.
41. Gown AM, Vogel AM, Hoak D, et al: Monoclonal antibodies specific for melanocytic tumors distinguish subpopulations of melanocytes. *Am J Pathol* 123:195–203, 1986.
42. Makin CA, Bobrow LG, Bodmer WF: Monoclonal antibody to cytokeratin for use in routine histopathology. *J Clin Pathol* 37:975–983, 1984.
43. Gullick WJ, Berger MS, Bennett PL, et al: Expression of the c-*erb* B_2 protein in normal and transformed cells. *Int J Cancer* 40:246–254, 1987.
44. Elder DE: Metastatic melanoma. In Elder DE (ed): *Pigment Cell*, vol 8. Basel, Karger, 1987, pp. 182–204.
45. Weinstock MA, Sober AJ: The risk of progression of lentigo maligna to lentigo maligna melanoma. *Br J Dermatol* 116:303–310, 1987.
46. Barnhill RL, Barnhill MA, Berwick M, Mihm MC Jr: The histologic spectrum of pigmented spindle cell nevus: A review of 120 cases with emphasis on atypical variants. *Hum Pathol* 22:52–58, 1991.
47. Coleman WP III, Loria PR, Reed RJ, Krementz ET: Acral lentiginous melanoma. *Arch Dermatol* 116:773–776, 1980.
48. Patterson RH, Helwig EB: Subungual malignant melanoma: A clinical-pathologic study. *Cancer* 46:2074–2087, 1980.
49. Saida T, Yoshida N, Ikegawa S, et al: Clinical guidelines for the early detection of plantar malignant melanoma. *J Am Acad Dermatol* 23:37–40, 1990.
50. Blessing K, Kernohan NM, Park KGM: Subungual malignant melanoma: Clinicopathological features of 100 cases. *Histopathology* 19:425–429, 1992.
51. Rigby HS, Briggs JC: Subungual melanoma: A clinicopathological study of 24 cases. *Br J Plast Surg* 45:275–278, 1992.
52. Saida T, Ohshima Y: Clinical and histopathologic characteristics of early lesions of subungual malignant melanoma. *Cancer* 63:556–560, 1989.
53. Clark WH Jr, Bernardino EA, Reed RJ, Kopf AW: Acral lentiginous melanomas including melanomas of mucous membranes. In Clark WH Jr, Goldman LI, Mastrangelo MJ (eds): *Human Malignant Melanoma.* New York, Grune and Stratton, 1979, pp. 109–124.
54. Ohashi K, Nemoto T, Kasuga T: Cytological and histological features of mucosal malignant melanoma (abstract). International Pigment Cell Society Meeting, London, September, 1993.
55. Conley J, Lattes R, Orr W: Desmoplastic malignant melanoma (a rare variant of spindle cell melanoma). *Cancer* 28:914–936, 1971.
56. Reiman HM, Goellner JR, Woods JE, Mixter RC: Desmoplastic melanoma of the head and neck. *Cancer* 60:2269–2274, 1987.
57. Egbert B, Kempson R, Sagebiel R: Desmoplastic malignant melanoma. A clinicohistopathologic study of 25 cases. *Cancer* 62:2033–2041, 1988.
58. Walsh NM, Roberts JT, Orr W, Simon GT: Desmoplastic malignant melanoma. A clinicopathologic study of 14 cases. *Arch Pathol Lab Med* 112:922–927, 1988.
59. Beenken S, Byers R, Smith JL, et al: Desmoplastic melanoma. Histologic correlation with behavior and treatment. *Arch Otolaryngol Head Neck Surg* 115:374–379, 1989.
60. Jain S, Allen PW: Desmoplastic malignant melanoma and its variants. A study of 45 cases. *Am J Surg Pathol* 13:358–373, 1989.
61. Smithers BM, McLeod GR, Little JH: Desmoplastic, neural transforming and neurotropic melanoma: A review of 45 cases. *Aust NZ J Surg* 60:967–972, 1990.
62. Cerio R, Anstey A, Smith NP, et al: Desmoplastic malignant melanoma—Clinicopathological and immunohistochemical study of 23 cases (abstract). *J Cutan Pathol* 17(5):289, 1990.
63. Skelton HG, Smith KJ, Laskin W, et al: Desmoplastic malignant melanoma (abstract). *J Cutan Pathol* 17(5):317, 1990.
64. Bryant E, Ronan SG, Felix EL, Manaligod JR: Desmoplastic malignant melanoma. A study by conventional and electron microscopy. *Am J Dermatopathol* 4:467–474, 1982.
65. From L, Hanna W, Kahn HJ, et al: Origin of the desmoplasia in desmoplastic malignant melanoma. *Hum Pathol* 14:1072–1080, 1983.
66. Labrecque PG, Hu C, Winkelmann RK: On the nature of desmoplastic melanoma. *Cancer* 38:1205–1213, 1976.
67. Valensi QJ: Desmoplastic malignant melanoma: A report of two additional cases. *Cancer* 39:286–292, 1977.
68. Valensi QJ: Desmoplastic malignant melanoma: A light and electron microscopic study of two cases. *Cancer* 43:1148–1155, 1979.

69. Valensi QJ: Desmoplastic malignant melanoma: Study of a case by light and electronmicroscopy. *J Dermatol Surg Oncol* 5:31–35, 1979.
70. Bruijn JA, Mihm MC Jr, Barnhill RL: Desmoplastic melanoma. *Histopathology* 20:197–205, 1992.
71. Bruijn JA, Salasche SJ, Sober AJ, et al: Desmoplastic melanoma: Clinicopathologic aspects of six cases. *Dermatology* 185:3–8, 1992.
72. Carlson JA, Dickerson GR, Sober AJ, Barnhill RL: Desmoplastic neurotropic melanoma: A clinicopathologic analysis of 28 cases. *Cancer* (in press, 1994).
73. Reed RJ, Leonard DD: Neurotropic melanoma: A variant of desmoplastic melanoma. *Am J Surg Pathol* 3:301–311, 1979.
74. Kossard S, Doherty E, Murray E: Neurotropic melanoma. A variant of desmoplastic melanoma. *Arch Dermatol* 123:907–912, 1987.
75. Gartner MFRM, Fearns C, Wilson EL, et al: Unusual growth characteristics of human melanoma xenografts in the nude mouse: A model for desmoplasia, dormancy and progression. *Br J Cancer* 64:487–490, 1992.
76. Fearns C, Dowdle EB: The desmoplastic response: Induction of collagen synthesis by melanoma cells in vitro. *Int J Cancer* 50:621–627, 1992.
77. Mihm MC, Googe PB: Problems in various subtypes of malignant melanoma. In Mihm MC, Googe PB (eds): *Problematic Pigmented Lesions—A Case Method Approach.* Philadelphia, Lea & Febiger, 1990, pp. 279–370.
78. Barr RJ, Morales RV, Graham JH: Desmoplastic nevus: A distinct histologic variant of mixed spindle cell and epithelioid cell nevus. *Cancer* 46:557–564, 1980.
79. Barnhill RL, Mihm MC: Cellular neurothekeoma: A distinctive variant of neurothekeoma mimicking nevomelanocytic tumors. *Am J Surg Pathol* 14:113–120, 1990.
80. Warner TF, Lloyd RV, Hafez GR, Angevine JM: Immunocytochemistry of neurotropic melanoma. *Cancer* 53:254–257, 1984.
81. Wick MR, Swanson PE, Rocamora A: Recognition of malignant melanoma by monoclonal antibody HMB-45: An immunohistochemical study of 200 paraffin-embedded cutaneous tumors. *J Cutan Pathol* 15:201–207, 1988.
82. Reed RJ, Ichinose H, Clark WH Jr, Mihm MC Jr: Common and uncommon melanocytic nevi and borderline melanomas. *Semin Oncol* 2:119–147, 1975.
83. Reed RJ: Consultation case. *Am J Surg Pathol* 2:215–220, 1978.
84. Hendrickson MR, Ross JC: Neoplasms arising in congenital giant nevi: Morphologic study of seven cases and a review of the literature. *Am J Surg Pathol* 5:109–135, 1981.
85. Muhlbauer JE, Margolis RJ, Mihm MC Jr, Reed RJ: Minimal deviation melanoma: A histologic variant of cutaneous malignant melanoma in its vertical growth phase. *J Invest Dermatol* 80(suppl):63S–65S, 1983.
86. Phillips ME, Margolis RJ, Merot Y, et al: The spectrum of minimal deviation melanoma: A clinicopathologic study of 21 cases. *Hum Pathol* 17:796–806, 1986.
87. Reed RJ: Minimal deviation melanoma. In Mihm MC Jr, Murphy GF, Kaufman N (eds): *Pathobiology and Recognition of Malignant Melanoma.* Baltimore, Williams & Wilkins, 1988, pp. 110–152.
88. Reed RJ, Webb S, Clark WH Jr: Minimal deviation melanoma (Halo nevus variant). *Am J Surg Pathol* 14:53–68, 1990.
89. Larsen TE, Grude TH: A retrospective histologic study of 669 cases of primary cutaneous malignant melanoma in clinical stage I: II. The relation of cell type, pigmentation, atypia, and mitotic count to histologic type and prognosis. *Acta Pathol Microbiol Scand [A]* 86:513–522, 1978.
90. Day CL, Harrist TJ, Lew RA, Mihm MC Jr: Classification of malignant melanoma according to the histologic morphology of melanoma nodules. *J Dermatol Surg Oncol* 8:874–875, 900, 1982.
91. Baak JP, Tan G: The adjuvant prognostic value of nuclear morphometry in stage I malignant melanoma of the skin: A multivariate analysis. *Anal Quant Cytol Histol* 68:241–244, 1986.
92. Sorensen FB: Objective histopathologic grading of cutaneous malignant melanomas by stereologic estimation of nuclear volume. *Cancer* 63:1784–1798, 1989.
93. Schmoeckel C, Castro CE, Braun-Falco O: Nevoid malignant melanoma. *Arch Dermatol Res* 277:362–369, 1985.
94. Steiner A, Konrad K, Pehamberger H, Wolff K: Verrucous malignant melanoma. *Arch Dermatol* 124:1534–1537, 1988.
95. Levene A: On the histological diagnosis and prognosis of malignant melanoma. *J Clin Pathol* 33:101–124, 1980.
96. Suster S, Ronnen M, Bubis JJ: Verrucous pseudonevoid melanoma. *J Surg Oncol* 36:134–137, 1987.
97. Kuehnl-Petzoldt Ch, Berger H, Wiebelt H: Verrucous-keratotic variations of malignant melanoma: A clinicopathological study. *Am J Dermatopathol* 4:403–410, 1982.
98. Blessing K, Evans AT, Al-Nafussi A: Verrucous naevoid and keratotic malignant melanoma: A clinicopathological study of 20 cases. *Histopathology* 23:453–458, 1993.
99. Okun M, Bauman L: Malignant melanoma arising from an intradermal nevus. *Arch Dermatol* 92:69–72, 1965.
100. Okun MR, Di Mattia A, Thompson J, Pearson SH: Malignant melanoma developing from intradermal nevi. *Arch Dermatol* 110:599–601, 1974.
101. Benisch B, Peison B, Kannerstein M, Spivack J: Malignant melanoma originating from intradermal nevi: A clinicopathologic entity. *Arch Dermatol* 116:696–698, 1980.
102. Ball NJ, Golitz LE: Melanocytic nevi with focal atypical epithelioid cell components: A review of 73 cases. *J Am Acad Dermatol* 30:724–729, 1994.
103. Kwittken J, Negri L: Malignant blue nevus: Case report of a Negro woman. *Arch Dermatol* 94:64–69, 1966.
104. Merkow LP, Burt RC, Hayeslip DW, et al: A cellular and malignant blue nevus: A light and electron microscopic study. *Cancer* 24:888–896, 1969.
105. Hernandez JF: Malignant blue nevus: A light and electron microscopic study. *Arch Dermatol* 107:741–744, 1973.
106. Rubinstein N, Kopolovic J, Wexler MR, Peled IJ: Malignant blue nevus. *J Dermatol Surg Oncol* 11:921–923, 1985.
107. Wetherington GM, Norin AL, Sadove AM: Locally invasive cellular blue nevus of the scalp. *Plast Reconstr Surg* 79:114–117, 1987.

108. Temple-Camp CRE, Saxe N, King H: Benign and malignant cellular blue nevus: A clinicopathologic study of 30 cases. *Am J Dermatopathol* 10:289–296, 1988.
109. Goldenhersh MA, Savin RC, Barnhill RL, Stenn KS: Malignant blue nevus. Case report and literature review. *J Am Acad Dermatol* 19:712–722, 1988.
110. Connelly J, Smith JL Jr: Malignant blue nevus. *Cancer* 67:2653–2657, 1991.
111. Rodriguez HA, Ackerman LV: Cellular blue nevus. *Cancer* 21:393–405, 1968.
112. Avidor I, Kessler E: "Atypical" blue nevus—A benign variant of cellular blue nevus. *Dermatologica* 154:39–44, 1977.
113. Enzinger FM: Clear-cell sarcoma of tendons and aponeuroses: An analysis of 21 cases. *Cancer* 18:1163–1174, 1965.
114. Chung EB, Enzinger FM: Malignant melanoma of soft parts: A reassessment of clear-cell sarcoma. *Am J Surg Pathol* 7:405–413, 1983.
115. Swanson PE, Wick MR: Clear cell sarcoma: An immunohistochemical analysis of six cases and comparison with other epithelioid neoplasms of soft tissue *Arch Pathol Lab Med* 113:55–60, 1989.
116. Sara AS, Evans HL, Benjamin RS: Malignant melanoma of soft parts (clear cell sarcoma): A study of 17 cases, with emphasis on prognostic factors. *Cancer* 65:367–374, 1990.
117. Zucman J, Delattre O, Desmaze C, et al: EWS and ATF-1 gene fusion induced by t(12;22) translocation in malignant melanoma of soft parts. *Nature Genetics* 4:341–345, 1993.
118. McGovern VJ, Shaw HM, Milton GW: Prognostic significance of a polypoid configuration in malignant melanoma. *Histopathology* 7:663–672, 1983.
119. Giuliano AE, Cochran AJ, Morton DL: Melanoma from unknown primary site and amelanotic melanoma. *Semin Oncol* 9:442–447, 1982.
120. Peters MS, Su WPD: Balloon cell malignant melanoma. *J Am Acad Dermatol* 13:351–354, 1985.
121. Kao GF, Helwig EB, Graham JH: Balloon cell malignant melanoma of the skin: A clinicopathologic study of 34 cases with histochemical, immunohistochemical, and ultrastructural observations. *Cancer* 69:2942–2952, 1992.
122. Okun MR: Melanoma resembling spindle and epithelioid cell nevus. *Arch Dermatol* 115:1416–1420, 1979.
123. Nakhleh RE, Wick MR, Rocamora A, et al: Morphologic diversity in malignant melanomas. *Am J Clin Pathol* 93:731–740, 1990.
124. Sarode VR, Joshi K, Ravichandran P, Das R: Myxoid variant of primary cutaneous malignant melanoma. *Histopathology* 20:186–187, 1992.
125. Prieto VG, Kanik A, Salob S, McNutt NS: Primary cutaneous myxoid melanoma: Immunohistologic clues to a difficult diagnosis. *J Am Acad Dermatol* 30:335–339, 1994.
126. Clark WH Jr, Elder DE, Guerry D IV: Dysplastic nevi and malignant melanoma. In Farmer ER, Hood AF (eds): *Pathology of the Skin.* Norwalk, Conn, Appleton and Lange, 1990, pp. 684–756.
127. McGovern VJ: Melanoma—Growth patterns, multiplicity and regression. In *Melanoma and Skin Cancer. Proceedings of the International Cancer Conference, Sydney.* Sydney, VCN Blight, Government Printer, 1972, pp. 95–106.
128. Blessing K, McLaren KM: Histological regression in primary cutaneous melanoma: Recognition, prevalence and significance. *Histopathology* 20:315–322, 1992.
129. McGovern VJ, Shaw HM, Milton GW: Prognosis in patients with thin malignant melanoma: Influence of regression. *Histopathology* 7:673–680, 1983.
130. Pack GT, Miller TR: Metastatic melanomas with indeterminate primary site. *JAMA* 176:55–56, 1961.
131. Smith JL Jr, Stehlin JS Jr: Spontaneous regression of primary malignant melanomas with regional metastases. *Cancer* 18:1399–1415, 1965.
132. Tefany FJ, Barnetson RS, Halliday GM, et al: Immunocytochemical analysis of the cellular infiltrate in primary regressing and non-regressing malignant melanoma. *J Invest Dermatol* 97:197–202, 1991.
133. Kang S, Barnhill RL, Mihm MC, Sober AJ: Regression in malignant melanoma: An interobserver concordance study. *J Cutan Pathol* 20:126–129, 1993.
134. Barnhill RL, Fandrey K, Levy MA, et al: Angiogenesis and tumor progression of melanoma: Quantification of vascularity in melanocytic nevi and cutaneous malignant melanoma. *Lab Invest* 67:331–337, 1992.
135. Barnhill RL, Mihm MC Jr: Histopathology of malignant melanoma and its precursor lesions. In Balch CM, Houghton AN, Milton GW, Sober AJ, Soong S-J (eds): *Cutaneous Melanoma* (ed 2). Philadelphia, Lippincott, 1992, pp. 234–263.
136. Cullity G: Intra-epithelial changes in childhood nevi simulating malignant melanoma. *Pathology* 16:307–311, 1984.

11

Metastatic Malignant Melanoma

SITES OF METASTASES

Melanoma can spread hematogenously, through lymphatic channels, or by direct local invasion and thus may occur in any site of the body. Metastases are more frequent to skin, subcutaneous tissue, and lymph nodes (nonvisceral sites) than to visceral organs.[1–3]

Cutaneous Metastases

Nearly half the patients with metastatic melanoma develop skin metastases,[2,3] which may occur in the area of locoregional lymphatic drainage or at a remote location. Two subtypes of regional cutaneous metastases have been described, and they are arbitrarily distinguished by their distance from the primary melanoma: cutaneous satellites and in-transit metastases.[4]

Cutaneous Satellites. Satellites of primary melanomas are defined as discontinuous tumor foci. They are tumor cell aggregates that are located in the dermis and/or subcutis within a 5-cm distance from the primary tumor mass. Their possible presence in the skin adjacent to a primary tumor has been used to argue in favor of wide local excision of melanomas. A study on reexcisions of melanomas revealed that satellites were found in 22 percent of tumors thicker than 2-mm.[5] Their presence indicates a greater risk of subsequent recurrences[6] and nodal metastases.[7]

Cutaneous In-Transit Metastases. In-transit metastases are regional tumor nests located more than 5 cm away from the primary melanoma. Such metastases were found in 4.3 percent of stage I melanomas thicker than 1 mm[8] and in 24 percent melanomas thicker than 2 mm.[5] The finding of in-transit metastases has poor prognostic implications, since the majority of patients with such lesions develop disseminated metastatic disease.[4]

Subcutaneous Metastases

In a study of 53 patients with metastatic melanoma,[9] all patients with subcutaneous metastases (38 percent) had primary lesions classified as Clark level IV or V. Five patients (11 percent) had subcutaneous nodules as the only indication of metastatic disease. The location of the subcutaneous nodules could not be predicted consistently from the anatomic site of the known primary tumor. Only half the patients with subcutaneous metastatic nodules had them at sites adjacent to the primary lesion or along lymphatic drainage pathways. Several patients had subcutaneous nodules remote from the site of primary malignancy with no evidence for metastases in the intervening subcutaneous tissue.

Lymph Node Metastases

Lymph nodes represent the most common site of metastatic melanoma. Between 60 and 80 percent of patients with metastatic melanoma have lymph node metastases.[3,10] The lymph node groups most commonly involved by metastatic melanoma are the ilioinguinal, axillary, intraparotid, and cervical lymph nodes.[11] The metastatic tumor may be clinically apparent (macroscopic metastasis) due to enlargement and induration of a node, or it may represent only small nests of tumor cells in the subcapsular sinus of a node detected on careful histologic examination (microscopic metastasis).

Visceral Metastases
In a number of autopsy series, the distribution of visceral metastases has been studied. While virtually any organ can be involved, certain sites are preferred for metastatic spread. As reviewed by Lee,[12] involvement of the lungs is seen most commonly. It has been documented to occur in 70 to 87 percent of postmortem examinations of individuals with metastatic melanoma. Next in frequency are liver (54 to 77 percent), brain (39 to 54 percent), bone (23 to 49 percent), intestine (26 to 58 percent), heart (40 to 45 percent), pancreas (38 to 53 percent), adrenals (36 to 54 percent), kidney (35 to 48 percent), and thyroid (25 to 39 percent).[1,12,13] To the clinician, the information as to which organ site the first metastases can be expected may be more relevant than the clinically end-stage or postmortem anatomic distribution of metastases. The most common first sites of visceral metastases reported in clinical studies are lung (14 to 20 percent), liver (14 to 20 percent), brain (12 to 20 percent), bone (11 to 17 percent), and intestine (1 to 7 percent), while first metastases at other sites are very rare (< 1 percent).[1]

HISTOLOGIC DIAGNOSIS OF METASTATIC MELANOMA

Confronted with the possibility of a malignant melanoma, the pathologist has to decide whether a lesion is truly metastatic and/or truly melanocytic. The histologic diagnosis of a melanocytic lesion as metastatic melanoma is usually straightforward, especially in the context of a well-documented clinical history and pathology of the primary tumor.

Typical Morphology of Metastatic Melanomas
Features commonly seen in metastatic malignant melanoma are listed in Table 11-1. Metastatic melanoma has a tendency to grow in nests, sheets, or fascicles (Figs. 11-1 and 11-2). The tumor may be nodular, circumscribed, or infiltrative. An infiltrative border, pleomorphism, mitoses, and necrosis are features often seen in metastatic melanomas. However, these are features of malignant tumors in general and help only in identifying a tumor as malignant.

Cytologically, epithelioid and/or spindle cells are found commonly in metastatic melanoma. In particular, a combination of both cell types (see Fig. 11-2) is typical of melanoma and is seen in few other tumors, such as meningiomas or a number of soft-tissue tumors. Rarer, more unusual cytologic forms can be found and are listed in Table 11-2. The epithelioid cells usually exhibit abundant cytoplasm (see Fig. 11-1*B*). They often show nuclear pleomorphism (Fig. 11-3). Their nuclei typically have irregular contours and a variable chromatin pattern. Often, a prominent eosinophilic or amphophilic nucleolus is seen (see Fig. 11-1*B*). Nuclear cytoplasmic pseudoinclusions are not uncommon (see Fig. 11-3). Such cytologic features are suggestive of melanoma in an appropriate cellular environment. They are, however, seen in a variety of other tumors and are therefore not specific.

Melanin pigment may be apparent (see Fig. 11-2), subtle, or absent (amelanotic melanoma). The presence of melanin greatly facilitates the recognition of a metastatic melanoma.

TABLE 11-1
Histologic Features of Metastatic Melanoma

Location: Melanocytic growth in unexpected sites (e.g., subcutis, lymph nodes, viscera)
Growth pattern: Nodular, circumscribed, or infiltrative
Cellular arrangements: Nests, sheets, or fascicles
Cytology
- Melanin pigment
- Epithelioid and/or spindle cells
  - Nuclear pseudoinclusions
  - Large eosino- or amphophilic nucleoli

Host response
- Sparse lymphocytic infiltrate
- Mild fibrosis

Diagnostic Problems Concerning Metastatic Melanoma
Several situations may arise in which the diagnosis of metastatic melanoma is not straightforward. The problem may lie in the identification of a metastatic-appearing lesion as melanocytic or in the distinction between a primary and secondary melanoma.

Melanoma Simulating Other Neoplasms. Metastatic melanoma may assume a great variety of morphologic appearances and may mimic a number of nonmelanocytic tumors, such as lymphoma, undifferentiated carcinoma, adenocarcinoma, a variety of sarcomas, and many others.[14] The differential diagnosis is particularly difficult in the presence of an amelanotic melanoma. Often, additional studies are needed, such as melanin stains, immunohistochemistry using a panel of antibodies, and electron microscopy (see Chap. 2), to identify conclusively a metastatic tumor as melanocytic.

When melanoma assumes an undifferentiated or unusual morphology, a major danger lies in the fact that the possibility of a melanoma may not be considered at all in the differential diagnosis. A variety of morphologic features that have been reported to occur in metastatic melanoma and the respective tumors and which may be mimicked are listed in Table 11-2.[14,15]

Epithelioid cell morphology is the most common appearance of melanomas in metastases (see Figs. 11-1, 11-2, 11-3,

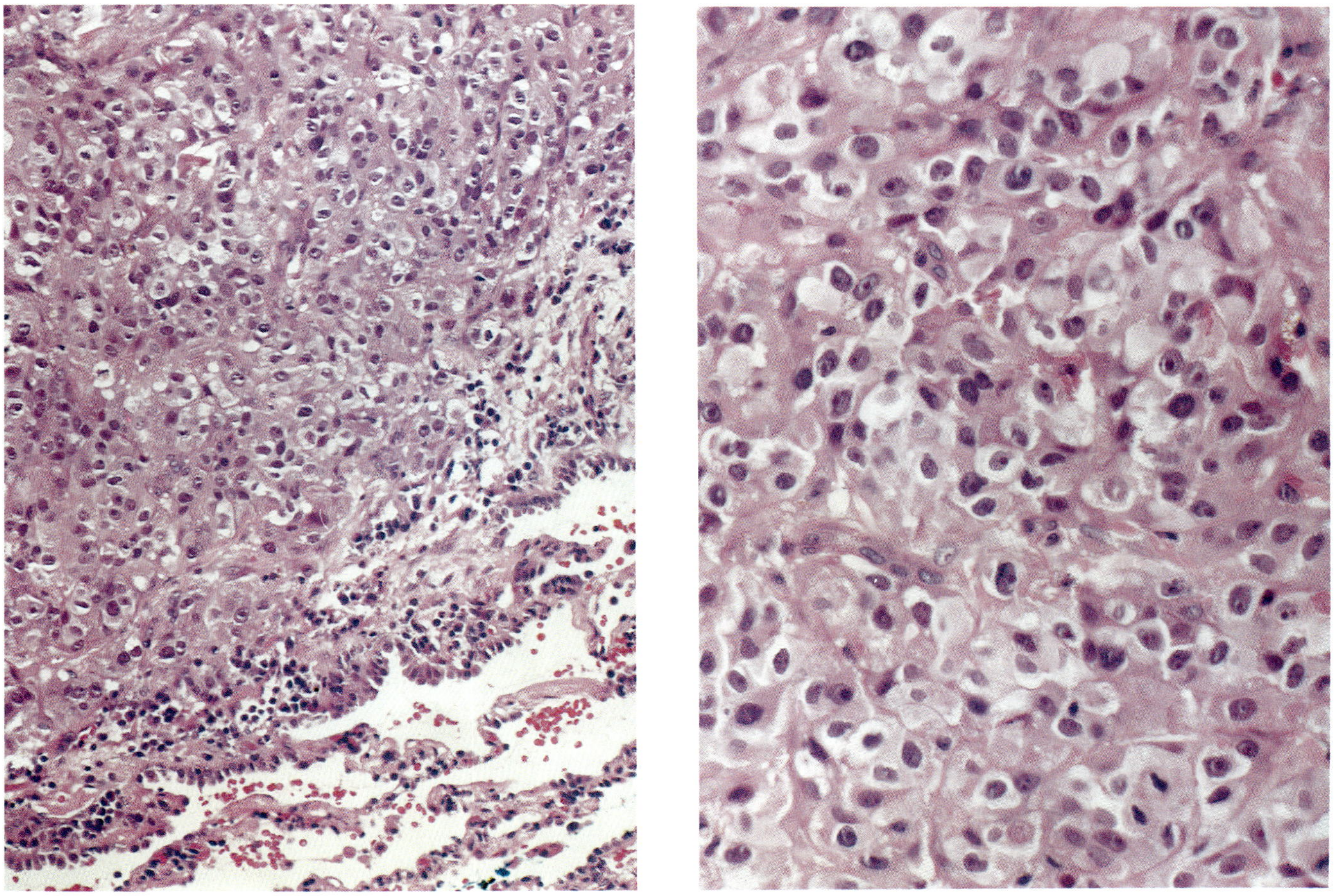

A B

FIGURE 11-1

Malignant melanoma metastatic to lung. (A) Nests of metastatic epithelioid cells are seen in lung parenchyma (H&E, × 400). (B) Many of their nuclei show prominent nucleoli (H&E, × 400). Immunoreactivity for S-100 (C) and HMB-45 (D) is illustrated (H&E, × 200).

11-6, 11-7, and 11-9). This type of melanoma needs to be distinguished from poorly differentiated carcinomas of various primary sites. The distinction can be accomplished by the identification of cytoplasmic melanin (see Fig. 11-1*B*) and/or by immunohistochemical studies (see Chap. 2) using epithelial (cytokeratins) or melanocytic (S-100, HMB-45) markers (see Fig. 11-1*C* and *D*).

Prominent or, in particular, exclusive *spindle cell morphology* of metastatic melanoma gives rise to a number of diagnostic possibilities (peripheral nerve-sheath tumors, fibrous, smooth-muscle or myofibroblastic neoplasms, spindle cell carcinomas, meningiomas, or sex cord stromal cell tumors).[15-18] The identification of scattered inconspicuous epithelioid cells and cytologic features of melanoma, such as nuclear pseudoinclusions or "dusty" melanin pigment, may greatly facilitate the differentiation from other spindle cell neoplasms. Otherwise, the final diagnosis rests on the expression of phenotypic markers or electron microscopic features. A particular differential diagnostic problem lies in the distinction of metastatic melanomas from a primary or metastatic pigmented peripheral nerve-sheath tumor, since both types of tumors may show fascicles and nests of spindle cells with or without occasional epithelioid cells, both may be melanotic, and both may display the same profile of immunoreactivity. Here, the distinction may be made at the ultrastructural level if features characteristic of schwannomas such as interdigitating processes, basal lamina, and long spacing collagen can be discerned.[19] In a few cases, cytogenetics may provide the final diagnosis of spindle and epithelioid cell tumors and their distinction from a metastatic melanoma. Such tumors are synovial

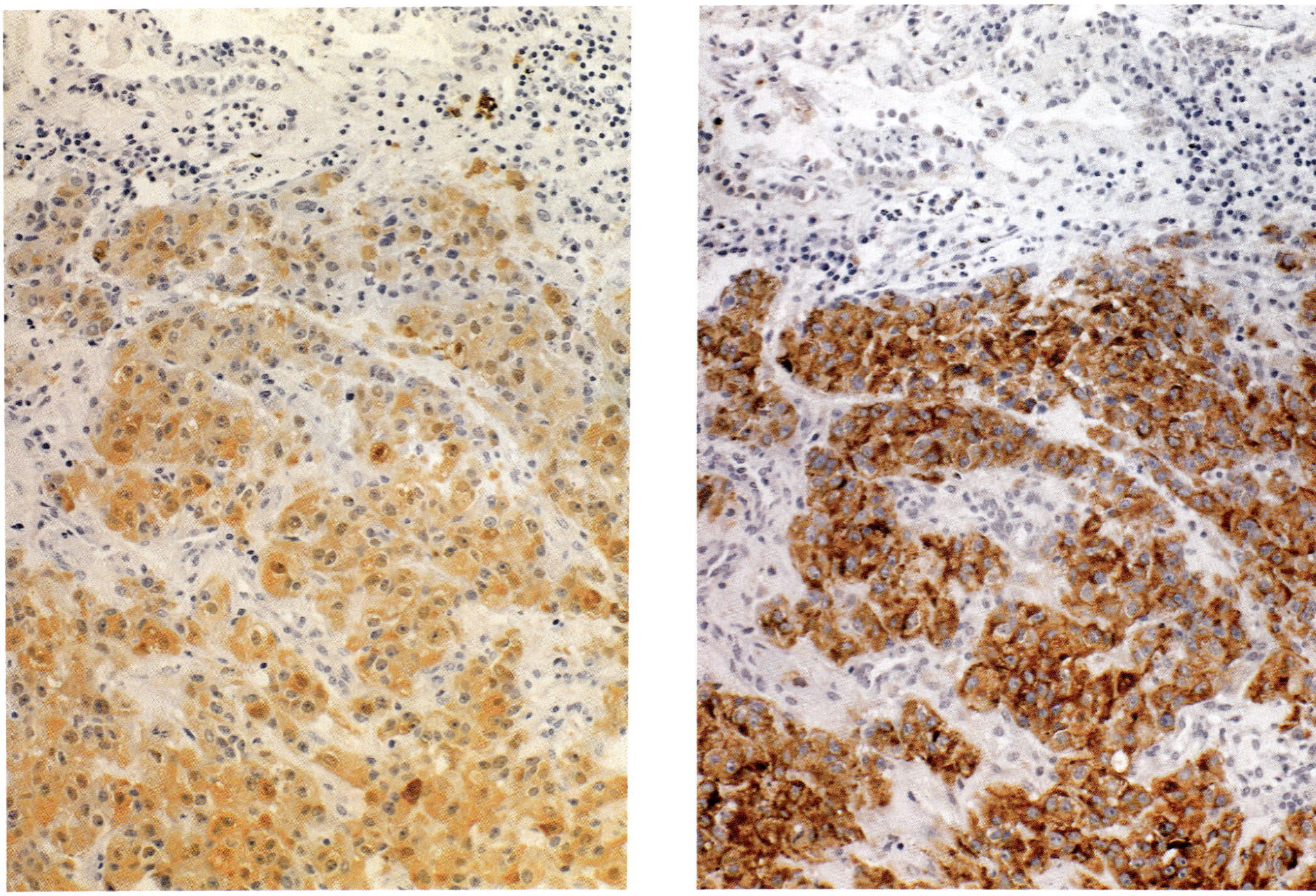

C D

FIGURE 11-1 *(Continued)*

sarcoma with its typical t(X,18) translocation[20] and melanoma of soft parts or clear cell sarcoma with its characteristic t(12,22) translocation.[21] In particular, the latter tumor is notorious for mimicking metastatic melanoma (Fig. 11-4).

Signet-ring cell morphology is seen in some primary or metastatic melanomas (Fig. 11-5), sometimes even with diastase-resistant PAS-positive material.[14,22] Mucicarmine stains are typically negative in such cases. The differential diagnostic workup primarily needs to rule out adenocarcinoma and signet-ring cell lymphoma. Typically, the tumor cells of signet-ring cell melanomas are negative for keratin, carcinoembryonic antigen, and leukocyte common antigen but at least weakly positive for S-100 and/or HMB-45.

Balloon cell morphology has been reported to occur in metastatic melanoma.[23–25] If macrovacuolar cytoplasmic changes are well developed, the presence of a liposarcoma may be suggested.[26] Prominent cytoplasmic clear cell appearance may resemble a metastatic renal cell carcinoma.[23]

Disassociation of tumor cells with adherence of tumor cells to the surrounding fibrovascular stroma may architecturally mimic alveolar rhabdomyosarcoma.[15] Large sheets or lobules of discohesive tumor cells may mimic malignant lymphoma.[15] Dissociation of tumor cells also may lead to irregular empty spaces and sometimes an adenoid/pseudopapillary pattern.[14]

Some metastatic melanomas may develop a prominent *myxoid stromal reaction*, as seen in various myxoid tumors (myxoid variants of MFH, liposarcoma, chondrosarcoma, rhabdomyosarcoma, malignant sweat gland tumors, pleomorphic adenoma or others).[27–29] A *"staghorn"-like vascular pattern* of prominent branching, thin-walled blood vessels, resembling the vascular pattern of a hemangiopericytoma, may occur in some metastatic melanomas.[14]

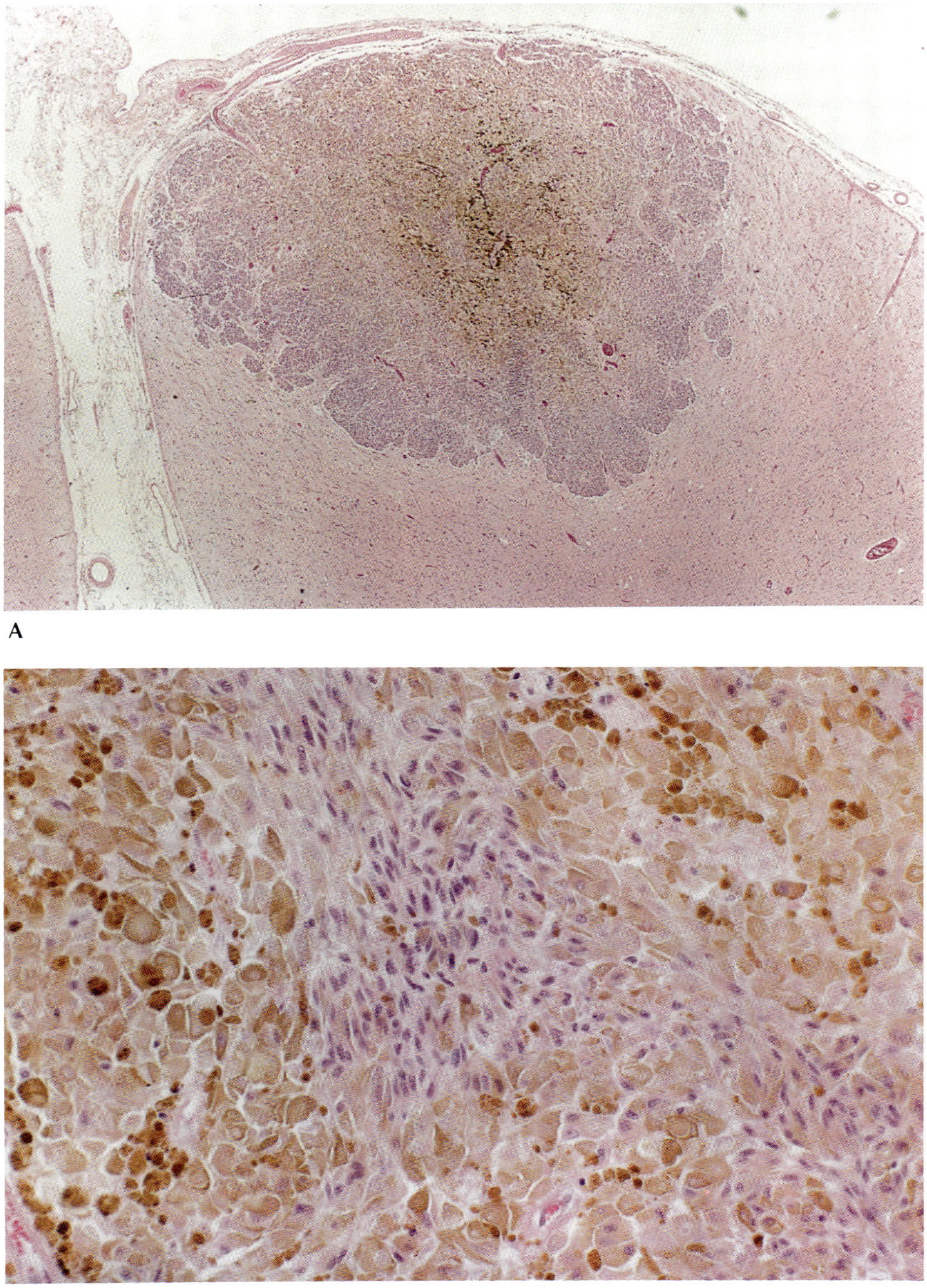

A

B

FIGURE 11-2

(A) Malignant melanoma metastatic to brain (H&E, × 40). (B) The metastatic lesions are composed of both spindle and epithelioid cells (H&E, × 400). Abundant melanin is present.

TABLE 11-2
Metastatic Melanoma Simulating Other Neoplasms

Morphologic Feature of Tumor Cells	*Differential Diagnosis*
Epithelioid cell	Carcinomas Ki-1 lymphoma Angiosarcoma
Spindle cell	Peripheral nerve-sheath tumors Fibrous tumors Fibrohistocytic tumors Smooth-muscle tumors Clear cell sarcoma Spindle cell carcinomas Meningiomas Kaposi's sarcoma Angiosarcoma Ovarian stromal tumors
Signet-ring cell	Adenocarcinoma Lymphoma Sarcoma
Balloon cell Macrovacuolization Clear cell changes	Liposarcoma Renal cell carcinoma
Disassociation of tumor cells Sheetlike/lobular Pseudoalveolar Adenoid/pseudopapillary	Lymphoma Alveolar rhabdomyosarcoma Adenocarcinoma, mesothelioma
Myxoid stromal changes	Myxoid variants of sarcomas Pleomorphic adenoma Malignant sweat gland tumor
"Staghorn" vascular pattern	Hemangiopericytoma

A number of other unusual patterns have been described in primary melanomas but not yet in secondary tumors. Such appearances include a small cell variant of melanoma[14] and melanoma with organoid features resembling neuroendocrine carcinoma.[30] It is possible that such features also might be seen in metastatic lesions.

Primary Cutaneous versus Cutaneous Metastatic Melanoma. The distinction between a primary cutaneous melanoma and a skin metastasis has obvious prognostic significance. A number of features have been suggested to differentiate histologically a cutaneous metastasis from a primary tumor (Table 11-3).

Cutaneous metastases usually lie within the reticular dermis or subcutis and only rarely involve the overlying epidermis (Fig. 11-6), while primary cutaneous melanomas typically have tumor cells located in the epidermis, which often account for a significant portion of the overall tumor mass.[4,15] In those cases of metastatic melanoma which do show epidermotropism,[31] the volume of the epidermal component is usually relatively small compared with the dermal mass (Fig. 11-7). However, metastases may be localized entirely to the epidermis, dermis, or both sites. In general, the intraepidermal component of many primary melanomas tends to extend laterally beyond the dermal component, whereas the dermal component of epidermotropic metastases often extends laterally beyond the intraepidermal component. If the dermal metastasis is very superficially located, the overlying epidermis may be thinned, and the lateral borders may show hyperplastic, elongated rete ridges turned inward and forming a *collarette*. Tumor cells within vascular lumina are more likely to be found in and around a metastatic lesion than near a primary tumor.[31]

Another important discriminating feature is overall size. Primary melanomas are almost always greater than 0.4 cm and usually greater than 1.0 cm in diameter. In contrast, melanoma metastases may be small, i.e., commonly less than 1 cm and in some instances less than 0.4 cm in diameter.

After evaluating the location and architecture of the lesion, the cytologic features of the tumor cells may provide additional clues in making a distinction between a primary and secondary tumor.[32] Primary tumors generally display more pleomorphism than metastatic lesions,

TABLE 11-3
Primary Cutaneous Melanoma versus Cutaneous Metastasis

	Primary Melanoma	*Cutaneous Metastasis*
Location of tumor	Usually both dermis and epidermis	Dermis and/or subcutis
If epidermal involvement	Usually prominent; pagetoid horizontal and vertical spread commonly present; usually epidermal component extends laterally beyond dermal component	Usually dermal component extends laterally beyond epidermal component; pagetoid spread less common
Size	Nearly always >0.4 cm and usually >1.0 cm	Often small; may be <1.0 cm and occasionally <0.4 cm
Epidermal collarette	Usually less common	More likely present
Cytology	Usually pleomorphic	Usually monotonous
Reactive fibrosis	May be marked	Usually mild
Vascular invasion	Rarely seen	More likely present

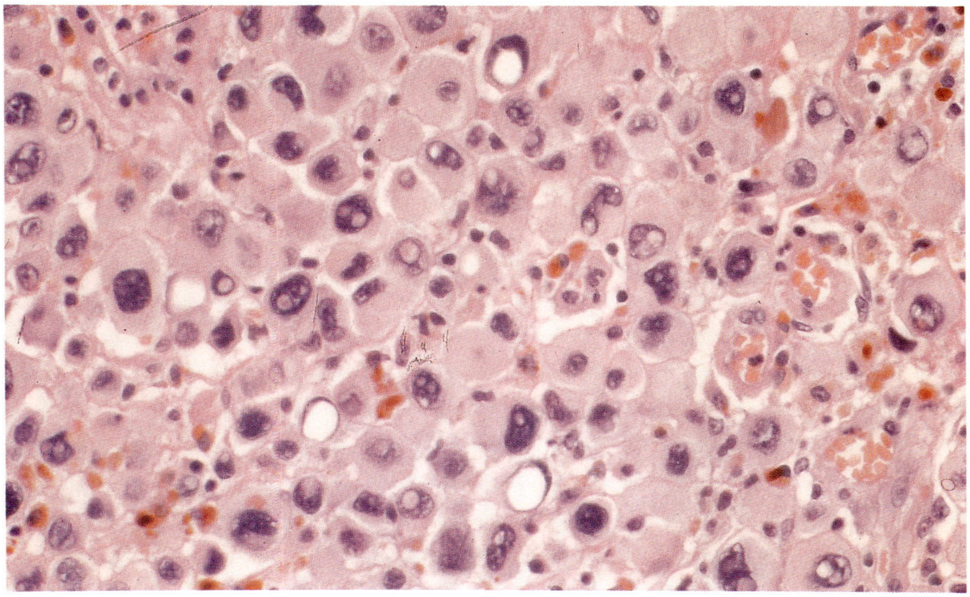

FIGURE 11-3
Malignant melanoma metastatic to brain (H&E, × 400). Pleomorphic epithelioid cells are present exhibiting marked irregularity in nuclear shape, size, and chromaticity. Many cells have nuclear pseudoinclusions, and some show signet-ring morphology.

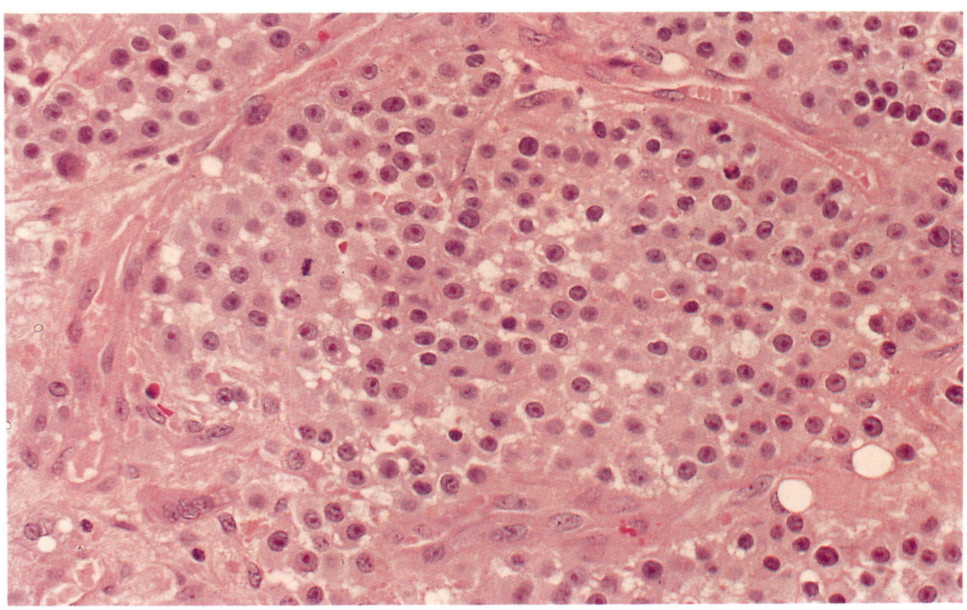

FIGURE 11-4
Malignant melanoma of soft parts (clear cell sarcoma) metastatic to bone. Epithelioid cells, some of which have clear cytoplasm, are arranged in nests. Their nuclei show prominent nucleoli (H&E, × 200).

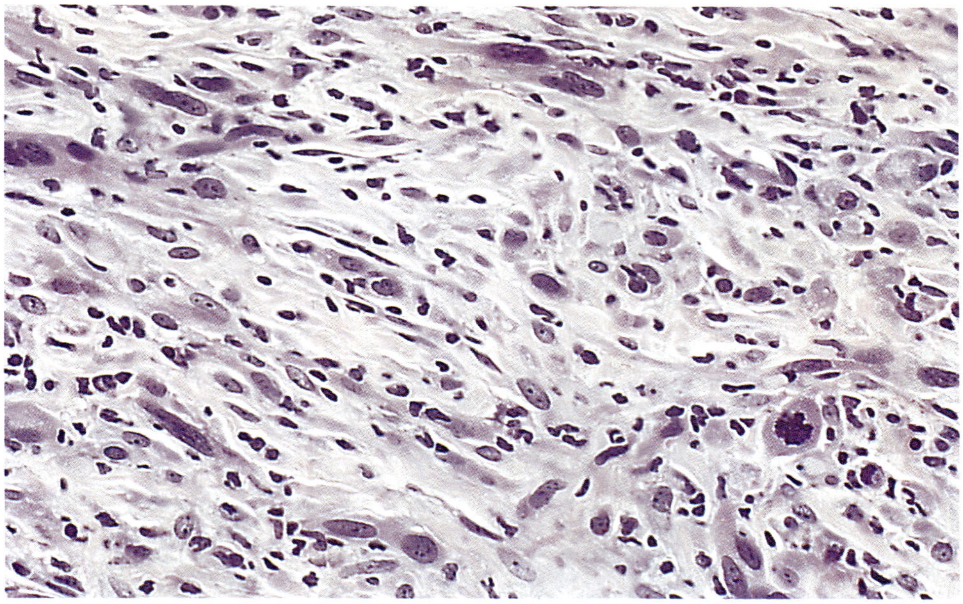

FIGURE 11-5
Metastatic melanoma with spindle cell morphology. Amelanotic malignant spindle cells and a few epithelioid cells with mitoses are present (H&E, × 400).

which often appear as an atypical but rather monomorphous population of cells. Primary tumors tend to show more variation in the overall composition of the lesion. There is often more fibrosis and more of an inflammatory host response.

The reliability of the guidelines listed in Table 11-3 has been questioned for a number of cases in which the histologic features of a presumed primary lesion did not fit the patient's clinical history.[33] When deciding whether a melanocytic tumor is a metastasis or a primary lesion, it is always important to weigh the histologic appearance against a careful and detailed clinical history to arrive at the correct diagnosis.

Sometimes a cutaneous metastasis must be distinguished from a dermal or compound nevus. For the latter discrimination, the pathologist must assess the lesion carefully for cytologic atypia, presence or absence of maturation, mitotic figures, particularly atypical ones, and the other features described above.

Melanocytic Aggregates versus Micrometastases. Collections of small melanocytes are occasionally seen within lymph nodes draining the skin (Fig. 11-8). These melanocytic or nevus cell aggregates[34] are usually small and inconspicuous. However, they may occupy as much as one-third of a lymph node.[35,36] They are usually located in the fibrous capsule of the node rather than in the marginal sinus,[37] but rarely they can be found in the lymphatic tissue proper.[36] They usually resemble architecturally and cytologically melanocytes of dermal nevi. Their bland appearance and their location in the fibrous capsule of the lymph node help to distinguish them from micrometastases. However, especially in frozen sections or in the rare situation of intranodal location, the presence of melanocytic aggregates in lymph nodes may lead to diagnostic confusion. Distinction from metastatic carcinoma may require a careful dermatologic examination. The prevalence of melanocytic aggregates in axillary lymph nodes of melanoma patients is an order of magnitude higher than in patients with breast carcinoma.[38,39]

Whether these nodal melanocytic lesions derive from aberrant migration of melanoblasts from the neural crest during embryogenesis or represent lymphatic spread from a benign cutaneous nevus has been the subject of much debate. The proponents of the theory of aberrant migration point out that the melanocytic aggregates are usually located in the fibrous capsule rather than intranodally.[40] The view that lymphatic spread may account for the phenomenon of melanocytic nodal aggregates,[36] is usually defined by the argument that intranodal deposition of a variety of extranodal tissue, such as endometrium,

has been suggested. Before a diagnosis of multiple primary melanomas is made, the possibility of metastatic lesions needs to be excluded.[43] Histologic guidelines (see Tables 11-1 and 11-3) assist in the diagnostic decision. However, they are not absolute. The final diagnosis depends on a good clinicopathologic correlation, taking into account not only the morphologic features of the tumor but also the time course of their development and their anatomic distribution.

Metastatic Melanoma with Unknown Primary Site

In as many as 4 to 12 percent of melanoma cases, a metastatic lesion is found without a clinically apparent primary tumor.[44-46] While it is possible that some melanomas may arise de novo within a lymph node or visceral site, it is generally believed that the phenomenon of an unidentified primary site is related to complete regression of a cutaneous melanoma that becomes clinically undetectable.[47,48] Metastatic melanomas with unknown primary site are twice as common in men as in women, which is in agreement with the observation that tumor regression is observed more commonly in men than in women.[49]

The most common site of presentation in one large series[50] has been reported to be in lymph nodes (64 percent) (Fig. 11-9), in particular in the axillary, inguinal, and neck regions. Another site is the subcutis (15 percent), most often on the trunk. Twenty-one percent of the cases presented with visceral metastases, most often to the lung and brain.[1,44,45,50]

A diagnosis of metastatic melanoma with unknown primary site obviously should only be rendered after careful diagnostic evaluation has failed to disclose a primary cutaneous, mucosal, or ocular melanoma or melanomas of other sites. The search for potential cutaneous primary sites can be facilitated by a Wood's lamp examination to detect areas of depigmentation. Ophthalmoscopic and radiographic studies may be indicated if the clinical situation suggests a potential extracutaneous primary melanoma. The relative frequencies of sites of primary extracutaneous melanoma according to the Third National Cancer Survey of the United States[51] were: eye (78.9 percent), vulva (7.2 percent), soft tissues (2.5 percent), anorectum (2.3 percent), vagina (2.1 percent), upper respiratory tract (1.6 percent), gums and mouth (1.2 percent), and gastrointestinal tract (0.7 percent). Other visceral sites accounted for less than 0.5 percent each.

Melanosis in Metastatic Melanoma

Cutaneous or generalized melanosis is a rare complication of metastatic melanoma.[1,52,53] Hyperpigmentation may be focal or diffuse, limited to the skin or generalized, and involving internal organs. Diffuse melanosis is thought to be a terminal event. In some patients, melanosis is accompanied by melanuria, melanoptysis, and dark-brown discoloration of the serum.[54] The majority of patients who develop diffuse hyperpigmentation in association with melanoma have widespread metastases.[1] Histologically, the involved skin may show hyperpigmentation of the epidermis and/or increased pigment deposition in the dermis and subcutis, predominantly within histiocytes.[52,53] It is thought that both increased production by epidermal melanocytes and lysis of heavily pigmented tumor cells play a role in melanosis.[55] Tumor-derived pigment is presumably carried and deposited via the circulation.[52,53]

REFERENCES

1. Balch CM, Milton GW: Diagnosis of metastatic melanoma at distant sites. In CM Balch, Milton, HM Shaw, S-J Soong, (eds): *Cutaneous Melanoma. Clinical Management and Treatment Results Worldwide.* Philadelphia, Lippincott, 1985, pp. 221–250.
2. McNeer G, Das Gupta T: Life history of melanoma. AJR 93:686–694, 1956.
3. Peterson N, Bodenham D, Lloyd O: Malignant melanoma of the skin: A study of the origin, development, etiology, spread, treatment and prognosis. *Br J Plast Surg* 15:49–116, 1962.
4. Elder DE, Murphy G: Metastatic malignant melanoma. In Elder DE, Murphy G (eds): *Melanocytic Tumors of the Skin.* Washington, American Registry of Pathology, Armed Forces Institute of Pathology, 1991, pp. 191–205.
5. Elder DE, Guerry DI, Heiberger R, et al: Optimal resection margins for cutaneous malignant melanoma. *Plast Reconstr Surg* 71:66–72, 1983.
6. Kelly J, Sagebiel R, Calderon W, et al: The frequency of local recurrence and microsatellites as a guide to reexcision margins for cutaneous malignant melanomas. *Ann Surg* 200:759–763, 1984.
7. Harrist TJ, Rigel DS, Day CL, et al: "Microscopic satellites" are more highly associated with regional lymph node metastases than is primary melanoma thickness. *Cancer* 53:2183–2187, 1984.
8. Roses D, Harris M, Rigel D, et al: Local and in-transit metastases following definitive excision for primary cutaneous malignant melanoma. *Ann Surg* 198:65–69, 1983.
9. Patten R, Shuman W, Teefey S: Subcutaneous metastases from malignant melanoma. AJR 152:1009–1012, 1989.
10. Barnhill RL, Mihm MC, Fitzpatrick TB, Sober AJ: Neoplasms: Malignant melanoma. In Fitzpatrick TB, Eisen AZ, Wolff K, et al (eds): *Dermatology in General Medicine,* vol 1. New York, McGraw-Hill, 1993, pp. 1078–1115.
11. Balch CM, Ursit MM, Maddox WA, et al: Management of regional metastatic melanoma. In Balch CM, Milton GW, Shaw HM, Soon S-J (eds): *Cutaneous Melanoma: Clinical Management and Treatement Results Worldwide.* Philadelphia, Lippincott, 1985, pp. 93–130.
12. Lee Y: Malignant melanoma. Patterns of metastasis. *Ca J Physicians* 30:69–75, 1980.
13. Elder DE: Metastatic melanoma. *Pigment Cell* 8:182–204, 1987.

14. Nakhleh R, Wick M, Rocamora A, et al: Morphologic diversity in malignant melanoma. *Am J Clin Pathol* 93:731–740, 1990.
15. Mooi WJ, Krausz T: Cutaneous melanoma. In Mooi WJ, Krausz T: *Biopsy Pathology of Melanocytic Disorders.* London, Chapman and Hall, 1992, pp. 215–303.
16. Wick M, Fitzgibbon J, Swanson P: Cutaneous sarcomas and sarcomatoid neoplasms of the skin. *Semin Diagn Pathol* 10:148–158, 1993.
17. Silvis N, Swanson P, Manviel J, et al: Spindle-cell and pleomorphic neoplasms of the skin. *Am J Dermatopathol* 10:9–19, 1988.
18. Fitzgibbons P, Martin S, Simmons T: Malignant melanoma metastatic to the ovary. *Am J Surg Pathol* 11:959–967, 1987.
19. Dickersin GR: Schwannoma and other nerve sheath neoplasms. In Dickersin GR (ed): *Diagnostic Electron Microscopy.* New York: Igaku-Shoin, 1991, p. 238.
20. Fletcher J, Kozakewich H, Hoffer F, et al: Diagnostic relevance of clonal cytogenetic aberrations in malignant soft tissue tumors. *N Engl J Med* 324:436–443, 1991.
21. Peulve P, Michot C, Vannier J-P, et al: Clear cell sarcoma with t(11;22) (q13-14;q12). *Genes Chrom Cancer* 3:400–402, 1991.
22. Sheibani K, Battifora H: Signet-ring cell melanoma. *Am J Surg Pathol* 12:28–34, 1988.
23. Akslen L, Myking A: Balloon cell melanoma mimicking clear cell carcinoma. *Pathol Res Pract* 184:548–550, 1989.
24. Gardner W, Vazquez M. Balloon cell melanoma. *Arch Pathol* 89:470–472, 1970.
25. Peters M, Su W: Balloon cell malignant melanoma. *J Am Acad Dermatol* 13:351–354, 1985.
26. Lodding P, Kindblom L, Angervall L: Metastases of malignant melanoma simulating soft tissue sarcoma: A clinico-pathological, light ane electron microsocpic and immunohistochemical study of 21 cases. *Virchows Arch [A]* 417:377–388, 1990.
27. Urso C, Gianotti B, Bondi R: Myxoid melanoma of the skin. *Arch Pathol Lab Med* 114:527–528, 1990.
28. Nottingham J, Slatter D: Malignant melanoma: A new mimic of colloid adenocarcinoma. *Histopathology* 13:576–578, 1988.
29. Bhuta S, Mirra J, Cochran A: Myxoid malignant melanoma. *Am J Surg Pathol* 10:203–211, 1986.
30. Levene A: On the histological diagnosis and prognosis of malignant melanoma. *J Clin Pathol* 33:101–124, 1980.
31. Kornberg R, Harris M, Ackerman A: Epidermotropically metastatic malignant melanoma. *Arch Dermatol* 114:67–69, 1978.
32. Elder DE, Ainsworth A, Clark W: The surgical pathology of cutaneous malignant melanoma. In Clark W (ed): *Human Malignant Melanoma.* New York: Grune and Stratton, 1979, pp. 55–108.
33. Bengoechea-Beeby M, Velasco-Oses A, Fernandez F, et al: Epidermotropic metastatic melanoma. *Cancer* 72:1909–1913, 1993.
34. Stewart F, Copeland M: Neurogenic sarcoma. *Am J Cancer* 15:1235–1320, 1931.
35. Von Alberti M: About a case of neuronevus with lymph node metastasis of the same type. *Bull Soc Fr Dermatol Syphilol* 42:1273–1278, 1935.
36. McCarthy S, Palmer A, Bale P, Hist E: Nevus cells in lymph nodes. *Pathology* 6:351–358, 1974.
37. Johnson W, Helwig E: Benign nevus cells in the capsule of lymph nodes. *Cancer* 23:747–753, 1969.
38. Ridolfi R, Rosen P, Thaler H: Nevus cell aggregates associated with lymph nodes: Estimated frequency and clinical significance. *Cancer* 39:164–171, 1977.
39. Andreola S, Clemente C: Nevus cells in axillary lymph nodes from radical mastectomy specimens. *Pathol Res Pract* 179:616–618, 1985.
40. Epstein J, Erlandson R, Rosen P: Nodal blue nevi: A study of three cases. *Am J Surg Pathol* 8:907–915, 1984.
41. Eckert F, Schmidt U, Lennert K: Immunohistologische charakterisierung sogenannter naevuszellnester in lymphknoten. *Pathologe* 8:81–84, 1987.
42. Moseley H, Guiliano A, Storm F, et al: Multiple primary melanoma. *Cancer* 43:939–944, 1979.
43. Warner T, Gilbert E, Ramirez G: Epidermotropism in melanoma. *J Cutan Pathol* 7:50–54, 1980.
44. Das Gupta T, Bowden L, Berg J: Malignant melanoma of unknown primary origin. *Surg Gynecol Obstet* 117:341–345, 1963.
45. Giuliano A, Cochran AJ, Morton D: Melanoma from unknown primary site and amelanotic melanoma. *Semin Oncol* 9:442–447, 1982.
46. Mooi W, Krausz T: Prognostic factors in cutaneous melanoma. In Mooi W, Krausz T (eds): *Biopsy Pathology of Melanocytic Disorders.* London, Chapman and Hall, 1992, pp. 304–330.
47. Pellegrini A: Regressed primary malignant melanoma with regional metastases. *Arch Dermatol* 116:585–586, 1980.
48. Smith J, Stehlin J: Spontaneous regression of primary melanomas with regional metastases. *Cancer* 18:1399–1415, 1965.
49. Chang P, Knapper W: Metastatic melanoma of unknown primary. *Cancer* 49:1106–1111, 1982.
50. Reintgen D, McCarty K, Woodard B, et al: Metastatic malignant melanoma with an unknown primary. *Surg Gynecol Obstet* 156:335–340, 1983.
51. Scotto J, Graumen J, Lee J: Melanomas of the eye and other noncutaneous sites: Epidemiologic aspects. *J Natl Cancer Inst* 56:489–491, 1976.
52. Silberberg I, Kopf A, Gumport S: Diffuse melanosis in malignant melanoma. *Arch Dermatol* 97:671–677, 1968.
53. Pierard G: Melanophagoic dermatitis and panniculitis. A condition revealing an occult metastatic malignant melanoma. *Am J Dermatopathol* 10:133–136, 1988.
54. Eide J: Pathogenesis of generalized melanosis with melanuria and melanoptysis secondary to malignant melanoma. *Histopathology* 5:285–294, 1981.
55. Rowden G, Sulicca V, Butler T, Manz H: Malignant melanoma with melanosis. Ultrastructural and histological studies. *J Cutan Pathol* 7:125–139, 1980.

12

Prognostic Factors in Cutaneous Malignant Melanoma

Over the past 20 to 30 years, there has been considerable refinement in the ability to predict survival from malignant melanoma of the skin. The principal reasons for the improved ability to assess prognosis are related to better histopathologic characterization of melanoma, the development of large databases with long-term follow-up of at least 8 to 10 years, proper coding of prognostic variables, and the use of powerful techniques of multivariate analysis.[1-6]

However, the results of many published studies to date must be interpreted cautiously, since all too frequently they have involved too few patients who have been followed for insufficient periods of time.[2] Thus studies with relatively short periods of follow-up probably do little more than yield confusing data. Another important characteristic of melanoma that must be considered in determining prognosis is the tendency of melanoma to recur after long intervals of time, even beyond 10 years.[2]

Although this chapter will address most prognostic factors in all stages of melanoma, the emphasis will be on pathologic factors for stage I (localized) melanoma (Table 12-1).

PROGNOSTIC FACTORS FOR STAGE I MELANOMA

Although numerous variables (Table 12-2) have been analyzed and new prognostic factors continue to be studied, it is apparent from the various studies conducted thus far that tumor thickness is the single most important prognostic factor in stage I melanoma.[1-7] Furthermore, it has been shown that many other prognostic variables derive much of their effect from a correlation with tumor thickness.[7] However, various combinations of prognostic factors may provide more precise estimates of prognosis than estimations from tumor thickness alone.[3] Thus, in recent years, considerable effort has been spent on developing multifactorial prognostic models that attempt to predict various measures of clinical outcome with some degree of accuracy (see below).[1,3,6]

Pathologic Factors

Tumor Thickness. Virtually all studies of stage I malignant melanoma have confirmed the overriding prognostic significance of tumor thickness.[1-13] As mentioned earlier, it was originally appreciated by Allen and Spitz[14] that superficial melanomas were associated with a better prognosis than more deeply invasive tumors. Subsequently, a number of observers established an inverse relationship between survival and depth of invasion of melanoma[15-18] (Table 12-3). Clark and colleagues[19] refined this method and correlated depth of tumor invasion with prognosis (see below).

In an effort to provide a more reproducible and more quantitative method of measuring the extent of tumor invasion, Breslow[8] introduced his method of directly measuring vertical tumor thickness with an ocular micrometer (Fig. 12-1). According to this technique, tumor invasion is measured vertically from the granular cell layer of the epidermis to the deepest penetration of melanoma into the dermis or subcutaneous fat.

For many years, it was believed that the relationship between melanoma thickness and prognosis was not linear. Breslow[8] reported that patients with tumors less than 0.76 mm thick had an almost 100 percent 5-year survival,

TABLE 12-1
Clinical and Histologic Stages of Melanoma

	Clinical	*Histologic*
Stage I	Localized disease (no clinically palpable nodes)	Absence of histologic evidence of tumor in regional lymph nodes
Stage II	Palpable regional lymph nodes	Histologic evidence of melanoma in regional lymph nodes
Stage III	Presence of distant metastases	Histopathologic documentation of distant metastases

whereas those with tumors greater than 3 mm thick had a poor prognosis. Subsequently, other authors have proposed additional "breakpoints" in melanoma thickness that mark stepwise increases in rates of metastasis and mortality (reviewed in ref. 20) (Table 12-4). For example, Day and colleagues[21] reported natural breakpoints of less than 0.86 mm, 0.86 to 1.69 mm, 1.7 to 3.64 mm, and 3.65 mm or greater that correlated with progressively worse prognoses. The recent use of larger databases and longer periods of follow-up evaluation has suggested that the relationship between tumor thickness and prognosis is almost certainly linear as originally proposed by Breslow, rather than interrupted or stepwise.[4,22]

Because tumor thickness does not always predict biologic behavior in melanoma, there has been a continued search for other prognostic factors or combinations of prognostic factors that more accurately predict outcome.[3]

TABLE 12-2
Prognostic Factors in Stage I Malignant Melanoma

Pathologic Factors	*Effect on Prognosis*
Thickness	Worse prognosis with increasing thickness
Level	Worse prognosis with deeper levels
Ulceration	Worse prognosis with presence of ulceration
Mitotic rate	Worse prognosis with increasing mitotic rate
Growth phase	Greater likelihood of metastasis with vertical growth phase
Regression	Increased risk for metastasis in tumors < 1.0 mm with marked regression
Tumor vascularity	Unsettled at this time
Microscopic satellites	Worse prognosis and increased risk for local, regional, and distant recurrences when present
Host lymphoid response	Worse prognosis with diminished lymphoid infiltrates
Histogenetic type	Better prognosis for lentigo maligna, worse prognosis for acral lentiginous melanoma
Cell type	Better prognosis for tumors composed of spindle cells versus other cell types
Tumor volume	Worse prognosis with increasing volume
Cross-sectional profile	Worse prognosis with polypoid or verrucous configuration
Clinical Factors	*Effect on Prognosis*
Age	Worse prognosis with increasing age
Anatomic site	Extremity lesions have more favorable prognosis versus head and neck areas, palms, and soles
Pregnancy	No clear effect
Gender	Women have better prognosis than men
Stage	Worse prognosis with more advanced stage
Other Factors	*Effect on Prognosis*
Volume-weighted mean nuclear volume	Worse prognosis with increasing nuclear volume
DNA content	Worse prognosis with increasing DNA aneuploidy
Nucleolar organizer regions	Worse prognosis with increasing AgNOR counts
Proliferation and tumor cell motility indices	Worse prognosis with increased values of these indices

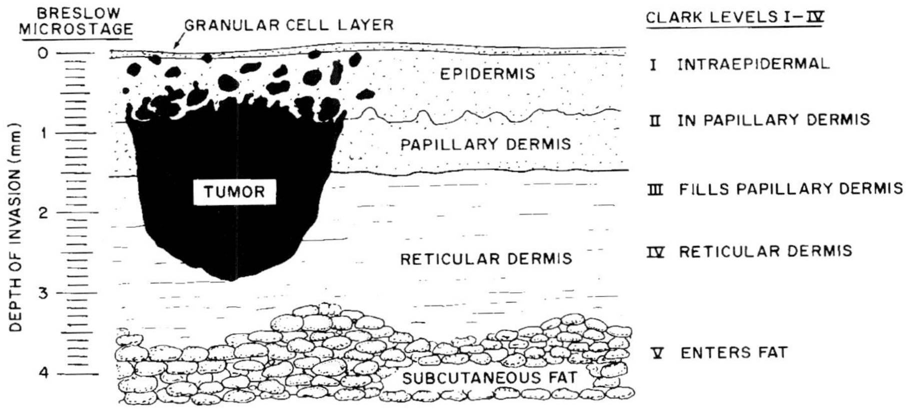

FIGURE 12-1

Breslow thickness and anatomic levels of invasion. As described by Breslow, the greatest depth of melanoma invasion is measured in the vertical dimension from the granular layer (or top of an ulcerated surface) to the point of deepest tumor invasion. The anatomic level of invasion (Clark) refers to the extent of melanoma incursion into the papillary dermis, reticular dermis, and subcutaneous fat.

TABLE 12-3
Early Studies Concerning Depth of Tumor Invasion and Prognosis

Author	*Depth of Invasion*	*Five-Year Survival*
Allen and Spitz, 1953[14]	Superficial	74.1% (5–12 years)
Lund and Ihnen, 1955[15]	Superficial	75%
Lane, Lattes, and Malm, 1958[16]	Invasion of reticular dermis	28%
Petersen, Bodenham, and Lloyd, 1962[17]	Superficial	
	Stage 1 (in situ)	100%
	Stage 2 (invasive without "tumor" formation)	82.3%
	Stage 3 (invasive with "tumor" formation)	50.7%
Mehnert and Heard, 1965[18]	Stage 1 (superficial invasion)	77.6%
	Stage 2 (invasion of reticular dermis)	38.6%
	Stage 3 (invasion of subcutaneous fat)	8.0%

For example, approximately 5 percent of patients with thin melanomas (under 1 mm) develop metastases.[3] Similarly, a small percentage of patients with melanomas greater than 4 mm in thickness remain disease-free on long-term follow-up evaluation.[3]

It also should be pointed out that tumor thickness has predictive value in stage II (nodal metastases) melanoma[2,23,24] and thus also may correlate with survival in patients with stage II disease.

Anatomic Level. In a study appearing in 1969, Clark and colleagues[14] defined five levels of melanoma invasion

TABLE 12-4
Five-Year Survival Based on Primary Tumor Thickness and Anatomic Levels of Invasion for Clinical Stage I Melanoma

<0.85 mm	99%	II	99%
0.85–1.69	94%	III	95%
1.70–3.64	78%	IV	75%
>3.65	42%	V	39%

Source: Day CL Jr, Lew RA, Mihm MC Jr, et al: The natural breakpoints for primary tumor thickness in clinical stage I melanoma (letter). *N Engl J Med* 305:1155, 1981.

(see Fig. 12-1) and showed that increasing level of invasion correlated inversely with survival (see Table 12-4).[19] Level of invasion is a significant prognostic factor on univariate analysis and retains much of this power on multivariate analysis.[1-7] However, virtually all multivariate analyses have confirmed the predominance of tumor thickness over anatomic level.[2] It also should be noted that there is considerable heterogeneity within each level category.[4,9] Thus, a thick level III polypoid melanoma may have a considerably worse prognosis than a thin level III tumor. However, in some instances, levels of invasion may more accurately depict the stage of tumor progression.[3] For example, a level II melanoma may have little or no metastatic potential regardless of tumor thickness, whereas level IV invasion may indicate more aggressive properties and a worse prognosis than a level III tumor of the same thickness.[9]

One particular problem in assessing level (in comparison with tumor thickness) has been its subjectivity. For example, determination of the papillary-reticular dermal boundary is particularly difficult for acral skin and not possible for submucosal locations.[25] Furthermore, it has been shown that anatomic level is one of the least reproducible parameters among pathologists when evaluating pathologic features of melanoma. In the study of Larsen et al.,[26] the overall rate of agreement for each of the levels was as follows: level I, 71.6 percent; level II, 66.7 percent; level III, 67.3 percent; level IV, 69.1 percent; and level V, 80 percent.

Ulceration. Histopathologic ulceration is an independent prognostic factor in some, but not all, multifactoral studies of stage I melanoma.[1-7,25,27] Approximately 20 to 25 percent of stage I melanomas are ulcerated.[4] In the population of patients with localized melanoma from the University of Alabama and Sydney Melanoma Unit, patients with ulcerated melanomas had a 50 percent survival rate at 10 years versus a 79 percent rate of survival at 10 years for nonulcerated melanomas.[4] One particular problem, already mentioned, is that ulceration is strongly associated with tumor thickness.[2] Thus some of the prognostic significance of ulceration may be confounded by this relationship with tumor thickness. Nonetheless, ulceration has still been shown to be an independent prognostic factor after adjustment for thickness in some multivariate analyses.[4,27] Ulceration also has an association with anatomic site of the melanoma and gender, since men tend to have thick, ulcerated melanomas on the trunk and women commonly have thinner, less frequently ulcerated cutaneous malignant melanoma (CMM) on the extremities.[4,27,28]

The prevalence of ulceration is probably also related to gross morphology of the primary CMM (polypoid versus flat profile), location on exposed surfaces that are subject to trauma, mitotic or proliferative rate, and intrinsic aggressive attributes.

Mitotic Rate. The mitotic rate of the invasive dermal component of CMM reflects the proliferative rate of the tumor and correlates inversely with survival. [2,29] The method of recording mitotic rate for melanoma has not been standardized. Older methods have included counting mitoses per 1, 5, or 10 high-power fields. More recently, there has been an emphasis on recording mitoses per square millimeter for the vertical growth phase only. Although mitotic activity is strongly related to tumor thickness,[2] some observers have demonstrated an independent effect on multivariate analysis.[3] In their study of 264 patients with vertical growth phase melanoma, Clark and colleagues[3] noted a 95 percent 8-year survival for patients with no observed mitoses, 79.4 percent survival at 8 years with a mitotic rate under 6 per square millimeter, and a 38.2 percent survival at 8 years in patients with melanomas having greater than 6 mitoses per square millimeter. When analyzed as a continuous variable, survival is inversely correlated with increasing mitotic rate.

In an attempt to improve the prediction of outcome, Schmoeckel and Braun-Falco[30] derived a so-called prognostic index (PI) which was the product of mitotic rate and tumor thickness. Indeed, PI was noted to have more prognostic significance than either of the factors alone. Patients with a PI of less than 10 had survival rates of 65 percent at 5 years versus 21 percent for those with a PI of greater than 10. More recently, Kopf et al.[31] reported that the PI had significant discriminative power for CMM in the thickness range 1.5 to 3.99 mm. Patients with a PI of greater than 19 had survival rates of 23 percent versus 85 percent survival for patients with a PI of less than 19. Based on the discrepancies in the latter three studies, it is still unclear whether mitotic rate significantly improves prediction of prognosis beyond that of thickness.

One particular issue related to recording mitotic rate is sampling error. In order to circumvent this problem, melanomas should be scanned for "hot spots" with the greatest mitotic activity before the number of mitoses are recorded.

Phase of Tumor Progression. As mentioned previously, the radial and vertical growth phases correlate with tumor thickness and level of invasion.[3,32] However, Clark and colleagues[3,32] believe that the presence of the vertical growth phase may signify the capacity for metastasis, whereas the radial growth phase only does not. These investigators have recorded survival rates of 100 percent at 8 years for patients with CMM of less than 1 mm in thickness and in the radial growth phase only. According to these authors, thin melanomas associated with metastasis and regression have shown evidence of the vertical growth phase (VGP) on histopathologic review. Since only 30 percent of CMMs exhibiting the VGP in the database of Clark et al. have metastasized, the utility of the VGP in predicting survival beyond tumor thickness might be called into question.[3,20]

A potential pitfall in assessing phase of tumor progression is the ability of pathologists to reliably distinguish the radial versus the vertical growth phase.

Regression. There has been considerable controversy surrounding the issue of regression and prognosis in CMM.[33–47] Since the report of Gromet et al.,[34] there has been a long-standing impression that thin CMMs (< 0.76 mm) showing histologic regression may have some potential for metastasis[1,3,35] (Table 12-5). However, some authors have reported that on long-term follow-up examination (i.e., 8 to 10 years) there are similar rates of metastasis in both regressing and nonregressing thin melanomas.[40,45] Recent observers have nonetheless maintained that there are higher rates of metastasis in thin melanomas with extensive regression.[42–44,46,47] Ronan and colleagues[44] reported that thin melanomas showing an area of regression greater than 77 percent of the tumor had significantly greater rates of metastasis than melanomas with lesser degrees of regression. Particular problems related to interpreting previously published reports concerning regression and prognosis are the lack of standardized criteria for recording histologic regression, variable periods of follow-up evaluation among published studies, and small sample sizes. A related issue has been the failure of most authors to distinguish almost entirely regressed thin melanomas associated with a residual thick zone of fibrosis from thin "evolving" melanomas with active lymphoid response or small focal or multifocal areas of regression.[39] Based on the results of recent studies, it appears that extensive or severe regression (regression of virtually the entire CMM) may have prognostic significance.

Vascular Invasion. The presence of melanoma cells within vascular or lymphatic spaces correlates with reduced survival—35.3 percent at 8 years for CMM in VGP versus 73.9 percent for comparable CMM without vascular invasion.[3] However, this effect usually disappears on multivariate analysis. Furthermore, the usefulness of this

TABLE 12-5
Frequency of Histologic Regression in Thin Melanomas and Its Effect on Prognosis

				Metastasis		
Author	*Number of Patients*	*No. with Regression*	*No. without Regression*	*Regression*	*No Regression*	*Effects of Regression on Prognosis*
Gromet, 1978[34]	121	23 (19%)	98	5 (21.7%)	2 (2%)	Adverse
Paladagu, 1983[35]	36	11 (30%)	25	5 (45.5%)	3 (12%)	Adverse
Trau, 1983[36]	116	41 (36.3%)	75	1 (1.3%)	0	None
McGovern, 1983[37]	353	205 (58%)	148	17 (8%)	8 (5%)	None
Briggs, 1984[38]	90	NA	NA	3/8	5/8	None
Cooper, 1985[39]	48 extremities	11 (23%)	37	0	0	None
Kelly, 1985[40]	251	69 (27%)	185	5 (7.2%)	7 (3.8%)	None
Sondergaard, 1985[42]	486	85 (17%) slight active 66 (14%) marked active 122 (25%) past	213	NA	NA	Adverse (79% 10-year survival for past regression versus 95% for no regression)
Naruns, 1986[43]	649	NA	NA	17/20	3	Adverse
Ronan, 1987[44]	103	30 (29%)	73	6 (>77% regression)	0	Adverse
Shaw, 1987[45]	846	518 (61%)	328	41 (7.9%)	20 (6.1%)	None
Slingluff, 1988[46]	681	Mild 14.6% Moderate 18.2% Severe 19.8%		40%	17%	Adverse for severe regression
Blessing, 1990[47]	555	13/26 Metastasis 1/40 No recurrence		NA	NA	Adverse

Note: NA, not available.

variable is further diminished because of its uncommon occurrence and frequent false-positive results due to tissue-shrinkage artifacts.[25]

Microscopic Satellites. Cohesive aggregates of tumor cells (arbitrarily defined as > 0.05 mm in diameter) in the reticular dermis, subcutaneous fat, or vessels that are separated from the main portion of the tumor by normal tissue presumably represent local extension of tumor or microscopic metastasis[48,49] (Fig. 12-2). This feature is probably closely related to vascular invasion. On univariate analysis, microscopic satellites are associated with significantly diminished survival, e.g., 40 percent at 8 years compared with 75.2 percent for VGP CMM without satellites.[3] However, this prognostic value is lost after statistical adjustment for the other prognostic factors. This parameter also may have significant predictive value for lymph node metastases. Patients in whom microscopic satellites were present had an incidence of nodal metastasis (53 percent) significantly greater than that of patients without this feature (12 percent).[49] These satellites also strongly correlate with visceral or bony metastasis.

In a recent study, the prognostic significance of microscopic satellites was reexamined; 30 CMMs exhibiting microscopic satellites were matched with 77 CMMs lacking satellites for thickness and five other prognostic parameters.[50] The presence of microscopic satellites correlated with significantly decreased survival and predicted an increased frequency of local and nodal metastases (though not statistically significant).

A particular problem with microscopic satellites has been the difficulty in establishing whether such foci are truly separate from the melanoma itself or merely extensions of the tumor not clearly demonstrated on sectioning.

Host Response/Lymphocytic Infiltration. As with regression, there has been largely no consistent or objective method of recording host response for prognostic purposes.[51] Various investigators have assessed mononuclear cell infiltrates at the tumor base, at the tumor periphery, and infiltrating the tumor. Host response also has been graded irrespective of radial or vertical growth phase. Consequently, as one might expect, many of these studies have been contradictory.[23,25,49,52–57] Despite the lack of a standardized approach to evaluating host response, there is some evidence that the presence of a lymphoid infiltrate at the base of a melanoma is a favorable prognostic factor versus a diminished or absent infiltrate indicating a worse outcome.[3,4,58] However, as reported by McGovern and colleagues,[59] lymphocytic infiltrates at the tumor base diminish with increasing tumor thickness. Thus lymphoid response may be inversely correlated with tumor thickness and may have no independent predictive value.[58,60] Other cell types reported to influence prognosis adversely have been the presence of plasma cells[61] and the presence of mature macrophages.[62]

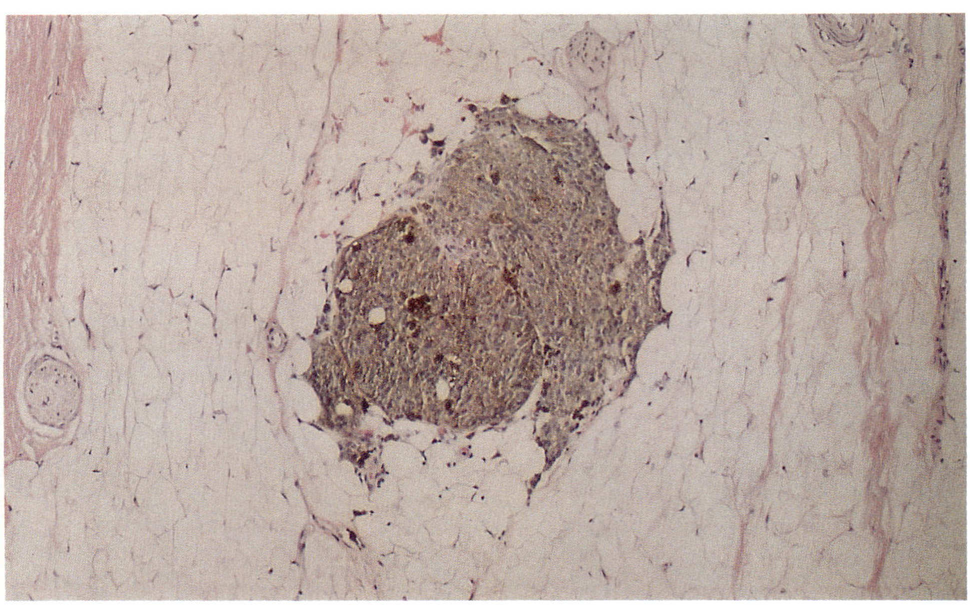

FIGURE 12-2
Microscopic satellite in subcutaneous fat. The primary melanoma measured 8.19 mm in thickness (H&E, × 100).

The presence of tumor-infiltrating lymphocytes (TILs) recently has been reported as a significant prognostic factor, even after adjustment for other variables including thickness.[3] The TILs were defined as "brisk" if lymphocytes permeated the VGP nodule and infiltrated the entire base of the VGP. The presence of "brisk" TILs was one of the most significant prognostic parameters in Clark's model (see below). A particular problem that must be addressed is the reproducibility of this histologic finding among different histopathologists.

Using computerized image analysis, Pastorfide et al.[63] recently quantified lymphocytic infiltration both within and subjacent to metastasizing versus nonmetastasizing CMM in the thickness range of 1.00 to 2.50 mm. The only significant difference noted between the latter two groups was the width of the lymphocytic infiltrate at the tumor base relative to tumor width. However, when regression analysis was applied to the group of metastasizing CMM only, a number of quantitative parameters of lymphocytic infiltration correlated with longer intervals to metastasis and improved survival. In particular, number of TILs per area of tumor was associated with both longer intervals to metastasis and greater length of survival.

Histogenetic Type. For some time after the description of the histogenetic subtypes of melanoma by Clark, it was reported that lentigo maligna melanoma (LMM) carried a more favorable prognosis than superficial spreading melanoma (SSM), and pari passu SSM, a better prognosis than nodular melanoma.[10,19] However, recent evidence suggests that differences in prognosis among histogenetic subtypes may simply reflect differences in thickness.[2–4,64] For example, the general trend for tumor thicknesses among histogenetic types is as follows: nodular melanoma > superficial spreading melanoma > lentigo maligna melanoma.[58]

When melanomas of equivalent thickness are stratified by histogenetic type, patients with LMM have significantly greater survival at 10 years compared with patients with SSM and nodular melanoma.[4] Similarly, patients with acral lentiginous melanoma (ALM) have a worse prognosis compared with persons with SSM and nodular melanoma.[4] Recently, Slingluff et al.[65] have shown that the poor prognosis of ALM is related primarily to location of the melanoma on glabrous (non-hair-bearing) skin, irrespective of the histologic type of melanoma.

Tumor Cell Type. Various observers have analyzed the prognostic significance of the predominant cell type or types composing the invasive component of melanoma, such as, for example, spindle cell, epithelioid cell, and nevoid or nevus-like (small) cell.[66–69] Some investigators have found that melanomas composed of predominantly spindle cells are associated with a significantly better prognosis than those containing mainly epithelioid or other cell types.[1,70,71] Sondergaard and Schou[1] and recently Heenan et al.[71] noted that the presence of a predominantly spindle cell invasive component continued to have prognostic significance even after adjustment for other prognostic factors. However, this result has not been confirmed consistently by other investigators on multivariate analysis.[3,25]

It should be noted that the cell type in the VGP has not been studied systematically for its prognostic significance. The concept of minimal-deviation melanoma suggests that this prognostic factor merits further investigation, since it is possible that well-differentiated or low-grade melanomas may have less aggressive courses. The use of histomorphometry, image analysis, or stereologic methods to quantify cell type or morphology has been reported recently in preliminary studies.[72]

Particular problems in evaluating cell type in the invasive component of melanoma are the prominent heterogeneity in many tumors and the lack of standardized definitions for recording cell type.

Tumor Vascularity. Folkman[73] has emphasized that the development of an adequate blood supply (angiogenesis) is necessary for the further growth of solid tumors beyond an approximate size of 1 to 2 mm.[73,74] A recent study has provided preliminary evidence that tumor vascularity may be a prognostic factor in malignant melanoma.[75] In this study, metastasizing melanomas in the thickness range of 1 to 2.50 mm had significantly greater vascularity than nonmetastasizing CMMs. Percent vascular area was a significant predictor of metastasis, whereas number of microvessels failed to correlate with risk for metastasis. However, a subsequent study examining CMMs 0.85 to 1.25 mm in thickness failed to show a significant prognostic effect for tumor vascularity.[76]

Tumor Volume. Although measurement of melanoma thickness was a significant advance in assessing the prognosis of CMM, Breslow's original objective was to measure melanoma volume as a prognostic factor. Because of the difficulty of determining tumor volume, he recorded tumor thickness instead as a surrogate of volume.[8]

In a small study of 35 patients with localized melanoma, Friedman and colleagues[77] reported that tumor volume was more discriminatory than tumor thickness in predicting survival. Patients with a tumor volume of less than 200 mm^3 had a 91.4 percent survival versus 16.7 percent for patients with melanoma tumor volumes greater than 200 mm^2. Although improved computer technology may facilitate measuring tumor volume, the calculation of tumor volume would seem rather impractical for routine use.

Cross-Sectional Profile. The *cross-sectional profile* refers to the surface topography of a CMM, i.e., relatively flat, dome-shaped, verrucous, or polypoid, on histopathologic examination. Some investigators have noted that a polypoid or verrucous surface is associated with reduced survival on multivariate analysis.[71] However, much of this effect is probably derived from a correlation with tumor thickness.[78]

Clinical Factors

Age. Although tumor thickness increases with age,[79] some observers have reported an independent effect of increasing age on prognosis even after adjustment for other factors, including tumor thickness.[80] However, this independent effect has not been confirmed in other prognostic models.[3,4]

Anatomic Site. For many years, various authors have reported that the location of a primary melanoma probably has an independent effect on prognosis.[2-4] It is important to point out that anatomic site is very closely related to gender and to a lesser extent also to thickness and ulceration.[2] Because of the close relationship between anatomic location and gender, usually only one of these two factors demonstrates an independent prognostic effect when subjected to multivariate analysis.[81] However, recent large multivariate analyses have confirmed an independent effect of anatomic site on survival.[3,4] In general, extremity melanomas are associated with a better prognosis than melanomas located on the trunk, head and neck, and palmar, plantar, subungual sites.[3] The greater survival associated with extremity melanomas may be explained potentially by a higher proportion of local and regional metastases compared with melanomas located on the trunk and head and neck.[82] Local and regional recurrences are thus associated with a greater survival than are systemic metastases. Particular anatomic sites predict significantly reduced survival and include the scalp and glabrous (non-hair-bearing) skin of the extremities.[4,65]

A possible anatomic basis for high-risk locations of CMM that often overly bony prominences has been reported by Luria et al.[83] These observers found that the tissue overlying bony prominences often seems to lack an intact muscle-fascia layer, and thus these sites constitute neurovascular "windows" with an increased concentration of perforating neurovascular bundles. In preliminary studies, these investigators found that melanomas occurring in these sites developed metastases more frequently than melanomas arising in low-risk areas during the same period of follow-up study.

Gender. In recent multivariate analyses, the female gender has been established as an independent prognostic factor even after adjustment for tumor thickness and anatomic site.[3,4] Nevertheless, in a study of 832 stage I melanoma patients, Vossaert et al.[81] found that anatomic site rather than gender was a more significant prognostic factor. These observers pointed out that differences in survival attributed to gender are related primarily to disparities between men and women in melanoma thickness, ulceration, and anatomic site of the primary melanoma. Nonetheless, Clark and colleagues[3] reported that women had an overall threefold greater survival compared with men for melanomas that had entered the VGP. Balch et al.[4] found increased survival for women overall on multivariate analysis, but this effect was operative only for melanomas 2.50 to 3.99 mm in thickness and localized to the extremities.

Pathologic Stage. Microscopic involvement of lymph nodes with melanoma (micrometastases, occult metastases) even though clinically uninvolved (clinical stage I, pathologic stage II) is associated with markedly diminished survival (e.g., 42 percent 5-year survival)[7,23,24] compared with greater than 80 percent 5-year survival for all clinical stage I patients.[7] In comparison, patients with occult metastases to lymph nodes (clinical stage I, pathologic stage II) have a significantly better prognosis than patients with clinically involved nodes (clinical stage II, pathologic stage II), (5-year survival of 47 percent for CSI versus 21 percent for CSII disease).[84] Prognosis within this heterogeneous group is related to extent of lymph node involvement, e.g., number of lymph nodes, percentage of lymph nodes involved by tumor, and characteristics of the primary melanoma, in particular tumor thickness and ulceration.[23] In fact, Day et al.[23] observed that prognosis in patients with minimal nodal involvement (< 20 percent of nodes affected) is related primarily to tumor thickness, again emphasizing the primacy of tumor thickness in the prognosis of CMM.

Pregnancy Status. There has been considerable controversy surrounding pregnancy, hormonal effects, and prognosis in melanoma.[85-95] Various observers have reported a favorable effect, an adverse effect, or no effect of pregnancy on outcome of malignant melanoma. It must be pointed out that many previous reports have included only limited numbers of patients and often have failed to control for thickness. However, recent studies have failed to show an adverse effect of pregnancy on survival of stage I melanoma[91-95] (Table 12-6). Nevertheless, Slingluff et al.[94] have documented decreased disease-free intervals for women with melanomas developing during pregnancy compared with nonpregnant women with melanoma.

Other Factors

Volume-Weighted Mean Nuclear Volume. Using modern stereologic techniques, Sorensen and colleagues[96] calculated volume-weighted mean nuclear volume in 71 stage I melanoma patients and observed that the latter variable had greater prognostic significance than nuclear DNA content and tumor thickness. Binder et al.[97] applied this

TABLE 12-6
Prognostic Effect of Pregnancy on Outcome of Stage I Melanoma

Author	*Number of Patients*	*Five-Year Survival*	*Effect of Pregnancy on Survival*	*Effect of Pregnancy on Disease-Free Interval*	*Effect of Pregnancy on Interval to Nodal Metastasi*
Shiu, 1976[91]	20	80%	None	None	NA*
Wong, 1989[92]	66	86%	None	None	NA
McManamny, 1989[93]	23	~85%†	None	None	NA
Slingluff, 1990[94]	100	~82%†	None	Significantly shortened	Significantly shortened
MacKie, 1991[95]	92	~80%†	None	None	NA

*NA, not available.
†Estimate of 5-year survival rates from survival curves.

technique to 32 thin melanomas (<0.76 mm) and found that there was a significant correlation between nuclear volume and metastasis. These authors also showed that nuclear area and shape factors measured by two-dimensional image analysis failed to correlate with prognosis.

DNA Ploidy. The significance of DNA content as a prognostic factor in stage I melanoma is unsettled.[98-100] Variation in the results of these studies of DNA content are probably related to the use of flow versus image cytometry, fresh versus formalin-fixed paraffin-embedded tissue, differences in instrumentation, and differences in interpretation of data.[100] In a study of 145 stage I melanoma patients, DNA aneuploidy was shown to be a significant independent prognostic factor.[98] However, as discussed earlier, this result has not been verified in other studies.[100] Furthermore, only about two-thirds of primary malignant melanomas exhibit DNA aneuploidy. DNA aneuploidy also correlates with increasing tumor thickness and the presence of the VGP. A recent study employing fresh tissue from 14 primary and 16 metastatic melanomas was performed using image analysis cytometry of monolayer imprints.[99] There was a higher frequency of DNA aneuploidy in fresh versus paraffin-embedded tissue, and the frequency of DNA aneuploidy was comparable in both primary (78 percent) and metastatic (75 percent) tumors. Furthermore, DNA aneuploidy correlated with metastatic disease or death, although numbers of patients were small.

Nucleolar Organizer Regions. Nucleolar organizer regions (NORs) are circular fragments of chromosomal DNA within nucleoli that are visualized by silver stains as black dots and designated AgNORs.[101] Among 98 stage I melanoma patients, the mean number of AgNORs (2.792 ± 0.901) was significantly less in patients without metastases than the mean number (4.889 ± 1.403) in patients with metastases.[102] AgNOR counts greater than 3.62 were associated with an 82 percent probability of developing metastases in those patients. Further studies are needed to establish whether assessment of AgNORs is a reliable prognostic parameter.

Proliferation and Motility. Computerized image analysis techniques have been utilized recently to estimate the contributions of proliferation and motility as prognostic factors in melanoma.[103,104] Smolle and colleagues[104] used mitotic rate and immunoreactivity with the Ki67 monoclonal antibody as estimates of proliferation. Tumor invasiveness was assessed by the architectural profile of the melanoma-stroma interface. Neither proliferation nor pattern analysis of motility alone were significant prognostic factors, but when these factors were assessed together, there was a significant effect on both overall and disease-free survival.

PROGNOSTIC FACTORS FOR STAGE II MELANOMA

In general, survival after regional lymph node involvement decreases dramatically to approximately 30 to 50 percent at 5 years, but there is considerable heterogeneity depending on the extent of nodal involvement.[3,4,8,10,48,55,105-113]

The most important factors relate to the degree of lymph node involvement and some characteristics of the primary tumor—tumor thickness, ulceration, and anatomic site (Table 12-7). Number or percentage of positive nodes has proved to be the single most important variable for this stage of disease. For example, Callery et al.[24] found that stage II melanoma patients with three or fewer involved nodes had a 45 percent 5-year survival versus 21 percent 5-year survival for patients with four or more positive nodes. However, additional measures of tumor burden such as percentage of total metastasis diameter relative to total nodal diameter may provide additional

TABLE 12-7
Prognostic Factors for Clinical Stage II Melanoma (Regional Lymph Node Involvement)

Nodal Factors	*Effect on Prognosis*
Number of positive nodes	Worse prognosis with increasing number of positive nodes
Percentage of positive nodes ($<20\%$ versus $>20\%$)	Worse prognosis with increasing percentage of positive nodes
Micro versus macrometastases	Worse prognosis with macrometastases
Extent of nodal metastasis (limited by or invasion through capsule)	Worse prognosis with invasion through capsule
Total tumor diameter as percentage of total node diameter ($\leq 15\%$ versus $\leq 15\%$)	Worse prognosis with total tumor diameter $\geq 15\%$
DNA ploidy	Worse prognosis with DNA aneuploidy
Clonality (monoclonal versus polyclonal)	Worse prognosis with monoclonality
Primary Melanoma Factors	*Effect on Prognosis*
Tumor thickness (especially for minimal nodal disease)	Worse prognosis with increasing tumor thickness
Ulceration	Worse prognosis with ulceration
Clinical Factors	*Effect on Prognosis*
Anatomic site (axial versus extremity)	Worse prognosis with axial site
Age	Worse prognosis with increasing age

TABLE 12-8
Prognostic Factors for Clinical Stage III Melanoma

Prognostic Variable	*Effect on Prognosis*
Number of metastatic sites	Worse prognosis with increasing number of sites
Location of metastases	Worse prognosis for visceral sites (lung, liver, brain, bone) versus nonvisceral sites (skin, subcutaneous tissue, distant lymph nodes)
Presence of "resectable" metastases	Better prognosis for solitary resectable metastases
Sex	Worse outcome for males
Duration of remission	Shorter duration of remission associated with worse prognosis

prognostic information.[114] In addition, Cochran[115] has noted that presence of DNA aneuploidy and multiple clones in nodal metastases, determined by DNA image cytometry, correlates with diminished survival.

When nodal involvement is limited—occult metastases (clinical stage I, pathologic stage II) with less than 20 percent of nodes involved—the prognosis is primarily related to melanoma thickness and other features of the primary tumor according to Day et al.[23] Thus patients with melanomas 3.5 mm thick or less and less than 20 percent of their nodes positive had an 80 percent 5-year survival. On the other hand, nodal factors seem to dictate prognosis when the nodes are clinically involved and 20 percent or more are positive.

PROGNOSTIC FACTORS FOR STAGE III MELANOMA

Once metastases to distant sites have developed, median survival is about 6 months.[4,116] The only variables of prognostic significance are number of metastatic sites, surgical resectability, duration of remission, and location of metastases (Table 12-8). Survival is longer for one metastatic site versus two, and two sites are more favorable than three or more. Solitary "resectable" metastases as in sites such as the lungs, brain, or bowel may be associated with significantly prolonged survival.[4,116] Patients also have improved survival with nonvisceral sites (skin, subcutaneous tissue, distant lymph nodes) versus visceral sites (lung, liver, bone, brain). Another study has reported a more favorable outcome for females, metastases limited

TABLE 12-9
*Predicted 5-Year and 10-Year Survival Rates from Initial Diagnosis for Patients with Stage I (Localized) Melanoma**

Tumor Thickness (mm)	*Anatomic Site*	*Ulceration*	*Clark's Level*	*Sex*	*5-Year Survival Rate (%)*	*10-Year Survival Rate (%)*†
< 0.76 mm	Extremity	—	II	—	99	97
	Extremity	—	Other	—	97	94
	Axial	—	II	—	96	92
	Axial	—	Other	—	91	84
0.76–1.49	Extremity	No	II	—	98	97
	Extremity	No	Other	—	93	89
	Extremity	Yes	II	—	94	91
	Extremity	Yes	Other	—	82	72
	Axial	No	II	—	95	93
	Axial	No	Other	—	85	77
	Axial	Yes	II	—	88	81
	Axial	Yes	Other		64	49
1.50–2.49	Extremity	No	—	—	86	81
	Extremity	Yes	—	—	76	69
	Axial	No	—	—	76	67
	Axial	Yes	—	—	61	49
2.50–3.99	Extremity	No	—	F	80	72
	Extremity	No	—	M	73	62
	Extremity	Yes	—	F	74	64
	Extremity	Yes	—	M	64	51
	Axial	No	—	F	73	63
	Axial	No	—	M	63	51
	Axial	Yes	—	F	65	52
	Axial	Yes	—	M	53	39
4.00–7.99	—	No	II/III	—	80	73
	—	No	IV/V	—	68	58
	—	Yes	II/III	—	67	57
	—	Yes	IV/V	—	51	38
≥ 8.00	—	—	—	—	43	25

*The projected survival rates have been adjusted for the effects of surgical treatment in those subgroups in which it was a significant factor.
†The projected 10-year survival rate for an individual patient is considered as this patient's clinical score; for applications see ref. 6.
Source: Soong, S-J: A computerized mathematical model and scoring system for predicting outcome in patients with localized melanoma. In Balch CM, Houghton A, Sober AJ, et al (eds): *Cutaneous Melanoma* (ed 2). Philadelphia, Lippincott, 1992, pp 200–212.

to bone, sparing of the liver, and greater activity level of the patient.[117]

PROGNOSTIC MODELS

The purpose of prognostic models has been to identify the most important variables that characterize prognosis in melanoma but also to predict the probabilities for survival, recurrence, and metastases in individual patients. Soong[6,118] developed a mathematical model for stage I melanoma based on the coding of four clinical variables (age, sex, anatomic site, and initial surgical procedure) and four pathologic variables (tumor thickness, level of invasion, ulceration, and histogenetic subtype or growth pattern) from 4568 patients at the University of Alabama at Birmingham and the Sydney Melanoma Unit. The predicted 5- and 10-year survival rates generated by this model are depicted in Table 12-9.

Clark and colleagues also have developed a prognostic model for stage I melanoma based on recognition of stage of tumor progression (as described above).[3] According to their model, patients with melanomas only in the RGP, irrespective of thickness (generally under 1.00 mm) and other prognostic variables, have 100 percent survival at 8 years.[3] The other component of their model is based on the histologic recognition of the VGP, an aggregative nodule or plaque of melanoma cells partially or completely filling or expanding the papillary dermis.

TABLE 12-10
Probabilities of 8-Year Survival (Multivariable Logistic Regression Model)

			Female				*Male*			
Mitotic Rate/mm²	*TILs**	*Tumor Regression*	*Extremities*		*Axial, Subvol†*		*Extremities*		*Axial/Subvol†*	
0.0/mm²	Brisk	Absent	1.00	**0.99**	1.00	**0.98**	1.00	**0.98**	0.99	**0.95**
		Present	1.00	**0.99**	0.99	**0.95**	0.99	**0.96**	0.96	**0.86**
	Nonbrisk	Absent	1.00	**0.98**	0.98	**0.94**	0.99	**0.95**	0.96	**0.84**
		Present	0.99	**0.95**	0.96	**0.85**	0.97	**0.88**	0.89	**0.66**
	Absent	Absent	0.99	**0.94**	0.95	**0.82**	0.96	**0.85**	0.86	**0.60**
		Present	0.96	**0.86**	0.87	**0.61**	0.89	**0.67**	0.69	**0.35**
0.1–6.0/mm²	Brisk	Absent	1.00	**0.98**	0.98	**0.94**	0.99	**0.95**	0.95	**0.84**
		Present	0.99	**0.95**	0.96	**0.84**	0.97	**0.87**	0.88	**0.65**
	Nonbrisk	Absent	0.99	**0.95**	0.95	**0.82**	0.96	**0.86**	0.87	**0.61**
		Present	0.96	**0.86**	0.87	**0.62**	0.90	**0.68**	0.70	**0.36**
	Absent	Absent	0.95	**0.83**	0.84	**0.57**	0.87	**0.63**	0.65	**0.31**
		Present	0.88	**0.64**	0.66	**0.32**	0.71	**0.38**	0.40	**0.14**
> 6.0/mm²	Brisk	Absent	0.99	**0.94**	0.95	**0.81**	0.96	**0.85**	0.86	**0.60**
		Present	0.96	**0.85**	0.86	**0.61**	0.89	**0.67**	0.68	**0.35**
	Nonbrisk	Absent	0.95	**0.84**	0.84	**0.57**	0.88	**0.63**	0.65	**0.31**
		Present	0.88	**0.64**	0.66	**0.32**	0.72	**0.38**	0.40	**0.14**
	Absent	Absent	0.85	**0.59**	0.61	**0.28**	0.67	**0.33**	0.34	**0.12**
		Present	0.68	**0.34**	0.35	**0.12**	0.42	**0.15**	0.16	**0.04**

Note: Data for lesions < 1.70 mm thick (i.e., vertical growth phase, clinical stage I cases) are in regular face; data for lesions ≥ 1.70 mm (vertical growth phase, clinical stage I cases) are in boldface.
*Tumor-infiltrating lymphocytes.
†Axial/subvol includes head, neck, trunk, volar, and submucosal locations.
Source: Clark WH Jr, Elder DE, Guerry D IV, et al: Model predicting survival in stage I melanoma based on tumor progression. *J Natl Cancer Inst* 81:1893–1904, 1989.

Once the VGP is recognized, other clinical and histologic prognostic indicators are assessed and used to formulate prognosis at 8 years. Six variables were found to be independent predictors of survival after multivariate analysis of 23 factors. These 6 modifying factors in descending order of importance were mitotic rate (higher mitotic rates predicted reduced survival), TILs (the more extensive and dense the lymphocytes infiltrating the tumor, the higher the rate of survival), tumor thickness (< 1.70 mm associated with the greater survival), anatomic site (extremity sites associated with better survival compared with axial locations), sex (better prognosis for females), and regression (absence of regression associated with greater survival) (Table 12-10). Variables found to have no prognostic value were ulceration, microscopic satellites, levels of invasion, and pathologic stage of lymph nodes. The basis of this model assumes that the histomorphologic growth pattern defined as the VGP is highly correlated with propensity for metastasis. This proposition has not been rigorously validated, and it remains to be seen whether this model can improve prediction of survival beyond that of thickness alone in other databases.

REFERENCES

1. Sondergaard K, Schou G: Survival with primary cutaneous malignant melanoma, evaluated from 2012 cases. *Virchows Arch [A]* 406:179–195, 1985.
2. Vollmer RT: Malignant melanoma: A multivariate analysis of prognostic factors. *Pathol Ann* 24:383–407, 1989.
3. Clark WH, Elder DE, Guerry D, et al: Model predicting survival in stage I melanoma based on tumor progression. *J Natl Cancer Inst* 81:1893–1904, 1989.
4. Balch CM, Soong S-J, Shaw HM, et al: An analysis of prognostic factors in 8500 patients with cutaneous melanoma. In Balch CM, Houghton A, Sober AJ, et al (eds): *Cutaneous Melanoma* (ed 2). Philadelphia, Lippincott, 1992, pp. 165–187.
5. Balch CM, Cascinelli N, Drzewiecki KT, et al: A comparison of prognostic factors worldwide. In Balch CM, Houghton A, Sober AJ, et al (eds): *Cutaneous Melanoma* (ed 2). Philadelphia, Lippincott, 1992, pp. 188–199.
6. Soong S-J: A computerized mathematical model and scoring system for predicting outcome in patients with localized melanoma. In Balch CM, Houghton A, Sober AJ, et al (eds): *Cutaneous Melanoma* (ed 2). Philadelphia, Lippincott, 1992, pp. 200–212.
7. Rigel DS, Friedman RJ, Kopf AW, Silverman MK: Factors influencing survival in melanoma. *Dermatol Clin* 9(4):631–642, 1991.

8. Breslow A: Thickness, cross-sectional areas and depth of invasion in the prognosis of cutaneous melanoma. *Ann Surg* 172:902–908, 1970.
9. Balch CM, Murad TM, Soong S-J, et al: A multifactorial analysis of melanoma. Prognostic histopathological features comparing Clark's and Breslow's staging methods. *Ann Surg* 188:732–742, 1978.
10. Cascinelli N, Morabito A, Bufalino R, et al: Prognosis of stage I melanoma of the skin. *Int J Cancer* 26:733–739, 1980.
11. Balch CM, Soong S-J, Murad TM, et al: A multifactorial analysis of melanoma: II. Prognostic factors in patients with stage I (localized) melanoma. *Surgery* 86(2):343–351, 1979.
12. Balch CM, Smalley RV, Bartolucci AA, et al and the Southeastern Cancer Study Group: A randomized prospective clinical trial of adjuvant *C. parvum* immunotherapy in 260 patients with clinically localized melanoma (stage I): Prognostic factors analysis and preliminary results of immunotherapy. *Cancer* 49(6):1079–1084, 1982.
13. Balch CM, Soong S-J, Milton GW, et al: A comparison of prognostic factors and surgical results in 1786 patients with localized (stage I) melanomatreated in Alabama, USA, and New South Wales, Australia. *Ann Surg* 196(6):677–684, 1982.
14. Allen AC, Spitz S: Melanomas: Diagnosis and prognosis. *Cancer* 6:1–45, 1953.
15. Lund RH, Ihnen M: Malignant melanoma. Clinical and pathologic analysis of 93 cases. Is prophylactic lymph node dissection indicated? *Surgery* 38:652–659, 1955.
16. Lane N, Lattes R, Malm J: Clinicopathological correlations in a series of 117 malignant melanomas of the skin of adults. *Cancer* 11:1025–1043, 1958.
17. Petersen NC, Bodenham DC, Lloyd OC: Malignant melanomas of the skin. *Br J Plast Surg* 15:49–94, 1962.
18. Mehnert JH, Heard JL: Staging of malignant melanoma by depth of invasion. *Am J Surg* 110:168–176, 1965.
19. Clark WH, From L, Bernardino EA, Mihm MC Jr: The histogenesis and biologic behavior of primary human malignant melanomas of the skin. *Cancer Res* 29(3):705–727, 1969.
20. Green MS, Ackerman AB: Thickness is not an accurate guage of prognosis of cutaneous melanoma. *Am J Dermatopathol* 15:461–473, 1993.
21. Day CL Jr, Lew RA, Mihm MC Jr, et al: The natural break points for primary tumor thickness in clinical stage I melanoma (letter). *N Engl J Med* 305:1155, 1981.
22. Keefe M, MacKie RM: The relationship between risk of death from clinical stage I cutaneous melanoma and thickness of primary tumour: No evidence for steps in risk. *Br J Cancer* 64:598–602, 1991.
23. Day CL Jr, Sober AJ, Lew RA, et al: Malignant melanoma patients with positive nodes and relatively good prognoses: Microstaging retains prognostic significance in clinical stage I melanoma patients with metastases to regional nodes. *Cancer* 47:955–962, 1981.
24. Callery C, Cochran AJ, Roe DJ, et al: Factors prognostic for survival in patients with malignant melanoma spread to the regional lymph nodes. *Ann Surg* 196(1):69–75, 1982.
25. Ronan SG, Han MC, Das Gupta TK: Histologic prognostic indicators in cutaneous malignant melanoma. *Semin Oncol* 15(6):558–565, 1988.
26. Larsen TE, Grude TH: A retrospective histological study of 699 cases of primary cutaneous malignant melanoma in clinical stage I. *Acta Pathol Microbiol Scand [A]* 87:469–477, 1979.
27. Balch CM, Wilkerson JA, Murad TM, et al: The prognostic significance of ulceration of cutaneous melanoma. *Cancer* 45:3012–3017, 1980.
28. Vossaert KA, Silverman MK, Kopf AW, et al: Influence of gender on survival in patients with stage I malignant melanoma. *J Am Acad Dermatol* 26:429–440, 1992.
29. Eldh J, Boeryd B, Peterson LE: Prognostic factors in cutaneous malignant melanoma in stage I: A clinical, morphological and multivariate analysis. *Scand J Plast Reconstr Surg* 12:243–255, 1978.
30. Schmoeckel C, Braun-Falco O: Prognostic index in malignant melanoma. *Arch Dermatol* 114:871–873, 1978.
31. Kopf AW, Gross DF, Rogers GS, et al: Prognostic index for malignant melanoma. *Cancer* 59:1236–1241, 1987.
32. Clark WH, Elder DE, Guerry D, et al: A study of tumor progression: The precursor lesions of superficial spreading and nodular melanoma. *Hum Pathol* 15:1147–1165, 1984.
33. Smith JL Jr, Stehlin JS Jr: Spontaneous regression of primary malignant melanomas with regional metastases. *Cancer* 18:1399–1415, 1965.
34. Gromet MA, Epstein WL, Blois MS: The regressing thin malignant melanoma: A distinctive lesion with metastatic potential. *Cancer* 42:2282–2292, 1978.
35. Paladagu RR, Yonemeto RH: Biologic behavior of thin malignant melanomas with regressive changes. *Arch Surg* 118:41–44, 1983.
36. Trau H, Rigel DS, Harris MN, et al: Metastases of thin melanomas. *Cancer* 51(3):553–556, 1983.
37. McGovern VJ, Shaw HM, Milton GW: Prognosis in patients with thin malignant melanoma: Influence of regression. *Histopathology* 7:673–680, 1983.
38. Briggs JC, Ibrahim NBN, Hastings AG, Griffiths RW: Experience of thin cutaneous melanomas (< 0.76 mm and < 0.85 mm thick) in a large plastic surgery unit: A 5 to 17 year follow-up. *Br J Plast Surg* 37:501–506, 1984.
39. Cooper PH, Wanebo HJ, Hagar RW: Regression in thin malignant melanoma: Microscopic diagnosis and prognostic importance. *Arch Dermatol* 121:1127–1131, 1985.
40. Kelly JW, Sagebiel RW, Blois MS: Regression in malignant melanoma: A histologic feature without independent prognostic significance. *Cancer* 56:2287–2291, 1985.
41. Sagebiel R: Regression and other factors of prognostic interest in malignant melanoma (editorial). *Arch Dermatol* 121:1125–1126, 1985.
42. Sondergaard K, Hou-Jensen K: Partial regression in thin primary cutaneous malignant melanomas clinical stage I: A study of 486 cases. *Virchows Arch [A]* 408:241–247, 1985.
43. Naruns PL, Nizze JA, Cochran AJ, et al: Recurrence potential of thin primary melanomas. *Cancer* 57:545–548, 1986.
44. Ronan SG, Eng AM, Briele HA, et al: Thin malignant melanomas with regression and metastases. *Arch Dermatol* 123:1326–1330, 1987.

45. Shaw HM, McGovern VJ, Milton GW, et al: Malignant melanoma: Influence of site of lesion and age of patient in the female superiority in survival. *Cancer* 46:2731–2735, 1980.
46. Slingluff CL, Vollmer RT, Reintgen DS, Seigler HF. Lethal "thin" malignant melanoma: Identifying patients at risk. *Ann Surg* 208(2):150–161, 1988.
47. Blessing K, McLaren KM, McLean A, Davidson P: Thin malignant melanomas (< 1.5 mm) with metastasis: A histological study and survival analysis. *Histopathology* 17:389–395, 1990.
48. Day CL, Harrist TJ, Gorstein F, et al: Malignant melanoma. Prognostic significance of "microscopic satellites" in the reticular dermis and subcutaneous fat. *Ann Surg* 194:108–112, 1981.
49. Harrist TJ, Rigel DS, Day CL, et al: Microscopic satellites are more highly associated with regional lymph node metastasis than is primary melanoma thickness. *Cancer* 53:2183–2187, 1984.
50. Leon P, Daly JM, Synnestvedt M, et al: The prognostic implications of microscopic satellites in patients with clinical stage I melanoma. *Arch Surg* 126:1461–1468, 1991.
51. Breslow A, Macht S: Evaluation of prognosis in stage I cutaneousmelanoma. *Plast Reconstr Surg* 61:342–346, 1978.
52. Hansen MG, McCarten AB: Tumor thickness and lymphocytic infiltration in malignant melanoma of the head and neck. *Am J Surg* 128:557–561, 1974.
53. Elias EG, Didolkar MS, Goel JP: Clinicopathologic study of prognostic factors in cutaneous malignant melanoma. *Surg Gynecol Obstet* 144:327–334, 1977.
54. Day CL Jr, Lew RA, Mihm MC Jr, et al: A multivariate analysis of prognostic factors for melanoma patients with lesions > 3.65 mm in thickness: The importance of revealing alternative Cox models. *Ann Surg* 195:44–49, 1982.
55. Day CL Jr, Sober AJ, Kopf AW, et al: A prognostic model for clinical stage I melanoma of the trunk: Location near the midline is not an independent risk factor for recurrent disease. *Am J Surg* 142:247–251, 1981.
56. Schmoeckel C, Bockelbrink A, Bockelbrink H, Braun-Falco O: Low- and high-risk malignant melanoma: II. Multivariate analyses for a prognostic classification. *Eur J Cancer Clin Oncol* 19(2):237–243, 1983.
57. Drzewiecki KT, Andersen PK: Survival with malignant melanoma: A regression analysis of prognostic factors. *Cancer* 49:2414–2419, 1982.
58. Kopf AW, Welkovich B, Frankel RE, et al: Thickness of malignant melanoma: Global analysis of related factors. *J Dermatol Surg Oncol* 13:345–390, 401–420, 1987.
59. McGovern VJ, Shaw HM, Milton GW, Farago GA: Lymphocytic infiltration and survival in malignant melanoma. In Ackerman AB (ed): *Pathology of Malignant Melanoma.* New York, Masson, 1981, p. 341.
60. Rowden G: Immunology of melanoma. In Mihm MC Jr, Murphy GF, Kaufman N (eds): *Pathobiology and Recognition of Malignant Melanoma.* Baltimore, Williams & Wilkins, 1988, pp. 50–78.
61. Mascaro JM, Molgo M, Castel T, Castro J: Plasma cells within the infiltrate of primary cutaneous malignant melanoma of the skin: A confirmation of its histoprognostic value. *Am J Dermatopathol* 9:497–499, 1987.
62. Bröcker E, Zwadlo G, Suter L, et al: Infiltration of primary and metastatic melanomas with macrophages of the 25F9-positive phenotype. *Cancer Immunol Immunother* 25:81–86, 1987.
63. Pastorfide GC, Kibbi A-G, de Roa AL, et al: Image analysis of stage I melanoma (1.00–2.50 mm): Lymphocytic infiltrates related to metastasis and survival. *J Cutan Pathol* 19:390–397, 1992.
64. Koh HK, Michalik E, Sober AJ, et al: Lentigo maligna melanoma has no better prognosis than other types of melanoma. *J Clin Oncol* 2:994–1001, 1984.
65. Slingluff CL, Vollmer R, Seigler HF: Acral melanoma: A review of 185 patients with identification of prognostic variables. *J Surg Oncol* 45:91–98, 1990.
66. Schmoeckel C, Bockelbrink A, Bockelbrink H, et al: Low- and high-risk malignant melanoma: I. Evaluation of clinical and histological prognosticators in 585 cases. *Eur J Cancer Clin Oncol* 19:227–235, 1983.
67. Huvos AG, Shah JP, Mike V: Prognostic factors in cutaneous malignant melanoma: A comparative study of long term and short term survivors. *Hum Pathol* 5:347–357, 1974.
68. Hacene K, Le Doussal V, Bruner M, et al: Prognostic index for clinical stage I cutaneous malignant melanoma. *Cancer Res* 43:2991–2996, 1983.
69. Shaw HM, Balch CM, Soong S-J, et al: Prognostic histopathological features in malignant melanoma. *Pathology* 17:271–274, 1985.
70. Van der Esch EP, Cascinelli N, Preda F, et al: Stage I melanoma of the skin: Evaluation of prognosis according to histologic characteristics. *Cancer* 48:1668–1673, 1981.
71. Heenan PJ, English DR, Holman CDJ, Armstrong BK: Survival among patients with clinical stage I cutaneous malignant melanoma diagnosed in Western Australia in 1975/1976 and 1980/1981. *Cancer*; 68:2079–2087, 1991.
72. Baak JP, Tan G: The adjuvant prognostic value of nuclear morphometry in stage I malignant melanoma of the skin. A multivariate analysis. *Anal Quant Cytol Histol* 68:241–244, 1986.
73. Folkman J: What is the evidence that tumors are angiogenesis dependent? *J Natl Cancer Inst* 82:4–6, 1990.
74. Barnhill RL, Fandrey K, Levy MA, et al: Angiogenesis and tumor progression of melanoma: Quantification of vascularity in melanocytic nevi and cutaneous malignant melanoma. *Lab Invest* 67:331–337, 1992.
75. Srivastava A, Laidler P, Davies RP, et al: The prognostic significance of tumor vascularity in intermediate-thickness (0.76–4.0 mm thick) skin melanoma: A quantitative histologic study. *Am J Pathol* 133:419–423, 1988.
76. Carnochan P, Briggs JC, Westbury G, Davies AJS: The vascularity of cutaneous melanoma: A quantitative histological study of lesions 0.85–1.25 mm in thickness. *Br J Cancer* 64:102–107, 1991.
77. Friedman RJ, Rigel DS, Kopf AW, et al: Volume of malignant melanoma is superior to thickness as a prognostic indicator: Preliminary observations. *Dermatol Clin* 9:643–648, 1992.

78. McGovern VJ, Shaw HM, Milton GW: Prognostic significance of a polypoid configuration in malignant melanoma. *Histopathology* 7:663–672, 1983.
79. Levine J, Kopf AW, Rigel DS, et al: Correlation of thickness of superficial spreading malignant melanoma and ages of patients. *J Dermatol Surg Oncol* 7:311–316, 1981.
80. Cohen HJ, Cox E, Manton K, Woodbury M: Malignant melanoma in the elderly. *J Clin Oncol* 5:100–106, 1987.
81. Vossaert KA, Silverman MK, Kopf AW, et al: Influence of gender on survival in patients with stage I malignant melanoma. *J Am Acad Dermatol* 26:429–440, 1992.
82. Reintgen DS, Volmer RT, Tso CY, Seigler HF: Prognosis for recurrent stage I malignant melanoma. *Arch Surg* 122:1338–1342, 1987.
83. Luria LW, Proper SA, Burnett SM, et al: An anatomical basis for prognosis of malignant melanoma. *Plast Reconstr Surg* 90:263–269, 1992.
84. Roses DF, Provet JA, Harris MN, et al: Prognosis of patients with pathologic stage II cutaneous malignant melanoma. *Ann Surg* 201:103–107, 1985.
85. Holly EA, Weiss NS, Liff JM: Cutaneous melanoma in relation to exogenous hormones and reproductive factors. *J Natl Cancer Inst* 70:827–831, 1983.
86. Holly EA: Current issues in melanoma research: Exogenous hormones,pregnancy. Cutaneous melanoma and oral contraceptives: A review of case-control and cohort studies. *Canc Res* 102:108–117, 1986.
87. Holly EA: Melanoma and pregnancy. *Cancer Res* 102:118–126, 1986.
88. Reintgen DS, McCarty KS Jr, Vollmer R, et al: Malignant melanoma and pregnancy. *Cancer* 55:1340–1344, 1985.
89. Beattie CW, Ronan SG, Amoss MS Jr: Estrogens influence the natural history of Sinclair swine cutaneous melanoma. *Canc Res* 51:2025–2028, 1991.
90. Walker MJ, Ronan SG, Han MC, et al: Interrelationship between histopathologic characteristics of melanoma and estrogen receptor status. *Cancer* 68:184–188, 1991.
91. Shiu MH, Schottenfeld D, MacLean B, Fortner JG: Adverse effect of pregnancy on melanoma: A reappraisal. *Cancer* 37:181–187, 1976.
92. Wong JH, Sterns EE, Kopald KH, et al: Prognostic significance of pregnancy in stage I melanoma. *Arch Surg* 124:1227–1231, 1989.
93. McManamny DS, Moss ALH, Pocock PV, Briggs JC: Melanoma and pregnancy: A long-term follow-up. *Br J Obstet Gynaecol* 96:1419–1423, 1989.
94. Slingluff CL, Reintgen DS, Vollmer RT, Seigler HF: Malignant melanoma arising during pregnancy: A study of 100 patients. *Ann Surg* 211:552–559, 1990.
95. MacKie RM, Bufalino R, Morabito A, et al: Lack of effect of pregnancy on outcome of melanoma. *Lancet* 337:653–655, 1991.
96. Sorenson FB, Kristensen IB, Grymer F, Jakobsen A: DNA level, tumor thickness, and stereological estimates of nuclear volume in stage I cutaneous malignant melanomas: A comparative study with analysis of prognostic impact. *Am J Dermatopathol* 13:11–19, 1991.
97. Binder M, Dolezal I, Wolff K, Pehamberger H: Sterologic estimation of volume-weighted mean nuclear volume as a predictor of prognosis in "thin" malignant melanomas. *J Invest Dermatol* 99:180–183, 1992.
98. Kheir SA, Bines SD, Vonroenn JH, et al: Prognostic significance of DNA aneuploidy in stage I cutaneous melanoma. *Ann Surg* 207:455–461, 1988.
99. Herzberg AJ, Kevus BJ, Borowitz MJ, et al: DNA ploidy of malignant melanoma determined by image cytometry of fresh, frozen, and parrafin-embedded tissue. J Cutan Pathol 1991;18:440–448.
100. Herzberg AJ: Significance of DNA ploidy in cutaneous lesions. *Arch Dermatol* 128:663–672, 1992.
101. Friedman RJ, Grin CM, Heilmen E, et al: Distinguishing benign and malignant melanocytic lesions with the Ag-NOR method. *Dermatol Clin* 9:689–693, 1991.
102. Gambini C, Casazza S, Borgiani L, et al: Counting the nucleolar organizer region-associated proteins is a prognostic clue of malignant melanoma. *Arch Dermatol* 128:487–490, 1992.
103. Smolle J, Smolle-Juettner F-M, Stettner H, Kerl H: Relationship of tumor cell motility and morphologic patterns: I. Melanocytic skin tumors. *Am J Dermatopathol* 14:231–237, 1992.
104. Smolle J, Smolle-Juettner F-M, Kerl H: Prognostic significance of proliferation and motility in primary malignant melanoma of the skin. *J Cutan Pathol* 19:110–115, 1992.
105. Elder DE: Metastatic melanoma. In Elder DE (ed): *Pigment Cell,* vol 8. Basal, Karger, 1987, p. 182.
106. Day CL Jr, Mihm MC Jr, Sober AJ, et al: Prognostic factors for melanoma patients with lesions 0.76 mm–1.69 mm in thickness: An apprasial of "thin" level IV lesions. *Ann Surg* 195:30–34, 1982.
107. Breslow A: Tumor thickness, level of invasion and node dissection in stage I cutaneous melanoma. *Ann Surg* 182:572–575, 1975.
108. Day CL Jr, Mihm MC Jr, Sober AJ, et al: Predictors of late deaths among patients with clinical stage I melanoma who have not had bony or visceral metastases within the first 5 years after diagnosis. *J Am Acad Dermatol* 8:864–868, 1983.
109. Wanebo HJ, Fortner JG, Woodruff J, et al: Selection of the optimum surgical treatment of stage I melanoma by depth of microinvasion: Use of the combined microstage technique (Clark-Breslow). *Ann Surg* 182:302–315, 1975.
110. Day CL Jr, Sober AJ, Kopf AW, et al: A prognostic model for clinical stage I melanoma of the lower extremity: Location on foot as independent risk factor for recurrent disease. *Surgery* 89:599–603, 1981.
111. Day CL Jr, Sober AJ, Kopf AW, et al: A prognostic model for clinical stage I melanoma of the upper extremity: The importance of anatomic subsites in predicting recurrent disease. *Ann Surg* 193:436–440, 1981.
112. Day CL Jr, Mihm MC Jr, Lew RA, et al: Prognostic factors for patients with clinical stage I melanoma of intermediate thickness (1.51–3.99 mm): A conceptual model for tumor growth and metastasis. *Ann Surg* 195:35–43, 1982.

113. Balch CM, Soong S-J, Murad TM, et al: A multifactorial analysis of melanoma: III. Prognostic factors in melanoma patients with lymph node metastases (stage II). *Ann Surg* 193:377–388, 1981.
114. Cochran AJ, Lana AMA, Wen D-R: Histomorphometry in the assessment of prognosis in stage II malignant melanoma. *Am J Surg Pathol* 13:600–604, 1989.
115. Zeng QS, Fu YS, Cochran AJ: Nuclear DNA measurements of metastatic melanoma by a computerized digital imaging system. *Hum Pathol* 21:1112–1116, 1990.
116. Balch CM, Soong S-J, Murad TM, et al: A multifactorial analysis of melanoma: IV. Prognostic factors in 200 melanoma patients with distant metastases (stage III). *J Clin Oncol* 1:126–134, 1983.
117. Presant CA, Bartolucci AA, and the Southeastern Cancer Study Group: Prognostic factors in metastatic malignant melanoma: The Southeastern Cancer Study Group Experience. *Cancer* 49:2192–2196, 1982.
118. Soong S-J, Shaw HM, Balch CM, et al: Predicting survival and recurrence in localized melanoma: A multivariate approach. *World J Surg* 16:191–195, 1992.

Index